Springer
Berlin
Heidelberg
New York
Barcelona
Budapest
Hong Kong
London
Milan
Paris
Santa Clara
Singapore
Tokyo

Joseph Schatzker · Marvin Tile

The Rationale of Operative Fracture Care

Second Edition, Completely Revised and Enlarged

With Contributions by T.S. Axelrod, R. Hu,
and D.J.G. Stephen

With a Foreword by M.E. Müller

With 557 Figures in 1910 Separate Illustrations

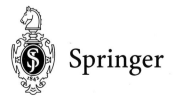 Springer

Joseph Schatzker, M. D., B. Sc. (Med.), F. R. C. S. (C)
Consulting Orthopaedic Surgeon
Professor of Surgery, University of Toronto

Marvin Tile, M. D., B. Sc. (Med.), F. R. C. S. (C)
Surgeon-in-Chief
Professor of Surgery, University of Toronto

Terry S. Axelrod, M. Sc., M. D., FRCS (C)
Orthopaedic Surgeon-in-Chief
Assistant Professor, University of Toronto

Richard Hu, M. D., F. R. S. C. (C)
Consulting Orthopaedic Surgeon
Assistant Professor, University of Toronto

David J. G. Stephen, M. D., F. R. S. C. (C)
Consulting Orthopaedic Surgeon
Lecturer, University of Toronto

Joint address:

Sunnybrook Health Science Center
Division of Orthopaedic Surgery
University of Toronto
A-315, 2075 Bayview Avenue
Toronto, Ontario, M4N 3M5
Canada

ISBN 3-540-59388-8 2nd Edition
Springer-Verlag Berlin Heidelberg New York

Corrected 2nd printing 1996

ISBN 3-540-10675-8 1st Edition
Springer-Verlag Berlin Heidelberg New York

Library of Congress Cataloging-in-Publication Data

Schatzker, Joseph. The rationale of operative fracture care/ Joseph Schatzker, Marvin Tile; with a foreword by M.E. Müller. – 2nd completely rev. and enlarged ed. p. cm. Includes bibliographical references and index. ISBN 3-540-59388-8 (hbk.: alk. paper) 1. Fractures – Surgery. I. Tile, Marvin. II. Title. RD 101.S28 1996 617.1´5 – dc20 95-39615 CIP

© Springer-Verlag Berlin Heidelberg 1987, 1996
a member of BertelsmannSpringer
Science+Business Media GmbH
Printed in Germany

The use of general descriptive names, registered names, trademarks, etc. in this publication does not imply, even in the absence of a specific statement, that such names are exempt from the relevant protective laws and regulations and therefore free for general use.

Product liability: The publishers cannot guarantee the accuracy of any information about the application of operative techniques and medications contained in this book. In every individual case the user must check such information by consulting the relevant literature.

Typesetting: Data conversion by Appl, Wemding
Printing and bookbinding: Appl, Wemding

SPIN: 10773956   24/3111 – 5 4
Printed on acid-free paper

Dedication

This second edition of our book
is dedicated to our families for their patience,
devotion, and understanding.

From Joseph Schatzker

To my late mother Helene Schatzker Schleifer
To my wife Valerie
To my children Erik, Adam, and Mark

From Marvin Tile

To my wife Esther
To my family: Gary, Rosemary, Katy, Sari, and Noah Tile
Stephen, Christine, David, Rachel, and Abby Tile
Steven, Deborah, Ian, and Annie Cass
Andrew Tile

Foreword to the Second Edition

Eight years have passed since the publication of the first edition of *The Rationale of Operative Fracture Care*. During this time, as I predicted, it has become the standard reference work for all concerned with the treatment of fractures: practicing surgeons, residents, and directors of academic units alike.

The second edition has been greatly expanded in scope. The original chapters have been completely reworked. Once again, Dr. Schatzker and Dr. Tile reveal their consummate understanding and mastery of the problems of trauma. They have included detailed discussions of all the conceptual changes in fracture treatment which have taken place since the publication of the original edition. Thus, indirect reduction, biological plating, indications for absolute and relative stability, as well as information on new implants, such as low contact plates, first and second generation reamed intramedullary nails, and the new unreamed nails and external fixation devices are critically discussed in appropriate sections of the book.

To fill the gaps in the first publication, Dr. Schatzker and Dr. Tile have turned to their colleagues and close collaborators at Sunnybrook Health Science Centre. Fractures of the wirst and hand, spine, and hip are now included and discussed in great detail in this new edition.

Although three new authors have contributed to this book, the second edition of *The Rationale of Operative Fracture Care* offers a uniformity of approach and method rarely encountered in similar efforts. The close collaboration and collegial scholarship which exists at Sunnybrook's famous trauma and orthopedic unit has produced this remarkable unity of thought and practice. This second edition will, I believe, be as popular as the first and provide a useful and inspiring reference to trauma surgeons throughout the world.

Berne, December 1995   MAURICE E. MÜLLER

Foreword to the First Edition

After the publication of the AO book *Technique of Internal Fixation of Fractures* (Müller, Allgöwer and Willenegger, Springer-Verlag, 1965), the authors decided after considerable discussion amongst themselves and other members of the Swiss AO that the next edition would appear in three volumes. In 1969, the first volume was published (the English edition, *Manual of Internal Fixation,* appeared in 1970). This was a manual of surgical technique which discussed implants and instruments and in which the problems of internal fixation were presented schematically without radiological illustrations. The second volume was to be a treatise on the biomechanical basis of internal fixation as elucidated by the work done in the laboratory for experimental surgery in Davos. The third volume was planned as the culminating effort based upon the first two volumes, treating the problems of specific fractures and richly illustrated with clinical and radiological examples. It was also to discuss results of treatment, comparing the results obtained with the AO method with other methods. The second and third volumes were never published.

The second edition of the AO *Manual* appeared in 1977. It dealt in greater detail with the problems discussed in the first edition, although it still lacked clinical examples and any discussion of indications for surgery. Like the first edition, it was translated into many languages and was well received.

Finally, after 22 years, the much discussed and much needed third volume has appeared. Two Canadian surgeons have successfully undertaken the challenging task of filling this gap in the AO literature.

Joseph Schatzker and Marvin Tile first came into contact with AO methods of internal fixation in 1965. Impressed by the results of the method, they set themselves to learn it in minute detail and before long became masters of the technique and strong exponents of its effectiveness. They appeared often as lecturers and instructors in AO courses in Switzerland, and North America. Their numerous publications and lectures have greatly contributed to the wide acceptance of the operative method of fracture care.

Joseph Schatzker translated the first and second editions of the *Manual* from German into English, and has, in addition to these excellent translations, achieved distinction as a teacher of the AO method. Both he and Marvin Tile participate annually as instructors in the instructional courses at the American Academy of Orthopedic Surgeons.

With their long association with AO techniques and tremendous clinical experience, these two distinguished surgeons were eminently qualified to undertake the monumental task of defining the specific indications for operative fracture care. In this book they present not only their own views but also a synthesis of the thoughts and writings of other AO members. The book is outstanding and far exceeds the goals originally envisaged for the projected third volume.

The authors have been careful in choosing examples and the appropriate radiological illustrations to delineate the mechanism of injury, the biomechanical problems, the indications for treatment, and the actual execution of surgical procedures. They always guide the reader to the essence of the problem, clearly emphasizing the principles of fracture treatment, a deductive approach through analysis to the clinical decision.

Schatzker and Tile speak of fractures having a "personality." This "personality" is a key concept requiring careful definition: it includes not only a careful analysis of the fracture and all of its soft tissue components, but also a thoughtful assessment of the patient, his or her age, occupation, health, and expectations of treatment, as well as a critical appraisal of the skill of the surgeon and the supporting surgical team and environment. This analysis, combined with the knowledge of what constitutes a reasonable result, allows the authors to formulate a guide to treatment. They also provide useful advice about avoiding technical difficulties and pitfalls, about planning correct postoperative care, and about the treatment of complications which may arise.

The book is superbly illustrated with many drawings skillfully employed to clarify and emphasize essential techniques. The style is easy to understand, clear and unambiguous, giving a lucid presentation of complex and difficult concepts. It will certainly become a standard reference work for everyone involved in the treatment of fractures.

Berne, July 1987   MAURICE E. MÜLLER

Preface to the Second Edition

As Professor Müller predicted in the foreword to the first edition, our book, which dealt with the challenging subject of surgical indications, rapidly filled the void left by the AO Manual which discussed mainly the surgical techniques of internal fixation and the associated instruments and implants. Thus, the *Rationale of Operative Fracture Care,* in dealing critically with the issues of surgical indications in addition to many other important aspects of fracture treatment, quickly became the standard reference for those involved in the treatment of musculoskeletal trauma – resident and practicing surgeon alike.

Eight years have passed since the publication of the first edition. During this time many changes have occurred in surgical philosophy and technique and in implants and instruments. Thus, in the preparation of our second edition, we have found it necessary to completely rework all the original chapters. We have dealt in great detail with the conceptual changes which have occurred in the principles of internal fixation and have made certain that the reader would see the relationship of these changes to the biological and biomechanical properties of the diaphyseal and end segments of bone. The reader will also rapidly become aware of the complexities of stable internal fixation achieved by means of compression and those of relatively stable fixation achieved by splintage and how these two diverse methods of internal fixation must be carefully adapted to the physiological and mechanical requirements of diaphyseal and intraarticular fractures. The new concepts, such as indirect reduction, biological plating, absolutely

stable and relatively stable fixation and their respective indications, as well as the new implants such as the low contact plates, the first and second generation reamed intramedullary nails and the new unreamed nails for the tibia and femur as well as the new designs of external fixateurs, are critically discussed in the appropriate segments of the book.

The second edition has also been greatly expanded in its scope. Voids which were left in the first edition have been carefully filled in the second. We have turned to our colleagues and close collaborators at Sunnybrook Health Science Centre to provide us with chapters which were omitted from the first edition. Thus T. Axelrod has written the chapter on the wrist, R. Hu the chapter on the spine, and D. Stephen the chapter on the foot. J. Schatzker has contributed a new chapter on fractures about the hip and M. Tile a chapter on the calcaneus. The close collaboration and unity of thought which exists between the members of the orthopedic unit at Sunnybrook has produced a remarkable unanimity of approach and execution rarely encountered in volumes written by more than one or two authors.

The second edition is thus an expanded and much more comprehensive treatise on the complexities of decision-making and surgical execution of fracture care. We are confident that it will once again enjoy popularity and bring guidance to the surgeons confronted with the difficult problems of their surgical practice.

Toronto, December 1995
JOSEPH SCHATZKER
MARVIN TILE

Acknowledgements

To the new generation of the Springer-Verlag team Udo Schiller, Gabriele Schröder, Sherryl Sundell, and Ute Pfaff for their professionalism, dedication, cooperation, and help in the publication of the second edition.

To our secretaries Shirley McGoveran and Carol Young for their continued support and help with this project.

To our research assistant Shirley Fitzgerald for her continued attention to detail in reading and editing the text.

To Maurice Müller for the Foreword and continuing support.

Preface to the First Edition

The purpose of this book is to describe our philosophy of fracture care, which reconciles both the closed and open methods of fracture treatment. We do not regard these two methods as representing opposing points of view, but as complementary to each other. Some surgeons, who tend to treat fractures by closed methods, often imply that the open method is dangerous. By "conservative treatment" they imply a nonoperative method and suggest that it is well thought out, tried, and safe, and will yield results equal to if not superior to those achieved by surgery. "Conservative" as defined by the Oxford dictionary means "characterized by a tendency to persevere or keep intact and unchanged." The surgeons who continue to view the open method of fracture treatment as the last resort, and who will do anything, no matter how extreme, to avoid opening a fracture, are indeed characterized by a tendency to keep unchanged an attitude whose prevalence was justified when the methods of internal fixation were inadequate and the results of surgical treatment often worse than those of nonoperative care.

However, the founding of the Swiss AO, an association for the study of problems in internal fixation, by Müller, Allgöwer, Willenegger and Schneider in 1958 ushered in a new era in fracture treatment. These pioneer surgeons developed new principles of stable internal fixation along with new implants. Their methods of open reduction and internal fixation, performed by atraumatic techniques, produced sufficient stability to allow early functional rehabilitation without an increase in the rate of malunion or nonunion. The results of treatment changed so dramatically that new standards of care and assessment had to be adopted. Nowadays, an excellent result means the full recovery of function, a painless extremity, a normal mechanical axis, and full joint stability with a normal range of motion. Anything less can no longer be considered excellent, as it has been in reports in the past. Operative fracture care has become safe, scientific, and predictable. It is now based on a firm foundation of biomechanical and clinical data.

Although it has become clear from clinical reviews that open fracture care in certain fractures gives far better results than closed treatment of that same fracture, we emphasize again and again that the indication for surgery for a particular patient must be based on a clear definition of the "personality of the fracture". The personality of a fracture depends upon many factors, including the age, medical condition, and expectations of the patient, the nature of the injury, and the skill of the health care team and surgical environment in which the fracture is to be treated.

Once the decision has been made that open reduction and stable fixation will afford the patient the best end result, we progress to the execution of the surgical procedure. We describe fully the methods of treatment that are best for each particular fracture based on the principles of stable internal fixation. The details of preoperative investigation and planning so essential to successful surgery are stressed. Technical details are also described, including the surgical approach, the selection of the best implant, the methods of inserting the implant, and the common pitfalls the surgeon may encounter.

Since the operative treatment of fractures demands so-called functional aftertreatment, the details of postoperative care have become as important as the steps of the operative procedure. We therefore describe not only the details of postoperative treatment, but also the danger signals of common complications and their treatment.

We hope that this book will become a guide for all surgeons treating fractures in this era of advanced technology, and that inadequate internal fixation, once so commonly encountered, will become history. Internal fixation should no longer be viewed as a last resort or as a more dangerous form of treatment, but as safe, scientific and predictable, and as the best form of treatment for those cases in which it is indicated.

Toronto, June 1987   JOSEPH SCHATZKER
MARVIN TILE

Acknowledgements

This book, a labor of love, could not have been completed without the unselfish support and hard work of many individuals. We are especially grateful to:

Our families for their patient understanding during this period

Valerie Schatzker for her help in the English editing

Our orthopedic teachers at the University of Toronto, who roused our interest in orthopedic trauma and have encouraged us to complete the task

Our orthopedic colleagues at Sunnybrook Medical Centre, Stanley Gertzbein, Jim Kellam, and Bob McMurtry, for contributing cases and helpful suggestions, and especially to Gordon Hunter, who read most of the manuscript, for his helpful criticism

The founding members of the AO-ASIF for recognition and support of our efforts

Maurice Müller for reading the manuscript and for his kind remarks in the Foreword

Instructional Media Services at the Wellesley Hospital and Sunnybrook Medical Centre in Toronto for their contribution, especially to Patsy Cunningham who did some of the artwork, and to Jim Atkinson and his staff in Medical Photography

The staff of Springer-Verlag, Heidelberg, for their efficiency and expertise in producing and publishing this volume

Mr. Pupp of Springer-Verlag, Heidelberg, to whom we are indebted for many of the new drawings in this book

Our secretaries, Shirley McGoveran and Joan Kennedy, for their constant support

Jan King and Ronda Klapp for typing the manuscript

Carol Young for typing the manuscript and helping with the index

Shirley Fitzgerald for her devotion to detail in both the editing and the completion of the index

Contents

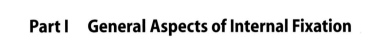

Part I General Aspects of Internal Fixation

1 Principles of Stable Internal Fixation

J. Schatzker

1.1 Introduction

1.1.1 Mechanical Properties of Bone

The principal mechanical function of bone is to act as a supporting structure and transmit load. The loads which bone has to withstand are those of pure compression, those of bending, which result in one cortex being loaded in tension and the other in compression, and those of torque, or twisting. Bone is strongest in compression and weakest in tension. Fractures as a result of pure compression are therefore rare and occur only in areas of cancellous bone with a thin cortical shell. Thus, we find pure compression fractures in such areas as the metaphyses, vertebral bodies, and the calcaneus. Transverse, oblique, and spiral are the fracture patterns commonly seen in tubular bone.

Transverse fractures are the result of a bending force (Fig. 1.1). They are associated with a small extrusion wedge which is always found on the compression side of the bone. If this extrusion wedge comprises less than 10% of the circumference, the fracture is considered a simple transverse fracture. If the extruded fragment is larger, the fracture is considered a wedge fracture and the fragment a bending or extrusion wedge. Because it is extruded from bone under load, it retains little of its soft tissue attachment and has therefore, at best, a precarious

blood supply. This must be kept in mind when planning an internal fixation. Attempts to secure fixation of such extruded fragments may result in their being rendered totally avascular. If very small they may be ignored. If larger, it is best to leave them alone and fill the defects created with cancellous bone.

Oblique fractures are also the result of a bending force. The extrusion wedge remains attached to one of the main fragments. The fissure between it and the main fragment is not visible on X-ray. If looked for at the time of an open reduction, it can be readily found. During closed intramedullary nailing this undisplaced extrusion wedge is often dislodged and becomes apparent on X-ray.

Spiral fractures are the result of an indirect twisting force (Fig. 1.1). They often occur in combination with wedge fragments of corresponding configuration. These fragments are larger and retain their soft tissue attachment. It is frequently possible to secure them with lag screws without disrupting their blood supply.

1.1.2 Types of Load and Fracture Patterns

Bone is a viscoelastic material. Fractures are therefore related not only to the force but also to the rate of force application. Much less force is required to break the bone if the force is applied slowly and over a long period

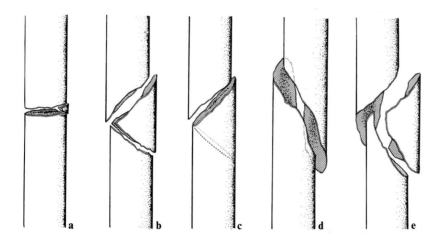

Fig. 1.1 a–e. Types of fracture patterns. A lateral bending force can result in transverse fracture (**a**), extrusion or bending wedge fractures (**b**), or oblique fractures (**c**) in which the extrusion wedge remains attached to one of the main fragments. A twisting or torsional force may result in a spiral fracture (**d**) or one with a single or multiple spiral wedge fragments (**e**)

Fig. 1.2. The scheme of the classification of fractures for each bone segment or each bone. Types: *A, B, C;* Groups *A1, A2, A3, B1, B2, B3, C1, C2, C3.* Subgroups: *.1, .2, .3.* The darkening of the arrows indicates the increasing severity of the fracture.
The small squares: The two first ones give the location, the next three the morphological characteristics of the fracture. (From Müller et al. 1990)

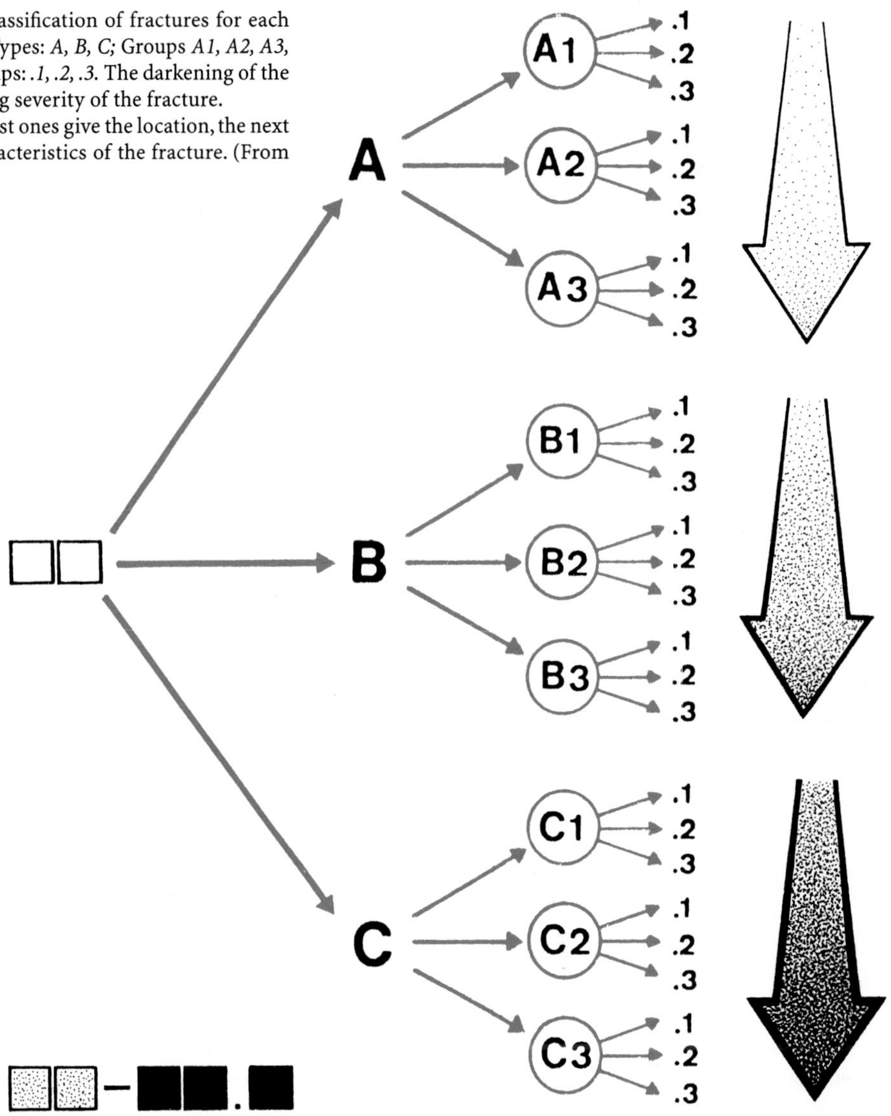

of time than if it is applied rapidly: bone is better able to withstand the rapid application of a much greater force. This force is stored, however, and when the bone can no longer withstand it and finally breaks, it is dissipated in an explosive fashion, causing considerable damage to the soft tissue envelope. A good example of this is the skier who walks away from a spectacular tumble, only to break his leg in a slow, twisting fall. We therefore distinguish between low- and high-velocity injuries.

Low-velocity injuries have a better prognosis. In high-velocity injuries the fractures are not only more fragmented but also associated with a much greater damage to the enveloping soft tissues, because of the higher energy dissipation and because of the direct application of force. Low-velocity injuries are more commonly spiral, without excessive comminution.

1.1.3 Classification of Fractures

The classification of fractures followed in this book is based on the *Comprehensive Classification of Fractures of Long Bones* (Müller et al. 1990). The unique feature of the this system of classification is that the principles of the classification and the classification itself are not based on the regional features of a bone and its fracture patterns nor are they bound by convention of usage or the popularity of an eponym. They are generic and apply to the whole skeleton. The philosophy guiding the classification is that a classification is worthwhile only if it helps in evolving the rationale of treatment and helps in the evaluation of the outcome of the treatment (Müller et al. 1990b). Therefore the classification must indicate the severity of the fracture, which in this classification

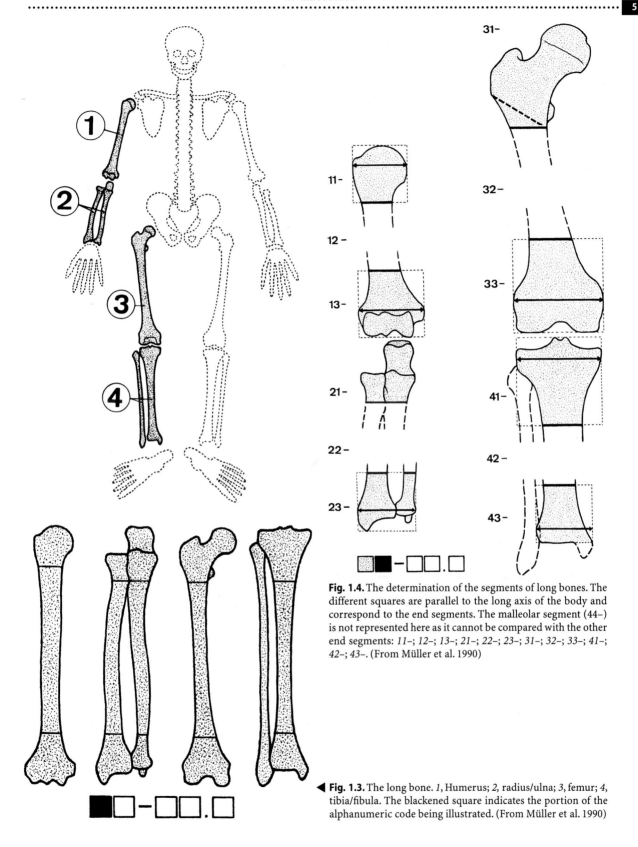

Fig. 1.4. The determination of the segments of long bones. The different squares are parallel to the long axis of the body and correspond to the end segments. The malleolar segment (44-) is not represented here as it cannot be compared with the other end segments: *11-; 12-; 13-; 21-; 22-; 23-; 31-; 32-; 33-; 41-; 42-; 43-.* (From Müller et al. 1990)

◀ **Fig. 1.3.** The long bone. *1,* Humerus; *2,* radius/ulna; *3,* femur; *4,* tibia/fibula. The blackened square indicates the portion of the alphanumeric code being illustrated. (From Müller et al. 1990)

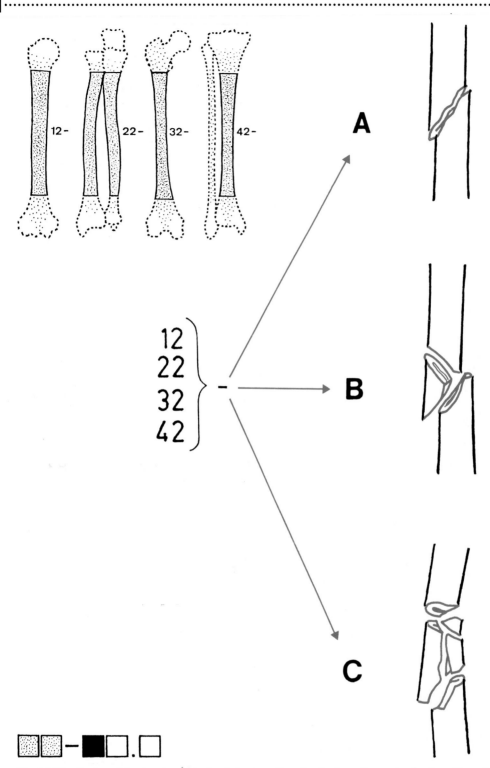

Fig. 1.5. The diaphyseal fracture types. *A*, simple fracture; *B*, wedge fracture; *C*, complex fracture. (From Müller et al. 1990)

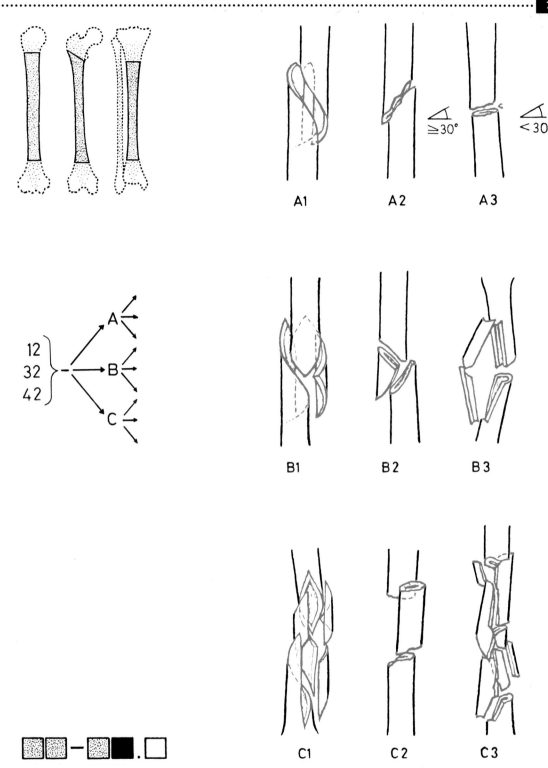

Fig. 1.6. The groups of the diaphyseal fractures of the numberus, femur, and tibia/fibula. *A1,* simple fracture, spiral; *A2,* simple fracture, oblique (≥30 °); *A3,* simple fracture, transverse (<30 °); *B1,* wedge fracture, spiral wedge; *B2,* wedge fracture, bending wedge; *B3,* wedge fracture, fragmented wedge; *C1,* complex fracture, spiral; *C2,* complex fracture, segmental; *C3,* complex fracture, irregular. (From Müller et al. 1990)

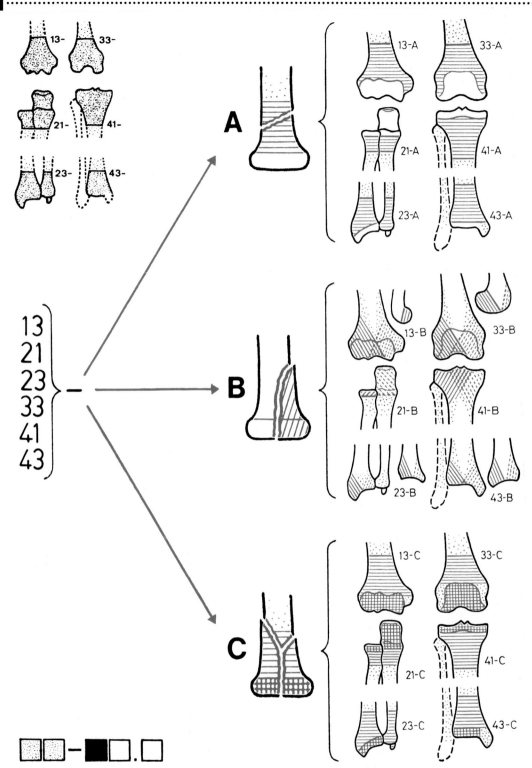

Fig. 1.7. The fracture types of the segments *13-* and *33-*, *21-* and *41-*, *23-* and *43-*. *A*, extra-articular fractures; *B*, partial articular fracture; *C*, complete articular fracture. (From Müller et al. 1990)

indicates the morphological complexity of the fracture, the difficulties to be anticipated in treatment, and its prognosis. This has been accomplished by formulating the classification on the basis of three fracture types A, B, and C, and their respective groups and subgroups. A, B, and C represent fracture types in ascending order of severity. Each fracture type has three groups, A1, A2, and A3, B1, B2, and B3, and C1, C2, and C3 and each group three subgroups, A1.1, A1.2 etc. The groups and the subgroups of each are also organized in an ascending order of severity (please see Fig. 1.2.) This organization of fractures in the classification in an ascending order of severity has introduced great clinical significance to the recognition of a fracture type.

The classification considers a long bone to have a diaphyseal segment and two end segments (Fig. 1.3, 1.4). Because the distinction between the diaphysis and the metaphysis is rarely well defined anatomically, the classification makes use of the rule of squares to define the end segments with great precision (Fig. 1.4). The location of the fracture has also been simplified by noting the relationship which the center of the fracture bears to the segment.

The authors of the *Comprehensive Classification of Fractures of Long Bones* have also developed a new terminology which is so precise that it is now possible to describe a fracture so accurately that its pictorial representation is superfluous. The new precise terminology divides fractures into simple and multifragmentary (Fig. 1.5). The multifragmentary fractures are further subdivided into wedge and complex fractures, not on the basis of the number of fragments, but rather on whether after reduction the main fragments have retained contact or not. In treatment this is, indeed, the essence of severity. Thus, a multifragmentary fracture with some contact between the main fragments is considered a wedge fracture. It has a recognizable length and rotational alignment. This is lost in a complex fracture where contact between the main fragments cannot be established after reduction (Fig. 1.6). Articular fractures are defined as those which involve the articular surface regardless of whether the fracture is intracapsular or not. A further distinction exists between partial and complete articular fractures (Fig. 1.7).

The diagnosis of a fracture is given by coupling the location of the fracture with its morphologic complexity. To facilitate computer entry and retrieval of the cases, an alphanumeric code has been created. The bones of the skeleton have been assigned numbers (Fig. 1.8). The segments are numbered from one to three proceeding from proximal to distal. Thus it is possible to express the location of a fracture by combining the number of the bone with the number expressing the involved segment: for instance, a fracture of the proximal segment of the humerus would be 11- and a fracture of the

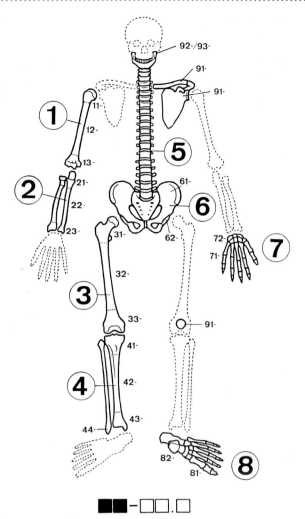

Fig. 1.8. The bones and their segments. An overview of the whole skeleton. *1,* Humerus and its three segments; proximal, diaphyseal, and distal; *2,* radius/ulna and its three segments; proximal, diaphyseal, and distal; *3,* femur and its three segments; proximal, diaphyseal, and distal; *4,* tibia/fibula and its four segments; proximal, diaphyseal, distal, and malleolar; *5,* spine and its three segments: cervical, thoracic, and lumbar; *6,* pelvis and its two segments: extra-articular and the acetabulum; *7,* hand; *8,* foot; *9,* other bones: *91.1,* patella, *91.2,* clavicle, *91.3,* scapula, *92,* mandible; *93,* facial bones and skull. (From Müller et al. 1990)

distal femur would be 33-. The morphological nature of the fracture is expressed by the combination of the letters A, B, and C and the numbers 1, 2, and 3, which when combined in a specific manner express the fracture type, group, and subgroup. The diagnosis can be coded using an alpha-numeric code (Fig. 1.9). As stated, this alphanumeric code is intended strictly for computer entry and retrieval and not for use in verbal communication. In verbal communication the clinician should use terminology which is so precise that it describes the full

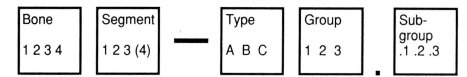

Fig. 1.9. The coding of the diagnosis

essence of the fracture, making a pictorial representation of the fracture no longer necessary.

We have validated this fracture classification in two separate clinical studies (Schatzker and Lichtenhahn, unpublished data; Schatzker and Tornkvist, unpublished data). The inter- and intraobserver concordance has been evaluated for fracture types, groups, and subgroups. Concordance for fracture types was close to 100%, for fracture groups between 80% and 85%, but for fracture subgroups only between 50% and 60%. We feel, therefore, that the clinician should rely principally on the recognition of the fracture types and groups. Classification into fracture subgroups should be reserved only for research studies.

The classification of the soft tissue injury associated with open fractures continues to be a problem which requires further elaboration. Many observers have attempted to grade open fractures (Allgöwer 1971; Gustilo and Andersson 1976; Tscherne and Gotzen 1984; Lange et al. 1985). A further classification of the soft tissue component of an injury was presented in the third edition of the *Manual of Internal Fixation* (Müller et al. 1991). In this most recent attempt a code for the injury is assigned to each of the elements of the soft tissue envelope rather than using an existing classification system. A new classification scheme which would characterize the morphological components of the soft tissue injury, identify its severity, and indicate the potential functional loss in a simple and comprehensive manner, and which could be expressed in a simple code, would be of great value clinically and in research.

1.1.4 Effects of Fracture

When a bone is fractured, it loses its structural continuity. The loss of the structural continuity renders it mechanically useless because it is unable to bear any load.

1.1.5 Soft Tissue Component and Classification of Soft Tissue Injuries

We have alluded to the poorer prognosis of high-velocity injuries because of the greater damage to the soft tissue envelope. Long-term disability following a fracture

is almost never the result of damage to the bone itself; it is the result of damage to the soft tissues and of stiffness of neighboring joints.

In a closed fracture the injury to the surrounding tissue evokes an acute inflammatory response, which is associated with an outpouring of fibrinous and proteinaceous fluid. If, after the injury, the tendons and muscles are not encouraged to glide upon one another, inflammation may develop and lead to the obliteration of tissue planes and to the matting of the soft tissue envelope into a functionless mass.

In an open fracture, in addition to the possible scarring from immobilization, there is direct injury to the muscles and tendons and in such cases the effects of infection must be reckoned with. Indeed, infection is the most serious complication of trauma because, in addition to the scarring related to the initial trauma, infection compounds the fibrosis as a result of the associated tissue damage and because of the prolonged immobilization which is frequently necessary until the infection is cured.

Stiffness in adjacent joints in nonarticular fractures is also the result of immobilization. Prolonged immobilization leads to atrophy of the articular cartilage, to capsular and ligamentous contractures, and to intra-articular adhesions. The joint space normally filled with synovial fluid becomes filled with adhesions which bind the articular surfaces together. Added to the local effects is, of course, the tethering effect of the scarred soft tissues.

Although the significance of the soft tissue component of open fracture injuries has been recognized for a long time, the soft tissue component of closed injuries has only recently been classified (Tscherne and Brüggemann 1976; Tscherne and Östern 1982; Tscherne and Gotzen 1984; Müller et al. 1991).

1.2 Aims of Treatment

The loss of function of the soft tissue envelope due to scarring and secondary joint stiffness can only be prevented by early mobilization. Thus, modern fracture treatment does not focus on bone union at the expense of function but addresses itself principally to the restoration of function of the soft tissues and adjacent joints. A deformity or a pseudarthrosis is relatively easy to correct in the presence of good soft tissue function, while scarring, obliteration of the soft tissue gliding planes, and joint stiffness are often permanent. The modern fracture surgeon will therefore direct treatment to the early return of function and motion, with bone union being considered of secondary importance.

Modern functional fracture treatment does not denote only operative fracture care. It makes use of specialized splinting of the bone in special braces which allow an early return of function and motion. There are, however, limitations to the nonoperative system, which we will address as we discuss the different fractures. It can be applied to fractures where angulation, rotation, and shortening can be controlled. Thus, it is limited only to certain long bone fractures. Its application to intra-articular and periarticular fractures is very limited.

Early return of full function following fracture can be achieved only by sufficiently stable internal fixation which will abolish fracture pain and which will allow early resumption of motion with partial loading without the risk of failure of the fixation and resultant malunion or nonunion. With nonfunctional methods full return of function is rarely achieved and then only after a prolonged rehabilitation period.

1.3 Previous Experience with Internal Fixation

Internal fixation is not a new science. The past 50 years have provided us with ample documentation of the results of unstable internal fixation. Surgery has frequently proved to be the worst form of treatment. It destroyed the soft tissue hinges, interfered with biological factors such as the blood supply and the periosteum, and was never sufficiently strong or stable to permit active mobilization of the limbs with partial loading. Supplemental external plaster fixation was often necessary. The emphasis was on bone healing and not on soft tissue rehabilitation. Healing became evident when callus appeared. Unfortunately, unstable internal fixation was unpredictable and uncertain, and it frequently resulted in delayed union, nonunion, or deformity. When union did occur, instead of signifying the end of treatment it merely signaled the beginning of a prolonged phase of rehabilitation designed to regain motion in the soft tissue envelope and in the stiff joints. The ravages of this prolonged nonfunctional form of treatment were such that open reduction and internal fixation were looked upon as the last resort in the treatment of a fracture.

1.4 Rigidity and Stability

It is important to distinguish between rigidity and stability. Rigidity is the physical property of an implant. It refers to its ability to withstand deformation. Thus, in an internal fixation the fixation devices employed may be rigid but the fixation of the fragments may be unstable.

The introduction of compression introduced stability. Stability was achieved not by rigidity of the implant, but rather by impaction of the fragments. The intimate contact of the fragments brought about by compression restored structural continuity and stability and permitted the direct transfer of forces from fragment to fragment rather than via the implant. Stable fixation restores load-bearing capacity to bone. This greatly diminishes the stresses borne by the implant and protects the implant from mechanical overload or fatigue failure.

Key (1932) and Charnley (1953) were the first to make use of compression in order to achieve stable fixation. Both applied it to broad cancellous surfaces by means of an external compression clamp. Similar attempts to achieve union of the cortex failed. The resorption around the pins of the external fixator employed to stabilize the cortical fragments was thought to be due to pressure necrosis of the cortex. Cancellous surfaces under compression united rapidly, and it was thought initially that compression provided an osteogenic stimulus to bone. The failure of the cortex to unite led to general acceptance of the thesis that cancellous and cortical bone behaved differently and that they probably united by different mechanisms.

Since then it has been demonstrated that, under conditions of absolute stability, both cancellous and cortical fragments heal by primary direct or vascular bone union (primary bone healing). The simple external fixator of Charnley, applied closely to broad, flat cancellous surfaces of an arthrodesis, was able to achieve absolute stability. The same system applied to diaphyseal bone, where tubular fragments rather than broad, flat surfaces were in contact, resulted in a system of relative instability with micromotion between the fragments. The resorption around the pins and at the fracture was due to motion and not due to pressure necrosis.

Danis in 1949 (Müller et al. 1970) was the first to demonstrate that cortical fragments stabilized by a special plate, which was able to exert axial compression and bring about absolute stability at the fracture, united without any radiologically visible callus. Danis referred to this type of union as "primary bone healing." Studies on experimental models by Schenk and Willenegger (1963) revealed a different type of union than that commonly associated with the healing of fractures. Union occurred by direct formation of bone rather than by callus and endochondral ossification. Different events were seen where bone was in contact and where gaps were present.

In areas of contact the healing was seen to be the result of proliferation of new osteons which arose from remaining open haversian systems. The osteons grew parallel to the long axis of the bone, through the necrotic bone ends, and then across the fracture. These osteons can be viewed as a myriad of tiny bone dowels which reestablished the continuity of bone. The capillary buds which sprang from the capillaries became cutting cones. These consisted of osteoclasts, followed by the capillary bud, surrounded by a cuff of osteoblasts which were laying down bone. In this way, there was simultaneous bone resorption and deposition. This bridging of a fracture line by osteons, which gives rise to an osteonal union, can occur only where bone is in direct contact and where there is absolute stability of the fragments without any movement at the interface. In this type of union there is no net resorption at the fracture interface. For every bit of bone removed, new bone is laid down. Under these circumstances, internal fixation does not lead to a relative distraction of the fragments, because no absolute resorption occurs.

Areas of bone separated by gaps demonstrated first of all an invasion of the gaps by blood vessels with surrounding osteoblasts. The osteoblasts laid down osteoid which served to bridge the gaps and to permit stage two to begin. Stage two is identical to contact healing, described above. Examination of human material (R. Schenk, personal communication) from autopsies of patients who had had fractures operated upon revealed that the experimentally noted phenomena of contact and gap healing also occurred clinically. The study of material from patients whose fractures had zones of comminution revealed that, although healing seemed undisturbed, free fragments whose blood supply had been interfered with lagged very much behind in the degree of revascularization and remodeling. Thus, the rate of revascularization and union was seen to be influenced by the severity of comminution, the degree of initial displacement – for this has a bearing on the severity of devitalization of the fragments – and by the presence and degree of severity of the soft tissue lesion. This last observation is of particular importance with regard to implant removal, for not every fracture, nor all areas of the same fracture, will have advanced to the same degree of remodeling at a given time from injury. With primary bone healing we see a biological phenomenon which is different from healing under conditions of relative stability which is associated with the formation of callus. Primary bone healing is not necessarily better, and certainly in the early stages of healing it is weaker than bone bridged by a peripheral concentric callus.

1.5 Methods of Stable Fixation

1.5.1 Lag Screw

Compression exerts its beneficial effect on bone union by creating an environment of absolute stability where no relative micromotion exists between the bone fragments. Healing is by primary union. Therefore, viability of the bone fragments is not a prerequisite to union. As long as absolute stability is maintained, the fragments

Fig. 1.10 a, b. The lag screw. **a** The hole next to the screw head is larger than the diameter of the thread. This is the *gliding hole*. The hole in the opposite cortex is the *thread hole*. As the screw is tightened the two fragments are pressed together. **b** Both holes are *thread holes*. The fragments cannot be compressed. (From Müller et al. 1979)

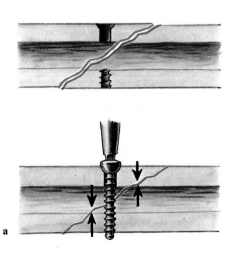

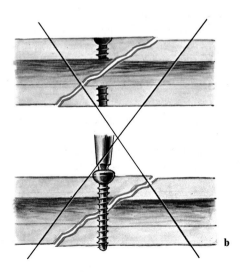

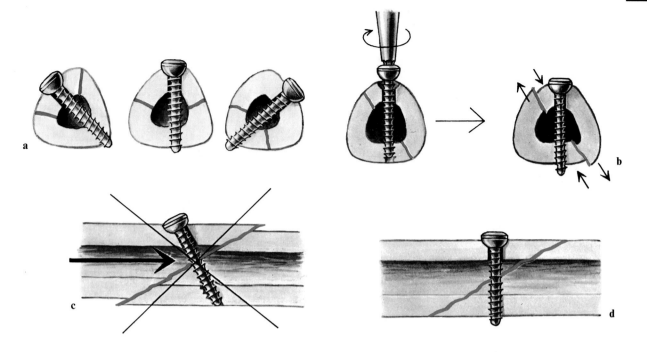

Fig. 1.11. a, b In order to exert the most efficient degree of compression, lag screws must be inserted into the center of the fragments and at right angles to the fracture plane. If they are off-center or angled, the fragments may displace on tightening of the screw, and reduction will be lost. **c** A lag screw inserted at a right angle to the fracture plane results in the best compression but does not provide the best stability under axial load, because the fragments may glide upon one another as the screw tips in the thread hole. **d** A lag screw at right angles to the long axis of the bone may cause tendency for the fragments to displace as the screw is tightened, but it provides the best resistance to displacement under axial load. Displacement can occur only if the thread rips out of the thread hole or the screw head sinks into the gliding hole. (From Müller et al. 1979)

will be revascularized and remodeled and primary bone union will occur. Articular cartilage also benefits from compression because absolute stability is necessary for articular cartilage regeneration and healing (Mitchell and Shepherd 1980). Interfragmental compression results in impaction of the fragments and in a marked increase in frictional resistance to motion. It is therefore the most important and efficient method of restoring functional and structural continuity to bone. It also greatly diminishes the forces borne by an internal fixation because the load transfer occurs directly from fragment to fragment. Stability is thus achieved, not by rigidity of the implant, but rather by compression and bone contact.

The simplest way of compressing two fragments of bone together is to lag them together with a *lag screw*. The lag screw is the simplest and most efficient implant

in use for securing interfragmental compression (Fig. 1.10).

The insertion of a screw into bone results in local damage which triggers the mechanisms for immediate repair. This is seen histologically as the formation of new bone which closely follows the profile of the screw threads. Thus, after the insertion of a screw, as healing occurs, the holding power of the screw increases, reaching its peak between the sixth and eighth weeks. The holding power then gradually declines to a level well above what it was at the time of insertion (Schatzker et al. 1975 b). This occurs because, as the bone matures and becomes organized, much of the newly laid-down woven bone around the screw is resorbed.

Screws may be either self-tapping or non-self-tapping. It was formerly thought that self-tapping screws provided a poorer hold in bone because they created more damage at the time of insertion and became embedded in fibrous tissue rather than in bone (Müller et al. 1979). This has been shown to be incorrect. The fibrous tissue forms as a result of instability and motion between the implant and bone. Instability is seen histologically as bone resorption and the formation of fibrous tissue, with occasional islands of cartilage and synovial-like cells (Schatzker et al. 1975 a). Size for size, the different thread profiles of self-tapping and non-self-tapping screws have almost the same holding power. The advantage of the non-self-tapping screws is that they can be inserted into bone with far greater ease and precision, particularly when the screw comes to lie obliquely through thick cortex, which it often does when used to lag fragments. Self-tapping screws offer the advantage of speed and are best suited for the fixation of plates to bone.

In order to exert the most efficient degree of inter-fragmental compression, lag screws must be inserted into the center of fragments and at right angles to the fracture plane (Fig. 1.11). A single lag screw is never strong enough to achieve stable fixation of diaphyseal fragments. A minimum of two, and preferably three screws are required. This means that only long oblique and long spiral fractures can be stabilized with lag screws alone and only in short tubular bones such as phalanges, metacarpals, metatarsals, or malleoli. If lag screws alone are used for the fixation of long bones such as the femur or the humerus, they almost always end in early failure because of mechanical overload. Therefore, the most common use of lag screws in the fixation of shaft fractures is in combination with neutralization, buttress, or tension-band plates which protect the screw fixation from mechanical overload.

1.5.2 Lag Screw, Neutralization, and Buttressing

Neutralization plates or *protection plates* are used to protect the primary lag screw fixation. They conduct part or all of the forces from one fragment to the other. In this way they protect the fracture fixation from the forces of bending shear and rotation (Fig. 1.12).

In metaphyseal areas the cortex is very thin, and if subjected to load it can fail. Such failures result in deformity and axial overload of the joint. Therefore, internal fixation in metaphyseal areas requires protection with plates which support the underlying cortex. These are referred to as *buttress plates* (Fig. 1.13). Buttressing may also be achieved with external fixation.

1.5.3 Tension Band Plate

Short oblique or transverse fractures do not lend themselves to lag screw fixation. In diaphyseal regions of the tibia and femur and occasionally the humerus, as will be seen in the section on splinting, we prefer intramedullary nailing for fixation. There are many transverse or short oblique fractures of diaphyses, such as of the radius and ulna, of the humerus, or of long bones close to or involving the metaphyses, which do not lend themselves to intramedullary nailing. Yet these fractures require stable fixation. Such fracture patterns can be stabilized by compression, but the compression has to be in the long axis of the bone. Such compression can be generated only by a plate. If a fracture is reduced and a plate is applied to the bone in such a way that axial compression is generated, either by means of the tension device or by the self-compressing principle of the dynamic compression (DC) plates or LC DCP, the plate is referred to as a *compression plate* (Fig. 1.14a, b).

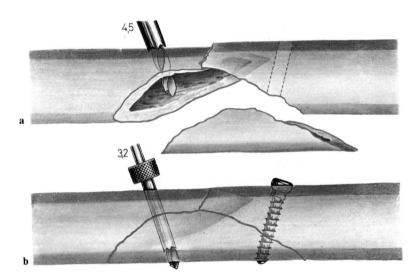

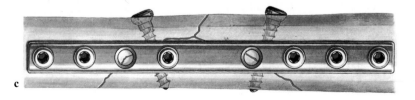

Fig. 1.12 a–c. The neutralization plate. The two lag screws provide interfragmental compression (**a, b**). The neutralization plate in **c** bridges the fracture zone and protects the lag screw fixation from bending and torsional forces. (From Müller et al. 1979)

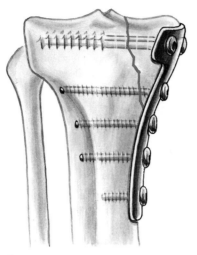

Fig. 1.13. The buttress plate. The T plate buttresses the cortex and prevents axial displacement. (From Müller et al. 1979)

Certain bones such as the femur are eccentrically loaded. This results in one cortex being under compression and the other under tension (Müller et al. 1979; Schatzker et al. 1980). If a plate is applied to the tension side of a bone and placed under tension which causes the cortex under the plate to be compressed, such a plate

not only achieves stability because of the axial compression it generates, but also, because of its location on the tension side of the bone, as bending forces are generated under load, it is capable of increasing the amount of axial compression. Such a plate is referred to as a *tension band plate* (Fig. 1.15).

1.6 Methods of Relative Stability or Splinting

1.6.1 External Skeletal Fixation

As we have seen from the classical experiments of Key (1932) and Charnley (1953), axial compression can be applied by means of pins which traverse bone and are then squeezed together. This type of fixation is stable over only a short length of the bone and only when broad, flat, cancellous surfaces are being compressed. When applied to tubular bone, such fixation is relatively unstable. Although not absolutely stable, the external fixator, either as a full frame or as a half frame, is extremely useful under certain clinical circumstances, such as in the treatment of open fractures not suitable for internal fixation, or in the treatment of infected fractures or infected nonunions or in the treatment of closed fractures of the end segment such as the distal radius, or

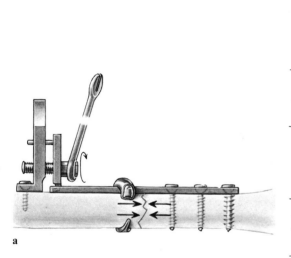

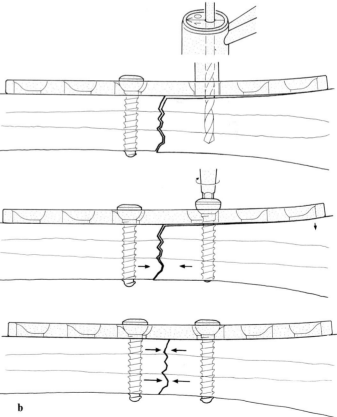

Fig. 1.14. a As the tension device is tightened, the plate is brought under tension and the bone under compression. (From Müller et al. 1979). **b** The dynamic compression plate. As the load screw is tightened it moves from its eccentric position to the center of the screw hole. This movement of screw and bone toward the fracture results in axial compression. (From Allgöwer et al. 1973)

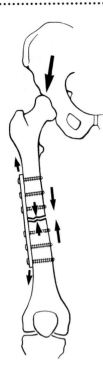

Fig. 1.15. Tension band plate. In an eccentrically loaded bone, not only does a compression plate secure a degree of compression at rest, but also, when the bone is loaded, the bending force so generated is converted by the action of the plate into further compressive stresses. Such a plate is called a "tension band plate" and the force generated "dynamic compression." The essence of dynamic compression is that although the compressive force fluctuates in magnitude it never reverses direction

when one wishes to delay the metaphyseal reconstruction because of the severity of the closed soft tissue injury. Under these circumstances the external fixator provides sufficient stability to permit functional use of the extremity while maintaining the bones in their reduced position. The stability is sufficient in fresh fractures to render the extremity painless and encourage soft tissue rehabilitation. Because external skeletal fixation does not result in absolute stability, it behaves similarly to unstable internal fixation in retarding or discouraging bone union. Therefore, when it is used as the definitive mode of fixation of open diaphyseal fractures it should almost always be combined with bone grafting.

1.6.2 Intramedullary Nailing

The manner in which an intramedullary nail splints and bestows stability is best likened to a tube within a tube. The nail is therefore dependent upon the length of contact for its resistance to bending and upon friction and the interdigitation of fracture fragments for rotational stability. Intramedullary reaming is frequently employed to enlarge the area of contact. This enlarges the medullary canal sufficiently to permit the insertion of a nail which is not only large enough to provide stability but also strong enough to take over the function of the bone. Old small nails adapted to the size of the medullary canal were frequently limited in size to the diameter of the isthmus, which in young patients is frequently narrow. As a result, they were rarely strong

enough and usually too flexible. Their use led to complications such as nail migration, nail bending, nail fracture, delayed union, and nonunion.

The biological expression of unstable fixation is the formation of external callus. The instability associated with intramedullary nailing is reflected in the amount of callus produced. A large intramedullary nail may, when tightly wedged, provide sufficient stability to result in primary bone healing without discernible callus. Most often, however, a variable amount of periosteal callus is seen.

As a mode of fixation of weight-bearing extremities, intramedullary nailing has distinct advantages. Because it is a load-sharing device and much stronger than a plate, weight bearing can be resumed much earlier after intramedullary nailing than after other means of fixation.

An intramedullary nail, because of the mode of application and the manner in which it renders stability, is best suited for fractures which occur in the middle one third of the femur and of the tibia. The proximal and distal ends of tubular bones widen into broad segments of cancellous bone. In these areas the nail can provide neither angular nor rotational stability. Axial stability of a nailed fracture depends on cortical stability and on the ability of the cortex to withstand axial loads. Thus, certain fracture patterns are not ideally suited for intramedullary nailing. These are: long oblique and long spiral fractures, and comminuted fractures in which the cortex in contact is less than 50 % of the diameter of the bone at that level.

An intramedullary nail has distinct mechanical and biological advantages. Because of its design and mode of application it is much stronger than a plate. Consequently, it will withstand loading for a much longer period of time than a plate will before failure. Reaming combined with closed insertion of the nail without disturbing the soft tissues surrounding the fracture has been associated with a much more rapid and more abundant appearance of callus. Thus, it is an ideal device for tubular bones.

The limitations imposed on the conventional nail by the location of a fracture and its pattern have given rise to the development of the interlocking nail (Kempf et al. 1985). The first-generation interlocked nails greatly extended the indications for intramedullary nailing to fractures of the proximal and distal part of the diaphyseal segment of the femur and tibia. Certain fractures of the proximal femur, such as subtrochanteric fractures involving the lesser trochanter or associated with intertrochanteric fractures, could not be stabilized with the first-generation nails. This stimulated the development of the second generation nails such as the reconstruction nail (Smith Newphew Richards, Memphis, TN, USA) or the short and long gamma nail (Howmedica).

For many years intramedullary reaming was considered an essential component of modern intramedullary nailing techniques because it not only improved the stability of the fixation, but, more importantly, surgeons were able to use larger nails, thus avoiding the complications of nail bending and breakage. A number of studies (Rhinelander 1973; Perren 1991; Waelchli-Suter 1980) demonstrated that reaming produces extensive damage to the endosteal blood supply of bone. The desire to use intramedullary nailing for the fixation of open fractures and recognizing the fact that dead bone would further infection led to the development of unreamed nails. Metallurgical and technical advances have overcome many of the early problems of bending and fracture with small-diameter nails. Recent experimental evidence that hollow nails appear to support infection has given rise to the development of solid unreamed nails for the femur and for the tibia (Synthes USA, Paioli, PA, USA). The unreamed solid nail for the femur (Synthes) is a second-generation implant which embodies a number of very elegant proximal locking techniques.

1.6.3 Bridge Plating

Once reduction is achieved a fracture has to be immobilized. The approach of the early AO/ASIF school in the treatment of a multifragmentary fracture was to secure stable fixation of each of the fragments (Fig. 1.16) and in this way convert the many pieces into a solid block of bone. The emphasis was on absolute stability and primary union of bone was the object of an internal fixation. Because multifragmentary fractures united very slowly, it was mandatory to bone graft them in order to prevent failure of the fixation with the resultant malunion or nonunion. Experience with closed locked intra-

medullary nailing strongly suggested that leaving the fragments alone preserved their blood supply and greatly accelerated their union.

Extramedullary splinting was tried with a plate (Heitemeyer and Hierholzer 1985). In this technique of plating the fracture is first reduced by means of indirect reduction. The zone of fragmentation is then bridged with a plate which is fixed to the proximal and distal main fragments. This maintains length, rotation, and axial alignment but reduction is not anatomical. This type of internal fixation is referred to as *bridge plating*. It is a form of splinting. It is not absolutely stable and union is by callus. Bridge plating is indicated only for the fixation of multifragmentary fractures. If one chooses to plate a simple transverse or oblique fracture, then absolute stability must be achieved by means of interfragmental compression or excessive strain at the fracture site will likely cause failure.

In stable fixation of a multifragmentary fracture, union depends on the revascularization of the dead fragments. As a result union is slow and failure to bone graft is the most common cause of failure of stable internal fixation. The bone graft is required to form a biological bridge opposite the plate and in this way protect the internal fixation. In bridge plating the union is rapid, and by callus. As a result the techniques of indirect reduction and bridge plating have made bone grafting of diaphyseal and metaphyseal multifragmentary fractures unnecessary. Bone grafting is now largely reserved for metaphyseal defects of articular fractures and for open fractures.

Not all fractures of long bones lend themselves to these techniques. Anatomical reduction of the diaphyses of the femur, of the tibia and of the humerus is not necessary. As long as length, rotation, and axial alignment are restored there will be no interference with function.

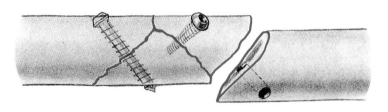

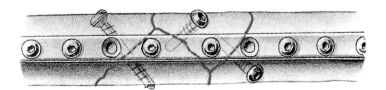

Fig. 1.16. Manual of internal fixation 1st ed 1969, pg 56, Fig. 49 c and d. In this manner of internal fixation each fragment is lagged to the other converting the many pieces into a solid block of bone. The necessary stripping robs these fragments of their blood supply

The radius and the ulna are an exception. Pronation and supination and normal elbow and wrist function depend on the preservation of the normal anatomical shape and relationship of these two bones. Therefore anatomical reduction of these two bones is mandatory and absolute stability of internal fixation is still the goal here. Thus a multifragmentary fracture of the radius and ulna, despite the use of indirect reduction techniques, requires bone grafting to accelerate union.

1.6.4 Methods of Reduction

Direct reduction is the direct manipulation of bony fragments during an open reduction of a fracture. As a prerequisite, the fracture site has to be exposed, which results in the stripping of soft tissue attachments and periosteum. The reduction is usually carried out with the help of surgical instruments such as levers and bone-holding clamps. It is a major cause of devitalization of bony fragments.

Indirect reduction is the reduction of a fracture by means of traction. In fractures which are being treated by closed methods, it is the principal method of securing reduction. Reduction of the fragments follows because of the application of an external force and because of the soft tissue attachments of the fragments. As traction is applied, the fragments tend to approximate themselves into reduction. Similar techniques have been adapted to open reduction in order to preserve the blood supply to the bony fragments and in order to simplify the reduction. Simple pull on a limb during an open reduction or the reduction of a fracture on a fracture table are classic examples of indirect reduction. The fragments are not manipulated directly, and their soft tissue attachment is not disturbed. As a result there is minimal interference with their blood supply.

Indirect reduction with the use of the distractor (Fig. 1.17) is a much more efficient technique because the distractor is fixed to the fragments being reduced. As a result the distraction is controlled and much less force is required. The distractor can be used alone to help in the reduction of a fracture (Fig. 1.18), as is most often the case in the reduction of diaphyseal fractures, but also most effectively in combination with plates in the reduction of metaphyseal fractures such as supracondylar fractures of the femur (Fig. 1.19). One can also use the articulating tension device in its distracting mode to secure indirect reduction, but this first requires the fixation of a plate to one of the main fragments of a fracture (Fig. 1.20). Lastly, the implant itself can be used to secure reduction of a fracture. The classic example of this is the reamed intramedullary nail. As the nail fills the medullary canal it secures axial realignment of the fracture. A straight plate, when properly contoured, can also be used to secure reduction (Fig. 1.21).

Indirect reduction techniques are very important because they not only help to preserve the blood supply to bone, but also because they make the reduction easier and therefore safer. It must be kept in mind, however, that indirect reduction alone will not bring about union. Whether the fracture is simple or multifragmentary,

Fig. 1.17. The femoral distractor. This type will allow distraction, interlocking, and manipulation of the proximal and distal fragment of the femur in all planes. (From Mast et al. 1989)

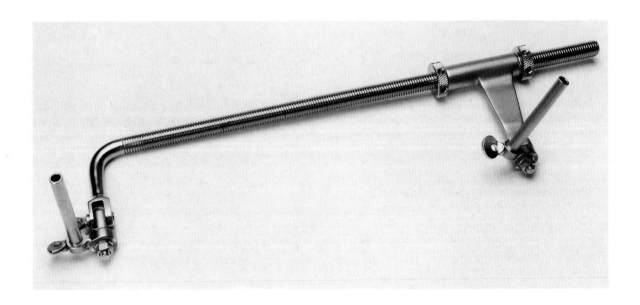

Fig. 1.18. a A simple fracture of the mid-shaft of the femur. Holes 4.5 mm in diameter are made in the proximal and distal fragments such that they will not interfere with the definitive implant after reduction. **b** With the femoral distractor attached, distraction of the fracture fragments is carried out. With distraction there is a tendency towards straightening of the femur and, if distraction forces are high, creating a deformity in the opposite direction from the distraction force – in this case a varus. **c** The tendency towards straightening may be corrected by carrying out the distraction over a bolster. The bolster acts as a fulcrum to maintain the antecurvatum of the femur. (From Müller et al. 1991)

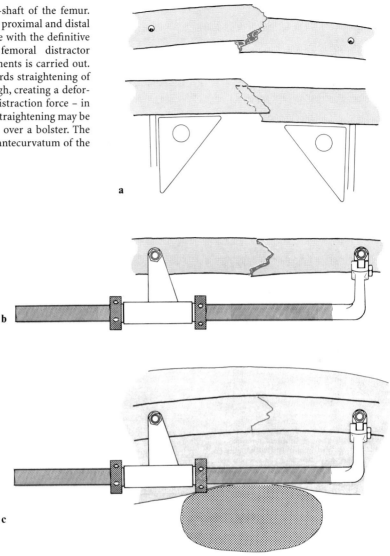

preservation of the blood supply to fragments greatly aids in union, but in order to achieve union the correct mode of fixation has to be chosen. As already outlined for simple fractures and articular fractures absolute stability is required. For multifragmentary fractures splinting by either a nail or a bridge plate is the method of choice.

1.7 Changes to the Early Concepts in Internal Fixation

At the time of the founding of the AO the prevailing schools of fracture treatment, such as the schools of Sir Reginald Watson-Jones in Great Britain and Böhler in continental Europe, concentrated on *bone union*. In contrast the AO concentrated on *function*. The AO group felt that immobilization resulted in *plaster disease* which was characterized by atrophy of the soft tissues, severe osteoporosis, thinning of articular cartilage, severe joint stiffness, and causalgic pain. To fight this disease the AO introduced "functional rehabilitation," a concept of fracture care based on the fact that if one achieved absolutely stable fixation of a fracture, then fracture pain would be completely abolished. This made it possible for the patient to move the extremity almost immediately after surgery.

This type of fracture treatment required the reduction to be anatomical and the fixation of the fracture not only sufficiently stable to abolish all pain, but also sufficiently strong and lasting to allow functional use without the danger of nonunion or malunion.

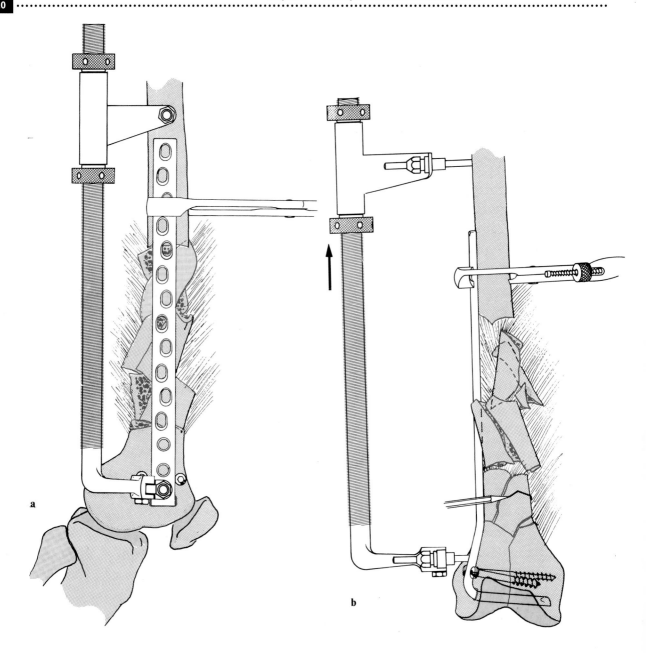

Fig. 1.19. a A severely comminuted fracture of the distal femoral shaft extending into the supracondylar and intracondylar area. The articular segment has been reconstructed and fixed. The blade plate has been inserted. The connecting bolt has been placed in the first hole of the plate, and the femoral distractor has spanned the comminuted area and portion of the femoral shaft to be plated. The plate is attached to the proximal fragment by means of a Verbrugge clamp. **b** Using a small instrument, such as a dental pick, comminuted fragments with their soft tissues attached are gently teased into approximate reduction. (From Mast et al. 1989)

Stability of the fixation was achieved by *compression* which recreated the structural continuity of the bone. The *lag screw* became the building block of stable internal fixation, and where necessary it was combined with *protection* or *neutralization plates or buttress plates.* Simple transverse or oblique fractures, because they could not be stabilized by means of lag screws, were brought under axial compression by means of *compression plates.* The emphasis in fracture treatment was on *mechanical stability* and the goal of internal fixation was to take many pieces of bone and convert them into a single solid block.

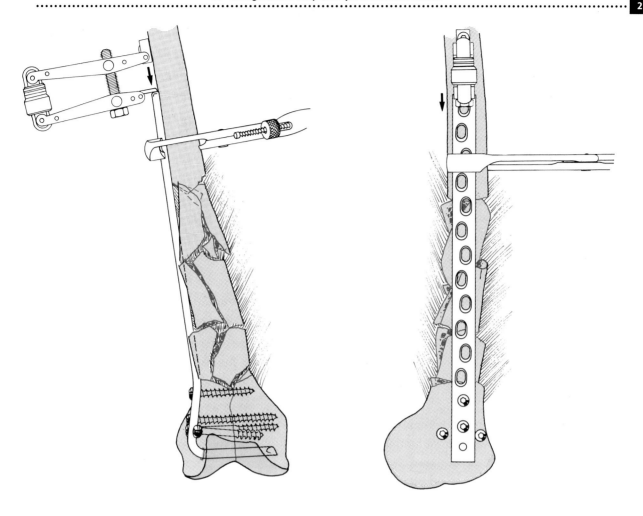

Fig. 1.20. The articulating tension device is placed as close as possible to the end of the plate and the tab turned to the distraction mode. The device is fastened to the bone by means of a uni- or bicortical screw, depending on the quality of the bone. Distraction is then carried out according to how much elongation of the segment is needed, determined in the preoperative plan. If the fracture morphology allows, the Verbrugge clamp may be tightened, the articulating tension device turned into compression mode, and an attempt made to load the fracture. It may be surprising, but using pointed reduction clamps in a couple of key places a comminuted fracture can be impacted and preloaded so that both mechanical stability and biological viability are achieved. Lag screws are inserted in the location previously occupied by clamps. However, in highly comminuted fractures this will be impossible and a pure buttress function of the plate is all that can be realized. (From Mast et al. 1989)

Simple fractures of the mid diaphysis of long bones such as the femur and tibia could also be treated by intramedullary nailing. Although this form of treatment, called *splinting*, achieved sufficient stability to allow functional aftertreatment, it did not provide absolute immobilization of fragments, which therefore healed with callus. In contrast, bone immobilized by means of interfragmental compression, and therefore stable, healed without the radiological evidence of callus by what was referred to as *primary bone union*.

Bone grafts were used frequently to ensure union of plated multifragmentary fractures and to fill defects in both cortical and metaphyseal bone. Indeed, failure to bone graft was the most frequent cause of failure of an internal fixation.

More than 30 years have passed since the formulation of the initial AO principles and methods. The initial goals of the AO – the improvement of fracture care with emphasis on the return of full function – have remained the same. There have been major changes, however, in principles, techniques, and implants. The most significant change has been a shift of emphasis from the mechanical to the biological aspects of internal fixation, with great emphasis on the preservation of the blood supply of bone and of soft tissue. A further development has been the recognition that absolute stability is necessary for revascularization and union of dead bone, and

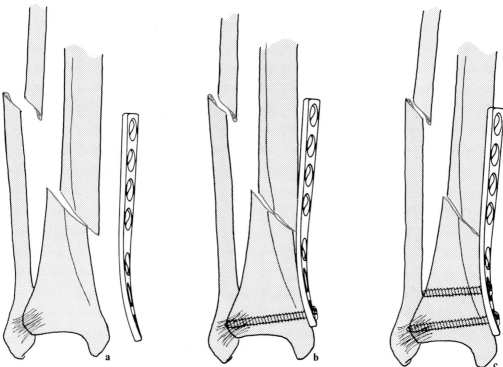

Fig. 1.21 a–c. Reduction of a distal third oblique fracture using an antiglide plate. **a** Following surgical exposure, a seven- to ten-hole plate, depending on the fracture, is selected. It is first twisted so that there is a torsion in the plate of approx. 25 °, then it is placed in a bending press and a mild concavity is pressed into its distal two thirds. This may be checked at surgery by using a marking pencil and a 20-cm length of suture thread to draw an arc on a flat surface against which the curve of the plate can be checked. The curvature may also be ascertained by a comparison AP X-ray of the opposite side. **b** The plate is then fixed to the distal fragment at the level of the buttress of the medial malleolus with one screw. Care must be taken not to enter thejoint with the screw because it is so low and because the curve of the plate has the natural tendency to direct the screw into the joint. There the normal 3.2-mm drill guide is used and a screw is inserted parallel with the joint. The screw is snugged but not definitively tightened. The plate is then rotated around the distal screw until its original orientation to the distal fragment is correct in the sagittal plane. The fit of the plate against the proximal fragment will be a little tight at this point. To accommodate this, the distal screw may need to be loosened slightly The tightness of the proximal end of the plate against the proximal fragment represents the plate–bone interference that in the end will reduce the fracture. With only the distal screw in place, the alignment of the fractures will be improved. At this time rotation should be corrected by gently twisting the patient's foot, and therefore the distal fragment, in the apropriate direction. **c** When little or no shortening is present, the next screw hole is drilled through the plate with a neutral drill guide. The screw length, which will be a little greater because the plate is not yet positioned snuggly against the bone, is measured and the screw is tapped and inserted. The distal screw and the second screw are then tightened together, but not definitively. The distal fragment of the fractured bone will be drawn in toward the plate. (From Mast et al. 1989)

that only living bone is capable of overcoming motion at the fracture and achieving union by the formation of callus. The appreciation of this difference is the key to choosing the correct technique of internal fixation of a fracture.

In the 1960 s and 1970 s the principles of internal fixation and stability were the same for articular fractures and for fractures of the diaphysis. In the years to follow we came to appreciate that the mechanical and biological requirements of articular and diaphyseal fractures are different. This has led to major alterations in the principles and methods of their treatment.

1.7.1 Articular Fractures

The principles of articular fracture surgery:

- Atraumatic anatomical reduction of the articular surface
- Stable fixation of the articular fragments
- Correction of axial deformity
- Metaphyseal reconstruction with bone grafting of defects
- Buttressing of the metaphysis
- Early motion

still apply today. What has changed is the timing of the different steps of the metaphyseal reconstruction.

Articular reconstruction must be undertaken as early as possible and with the least trauma to the tissues. A delay leads to permanent deformity because articular fragments unite rapidly and defy late attempts at reduction. Articular cartilage does not remodel. Any residual incongruity becomes permanent and can lead to posttraumatic arthritis (Llimas 1993, 1994). In contrast, the diaphysis and metaphysis have tremendous capacity for remodeling. Furthermore, any residual deformity can be relatively easily corrected by osteotomy.

The preservation of the viability and integrity of the soft tissue envelope of the metaphysis is the key to success (Marsh and Smith 1994; Stamer 1994). Thus, external fixation is frequently used as a temporary measure to achieve length and alignment of the metaphysis while the soft tissue envelope is recovering. The definitive reconstruction is then delayed for 2–3 weeks or longer if necessary. If the articular fragment is small and does not afford purchase for the external fixator, the joint is bridged temporarily with the external fixator to provide the necessary immobilization. Whenever the definitive reconstruction is carried out, either as a primary or delayed procedure, all measures are taken to minimize the damage to the blood supply of the soft tissue and bone. These measures include indirect reduction, minimal exposure, and percutaneous screw fixation of fragments. Buttressing continues to be important in preventing axial deformity, but the methods of buttressing today are designed to minimize soft tissue trauma. Thus, buttressing today may be in the form of plating or it may be achieved by means of an external fixation frame or it may be a combination of both.

1.7.2 Diaphyseal Fractures

The most notable change in the treatment of diaphyseal fractures has been the shift from the mechanical aspects of internal fixation, with absolute stability and primary bone union as the goal, to the biological aspects of internal fixation with splinting, relative stability, and healing with callus as the preferred method. Today the dominant theme in the fixation of fractures of the diaphysis is the biology of bone and the preservation of the blood supply to bony fragments. Absolute stability is no longer the object of internal fixation.

Whereas at one time the lag screw was the building block of stable internal fixation of fractures of the diaphysis, today the *locked intramedullary nail* has become the choice implant for the fixation of diaphyseal fractures. The development of locking of the main fragments onto the nail has greatly increased the scope of intramedullary nailing. Whereas before, multifragmentary fractures were a contraindication, today a multifragmentary fracture is *the* indication for using a locked

intramedullary nail. Locking has also made it possible to stabilize fractures of the proximal and distal third of the diaphysis and to treat subtrochanteric fractures with involvement of the lesser trochanter and ipsilateral fractures of the shaft and neck of the femur (Kyle 1994).

The biological and mechanical events associated with reaming or nail insertion and the consequent cardiopulmonary events have become the subject of major controversy among trauma surgeons. Reaming has been recognized as contributing significantly to the damage of the blood supply to the cortex. Reaming has also been recognized to cause a marked increase in the intramedullary pressure of bone (Stürmer 1993) and in a marked rise in the associated embolization of marrow contents to the lung (Wenda et al. 1993). These observations have resulted in the development of unreamed intramedullary nails for the tibia and femur, which as one might expect, however, have not eliminated the cardiopulmonary events. We are in the midst of a lively debate as to whether to nail the long bone fractures of polytrauma patients with a high Injury Severity Score, who have been in shock, and who have concomitant injuries to the thoracic cage and lung contusion (Pape et al. 1993). Long bone fractures in these patients should probably be either plated or stabilized initially by means of an external fixator (O. Trentz, personal communication).

Although locked intramedullary nailing is the preferred method for internal fixation of diaphyseal fractures, there continue to be many indications for plating. These will be discussed in detail in the ensuing chapters. Whenever plating is carried out the fracture is exposed. At this point the surgeon has the choice of carrying out either a direct or an indirect reduction. Direct reduction is the major cause of the devitalization of bony fragments. *Indirect reduction* techniques have been popularized to minimize on the damage to the blood supply of bone and of the soft tissue envelope (Mast et al. 1989). The method of reduction does not determine the degree of stability. Although stable fixation is usually practiced in association with direct reduction, indirect reduction techniques are equally applicable.

The method of *bridge plating* (Heitemeyer 1985) was developed to help prevent the devitalization of fragments of multifragmentary fractures (Perren 1991). In this technique of plating the fracture is first reduced by means of indirect reduction in order to minimize on the devitalization of fragments as bridge plating is very dependent on the viability of bone for the formation of callus and union. In this technique once length and rotation are reestablished, the zone of fragmentation is bridged with a plate which is fixed to the proximal and distal main fragments. The correct contouring of the plate reestablishes correct alignment. This type of internal fixation is a form of splinting. It is not absolutely stable and union is by callus. This technique of plating is

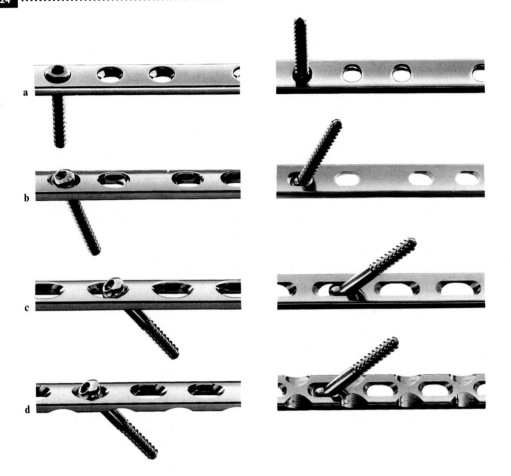

Fig. 1.22 a–d. The developments in AO internal fixation plates. In **a–d** upper *(left)* and lower *(right)* surfaces are shown. **a** The round hole plate (Müller et al. 1963). The conically undercut screw head allows for only a perpendicular position of the screw. The distance between the inner screw holes is larger. The plate undersurface is smooth. **b** The dynamic compression plate (DCP; Perren et al. 1969). The spherical contact geometry allows for 20 ° tilting of the screw along the long axis of the bone. **c** The dynamic compression unit (DCU; Klaue and Perren 1982). The completely symmetric screw holes are distributed at even distances throughout the plate. Symmetric screw holes with oblique undercut for improved range of inclination. **d** The limited-contact dynamic compression plate (LC-DCP; Perren et al. 1969) viewed from above; symmetric arrangement of the screw holes without a solid elongation between the innermost screw holes. The screw holes themselves are symmetric and are provided with two sloped cylinders. Lateral undercuts allow for bone formation at the plate (tension) side of the periosteal surface. Less damage to blood supply results, and the trapezoid cross section allows for easier and less traumatic removal of the plate. (From Müller et al. 1991)

indicated only for the fixation of multifragmentary fractures. If the surgeon chooses to plate a simple transverse or oblique fracture, then absolute stability must be achieved by means of interfragmental compression or excessive strain at the fracture site is likely to cause failure (Perren 1991).

The techniques of indirect reduction and bridge plating have made bone grafting of diaphyseal and metaphyseal multifragmentary fractures unnecessary. Bone grafting is now largely reserved for metaphyseal defects of articular fractures and for open fractures.

Anatomical reduction of the diaphyses of the femur, of the tibia, and of the humerus is not necessary. As long as length, rotation, and axial alignment are restored there will be no interference with function. The radius and the ulna are an exception. Pronation and supination and normal elbow and wrist function depend on the preservation of the normal anatomical shape and relationship of these two bones. Therefore anatomical reduction of these two bones is mandatory and stability should be achieved with an appropriate plating technique.

Preservation of the blood supply of the bony fragments has been achieved not only by indirect reduction and by changing the methods of internal fixation, but also by changes in the design of implants. The unreamed intramedullary nail was developed to minimize on the damage to the endosteal blood supply of long bones. The observation of Perren (1991; see also Gunst et al. 1979; Waelchli-Suter 1980) who studied the effects of plating on the blood supply of bone led to the discovery that the porosis of the cortex deep to the plates was not the result of stress protection but rather the result of local bone necrosis and its accelerated haversian remodeling. The degree of necrosis was determined by the degree of contact which the plate made with bone. This explained the seeming paradox that the so-called haversian remodeling was greater with flexible and elastic plates which were being used to overcome the stress protection of the stiffer metallic plates. The flexible plates made closer contact with the bone and interfered to a greater degree with the blood supply of the underlying cortex. These observations have led to the development of plates which have been designed in such a way as to minimize their contact with the underlying bone. The limited contact-dynamic compression plate (LC-DCP) is such a plate currently in use (Fig. 1.22). Its successor, the point contact plate or PCP, which is currently being developed, will be designed such that the plate will make absolutely no contact with the bone (S. Perren, personal communication). These methods of plating should eliminate any damage to the cortical blood supply and theoretically should make plating as advantageous as nailing in the treatment of fractures of the diaphysis.

1.8 Implant Failure and Bone Grafting

Metal plates or other devices, no matter how rigid or how thick and strong, will undergo fatigue failure and break if subjected to cyclical loading. Metal is best able to withstand tension; bone is best able to withstand compression. Thus, in an ideal internal fixation, the biomechanical arrangement should be such that the bone is loaded in compression and the metal in tension. If a defect is present in the cortex opposite the plate, and the bone is under bending load, the fulcrum will move closer and closer to the plate until it eventually falls within the plate (Fig. 1.23). Consequently, with repetitive loading, even if due only to muscular contraction, the implant is repeatedly cycled and may fail. Internal fixation can therefore be viewed as a race between bone healing and implant failure.

In order to prevent the possibility of implant failure after stable fixation, whenever there is comminution, whenever there is a defect in the cortex opposite the plate, whenever there is devitalization of fragments (as is frequently the case in high-velocity injuries), and whenever enormous forces have to be overcome, as in plating of femoral shaft fractures the fracture should be bone grafted. Such a graft, once it becomes incorporated into an osteoid bridge opposite the plate, rapidly hypertrophies and matures because it is subjected to compressive stresses. As soon as it reestablishes the continuity of bone opposite the plate it acts as a second plate and prevents the cycling and inevitable fatigue failure of the implant (Fig. 1.24).

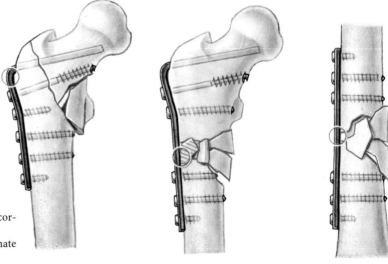

Fig. 1.23. Examples of deficiencies of the cortex opposite the plate which will result in cyclic bending of the plate and in its ultimate failure. (From Müller et al. 1979)

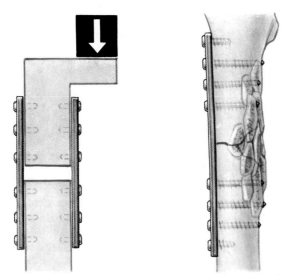

Fig. 1.24. Once it becomes incorporated into an osteoid bridge, a bone graft, if it is under compression, rapidly matures and hypertrophies. It reestablishes the continuity of the bone opposite the plate and prevents further cycling of the plate and its failure. (From Müller et al. 1979)

In stable fixation of a multifragmentary fracture union depends on the revascularization of the dead fragments. As a result union is slow and failure to bone graft is the most common cause of failure of stable internal fixation. In bridge plating union is rapid, and by callus. As a result the techniques of indirect reduction and bridge plating have made bone grafting of diaphyseal and metaphyseal multifragmentary fractures unnecessary. Bone grafting is now largely reserved for metaphyseal defects of articular fractures and for open fractures.

1.9 Implant Removal

Early on after fracture, bone which has united by primary bone healing is weaker than that united by callus. A callus, because of its spatial disposition, is further away from the central axis of bone than a plate and therefore in a mechanically more advantageous position to withstand force. The osteons of primary healing are closer to the central axis and the union is therefore mechanically weaker.

Primary bone healing is also weaker than that by callus because it undergoes a tremendous remodeling, which is manifested by a proliferation of haversian canals. Thus, such bone, although unchanged in its cross-sectional diameter, contains less bone per cross-sectional area because of the haversian proliferation. This continues until the accelerated remodeling ceases and the architecture gradually returns to normal. Based on their studies, Matter et al. (1974) suggested that the

intense remodeling subsides some 12 months or so after fracture. Factors which prolong the remodeling phase are the patient's age, the degree of comminution, the degree of devitalization, the size of the gaps, the accuracy of the reduction, the stability of the fixation, and whether the fracture was bone grafted. Furthermore, it is important to note whether there were any signs of instability during the time of healing or whether the fracture progressed uneventfully to union.

All these factors must be borne in mind when implant removal is being contemplated. If the implant is removed prematurely the bone will fail and refracture. We feel that most implants should be left in place for 2 years before their removal is contemplated. This timing may be modified by the factors indicated in the preceding paragraph.

Following removal of an implant the bone must be protected from overload. The screw holes act as stress raisers, and if the bone is suddenly loaded before the screw holes have filled in – a process which takes 6–8 weeks in experimental animals – the bone may fail. Similarly, the ridges which frequently develop on each side of the plate should not be osteotomized, as this further weakens the bone and may contribute to its failure.

Implant removal is carried out only if there are specific indications. It is a procedure with inherent risks and should not be entertained lightly.

References

Allgöwer M (1971) Weichteilprobleme und Infektrisiko der Osteosynthese. Langenbecks Arch Chir 329:1127

Allgöwer M, Matter P, Perren SM, Rüedi T (1973) The dynamic compression plate. Springer, Berlin Heidelberg New York

Charnley J (1953) Compression arthrodesis. Livingstone, Edinburgh

Gunst M, Suter C, Rahn BA (1979) Die Knochendurchblutung nach Plattenosteosynthese. Eine Untersuchung an der intakten Kaninchentibia mit Disulfinblau-Vitalfaerbung. Helvetica Chir Acta 46:171–175

Gustilo R, Andersson JP (1976) Prevention of infection in the treatment of one thousand and twenty-five open fractures of long bones. J Bone Joint Surg 58A:453

Heitemeyer U, Hierholzer G (1985) Die überbrückende Osteosynthese bei geschlossenen Stückfrakturen des Femurschaftes. Akt Traumatol 15:205–209

Kempf I, Grosse A, Beck G (1985) Closed locked intramedullary nailing. J Bone Joint Surg 67 A: 709–720

Key JA (1932) Positive pressure in arthrodesis for tuberculosis of the knee joint. South Med J 25:909–915

Klaue K, Perren SM (1982) Fixation interne des fractures par l'ensemble plaque-vis à compression conjuguée (DCU) Helv Chir Acta 49:77–80

Kyle RF (1994) Fractures of the Proximal Part of the Femur. J Bone Joint Surg 76A:924–950

Lange RH, Bach AW, Hansen ST, Johansen KH (1985) Open tibial fractures with associated vascular injuries: prognosis for limb salvage. J Trauma 25(3):203

Llinas A, McKellp HA, Marshall GJ, Sharpe F, Bin Lu MS, Kirchen M, Sarmiento A (1993) Healing and remodelling of articular incongruities in a rabbit fracture model. J Bone Joint Surg 75A:1508–1523

Llinas A, Lovasz G, Park SH (1994) Effect of joint incongruity on the opposing articular cartilage. Annual AAOS meeting, Los Angeles, CA

Marsh JL, Smith ST (1994) Outcome of severe tibial plateau fractures. Annual OTA meeting, Los Angeles, CA

Mast J, Jakob R, Ganz R (1989) Planning and reduction technique in fracture surgery. Springer, Berlin Heidelberg New York

Matter P, Brennwald J, Perren SM (1974) Biologische Reaktion des Knochens auf Osteosyntheseplatten. Helv Chir Acta [Suppl] 12

Mitchell N, Shepard N (1980)) Healing of articular cartilage in intraarticular fractures in rabbits. J Bone Joint Surg 62A:628–634

Müller ME, Allgöwer M, Willenegger H (1963) Technik der operativen Frakturenbehandlung. Springer, Berlin

Müller ME, Allgöwer M, Willenegger H (eds) (1970) Manual of internal fixation, 1 st edn. Springer, Berlin Heidelberg New York, p 10

Müller ME, Allgöwer M, Schneider R, Willenegger H (eds) (1979) Manual of internal fixation, 2 nd edn. Springer, Berlin Heidelberg New York

Müller ME, Nazarian S, Koch P, Schatzker J (1990) The comprehensive classification of fractures of long bones. Springer, Berlin Heidelberg New York

Pape H-C, Regel G, Dwenger A, Sturm JA, Tscherne H (1993) Influence of thoracic trauma and primary femoral intramedullary nailing on the incidence of ARDS in multiple trauma patients. Injury 24 (Suppl 3):82–103

Perren SM (1991) The concept of biological plating using the limited contact-dynamic compression plate (LC-DCP). Scientific background, design and application. Injury 22 (Suppl 1):5

Perren SM, Russenberger M, Steinemann S, Müller ME, Allgöwer M (1969) A dynamic compression plate. Acta Orthop Scand [Suppl] 125:31–41

Rhinelander FW (1973) Effects of medullary nailing on the normal blood supply of diaphyseal cortex. A.A.O.S. Instructional Course Lectures. Mosby, St. Louis, pp 161–187

Schatzker J, Horne JG, Sumner-Smith G (1975 a) The effects of movement on the holding power of screws in bone. Clin Orthop 111:257–263

Schatzker J, Sanderson R, Murnaghan P (1975 b) The holding power of orthopaedic screws in vivo. Clin Orthop 108:115

Schatzker J, Manley PA, Sumner-Smith G (1980) In vivo strain gauge study of bone response to loading with and without internal fixation. In: Uhthoff H (ed) Current concepts of internal fixation of fractures. Springer, Berlin Heidelberg New York, pp 306–314

Schenk R, Willenegger H (1963) Zum histologischen Bild der sogenannten Primärheilung der Knochenkompakta nach experimentellen Osteotomen am Hund. Experientia 19:593

Stürmer KM (1993) Measurements of intramedullary pressure in an animal experiment and propositions to reduce the pressure increase. Injury 24 (Suppl 3):7–21

Tscherne H, Brüggemann H (1976) Die Weichteilbehandlung bei Osteosynthesen, insbesondere bei offenen Frakturen. Unfallheilkunde 79:467

Tscherne H, Gotzen L (1984) Fractures with soft tissue injuries. Springer, Berlin Heidelberg New York Tokyo, pp 1–9

Tscherne H, Östern HJ (1982) Die Klassifizierung des Weichteilschadens bei offenen und geschlossenen Frakturen. Unfallheilkunde 85:111

Waelchli-Suter C (1980) Vascular changes in cortical bone following intramedullary fixation. In: Uhthoff HK (ed) Current concepts of internal fixation of fractures. Springer, Berlin Heidelberg New York, pp 411–415

Wenda K, Runkel M, Degreif J, Ritter G (1993) Pathogenesis and clinical relevance of bone marrow embolism in medullary nailing – demonstrated by intraoperative echocardiography. Injury 24 (Suppl 3):73–81

2 Intra-articular Fractures

J. Schatzker

2.1 Introduction

Intra-articular fractures may result in stiffness, deformity, pain, and post-traumatic arthritis. In order to avoid deformity and stiffness it is necessary to secure an anatomical reduction and begin early motion. Sir John Charnley stated that "perfect anatomical restoration and perfect freedom of joint movement can be obtained simultaneously only by internal fixation" (Charnley 1961). At the time that Charnley wrote *The Closed Treatment of Common Fractures*, sufficiently stable and sufficiently strong internal fixation which would allow early motion was not available. Indeed, the results of internal fixation were so discouraging because of stiffness, deformity, delayed union, and nonunion that Charnley argued in favor of nonoperative treatment. His sentiments were soon echoed by Stewart et al. (1966) and Neer et al. (1967), who published the results of treatment of a major intra-articular fracture, the supracondylar fracture of the femur in the adult. Even with limited criteria of excellence which today would be thought unacceptable, such as the acceptance of 70° knee flexion as satisfactory (Neer et al. 1967), both groups found the results of surgery to yield just over 50% acceptable results. Stewart et al. went on to state that it was the added trauma of surgery and the presence of metal in periarticular locations which directly contributed to stiffness. A review of the publications of these authors and others makes it evident that the techniques of internal fixation then in existence and the implants available were totally inadequate. Sufficient stability could never be achieved to permit early pain-free motion. If motion was permitted, not only did pain inhibit motion and result in stiffness, but displacement and loss of reduction were also very common. To prevent displacement, internal fixation was combined with plaster fixation, and this invariably resulted in permanent stiffness.

The publication of the Swiss AO/ASIF group in 1970 (Wenzl et al. 1970), our own review (Schatzker et al. 1974), and other reviews (Mize et al. 1982; Olerud 1972; Schatzker and Lampert 1979) of results of treatment of major intra-articular injuries utilizing the AO methods and implants indicated strongly that with the new principles, methods, and implants, stable fixation and early

motion after internal fixation was an attainable surgical goal, and that fractures – particularly intra-articular fractures – so treated did amazingly well.

The AO/ASIF methods of open reduction and internal fixation made strong, stable, and lasting fixation possible. Despite early, unprotected mobilization, accurate anatomical reduction of the joint and of the metaphyseal fractures could be maintained. Indeed, the patients were so completely free of pain that it was difficult to persuade them not to bear full weight and resume full function before union was complete.

The large number of patients who were treated nonoperatively (Schatzker et al. 1974, 1979) permitted us to make certain observations which we consider invaluable lessons in articular fracture treatment. Patients whose intra-articular fractures were immobilized in plaster for 1 month or longer ended with permanent marked stiffness of these joints. Patients with similar fractures which were treated by open reduction and internal fixation, but whose joints were subsequently immobilized in plaster, ended with far greater stiffness. Patients whose intra-articular fractures were treated by traction and early motion ended with varying degrees of joint incongruity, but invariably with a much better range of motion. This allowed us to formulate a principle of intra-articular fracture treatment: *Displaced intra-articular fractures which are not treated by open reduction and stable internal fixation should be treated by traction and early motion.*

Fractures which were treated by manipulation and traction often showed persistent displacement of some fragments. At surgery these fragments were always found to be firmly impacted into the metaphyseal cancellous bone and could be dislodged only by direct surgical manipulation. This permitted us to formulate the second principle of treatment: *Intra-articular fragments which do not reduce as a result of closed manipulation and traction are impacted and will not reduce as a result of further manipulation or traction.*

A number of cases of patients with intra-articular fractures which were initially treated closed but eventually operated on led to one further important observation: *Major intra-articular depressions do not fill with fibrocartilage to restore joint congruity and instability. If a joint is unstable because of major joint depression, the instability will become permanent unless the fragment is reduced surgically and held in position until union occurs.*

Pauwels (1961) postulated that in a normal joint there is a state of equilibrium between articular cartilage regeneration and articular cartilage destruction. Furthermore, he felt that articular cartilage wear occurred constantly, as a result of stress. As stress is the result of force acting on a specific surface area, i.e., $S=F/A$, it becomes clear that stress can be increased and the equilibrium tipped in favor of joint destruction either by decreasing the surface area of contact (A) or by increasing the force (F), or by both. F is increased above its physiologic level by axial overload, the result of a metaphyseal or diaphyseal deformity.

A consideration of the above led us to an inescapable conclusion: *Anatomical reduction of the joint is essential to restore joint congruity and increase the surface area of contact to the maximum possible, and metaphyseal and diaphyseal deformity must be corrected to prevent axial overload* (Fig. 2.1).

These are the principles of intra-articular fracture care enunciated by the AO (Müller et al. 1979), and we fully agree with them. The therapeutic validity of these principles is confirmed by the favorable results of modern operative treatment of intra-articular fractures.

What about articular cartilage damage sustained at the time of injury and the possibility of articular cartilage regeneration? In an elegant experiment, Mitchell and Shepard (1980) studied the effects of the accuracy of reduction and stable fixation. With the aid of histological methods and electron microscopy, they were able to show that anatomical reduction and stable fixation of intra-articular fragments by means of compression resulted in articular cartilage regeneration.

Salter et al. (1980, 1986) studied experimentally and clinically the effects of continuous passive motion on articular cartilage healing and regeneration. They demonstrated very convincingly that continuous passive motion stimulated both processes.

More recent investigations into stepoff defects (Llinas 1993, 1994) have delineated the limits of positive stepoff deformities, which should not exceed the thickness of the articular cartilage. These studies have also confirmed the limited ability of articular cartilage to remodel. They have further demonstrated the danger of a positive stepoff deformity to the opposing articular surface in causing rapid degenerative change.

Magnetic resonance imaging (MRI) investigation of closed joint injuries has revealed "bruising" of the subchondral bone and has allowed a correlation between certain MRI patterns of bruising and subsequent osteochondral fragmentation and the formation of articular defects (Vellet et al. 1991). Similar damage to articular cartilage and subjacent bone must also occur in association with fractures. This points to the shortcomings of visual evaluation of articular cartilage injury and indicates why caution should be exercised in the prognosis of articular injuries, since some aspects of the injury may escape detection and are not influenced by treatment.

These experimental and clinical studies permit us to enunciate the principles of intra-articular fracture treatment as follows:

1. Immobilization of intra-articular fractures results in joint stiffness.
2. Immobilization of articular fractures treated by open reduction and internal fixation results in much greater stiffness.
3. Depressed articular fragments which do not reduce as a result of closed manipulation and traction are impacted and will not reduce by closed means.
4. Major articular depressions do not fill with fibrocartilage, and the instability which results from their displacement is permanent.
5. Anatomical reduction and stable fixation of articular fragments is necessary to restore joint congruity.
6. Metaphyseal defects must be bone-grafted to prevent articular fragment redisplacement.
7. Metaphyseal and diaphyseal displacement must be reduced to prevent joint overload.
8. Immediate motion is necessary to prevent joint stiffness and to ensure articular cartilage healing and recovery. This requires stable internal fixation.

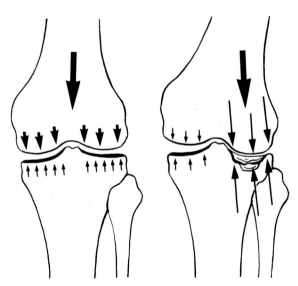

Fig. 2.1. Anatomical reduction of the joint and correction of metaphyseal and diaphyseal deformity greatly reduces the stress on articular cartilage

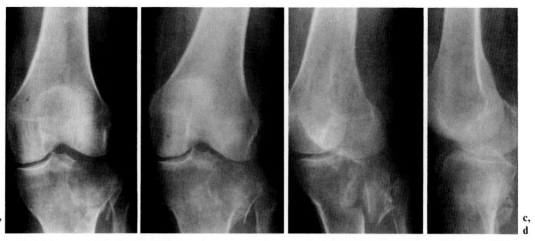

Fig. 2.2 a–d. Tibial plateau fracture roentgenograms. **a** Anteroposterior. **b** Oblique. **c** Oblique. **d** Lateral. Note particularly on the two oblique projections (**b, c**) the marked improvement in the definition of the lateral plateau comminution and depression

2.2 Clinical Aspects

The clinical aspects of intra-articular fractures are important in the decision-making process regarding the best mode of treatment for a particular injury. We emphasize repeatedly in this book the concept of the "personality" of the fracture. In order to define the personality, we must know not only such obvious factors as the violence involved in the injury, but also the patient's age, occupation, athletic pursuits, expectations of treatment, and similar details.

2.2.1 Physical Examination

Although radiological examination is indispensable in defining the fracture pattern, it does not shed light on the soft tissue components of the injury. Tenderness over the course of a ligament or its insertion may be the only available clue to a ligament disruption. Similarly, the presence of a neurological deficit, a compartment syndrome, or a vascular lesion is best established by physical examination.

2.2.2 Radiological Evaluation

An anterioposterior and a lateral radiograph are frequently insufficient to define precisely the pattern of injury (Fig. 2.2). We have found that oblique projections, as well as stress X-rays when indicated, add greatly to the definition of an injury. Often intra-articular detail is obscured because of distortion and overlap of fragments (Fig. 2.3). Plain tomography will help to define the detailed outline of intra-articular and metaphyseal fragments (Fig. 2.4), which will facilitate classification of the injury and determination of its prognosis and thus guide its treatment. Computerized axial tomography has been invaluable in some complex fractures such as acetabular injuries, pilon fractures, fractures around the knee, and some shoulder injuries (Fig. 2.5).

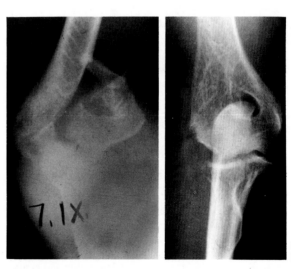

Fig. 2.3. a Anteroposterior roentgenogram of a supracondylar fracture of the humerus. The details of the fracture are almost completely obscured. **b** Anteroposterior roentgenogram of the opposite, uninvolved elbow to be used as template for preoperative planning

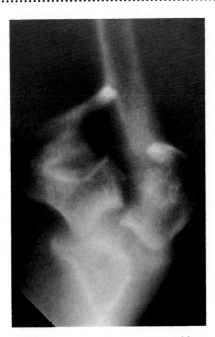

Fig. 2.4. Anteroposterior tomogram adds greatly to the precise definition of the injury

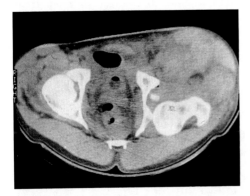

Fig. 2.5. Computed tomography (CT) scan of a posterior fracture–dislocation of the hip. Note the large intra-articular fragment which was not evident on a plain roentgenogram or plain tomography

2.3 Surgery

2.3.1 Timing

Certain intra-articular injuries, such as ankle and elbow fractures, should be treated as emergencies and operated on as soon as possible. The rapid swelling of a fracture–dislocation of an ankle or of a pilon fracture is the result of a rapidly developing hematoma. Immediate surgery allows the evacuation of such hematomas and the reduction of the distortion of the soft tissues. This vastly improves the circulation and minimizes subsequent swelling. In cases in which closure at the end of surgery is difficult because of tissue tension, once the joint is closed we leave the wounds open and close them secondarily after the swelling has subsided. This policy has permitted early safe surgery without incurring wound-edge necrosis or sepsis. We have found that elbow injuries should also be treated as emergencies, not only because of the swelling and possible vascular complications, but also because of the very high incidence of myositis ossificans associated with delays of 4 or 5 days from the time of injury (Fig. 2.6).

We have been delaying surgery of certain intra-articular fractures because of their complexity: among these are difficult supracondylar fractures of the femur, certain tibial plateau fractures, pilon fractures, and acetabular fractures. In acetabular fractures, delay has been caused not only by the complexity of the lesion and the time required for its exact definition, but also by associated injuries commonly present and the general condition of the patients. The high incidence of myositis ossificans seen in acetabular fractures operated on through the posterior approach may in part be the result of the delay, as it is in periarticular fractures of the elbow.

Our recommendations to delay immediate reconstruction of complex articular fractures have been reinforced by the more recent experience of other surgeons (Marsh et al. 1994; Stamer et al. 1994; Keppler et al. 1994). The complications encountered as result of early reconstruction of high-velocity articular fractures, particularly of subcutaneous joints such as the tibial plafond and the tibial plateau, have led to major changes in the timing of reconstruction, in the exposure techniques, and in the methods of fixation. We now recommend securing reduction of the articular surfaces as early as possible because articular fractures unite rapidly and defy attempts to perform late reduction or joint reconstruction. The timing of the reconstruction of the injury's metaphyseal component is based on the severity of injury to the soft tissue envelope. In high-velocity injuries we generally tend to delay the metaphyseal reconstruction and maintain length and alignment of the metaphysis by either traction or external fixation. The current guiding principle in the internal fixation of articular injuries is the preservation of the blood supply to the soft tissues and to all the bony fragments. Thus not only is the metaphyseal reconstruction carefully staged, but we also rely on techniques of indirect reduction, on the percutaneous insertion of lag screws, and, where indicated, on the buttressing of these fractures in hybrid frames in order to preserve the viability of tissues as much as possible.

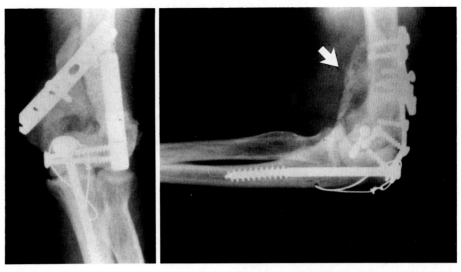

Fig. 2.6. Florid ossifying myositis *(arrow)* particularly in front of the elbow – a frequent complication of delayed surgery around the elbow

2.3.2 Approach and Technique

Once the personality of the fracture has been defined by painstaking clinical and radiological investigation, it is necessary to make a careful preoperative plan of the surgery. This includes a plan of the surgical approach as well as a detailed plan of the internal fixation and any bone-grafting required.

The exposure of the joint must be atraumatic, and yet it must be extensive so that all the components of the injury can be visualized and be made fully accessible to manipulation and fixation. (For detailed descriptions of such exposures, please refer to the chapters on the specific joint fractures.)

The surgical reconstruction of the joint begins with an anatomical reduction of the articular surface. This often requires that depressed portions of the articular cartilage be elevated from their impacted position in the metaphysis. This is best done by elevating the depressed fragments together with the impacted metaphyseal cancellous bone. Once elevated, the fragments must be held provisionally in their reduced positions using Kirschner wires. It is then necessary to bone-graft the metaphyseal defect which is invariably created when the articular fragments are disimpacted and elevated. Although some authors have described the use of cortical struts to hold up the articular surface, we prefer autogenous cancellous bone, which we compact with a bone punch. This allows good filling of the defects and helps to maintain the articular reduction. Next in order of importance is a careful reduction of the metaphyseal and diaphyseal components of the fracture.

Once the fractures are reduced, we secure fixation of the articular components by means of lag screws. These lag screws should not be inserted too close to the subchondral bone because they lead to its stiffening and to possible chondrolysis (Manley and Schatzker 1982). The metaphysis must be buttressed to prevent axial overload, and the diaphyseal components must be fixed so that early motion can be started. Prior to closure, certain intra-articular structures such as the menisci of the knee should be repaired if torn or peripherally detached. In-substance lesions of the cruciate ligaments are not repaired primarily nor substituted, as such repairs require postoperative immobilization, which we like to avoid. The only cruciate lesions we repair immediately are avulsions of the anterior or posterior cruciate ligament with a piece of bone; these can be fixed with lag screws or wire loops with sufficient stability to allow immediate mobilization. Any other cruciate deficiencies are repaired at a later stage, if indicated. This policy has allowed us to concentrate on the mobilization of the joints, which we feel is far more important than early anteroposterior stability. This policy does not, however, apply to lateral stability. All collateral ligaments are carefully repaired at the time of the initial surgery; collateral repair does not prevent early mobilization of the joint.

As already alluded to, the timing of the reconstruction of the metaphyseal component is frequently delayed in order not to prejudice the soft tissue envelope. This does not mean that a primary reconstruction cannot be carried out, but caution is the key. It is best to err on the side of delay rather than haste. Once the reconstruction is undertaken, all efforts are undertaken to minimize trauma in order to preserve the blood supply to the soft

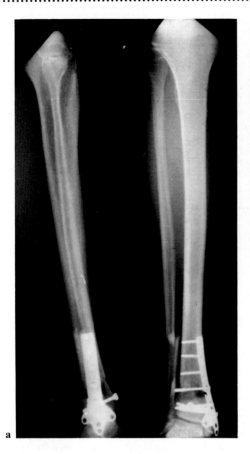

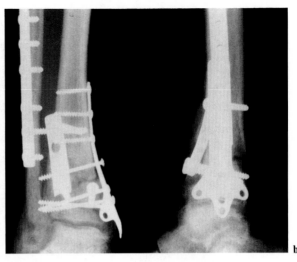

a

b

Fig. 2.7. a An intra-articular pilon facture at 6 weeks after surgery. A number of surgical principles have been violated. The fibula was not reduced, the metaphysis was not bone-grafted, and the lesion was not properly buttressed. **b** Note the excellent correction of the deformity achieved by reduction of the fibula, by bone-grafting of the metaphyseal defect created once the valgus was corrected, and by proper buttressing of the metaphysis

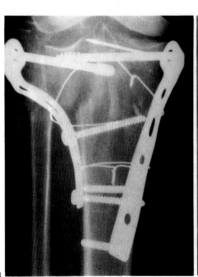

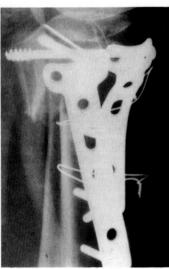

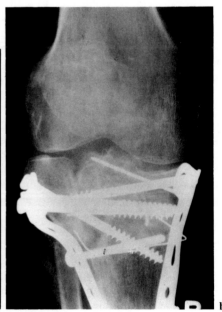

a

b

Fig. 2.8. a Serious malreduction of a difficult tibial plateau fracture. **b** Stability was restored by an intra-articular wedge excision of the depressed area. This allowed us to narrow the lateral plateau and reduce the remaining intact portion, which carried the meniscus under the lateral femoral condyle

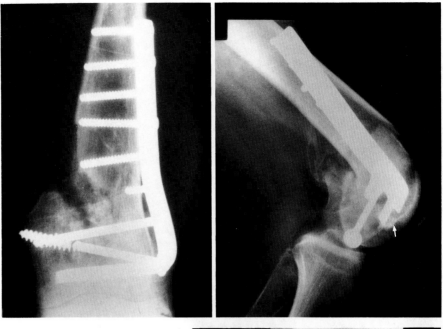

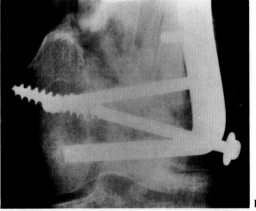

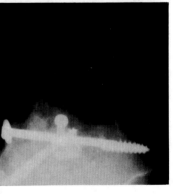

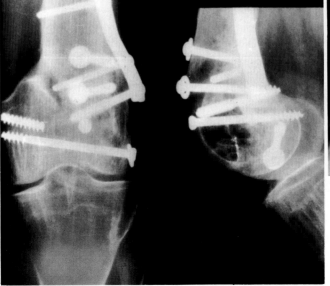

Fig. 2.9. a, b Malunion of the lateral femoral condyle and fracture of the cancellous screw. Note the double contour of the lateral femoral condyle, best seen in **b**. This malunion distorted the intercondylar groove and markedly restricted knee motion. **c** An intra-articular osteotomy was carried out. The excessive fibrocartilage and all callus were carefully excised, recreating the original fracture fragment. This allowed an anatomical reduction of the joint. Note the unorthodox position of a buttress plate on the posterolateral aspects of the distal femoral metaphysis. Anatomical reduction and stable fixation led to an excellent recovery of the joint

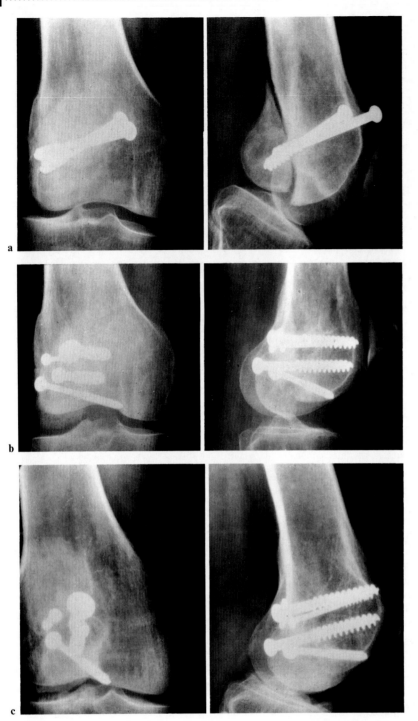

Fig. 2.10. a A 2-year-old nonunion of the lateral femoral condyle in an 18-year-old boy. **c** Note the excellent correction of the valgus deformity at 3 years after surgery, with union and an excellent preservation of joint function, despite the intra-articular step clearly evident in **b** soon after corrective surgery

tissue and bone. Thus techniques of indirect reduction are employed together with minimal exposure and the use of percutaneous lag screws where indicated. Most buttressing is still accomplished with plates, but where immediate surgery has to be undertaken, such as in open fractures or in closed fractures complicated by a vascular injury or an acute compartment syndrome, we rely on hybrid frames rather than plates. If the epiphyseal fragment is too small for a hybrid frame, then we are prepared to bridge the joint with an external fixateur. Necrosis of the soft tissue envelope is a preventable disaster. Some loss of motion is preferable to infection. If early operation is essential, the skin should never be closed under tension. We like to close the synovium and capsule to prevent dessication of the articular cartilage and to cover any exposed tendon or nerve. The remainder of the wound is left open and closed secondarily 5 or 6 days later.

2.4 Postoperative Care

The experiments of Salter et al. (1980) and Mitchell and Shepard (1980) have underlined the importance of early motion. Our clinical experience, as well as that of many other investigators, bears this out. After their reconstruction, all major intra-articular injuries are placed on a continuous passive motion machine; passive mobilization is started in the recovery room and is continued for 5–7 days. In late joint reconstructions this may be continued for up to 3 or 4 weeks.

It must be remembered that mobilization and its benefits need to be in balance with the degree of stability obtained at the time of surgery. At times, the degree of stability of the internal fixation is insufficient to permit unprotected mobilization. In these instances we have combined internal fixation with fracture bracing. The fracture brace can be applied on the first day or two without jeopardizing the internal fixation or wound care. Similarly, it must be remembered that in at least 25%–30% of cases major intra-articular fractures, particularly around the knee, are associated with major ligamentous disruptions, which must be repaired at the time of the initial surgery. The usual practice is to protect any ligamentous repair in plaster. As we have already pointed out, intra-articular fracture repair combined with plaster immobilization results in an unacceptable degree of stiffness. Therefore, we have always managed these combined injuries and repairs by protecting the ligamentous reconstructions by immediate fracture bracing and then carrying on with the usual mobilization on a continuous passive motion machine. Because in-substance cruciate ligament reconstructions require the surgeon to limit the excursion of the knee, we have deferred such reconstructions, but have always repaired collateral ligaments and cruciate avulsions with bone. Late cruciate insufficiency has been dealt with when necessary once the joint has been fully rehabilitated. Joint stiffness is one complication which must be avoided at all costs.

2.5 Late Intra-articular Reconstructions

Late intra-articular deformities arise either (a) as a result of failed nonoperative treatment, (b) because of incomplete surgical reduction of the fracture, or (c) because of loss of position due to unstable fixation. Such articular deformities have usually been considered as permanent and not amenable to any surgical reconstruction. We have subjected many such intra-articular deformities to late intra-articular reconstruction, at varying intervals from the time of injury (Figs. 2.7– 2.10). This has often required intra-articular osteotomies with meticulous excision of the fibrocartilage from the joint and of the callus from the metaphysis, in order to redefine the original fragments and permit an anatomical reconstruction. We have also treated a number of intra-articular nonunions. The principle followed with these, as with the malunions, has been meticulous reconstruction of the joint, stable fixation of the joint and of the metaphyseal component with bone-grafting where necessary, arthrolysis and soft tissue mobilization periarticularly to regain a satisfactory range of motion, and then mobilization of the joint on a continuous passive motion machine. Although we have never managed to achieve a return to a perfectly normal degree of joint function, we have been impressed with the successes attained and feel that unless there is evidence of serious post-traumatic arthritis, a late joint reconstruction should be undertaken if it is at all technically feasible. This is preferable to joint arthroplasty or arthrodesis.

References

Charnley J (1961) The closed treatment of common fractures. Livingstone, Edinburgh

Keppler P, Meining R, Suger G, Kinzl L (1994) Long term results of the operative reconstruction of the bicondylar tibial plateau fractures. Annual Orthopaedic Trauma Meeting, Los Angeles, CA

Llinas A, McKellop HA, Marshall GJ, Sharpe F, Bin Lu MS, Kirchen M, Sarmiento A (1993) Healing and remodelling of articular incongruities in a rabbit fracture model. J Bone Joint Surg 75A:1508–1523

Llinas A, Lovasz G, Park SH (1994) Effect of joint incongruity on the opposing articular cartilage. Annual AAOS meeting

Manley P, Schatzker J (1982) Replacement of epiphyseal bone with methylmethacrylate. Its effects on articular cartilage. Arch Orthop Traum Surg 100:3–10

Marsh JL, Smith ST, Do TT (1994) Outcome of severe tibial plateau fractures. Annual Orthopaedic Trauma Association meeting, Los Angeles, CA

Mitchell N, Shepard N (1980) Healing of articular cartilage in intra-articular fractures in rabbits. J Bone Joint Surg 62A:628–634

Mize RD, Bucholz RW, Grogan DP (1982) Surgical treatment of displaced comminuted fractures of the distal end of the femur. J Bone Joint Surg 64A:871–879

Müller ME, Allgöwer M, Schneider K, Willenegger H (1979) Manual of internal fixation, 2nd edn. Springer, Berlin Heidelberg New York

Neer C, Graham SA, Shelton ML (1967) Supracondylar fracture of the adult femur. J Bone Joint Surg 49A:591–613

Olerud S (1972) Operative treatment of supracondylar-condylar fractures of the femur. Technique and results in fifteen cases. J Bone Joint Surg 54A:1015–1032

Pauwels F (1961) Neue Richtlinien für die operative Behandlung der Coxarthrose. Verh Dtsch Orthop Ges 48:332–366

Salter RB, Simmonds DF, Malcolm BW, Rumble EJ, MacMichael D (1980) The biological effects of continuous passive motion on the healing of full thickness defects in articular cartilage: an experimental investigation in the rabbit. J Bone Joint Surg 62A:1232–1251

Salter RB, Hamilton HW, Wedge JH, Tile M, Torode IP, O'Driscoll SW, Murnaghan J, Saringer JH (1986) Clinical application of basic research on continuous passive motion for disorders and injuries of synovial joints: a preliminary report of a feasibility study. Techniques Orthopaed I(I):74–91

Schatzker J, Lampert DC (1979) Supracondylar fractures of the femur. Clin Orthop 138:77–83

Schatzker J, Horne G, Waddell J (1974) The Toronto experience with the supracondylar fractures of the femur 1966–1972. Injury 6:113–128

Schatzker J, McBroom R, Bruce D (1979) The tibial plateau fracture: the Toronto experience. Clin Orthop 138:94–104

Stamer DT, Schenk R, Staggers B, Aurori K, Aurori B, Behrens F (1994) Bicondylar tibial plateau fractures treated with a hybrid ring external fixator: a preliminary study. Annual Orthopaedic Trauma Association meeting. Los Angeles, CA

Stewart M, Sisk D, Wallace SL (1966) Fractures of the distal third of the femur. J Bone Joint Surg 48A:784–807

Vellet AD, Marks P, Fowler PJ, Munro TG (1991) Post-traumatic osteochondral lesions of the knee. Prevalence classification and short term sequela. Evaluation with MRI imaging. Radiology 178:271

Wenzl H, Casey PA, Hébert P, Belin J (1970) Die operative Behandlung der distalen Femurfraktur. AO Bulletin, Bern

3 Open Fractures

J. Schatzker and M. Tile

3.1 Introduction

In spite of the advances made in fracture care and in the prevention of and management of infection, open fractures remain a serious surgical problem. Even now an open fracture of the tibia with an associated vascular injury results in an amputation in 60 % of cases (Lange et al. 1985).

In past decades open fractures often resulted in the loss of life and/or the loss of limb (Billroth 1866). Tscherne (1984) has described the four major eras in the treatment of open fractures: the era of life preservation, the era of limb preservation, the era of avoidance of infection, and the era of the preservation of function. In the past two decades, because of advances in fracture care, most of the effort in managing open fractures has been devoted to the preservation of function. Preventing infection and ensuring union of the fracture, in the absence of good limb function, is no longer acceptable, except in circumstances in which a joint has been destroyed, or major muscle or nerve loss has occurred.

The aim of all fracture care is the return of the injured extremity to full function in the shortest possible period of time. In caring for an open fracture the surgeon should aim for no less. Other factors such as major bone loss, muscle injury, and nerve or tendon loss may make this goal unattainable; nevertheless, the goal should be strived for. A combined study from the University Hospital in Nottingham, UK, and Sunnybrook Medical Centre, Toronto, Canada (Beauchamp et al. 1984) showed that this is attainable. In 97 open fractures of the tibial shaft 89 % of patients achieved excellent functional results.

In this chapter we discuss only the general principles of open fracture management. The details of treatment as they apply to particular bones are found in the chapters dealing with the specific injuries in question.

3.2 Assessment of the Soft Tissue Wound

Many observers have attempted to grade open fractures (Allgöwer 1971; Gustilo and Andersson 1976; Oestern and Tscherne 1984); however, since each injury is unique, a clear description of each particular injury is more important than assigning it a numerical grade. The surgeon must look beyond the skin wound and carefully assess the state of the entire wound, including the amount of skin contusion, the apparent damage to subcutaneous tissue, muscle, fascia, vital structures, and bone. Most classifications define a grade I injury as a small puncture wound of less than 1 cm; however, the location of the wound may be more important than its size. For example, if it is on a subcutaneous border, it may have been caused by a relatively low-energy injury and therefore be associated with relatively little muscle damage. However, one must assume that to produce a similarly sized wound in an area of thick muscle belly, such as the posterior tibia or the femur the bone ends must have penetrated a large mass of muscle to reach the skin: therefore the amount of muscle damage is far greater (see Fig. 20.6). Failure to recognize this fact and consequent failure to resect all the necrotic tissue could lead to grave consequences for the patient, such as gas gangrene, amputation, or even death.

Careful assessment of the wound and, more importantly, the implications of the wound are therefore essential to good patient management.

3.3 Classification

Several grading systems have been proposed for open fractures. Some of these have gained widespread acceptance. Unfortunately though some of these overlap with one another. Allgöwer (1971) described three grades of open fracture: grade I, a small skin wound pierced from within by bone; grade II, a skin wound with skin contusion; grade III, an extensive skin wound with major damage to skin, muscle, and vital structures. Gustilo and Andersson (1976) used a similar classification, a grade I wound being less than 1 cm, a grade II wound more than 1 cm, and a grade III wound being extensive. Tscherne (1984) described four grades of soft tissue injury associated with open fracture. In his classification the size of the skin wound was not important, but the degree of soft tissue damage, the severity of the fracture, and the degree of contamination were important.

The following grading system from Lange et al. (1985) is widely used and is recommended:

- Grade I: a skin wound from within, usually less than 1 cm, with little or no skin contusion.
- Grade II: a skin wound of more than 1 cm, with skin and soft tissue contusion, but no loss of muscle or bone. A small wound over a major muscle mass should be considered a grade II open fracture.
- Grade III: a large, severe, open wound with extensive skin and subcutaneous contusion, muscle crush or loss, and severe bone communution. This grade is divided into four subgrades, all with severe soft tissue injury and the following:
- a: A comminuted fracture with bone exposed but covered by periosteum
- b: A comminuted fracture with loss of periosteal cover
- c: Vascular lesion and neurovascular lesion
- d: A traumatic amputation

3.4 Management

The goal in treating open fractures is to secure union and restore normal anatomy and early return of normal function. To achieve this goal one must prevent infection, which is the single most important cause of permanent disability in open fractures. Infection contributes to scarring and to loss of function of the soft tissue envelope, to stiffness of joints, to deformity, and to delayed union and nonunion.

3.4.1 Decision Making

Many factors must be considered in determining the method of treatment of an open fracture. These include general factors such as the age and general medical state of the patient, whether the patient is polytraumatized or the injury isolated to one limb, and the severity of the injury. The local factors include the extent of the soft tissue wound, the time elapsed between injury and definitive treatment, the fracture configuration, and the presence or absence of major injury to vital structures, especially vascular injuries. All of these factors must be considered, and the method of treatment selected must have a favorable risk-benefit ratio for the patient.

3.4.2 Immediate Treatment

Emergency treatment of open fractures seeks (a) to create an environment that denies bacteria which have gained access to the tissues sufficient opportunity to multiply and establish an infection and (b) to prevent further contamination. Therefore the first cardinal rule is to avoid further soft tissue injury. Fractures should be reduced on the scene to alleviate pressure on the injured ischemic soft tissues. Swelling and the spread of hematoma should be controlled by placing a sterile dressing over the wound, and the extremity must be splinted.

Rapid transport to a hospital and immediate treatment are essential. Tscherne (1984) found that the infection rate of open fractures delivered to the hospital by helicopter within 30 min of the accident is 3.5%, while that of fractures presenting for treatment after 10 h is 22.2%. Limiting contamination is also very important. Tscherne showed that maintaining the initial sterile dressing intact restricted the infection rate to 4.3%, whereas wounds without a sterile dressing developed a 19.2% infection rate (Table 3.1).

During resuscitation of the patient the dressing should not be removed. The patient should be given prophylactic antibiotics, usually a first-generation cephalosporin. In grade III injuries we also add an aminoglycoside. Antitetanus prophylaxis must also be administered.

3.4.3 Operative Treatment

3.4.3.1 Limb Salvage

The first decision to be made is whether the limb is salvageable or not (Chapman and Mahoney 1979; Chapman 1980). This decision depends upon many factors. If the open fracture is associated with a vascular injury in a polytraumatized individual, amputation may be life saving and must be considered, especially in the more distal regions of the extremities. Vascular repair may be a lengthy procedure, greatly prolonging the time a critically ill patient spends under anesthesia. In distal vascular injuries the chances for a good functioning extremity are remote. A recent study found that 60% of all open tibia fractures associated with vascular injury eventually require amputation (Lange et al. 1985). Many of the salvaged limbs had poor function. Therefore if the patient is polytraumatized, the risks of attempting limb salvage may be much greater than the benefit to the patient; the attempt may be costly indeed.

Table 3.1. Infection rates of open fractures, with and without continuous sterile covering from accident scene to operating room (from Tscherne 1984)

	With sterile dressing (*n*=16)	Without sterile dressing (*n*=77)
Infection rate	5 (4.3 %)	15 (19.2 %)

3.4.3.2 Cleansing

The skin should be cleansed with soap and shaved, the bone ends if they protrude through the wound brushed, and the wound irrigated with approximately 12 l Ringer's lactate solution. The skin may then be prepared with an antiseptic agent, such as chlorohexadine. A tourniquet should be applied but not used unless essential to stop massive bleeding.

3.4.3.3 Débridement

Living tissue offers the best defense against infection. Next to a hematoma, tissues that are poorly perfused or devitalized offer the best medium for bacterial proliferation. As Louis Pasteur said "The germ is nothing; the terrain on which it grows is everything." The next steps in the treatment are therefore aggressive excision of all dead and devascularized tissues and stabilization of the fracture using techniques which offer the least compromise to the blood supply to soft tissues and bone.

Thorough débridement must take into account the full zone of injury. The apparent zone of injury is often very small compared to the real extent. Unfortunately, there are no reliable tests for tissue viability. Godina (1986) and Byrd (1985) advised immediate radical excision of all suspected tissues, treating it as a pseudotumour and then carrying out immediate soft tissue reconstruction. Most surgeons are less radical and practice serial débridements. Initial débridement attempts to rid the wound of all dead soft tissue and bone. The patient is returned to the operating room at intervals 24–48 h for serial débridements until one can be certain that all dead tissue has been removed.

Débridement thus refers to the removal of all contamination and the meticulous excision of all devitalized tissue. The amount of débridement required depends on the severity of the soft tissue injury. In grade I injuries the location of the wound dictates the débridement. If the wound is a small puncture and over a subcutaneous bone, very little extension of the wound is required since muscle damage is minimal. However, if the puncture wound is over muscle, the wound must be extended sufficiently to reveal all the traumatized tissue so that an extensive and meticulous débridement can be executed.

All grade II and grade III open wounds must be carefully débrided (Bosse et al. 1984). Any tight compartments must be decompressed and the muscle viability assessed. The important factors in assessing the viability of muscle include bleeding, contractility, and color. Avulsed ends of muscle, skin, and subcutaneous tissue must be excised. In grades II and III the wound must also be extended to allow for easy access to the bone. The

exact method of extending the wound depends on the location of the wound and the decision as to the method of stabilization required. In some circumstances internal fixation is performed through the extended wound while in others a separate wound is preferable for the internal fixation. If external fixation is to be the method of stabilization, local extension of the wound will usually suffice.

All cortical fragments stripped of their muscle attachments should be removed because they are dead. An exception is a large fragment containing articular cartilage which is essential to the stability and function of the joint.

During the débridement, constant irrigation should be maintained to minimize on the damage to tissue from drying.

3.4.3.4 Choice of Fixation

Once again, decision making must depend upon a favorable risk-benefit ratio for the patient. If the indication for fixation is great, the risks are worthwhile.

Stabilization of the fracture decreases dead space, controls hematoma, decreases local irritation, improves the blood supply to the tissues, facilitates wound care, creates a better environment for soft tissue and bone healing, facilitates soft tissue envelope reconstruction, decreases infection, increases the speed of rehabilitation, and finally it leads to much better function.

Plaster immobilization interferes with the care of the soft tissue. It is occlusive. One cannot adequately care for a wound through a window in the plaster. Removal of the plaster for proper wound care leads to loss of reduction and further, repeated soft tissue damage. It is associated with a high complication rate of sepsis, delayed union and nonunion, and therefore poor outcome of treatment. Plaster also immobilizes the adjacent joints, which makes functional treatment impossible and therefore contributes to major joint stiffness. In classical experiments Rittman and Perven (1974) and subsequently Worlock (1994) demonstrated that stable fixation greatly reduces the likelihood of infection. Significantly larger quantities of bacteria were necessary to infect experimental fractures with stable fixation than those fixed in plaster. Furthermore, these experiments also demonstrated that stable fixation leads to union even in the presence of infection. Diaphyseal fractures which became infected and were immobilized in plaster failed to unite.

In open fractures involving joints and in open epiphyseal plate injuries in children internal fixation is necessary to maintain reduction and preserve function. The risks of internal fixation are therefore justified. As noted above, in open diaphyseal injuries other methods of stabilization, such as an external frame, may be preferable. Other important factors which may lead the surgeon to choose internal fixation include polytrauma in the patient and fractures associated with a vascular injury.

Studies of polytrauma patients with long bone fractures have demonstrated that immediate stabilization of long bones is a life-saving measure. Other studies, addressing the functional outcome of treatment, have clearly demonstrated the superiority of surgical stabilization of fracture over the results of plaster immobilization.

The choice of the method of stable fixation is complex and difficult but is of paramount importance in determining the outcome of treatment.

3.4.3.5 Implant Selection

Selecting an implant to stabilize an open fracture depends mainly on the fracture configuration and the extent of the soft tissue injury. The methods available are: (a) external skeletal fixation, (b) plating, and (c) intramedullary nailing, either with or without reaming. The correct choice of fixation is based on a combination of biomechanics and biology. On the one hand, one must consider the biomechanical requirements of the particular bone and of the fracture configuration. On the other, one must consider the potential damage to the blood supply of the bone by the method being considered, the existing damage to the soft tissue envelope, i.e., the size and the location of wounds and incisions, and the degree of further potential damage to the soft tissues as a result of the method of fixation.

External skeletal fixation is theoretically the ideal choice; it is least invasive and least traumatizing because the fixation of the bone is secured at a distance from the zone of injury. The problems encountered with external fixation include: (a) pin loosening and pin tract sepsis, (b) interference with soft tissue envelope reconstruction, (c) loss of reduction with deformity, (d) late deformity after removal of the frame, (e) delayed union, and (f) nonunion.

Conversion from external skeletal fixation to internal fixation in the event of complications has not been without problems. Studies have demonstrated that if conversion is undertaken because of pin loosening and pin tract sepsis, the incidence of sepsis following internal fixation is high. This is true for plating and particularly for intramedullary nailing. To minimize the incidence of sepsis in conversions surgeons have tried staged conversion, in which the external fixator is removed and the extremity immobilized in plaster until such time as all drainage from the pin sites has cleared. Others have reserved the conversion to cases in which the pin tracts were free of any drainage or inflammation. Despite these

precautions the incidence of sepsis remains around 20%, which is discouragingly high. Present recommendations are that if conversion to intramedullary nailing is being considered, it should be carried out as soon as possible after the external skeletal fixation and not after the first 3 weeks, and never if there has been pin tract drainage or anything to suggest sepsis.

The recent development of the pinless external fixator (Synthes, Paioli, PA, USA) will unquestionably greatly extend the indications for initial external fixation and then subsequent conversion to a more stable system of fixation once the danger of infection and further damage to the tissues has passed. This introduces, however, another aspect of external fixation which must be considered: the particular bone and segment in question. The pinless external fixator is applicable only to a subcutaneous bone such as the tibia. In considering the long bones and bone segments we see from these charts that external fixation is best suited for stabilizating fractures of the tibial diaphysis, the distal radius, and the distal tibia. Its use in other long bones such as the humerus, radius, ulna, and femur introduces many problems which greatly outweight its advantages. It is for this reason that its use in these areas is reserved for special circumstances.

Plating has been a very successful method in treating open fractures of the shaft of the humerus and the radius and ulna as these bones, particularly the radius and ulna, do not lend themselves to intramedullary nailing or external fixation (Moed 1986). Plating of fractures of the femoral shaft has been associated with a higher incidence of implant failure and nonunion than intramedullary nailing. The complication of plate failure is more common in open fractures of the femur as these take longer to unite. Plating, however, has been demonstrated to be a very successful method of treatment of the grades 1 and 2 open fractures of the tibia, with excellent functional results (Clifford et al. 1988).

Plating has far greater indications in the treatment of end segment fractures. Articular fractures involving the epiphysis are fixed with lag screws. Fractures involving the metaphysis are not suitable for intramedullary nailing as the distal segment is often too short. These are therefore fixed with plates which function either as buttress plates, bridge plates, or both. The proximal and distal humerus, the proximal radius and ulna, the distal radius, the proximal and distal femur, and the proximal and distal tibia are areas where lag screw fixation and plating is indicated. In some instances of fractures of the distal radius and distal tibia lag screw fixation of the joint fractures may be combined with external fixation, particularly if the soft tissue envelope has been severely traumatized. Where the metaphysis is under a good muscle cover such as the proximal humerus, and the proximal and distal femur this type of fixation has resulted in excellent function even if associated with the development of sepsis (E. Schemitch, personal communication 1991; Siliski 1989).

Recent advances in plate design have been directed towards the use of titanium, which is biologically inert, and towards new plate geometry, which greatly decreases the plate contact with the underlying bone and thus greatly diminishes the insult of plating on the circulation of the underlying cortex. These developments and the projected future development of the point contact plate will unquestionably further extend the indication for plating in the presence of open fractures.

Closed locked intramedullary nailing is biomechanically and biologically better than plating as a method of securing stable fixation of diaphyseal fractures of long bones. This has been shown to be particularly true for the multifragmentary fractures of the femur and tibia (Brumbach et al. 1989; Winquist et al. 1984). Locking has also made it possible to nail fractures of these bones which encroach on the proximal and distal segment.

Although in the past open fractures were considered as an absolute contraindication to intramedullary nailing because of the high incidence of sepsis and the greater difficulties in erradicating endosteal osteomyelitis, recent studies have shown the technique to be effective and as safe as other methods in carefully selected cases.

The difficulties encountered with external fixation and with plating of open fractures of the femur led surgeons to attempt locked reamed intramedullary nailing of the femur in grade 2 open fractures. The poor results of plating arose because of the incidence of implant failure, deformity, delayed union, and nonunion. Locked intramedullary nailing is biomechanically vastly superior as a method of internal fixation of diaphyseal fractures. The success achieved with grade 2 fractures led to the extension of the techniques to grade 3A and even to some grade 3B fractures. The good results affirmed the soundness of this technique. The femur is enveloped in a thick muscle envelope. This gives the cortex good cover and a rich and secure blood supply.

The subcutaneous position of one-third of the tibia, its relatively poor muscle cover, and sparse blood supply to the diaphysis suggested strongly that reamed intramedullary nailing of the tibia should not be attempted. The results of Lottes (1974) with unreamed intramedullary nailing of the tibia and the results of flexible intramedullary nailing of select stable fractures of the tibia suggested very strongly that unreamed intramedullary nailing of the tibia could prove to be a successful technique.

The results to date with unreamed locked intramedullary nailing of the tibia indicate that it is an ideal method of treatment. It minimizes the damage to the cortical blood supply and is biomechanically sound. The solid nail reduces the dead space and therefore the incidence of sepsis, and it is a suitable splint for stable and unstable fracture configurations. This technique, however, is not without problems, although most are technical or mechanical and will therefore be addressed with further refinements in the technique. The unreamed nail has not decreased the incidence of delayed union and nonunion of the open fractures. The fatigue failure of the locking screws is a common complication. The choice of the correct length of the nail is difficult, and axial alignment with the unreamed nail is difficult to achieve as the nail is a splint and has very limited contact with the endosteal bone. The nail has also limited applications in proximal and distal fractures.

Some authors have reported good results with reamed locked intramedullary nailing of open fractures of the tibia. (Court-Brown et al. 1991). These authors have limited the size of the nail to 11 mm or less, do not employ the tourniquet during reaming, emphasize the importance of a very meticulous débridement of the fracture, and early well-vascularized soft tissue cover.

The postulated damage to the endosteal circulation of the cortex as a result of reaming has been documented experimentally. There are systemic effects of reaming which have been noted particularly in patients with femoral shaft fractures and concomitant chest trauma (Pape et al. 1993). The higher incidence of adult respiratory distress syndrome in these patients has been attributed to thrombotic or embolic phenomena. This has resulted in the design of unreamed hollow or solid intramedullary nails for the femur. These are being used more and more frequently. The initial results are very encouraging, but final evaluation must await further studies.

3.4.3.6 Care of the Soft Tissue Wound

Primary

After the initial débridement and stabilization the wound of the injury must always be left open. Part of the surgical incision which was made as an extension of the wound to permit thorough débridement can be closed as long as the edges can be brought together without any tension. The open wound can either be packed with gauze soaked in various solutions such as acroflavine in oil, betadine solution, or normal saline, or it can be covered with skin substitutes such as epigard, which permit drainage but prevent the dessication of tissue. Another technique, popularized by Seligson, is also available. This consists of inserting into the wound down to the bone antibiotic-impregnated methyl methacrylate beads and then covering the wound with an adherent plastic drape such as vidrape. The principle of this technique depends on preventing dessication by capturing the exudate and turning it into a solution with an antibiotic concentration which then bathes the tissues and helps to prevent dessication and sepsis.

Whichever technique is employed, the patient must be returned to the operating room for serial débridements until such time as one can be certain that all dead tissue has been eradicated.

In our opinion, relaxing incisions and primary flaps should almost never be used in acute trauma because of the risk of losing the flap.

Secondary

The next step is to reconstruct the soft tissue envelope. The options available to the surgeon are: (a) secondary closure, (b) healing by granulation tissue and reepithelialzation, (c) healing by granulation tissue and thickness grafting, (d) closing the wound by means of local rotation flaps, and (e) free flap reconstruction. Secondary closure is possible only if the wound is over well-vascularized tissue, and if the soft tissue defect is so small that closure is possible without any undue tension.

Healing by granulation tissue and reepithelialization or split thickness skin grafting is possible if the floor of the wound is formed by well-vascularized tissue such as muscle or periosteum which becomes rapidly covered by granulation tissue. Once granulation tissue forms, one has the option of allowing the wound to reepithelialize, which takes a long time and results in considerable scarring, or securing cover by means of split-thickness skin grafting. Skin grafting is preferable because it is not only a faster cover, but the quality of the scar is superior. If the granulation tissue is over bone, whether allowed to reepithelialize or skin grafted, the scar becomes adherent and prone to frequent breakdown.

All open wounds which result in the exposure of bone, articular cartilage, tendon, and nerve require a rapid soft tissue reconstruction because these tissues are very sensitive to drying. Dessication causes death of the tissues and infection The most common clinical problem of this type is the wound over the subcutaneous border of the tibia with loss of tissue and exposure of bone which has lost its periosteal cover. If not rapidly covered within the first week, the bone dries out and dies, turns a yellowish brown color, and becomes rapidly infected.

In the proximal tibia coverage can be obtained by means of local myofascial rotation flaps using the gastrosoleus muscles. Great care must be exercised in carrying out such cover that the muscle which is rotated has not been part of the zone of injury. This danger is present particularly in crushing injuries. Attempts at advancing and rotating a damaged muscle frequently lead to its necrosis.

In the distal tibia and in other situations in which there is no available local muscle to rotate one should not resort to fasciocutaneous flaps as these are particularly dangerous during the first 4 weeks. These flaps rely on vessels which run from muscle fascia and then into the skin. Elevating the fasciocutaneous flap endangers its blood supply. A problem with these flaps is that they leave a cosmetic defect in the donor site.

In these situations where coverage must be obtained, and where one cannot use a local rotation flap, one must resort to free muscle flap harvested with its own vascular pedicle. Godina (1986) advocated radical excision of the zone of injury and immediate free flap reconstruction within 72 h of injury. In the majority of trauma centers today the practice is to débride the wound, have at least one if not two looks 2 days apart, and then when the wound is clean and stable carry out the free flap. Coverage should be obtained within one week. A delay leads to drying, death of tissue and unavoidable infection. The advantages of the free flap are numerous. The muscle conforms well to the defect and fills gaps well. It scavengers bacteria, is of definite benefit in healing of the underlying bone, and forms an excellent cover under which one can carry out cancellous bone grafting to reconstruct any missing bone. The disadvantage of free flap coverage is its resource intensiveness and cost, as well as its high failure rate in older individuals, heavy smokers, and diabetics.

3.4.3.7 Secondary Fracture Care

Early communication between the surgeon and patient is essential. The patient must be told that the primary stabilization is step 1 in the management of the fracture, that is, it is only the beginning. At the first dressing change the surgeon must also begin to decide on the follow-up management of the bony injury.

The more severe the open fracture, the less likely it is to go on to union. This is related to the interference with the endosteal and periosteal blood supply as well as to the extent of the soft tissue injury and its devitalization. The greater the force, the greater are the fragmentation of bone and the devitalization. In addition, open fractures are frequently associated with bone loss either as a result of bone loss at the time of the injury or as a result of the débridement in which all bone devoid of blood supply and soft tissue attachment must be removed. The only exception to this rule are major articular fragments which are necessary for the joint mechanics and stability.

All open fractures treated definitively in an external fixator are bone grafted to secure union. In fractures treated by plating or nailing the indications for bone grafting depend on the severity of the soft tissue wound and the fracture morphology. The timing of the bone graft varies with the severity of the open wound. Grade 1 and grade 2 fractures for the purpose of bone grafting are regarded in the same light as closed injuries. Therefore simple fractures and those associated with a spiral wedge wound are not grafted, nor is an extrusion wedge fracture if the extrusion wedge retains its blood supply and is retained in the wound. If the extrusion wedge had to be removed, and if there is very limited contact between the main fragments, the fracture is bone grafted to secure union and prevent implant failure. The timing of the bone graft depends on the severity and location of the soft tissue defect. If the wound is such that either secondary closure is possible or simple skin graft over a healthy granulating surface, the grafting is performed early at the time of the wound closure. If the wound was such that either a rotation myofascial flap or a free muscle flap was necessary, the bone graft is carried out after 5–7 weeks, once a stable soft tissue envelope has been secured. Early bone grafting is associated with increased infection rate, graft failure, and flap failure.

Certain type B wedge fractures and most type C complex fractures result in a segmental bone defect. Initially, at the time of the definitive fixation, the defect is either ignored or, preferably, filled with either antibiotic-impregnated methyl methacrylate beads or an antibiotic-impregnated methyl methacrylate bone plug. Bony reconstruction is undertaken after 5–7 weeks once a stable soft tissue envelope has been achieved. If the defect is less than 6 cm, autogenous cancellous bone graft is the usual choice (Christian et al. 1989). If the defect is greater than 6 cm, a free vascularized bone pedicle is employed. Welland (1981) has reported an 88% success rate with this technique using the fibula as a free vascularized bone pedicle graft, although a secondary bone graft was frequently necessary.

The recent introduction of the circular frame external fixator with traction osteogenesis, as developed and recommended by Ilizarov, has led to the development of an ingenious protocol to deal with both the soft tissue and bone defects. Primary shortening of the extremity is carried out at the time of the primary débridement and stabilization. This facilitates closure of the soft tissue defect without the need for local rotational or distant free flaps. Once a stable soft tissue envelope is achieved a corticotomy is carried out, and the limb is then gradually lengthened to its original length. This may have to be combined with docking of the intervening segment with the distal main fragment if contact was not achieved at the time of the initial shortening. There are sparce reports on this technique in the literature. We have had no personal experience with it.

3.4.3.8 Open Joint Injuries

In the past 20 years the principles of treatment of intra-articular fractures has been very clearly defined:
1. Anatomic reduction of the joint surfaces is necessary to achieve the maximum surface area possible. This reduces stress and makes recovery of articular cartilage possible. Furthermore congruous joint surfaces are necessary to ensure normal mechanical function such as a range of movement and stability.
2. The work of Mitchell has proven that stable fixation of the joint surfaces is necessary for articular cartilage regeneration.
3. Reduction of the metaphyseal deformity and axial realignment is necessary to prevent joint overload.
4. Stable fixation of the metaphyseal component of the fractures is necessary to permit early motion.
5. The importance of motion in bringing about articular cartilage regeneration has been clearly shown by Salter (1980) in his investigations on continuous passive motion and intermittent active motion.

Anatomic reduction, stable fixation of the articular fracture and its metaphyseal component, and early motion can be achieved only if the fracture is treated by open reduction and stable internal fixation.

The principles governing the treatment of open joint fractures are very similar to those for treating open fractures of the diaphyseal segment. The emergency care, the initial assessment, and the débridement are the same. However, major joint fragments which are covered by articular cartilage, and which have become completely devitalized, but which are essential to the mechanical integrity of the joint are preserved even though this risks sepsis. This is done because they are essential to preserve function. A diaphyseal defect can be reconstructed at a later date. A joint defect is permanent.

All that has been said about the importance of stability applies also to articular fractures. However, one cannot resort to temporary splinting by means of an external fixator and delayed reconstruction. The articular fragments are supported by cancellous bone which unites rapidly. The longer that one delays the articular reconstruction, the more difficult it becomes to achieve. It is for this reason that we advise that at the time of the initial surgery one should carry out an anatomic reduction of the articular surfaces and their stabilization with the minimum of internal fixation. It is best to use lag screws as these provide the best stability and can be left as the definitive means of fixation. The exact method of fixation must be left to the judgement of the surgeon as long as the principle of minimum added trauma and minimum of internal fixation is kept in mind.

Whether one proceeds to a primary reconstruction of the metaphyseal component of the fracture depends entirely on the damage to the soft tissue envelope. This is particularly true of subcutaneous joints such as the tibial pilon. One must remember that the zone of injury extends well beyond the apparent damage. In evaluating the extent of the zone of injury one must take into account the mechanism of injury and the potential amount of energy involved. If there is any doubt as to the integrity of the soft tissue envelope beyond the wound and the surgical incisions made, it is best to delay the reconstruction of the metaphysis and bridge the fracture with an external fixator. If the joint segment is too small to permit adequate purchase for the fixator, the joint is bridged. Treatment of the metaphyseal fracture depends whether there is a defect. If the initial bone loss or subsequent débridement has resulted in a segmental defect, it is advisable to pack the defect with antibiotic-impregnated methymethacrylate beads. Otherwise the metaphysis is left alone with the fracture reduced and realigned by means of ligamentotaxis.

The definitive reconstruction of the metaphyseal defect is undertaken 4–6 weeks later when a stable and healthy soft cover has been achieved. The metaphyseal component of the fracture is held with a plate which functions either as a buttress or a bridge plate or both. The defect is packed with autogenous cancellous bone. If plating cannot be carried out for technical reasons, or because the soft tissue envelope contraindicates the required dissecation and the insertion of more metal, the external fixation is left on and the metaphysis is bone grafted as indicated. External fixators can be left bridging major joints for 8–10 weeks with only moderate loss of ultimate motion (Bone et al. l993; Jakob 1985; Schatzker and Tile 1987).

If there is a good soft tissue cover, good tissue viability, low contamination, and no segmental defect, a primary reconstruction of the metaphysis is undertaken. If the fracture is simple, it is reduced and fixed. If the fracture is multifragmentary, one uses indirect reduction to minimize the devizalization of the fragments. If bone grafting is necessary, this should be delayed and carried out at the time when the wound is being closed.

All open fractures are left open. This also applies to open intra-articular fractures, with the following caveat. if left exposed, cartilage dessicates and becomes permanently damaged. Therefore the capsule should be closed, if at all possible, and the wound left open for subsequent closure by whatever means indicated. If there is a soft tissue defect with exposure of the joint, this must be dealt with in the same manner as exposed bone devoid of its periosteal cover. The tissue is kept moist with packing or with artificial skin such as Epigard, and a definitive soft tissue cover usually by means of a free muscle is obtained within the first week.

Early motion is as important in open fractures as it is in closed injuries. Motion should not be started, however, if it would compromise the healing of the wound, as this could result in sepsis. Once a stable soft tissue cover has been achieved, and the fracture is stabilized, vigorous mobilization of the joint must commence.

3.5 Summary

Open fractures continue to test the decision-making and technical skills of the orthopedic surgeon. The main principles of management in open fractures consist of immediate sterile bandaging of the wound to prevent further contamination followed by cleansing and débridement in the operating room. Where possible, stable fixation of the fracture using either external fixation, open reduction, and internal fixation, or combined methods is indicated. The wound should be left open primarily in all cases. Secondary wound inspection in the operating room must be carried out between the first and fifth days, depending on the degree of devitalization and contamination. Secondary wound management may be by secondary suture, split thickness skin graft, flaps, or free tissue transfers.

Secondary cancellous bone grafting is almost always necessary. Where extensive bone loss is present, free bone pedicle transfer may be necessary. The key to the care of an open wound is to observe the fracture closely and change the management as necessary. The most common and often the most serious error is to attempt definitive care of an open fracture in one step.

References

Allgöwer M (1971) Weichteilprobleme und Infektrisiko der Osteosynthese. Langenbecks Arch Chir 329:1127

Beauchamp CG, Clifford RP, Webb JK, Kellam JF, Tile M (1984) Functional results after immediate internal fixation of open tibial fractures. Presented at the Canadian Orthopaedic Association Meeting, Winnipeg, Canada, June 1984

Billroth T (1866) Die allgemeine und chirurgische Pathologie und Therapie in 50 Vorlesungen. Reimer, Berlin

Bone L, Stegemann P, McNamara K, Seibel R (1993) External fixation of severely comminuted and open tibial pilon fractures Clin Orthop Rel Res 292:101–107

Bosse MJ, Burgess AR, Brumback RJ (1984) Evaluation and treatment of the grade 3 tibia fracture. Adv Orthop Surg 8:3–17

Brumbach RJ, Ellison PS Jr, Poka A, Lakatos R, Bathon GH, Burgess AR (1989) Intrameduallary nailing of open fractures of the femoral shaft. J Bone Jt Surg Am 71:1324–1331

Byrd, HS, Spicer TE, Cierney G (1985) Management of open tibial fractures. Plast Reconstr Surg 76(5):719

Chapman MW, Mahoney M (1979) The role of early internal fixation in the management of open fractures. Clin Orthop 138:120–131

Chapman W (1980) The use of internal fixation in open fractures. Orthop Clin North Am 11:579–591

Christian EP, Bosse Mi, Robb G (1989) Reconstruction of large diaphyseal defects without free fibular transfer in grade 3B tibial fractures. J Bone Jt Surg Am 71:994–1004

Clifford RP, Beauchamp CG, Kellam JF, Webb JK, Tile M (1988) Plate fixation of open fractures of the tibia. J Bone Jt Surg Br 70:644–648

Court-Brown CM, McQueen MM, Quaba AA, Christie J (1991) Locked intramedullary nailing of open tibial fractures. J Bone Jt Surg Br 73:959–964

Godina M (1986) Early microsurgical reconstruction of complex trauma of the extremities. Plast Reconstr Surg 778:(3)285–292

Gustilo B, Andersson JP (1976) Prevention of infection in the treatment of one thousand and twenty-five open fractures of long bones. J Bone Joint Surg Am 58:453

Jakob R (1985) The use of the small external fixator on fractures of the wrist. Topics in Orthop Trauma 1:35–36

Lange RH, Bach AW, Hansen ST Jr, Johansen KH (1985) Open tibial fractures with associated vascular injuries: prognosis for limb salvage. J Trauma 25(3):203

Lottes JO (1974) Medullary nailing of the tibia with the tri-flange nail. Clin Orthop Rel Res 105:253–266

Moed BR, Kellam JF, Foster RJ, Tile M, Hansen ST Jr (1986) Immediate internal fixation of open fractures of the diaphysis of the forearm. J Bone Jt Surg Am 68(4):1008–1017

Oestern HJ, Tscherne H (1984) Pathophysiology and classification of soft tissue injuries associated with fractures. In: Tscherne H, Gotzen L (eds) Fractures with soft tissue injuries. Springer, Berlin Heidelberg New York, pp 1–9

Pape HC, Regel G, Dwenger A, Sturm JA, Tscherne H (1993) Influence of thoracic trauma and primary femoral intramedullary nailing on the incidence of ARDS in multiple trauma patients. Injury 24 [Suppl]:82–103

Rittmann WW, Perren SM (1974) Cortical bone healing after internal fixation and infection. Springer, Berlin, Heidelberg, New York

Salter RB, Simmonds DF, Malcolm BW et al (1980) The biological effect of continuous passive motion on the healing of full thickness defects in articular cartilage – an experimental investigation in the rabbit. J Bone Jt Surg Am 62(8):1232–1251

Schatzker J, Tile M (1987) The rationale of operative fracture care. Springer, Berlin, Heidelberg, New York

Siliski JM, Mahring M, Hofer HP (1989) Supracondylar intercondylar fractures of the femur. J Bone Jt Surg Am 71:95–104

Tscherne H (1984) The management of open fractures. In: Tscherne H, Gotzen L (eds) Fractures with soft tissue injuries. Springer, Berlin Heidelberg New York

Weiland AJ (1981) Current concepts review. Vascularized free bone transplants. J Bone Jt Surg Am 63:166–169

Winquist RA, Hansen ST Jr, Clawson DK (1984) Closed intramedullary nailing of femoral fractures. A report of five hundred and twenty cases. J Bone Jt Surg Am 66:529–539

Worlock P, Slack R, Harvey L, Mawhinney R (1994) The prevention of infection in open fractures: an experimental study of the effect of fracture stability. Injury 25(1):31–38

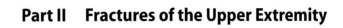

Part II   Fractures of the Upper Extremity

4 Fractures of the Proximal Humerus

M. TILE

4.1 Introduction

4.1.1 General Considerations

Since the publication of the first edition of this book, there has been considerable interest in the management of these fractures (Szyszkowitz et al. 1993; Rasmussen et al. 1992; Flatow et al. 1991), so we can no longer state that fractures of the proximal humerus have for years been relegated to the surgical scrap heap. The majority of these fractures occur in elderly individuals, are stable, and can be successfully treated by judicious neglect. Unfortunately, the same reasoning, and therefore the same treatment, is too often applied to the minority which occur in young individuals, are unstable, and have a poor prognosis. Operative techniques have become more standardized and are more often related to the type of fracture and the quality of the bone, as recommended in the first edition. Many of the technical difficulties have been solved, however, the problem of surgical care in osteoporotic bone remains. However, by applying the same principles of treatment of this particular fracture as to any other, a logical approach may be developed which will suit all groups of patients.

4.1.2 Anatomy

Codman (1934) recognized that fractures of the proximal humerus may separate into four major fragments (Fig. 4.1). The first fragment is the humeral head, consisting of that portion of the humerus superior to the anatomical neck. Since this head fragment is almost completely covered by articular cartilage and is devoid of soft tissue attachment, its blood supply is precarious. Therefore, if the head fragment is displaced following injury, avascular necrosis may be the inevitable result.

The second fragment consists of the lesser tuberosity with its attached subscapularis muscle. Avulsion of this fragment may allow undue external rotation of the head in the presence of a humeral neck fracture.

The third fragment is the greater tuberosity with its attached rotator cuff. Isolated avulsions of this fragment are equivalent to rotator cuff avulsions, while those asso-

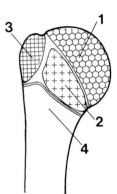

Fig. 4.1. The four major fragments of the proximal humerus. *1*, Humeral head superior to the anatomical neck; *2*, lesser tuberosity; *3*, greater tuberosity; *4*, shaft of the humerus

ciated with a surgical neck fracture may allow internal rotation of the head fragment.

The fourth fragment is created by a fracture through the surgical neck of the humerus and is the most common fracture in this area. As in other areas of metaphyseal bone, the behavior of this fragment differs according to the type of injury, be it compression, rendering the fracture stable, or shear, rendering it unstable. Also, the presence of ample soft tissue attachment to the large head fragment makes avascular necrosis most unlikely.

These anatomical considerations are of major clinical significance. Fractures of the upper end of the humerus may be compared to those of the upper femur. Fractures through the anatomical neck of the humerus are akin to intracapsular fractures of the femur, i.e., they are intracapsular. The fractured fragments are almost entirely covered by articular cartilage and are therefore devoid of a blood supply, leading to a high incidence of avascular necrosis for both (Fig. 4.2a, b). Fractures through the surgical neck of the humerus are more akin to intertrochanteric and pertrochanteric fractures of the femur, i.e., they are extracapsular, usually with an adequate blood supply and a relatively low incidence of avascular necrosis (Fig. 4.2 c,d).

4.1.3 Vascular Anatomy

As in the femoral head, the blood supply to the humeral head is precarious, because both are covered in articular

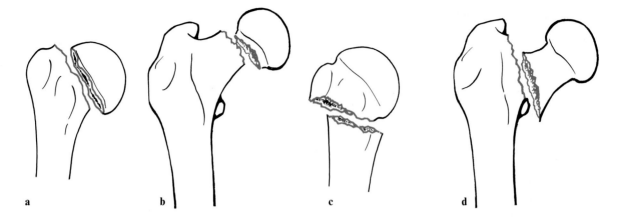

a   b   c   d

Fig. 4.2 a–d. Comparison of the intracapsular anatomical neck fracture of the humerus (**a**) with the intracapsular fracture of the neck of the femur (**b**). Both are almost entirely covered by articular cartilage and therefore devoid of blood supply, resulting in a high incidence of avascular necrosis for both. **c, d** Comparison of the extracapsular surgical neck fracture of the humerus (**c**) with the intertrochanteric extracapsular fracture of the proximal femur (**d**). Since they are extracapsular, the incidence of avascular necrosis is low

viability of the humeral head (see Fig. 4.17 a). The importance of maintaining the soft tissue attachment to this area cannot be overstated, as stressed by Szyszkowitz et al. (1993).

Other blood supply enters through the rotator cuff or branches of the posterior humeral circumflex artery, neither can normally maintain viability to the humeral head.

cartilage. A precise knowledge of the blood supply is essential to understanding the outcome of some of the injury patterns and also to avoid the distraction of any remaining blood to the humeral head during surgery. The main blood supply to the humeral head is from the anterior humeral circumflex artery (Fig 4.3). The arcuate artery arising from the anterior circumflex perfuses the humeral head. Fractures of the head often have a small, wedge-shaped portion of the metaphysis attached, which may contain the arcuate artery and maintain the

4.1.4 Four-Segment Classification

Neer (1970) expanded the anatomical considerations of Codman into a working classification based on the displacement of the fragments. The group of minimally displaced fractures which may be treated by closed means must, in his opinion, have no segment displaced more than 10 mm or angulated more than 45°. He further classified the displaced fractures according to the number of parts fractured, plus the presence of a dislocation.

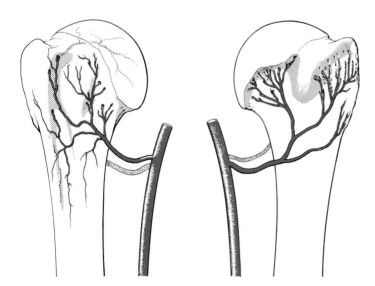

Fig. 4.3. Blood supply to the humeral head. The main blood supply to the humeral head is from the anterior humeral circumflex artery from which arises the arcuate artery entering the head from the small metaphyseal area on the inferior aspect of the head

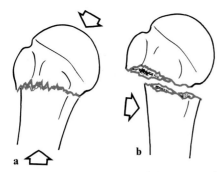

Fig. 4.4 a,b. Stable and unstable fractures of the proximal humerus. **a** Typical impacted stable fracture in which the shaft and head move as one unit. **b** An unstable fracture of the proximal humerus, characterized by movement between the shaft and head fragments

For example, the greater tuberosity fragment may be involved in a two-, three-, or four-part fracture, with or without a dislocation. Neer's classification, based on a study of 300 cases, has clarified the natural history of these various types. Once it became evident that some types treated by closed means were associated with dismal results, logical decision-making could follow.

4.1.5 Stability

In any classification, consideration should also be given to the stability of a given fracture, as well as to the number of segments involved. Cancellous bone may fail in compression, resulting in a stable impacted fracture or in tension or shear, resulting in an unstable fracture (Fig. 4.4). These two types of injury behave quite differently. The stable impacted types cause less pain, allowing earlier movement, and heal rapidly. In contrast, the unstable types cause severe pain, precluding early function; in addition, healing is often delayed. Therefore, to consider only the number of fracture segments irrespective of their stability may lead to poor management decisions, usually toward overtreatment. An impacted, stable, relatively painless fracture of the proximal humerus will have a very different outcome than will a fracture with the same number of segments but with inherent instability. Stability must be assessed by a careful clinical as well as a complete radiological investigation.

4.1.6 Surgical Difficulties

If surgery is the answer for some of the unstable fracture types identified as having a poor outcome if treated by nonoperative means, why has it not been universally adopted? The answer is obvious – surgery is not without

its own set of problems, such as: (a) osteoporotic bone, which greatly reduces the holding power of screws so that they may pull out prior to fracture healing (see Fig. 4.24); (b) comminution so severe that anatomical reduction may be impossible; (c) avascular necrosis of the humeral head; (d) difficult techniques and imperfect implants. We should not be deterred by these problems, but instead should rise to the challenge in order to improve the results of this difficult injury.

4.2 Classification

Any classification is useful only if it aids the surgeon in the management of a given injury. The proposed classification (Table 4.1), adapted from the previous reports of Codman and Neer, should, if followed, lead the surgeon to logical management based on the natural history of the various fracture types. The two major considerations in this classification are, first, the anatomical features of the fracture, i.e., whether the fracture is through the anatomical neck separating the head fragment (intracapsular) or through the surgical neck (extracapsular), and, second, whether the fracture is stable, i.e., the head and shaft are impacted and move together, or unstable.

Recently, the value of this particular classification and indeed all classifications have been questioned (Siebenrock and Gerber 1993; Burstein 1993; Sidor et al. 1993).

Table 4.1. Classification of fracture types

1. Stable
2. Unstable
  A. Minimally displaced
  B. Displaced
    1. Two-part
      (a) Lesser tuberosity
      (b) Greater tuberosity
      (c) Surgical neck
      (d) Anatomical neck
    2. Three-part – Surgical neck
      (a) Plus lesser tuberosity
      (b) Plus greater tuberosity
    3. Four-part – Anatomical neck
      Plus tuberosities
    4. Fracture-dislocation
      (a) Two-part – with greater tuberosity
      (b) Three-part – I. anterior, with greater
        tuberosity
      II. posterior, with lesser tuberosity
      (c) Four-part – I. anterior
            II. posterior
3. Articular
  (a) Head impaction – (Hill-Sachs)
  (b) Articular fractures
    1. Humeral head split
    2. Glenoid rim

Table 4.2. Fractures of the proximal humerus. Classification and treatment guidelines. Fractures in the red boxes should be considered for open reductions and internal fixation (see text)

	Lesser tuberosity	Greater tuberosity	Surgical neck	Anatomical neck
2 Part				
3 Part				
4 Part				
Fracture dislocation ant				
post				
articular impaction			head impaction	

In these studies, the rate of interobservor error was found to be unacceptably high, thereby invalidating the classification, sparking an angry response from many observors.

Do the studies mean that these concepts in the classification are invalid. This depends on one's view of classifications and their use in clinical medicine.

I believe that for decision making in individual cases, the classification should serve only as a guide to treatment. The surgeon must consider not only fracture factors, which may vary for each individual case, but patient factors, both of which comprise the "personality" of the fracture. The present classifications can serve as a guide but cannot be used as a "cookbook."

For clinical trials and studies, the classification is also used to compare cases from different centers. For this purpose, high interobservor error is disturbing; nevertheless, we must continually strive to understand existing classifications and change them when underated.

4.3 Natural History and Surgical Indications

A careful study of the natural history of each of the fracture types in the proposed classification will greatly aid the surgeon in his final decision-making process. Delayed union or nonunion and avascular necrosis are the major complications affecting proximal humeral fractures. By indicating those fractures which are likely to end in a poor result with closed methods, we hope the surgeon will, by deduction, come to open treatment as the preferred alternative. In general, those fractures where open reduction must be considered as a treatment option because of a poor prognosis with nonoperative care are marked in red in Table 4.2.

4.3.1 Stable Fractures

As in other areas of the body, stability must here be considered a relative and not an absolute concept. A stable fracture is one which cannot be displaced by physiological forces. A rigidly impacted fracture of the proximal humerus caused by compressive forces fulfills these criteria, no matter how many fragments may be present. Soft tissue hinges are most likely to be intact, so that avascular necrosis is improbable. Impaction of the cancellous bone allows early pain-free motion and rapid union, both contributing to a good functional result. The natural history of the stable fracture is usually favorable; therefore surgery, except in the most unusual circumstances, is meddlesome and dangerous.

Exceptions to this rule are *stable fractures with unacceptable displacement,* for example, an impacted stable fracture with excessive angulation in a young patient. Unacceptable displacement cannot be defined by a number, but can be ascertained only after a careful assessment of all the factors making up the personality of the injury.

4.3.2 Unstable Fractures

The state of the soft tissue envelope will determine the degree of instability present. A grossly unstable fracture will allow the fragments to move independently of each other, as noted in the clinical and radiographic assessment. Instability of the major fragments may result in pain, as well as in delayed union, both contributing to prolonged immobilization and a less than perfect result.

Displaced fractures of the articular fragment through the anatomical neck often result in avascular necrosis. Thus, the natural history of the unstable proximal inju-

Fig. 4.5 a, b. Unstable, minimally displaced three-part fracture of the proximal right humerus in a 67-year-old woman (**a**). Treatment consisted of a sling and a swathe for 3 weeks, until the pain subsided, and then a program of physiotherapy. At 8 weeks (**b**), the fracture had healed in a good position. Note the slight inferior subluxation, which is almost inevitable in these individuals. When rehabilitation is complete, the inferior subluxation usually reduces spontaneously

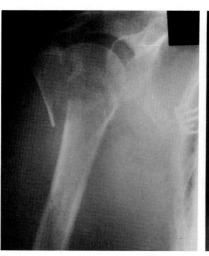

a

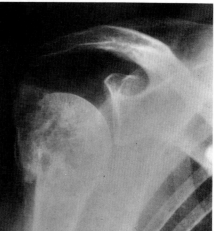

b

ry is markedly different from that of the stable injury and requires a different approach.

4.3.2.1 Minimal Displacement

A minimally displaced fracture usually implies a less violent force and the presence of some soft tissue hinges. Neer (1970) arbitrarily chose less than 1 cm of displacement as indicating some attached soft tissue. This must, of course, be confirmed by clinical examination, often with image intensification. If soft tissue hinges have been retained, the ultimate prognosis is good, no matter how many fragments are present. Vascularity of the head fragment is usually assumed, and surgery is virtually never indicated for this type of injury (Fig. 4.5).

4.3.2.2 Major Displacement

The fractures with major displacement will be considered according to the *anatomical* structures and the *number of segments* involved.

a) Two-Part

Displaced fractures may occur through any of the four segments previously described. The outcome of a single fracture through these segments will vary considerably, depending upon the retained soft tissue envelope.

Lesser Tuberosity. Pure avulsions of the lesser tuberosity are rare and are of little clinical significance. However, an isolated lesser tuberosity fracture should always alert the surgeon to the possibility of a *posterior dislocation* of the shoulder, with which it is frequently associated. Unless associated with some other major displaced fragment, closed treatment only is indicated.

Greater Tuberosity. A displaced isolated avulsion fracture of the greater tuberosity is indicative of a loss of function of the rotator cuff (Fig. 4.6 a). In the two-part pattern, the bony fragment may retract under the acromion, acting as a block to abduction. To correct both the mechanical block and the loss of rotator cuff function, surgery is mandatory. We regard the displaced retracted greater tuberosity fracture as an *absolute* indication for surgery.

Greater tuberosity fractures occur more commonly in association with anterior dislocation of the shoulder, and, as will be described in the section on fracture-dislocation, they rarely require open reduction in that particular situation (Fig. 4.6 b).

Surgical Neck Fractures. Impacted fractures through the surgical neck are common and usually minimally displaced, thus requiring only closed treatment. However, shearing forces may cause displacement and instability. The large proximal fragment usually has sufficient soft tissue attachment to ensure the viability of the humeral head. Associated undisplaced fractures into the tuberosities are common, but they do not alter the natural history because the soft tissues are retained. Avascular necrosis is rare, unless the blood supply is destroyed by injudicious surgery; however, union may be delayed because of the gross instability of the main fragments.

These grossly unstable fractures usually occur in young patients with strong cancellous bone and are usually caused by high-energy shearing forces. Severe pain and delayed union will require prolonged immobilization, which may lead to permanent stiffness in spite of lengthy rehabilitation. Open reduction and stable internal fixation, using standard techniques, will immobilize the fracture sufficiently to reduce pain, ensure rapid healing, and allow early motion with improved results. We regard this fracture as a *relative* indication for surgery, especially in young patients with good bone (Fig. 4.7).

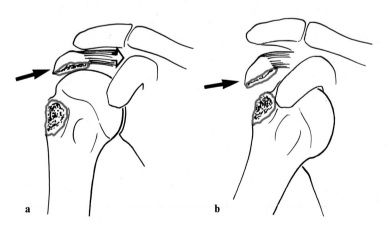

Fig. 4.6 a, b. Fracture of the greater tuberosity. **a** An avulsion-type fracture of the greater tuberosity. This is a true avulsion of the rotator cuff, in which the bone lodges under the acromion and acts as a mechanical block. Surgery is mandatory. **b** Fracture of the greater tuberosity has occurred at the time of anterior dislocation of the humeral head. In this situation, the tuberosity is in its correct position and does not retract. Therefore, reduction of the dislocation usually leads to an anatomical reduction of the tuberosity to the shaft, and surgery is rarely necessary

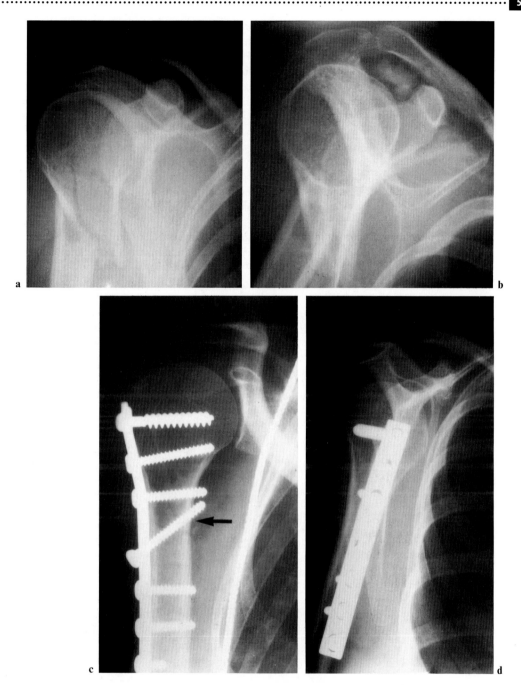

Fig. 4.7 a–d. Unstable three-part fracture through the proximal humerus. **a** Anteroposterior and **b** lateral radiographs showing an unstable oblique fracture in the upper humerus with an extension through the greater tuberosity. This fracture occurred when a 33-year-old woman was thrown from a horse and struck a tree. The fracture was grossly unstable on clinical examination, and, in consultation with the patient, treatment consisted of open reduction and internal fixation using a dynamic compression (DC) plate with a lag screw across the fracture through the plate (**c**, *arrow*; **d**). Excellent stability was obtained. The patient regained full shoulder motion within 10 days of injury

Anatomical Neck. Two-part fractures involving the anatomical neck are rare. Since the head segment is covered by articular cartilage, displaced fractures through the anatomical neck are associated with a high incidence of avascular necrosis (see Fig. 4.2 a). Because of the instability of the bone fragments, nonunion may also occur. In the two-part anatomical neck fracture with displacement, surgery should be performed if closed manipulation fails to restore the local anatomy. In such cases, care should be taken to preserve any remaining soft tissue attachments. If compression of the cancellous fracture is achieved by surgery, rapid healing of the cancellous fracture will ensue, but avascular necrosis will not be prevented. Some patients may manage reasonably well with an avascular head if the fracture has healed and the head revascularizes in time to prevent collapse.

b) Three-Part

The three-part fracture consists of a large displaced proximal fragment through the surgical neck, associated with an avulsion of either the lesser or greater tuberosity or both. Since the proximal fragment is large, some soft tissue envelope is usually retained. Avulsion of

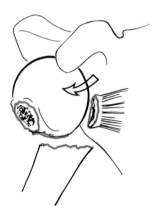

Fig. 4.8. Three-part fracture of the proximal humerus in which the lesser tuberosity is avulsed, allowing the proximal fragment to externally rotate. The radiological appearance of the head is that of a full moon on the anteroposterior view

Fig. 4.9. a Three-part fracture of the proximal humerus with avulsion of the greater tuberosity. In this particular case, the remaining attachment of the subscapularis through the lesser tuberosity internally rotates the proximal fragment 90°, again appearing radiographically as a full moon on the anteroposterior view. This is clearly seen in **b** ▼

either tuberosity diminishes the blood supply to the humeral head, but avascular necrosis is uncommon, although it occurs with greater incidence than in the two-part surgical neck fracture.

Of much greater clinical significance is the rotatory deformity of the proximal fragment caused by the avulsion of the tuberosities. If the *lesser tuberosity* containing the subscapularis is avulsed, the proximal fragment is externally rotated by the remaining rotator cuff, the supraspinatus, infraspinatus, and teres minor (Fig. 4.8). If the *greater tuberosity* is avulsed, the proximal fragment is internally rotated by the unopposed pull of the subscapularis (Fig. 4.9 a). In both instances, the unstable shafts may be driven into the mass of deltoid muscle and may be anterior to the proximal fragment. Poor bone contact will lead to delayed union or nonunion in most cases.

The presence of a round proximal fragment with the appearance of a full moon on the anteroposterior radiograph should alert the astute surgeon to this injury (Fig. 4.9 b). Open reduction and internal fixation should always be performed if delayed union and nonunion are to be prevented.

c) Four-Part

The four-segment fracture is the most difficult to treat and is associated with the poorest results. Added to the problems of the three-part fracture, namely delayed union or nonunion, is avascular necrosis of the humeral head. The pathognomonic feature is the small, crescentic, proximal articular fragment severed from the anatomical neck of the humerus. This fragment may be devoid of all soft tissue, making avascular necrosis a certainty, irrespective of treatment. Occasionally, some capsular attachments may remain; therefore, the presence of

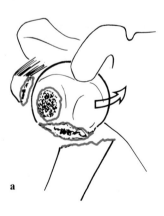

a

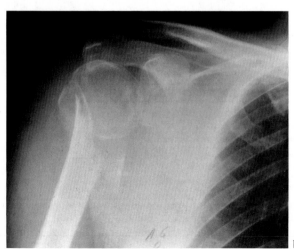

b

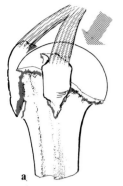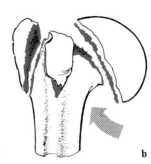

a   b

Fig. 4.10 a,b. Four-part fracture patterns. There are two types of four-part fracture patterns, each differing markedly in treatment and outcome. In the first type, the crescentic head fragment is impacted and stable (**a**), whereas in the other the head is unstable (**b**)

a small head fragment does not necessarily doom the head to avascularity.

There are two types of four part fracture patterns, each differing markedly in treatment and outcome. In the first type, the small crescentic head fragment is impacted and stable, whereas in the other, the head is unstable and not impacted. (Fig. 4.10 a,b).

Impacted Stable Type. This fracture pattern is caused by a fall on the outstretched arm in the abducted position. In this mechanism, the head is driven into the porotic neck, splitting the tuberosities. The soft tissue remains intact, usually maintaining the blood supply to the head, unless it is destroyed by injudicious surgery.

If the small head fragment is impacted and not acting as a mechanical block to movement, surgery should be avoided, as attempts at open reduction may destroy any remaining blood supply (Figs. 4.11, 4.12). The avulsed abductor mechanism, often in one large fragment consisting of the greater and lesser tuberosities with the intervening long head of biceps tendon, may be replaced without disturbing the impacted head. If the impacted fragment causes a block to motion during examination of the patient under anesthesia, then careful open reduction of the fracture is indicated. The technique must be atraumatic, so that any remaining blood supply to the humeral head is not compromised (Fig. 4.13, 4.14) (Jakob et al. 1991).

Unstable Type. This fracture is usually caused by a high-energy shearing force, tearing the soft tissue envelope, thereby commonly leaving the humeral head avascular.

If the head fragment is free, it must be reduced to a satisfactory position by either closed or open means, as will be described. A completely free head may have to be discarded during surgery and replaced with a prosthesis; however, in young patients, every effort should be made to retain the head fragment.

d) Fracture-Dislocation

Fracture-dislocations may be considered an extension of the two-, three-, and four-segment classifications. As in our previous discussion, the ultimate prognosis will depend upon the probability of nonunion or avascular necrosis of the fracture. Add to this the problems associated with the dislocation, such as irreducibility of the humeral head or impaction of its articular surface, and one can see why this injury has the worst prognosis of any in this region. In the two- and three-part fracture-dislocations, the proximal fragment is usually of sufficient size to retain capsular attachments, making avascular necrosis uncommon. The retention of at least one tuberosity almost always ensures viability of the humeral head. In the four-part fracture-dislocation, however, the head fragment is usually completely detached and avascular.

Two-Part. The two-part *anterior* fracture-dislocation is associated with an avulsed greater tuberosity (Fig. 4.15 a). In older patients with anterior humeral head dislocations, massive tears through the rotator cuff are more common than avulsions of the greater tuberosity and are often overlooked (Fig. 4.15 b). Satisfactory reduction is usually achieved by closed means with or without a general anesthetic. In almost all cases, closed reduction with no surgical intervention is indicated. In rare instances, the long head of biceps tendon may act as a block to reduction, causing either irreducibility of the dislocation or persistent displacement of the fracture (Fig. 4.15 c). In this situation, open reduction is indicated.

A two-part *posterior* fracture-dislocation is associated with an avulsed lesser tuberosity. Closed treatment is usually sufficient for this injury.

Three-Part. The major feature of the three-part dislocation is the large proximal fragment created by the fracture of the surgical neck of the humerus (Fig. 4.16 a). Some capsular tissue is almost always retained on the large head fragment, ensuring its viability. If the head fragment is displaced *anteriorly,* the greater tuberosity is usually fractured, whereas the lesser tuberosity is retained. In the *posterior* fracture-dislocation, the greater tuberosity is usually retained, whereas the lesser is avulsed.

In the three-part fracture-dislocation, closed manipulation with general anesthesia may restore the proximal fragment to an anatomical position. (Fig. 4.16 b-e) If the proximal fragment cannot be reduced because of soft tissue interposition, then open reduction is mandatory. If gross instability of the fracture remains after closed reduction of the dislocation, then open reduction

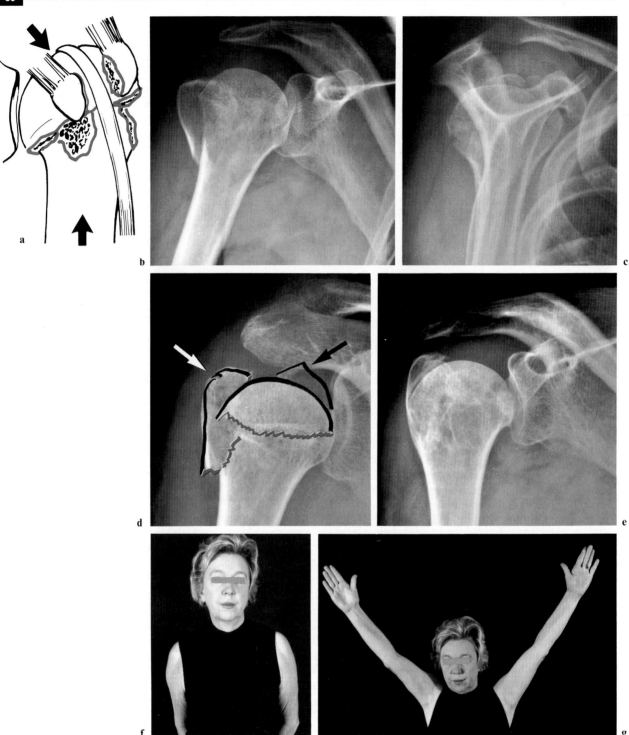

Fig. 4.11 a–g. Impacted four-part fracture of the proximal humerus with valgus position of head. **a** Extreme valgus position of the head driven into the soft cancellous bone by the abducted shoulder. Note the avulsion of both the greater and lesser tuberosities, which remain in their normal position. This is clearly seen on the anteroposterior and lateral radiographs (**b, c**) and is emphasized in **d**. The impacted valgus position of the head is clearly seen, as are the greater and lesser tuberosity avulsions, marked by the two *arrows*. This 49-year-old woman was taken to the operating room and the shoulder was manipulated under general anesthesia. Since there was no block to motion and the head and shaft fragments moved together, her injury was treated nonoperatively. At 1 year (**e**) the fracture has united with no evidence of avascular necrosis. The patient's range of motion is almost full (**f, g**) and she functions normally

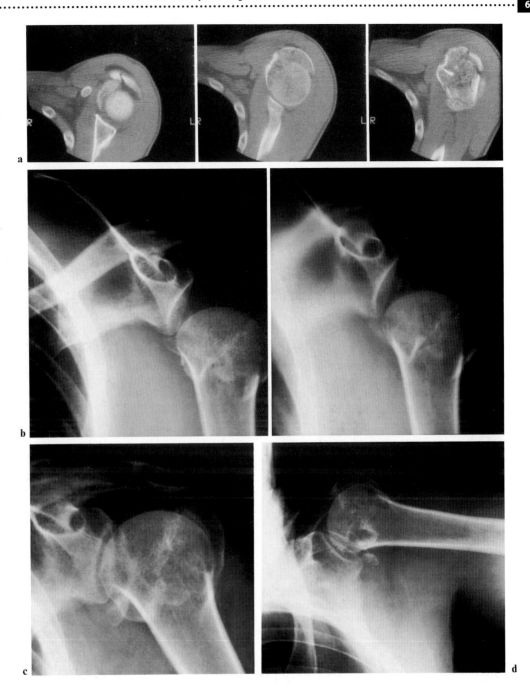

Fig. 4.12. a Anteroposterior tomograms demonstrating an impacted four-part fracture with the head in marked valgus and inferior subluxation in a 47-year-old male patient. Note the avulsion of the rotator cuff and the valgus position of the head in the CT scans (**b**). The patient was treated nonoperatively and the fracture has united (**c, d**). Note that the inferior subluxation has corrected and no avascular necrosis is present

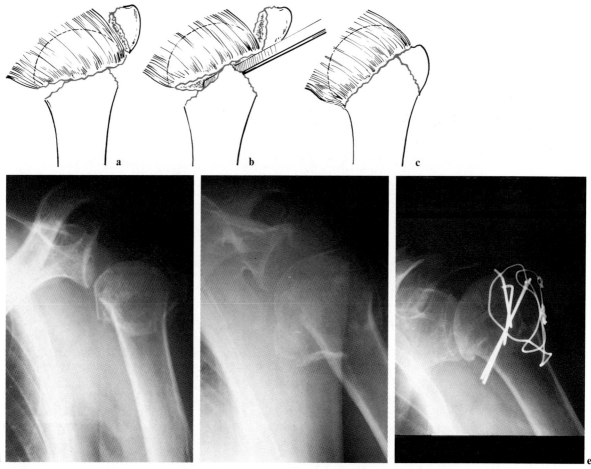

Fig. 4.13 a–f. Atraumatic dissection. **a** Three-part fracture of the proximal humerus. **b** Head fragment being reduced into its normal position with a periosteal elevator. The surgeon's finger is also an excellent reduction tool and may be less traumatic. **c** Reduction is complete. Note that the capsular attachment to

the proximal fragment has not been interfered with, thereby not interfering with the blood supply to the humeral head. **d** Anteroposterior and **e** lateral xray of 3 part fracture treated by this atraumatic method with an excellent result **f**

Fig. 4.14. a This 59-year-old woman sustained an impacted four-part type fracture of the proximal humerus. **b** Operative intervention and fixation resulted in an avascular necrosis of the humeral head. If this fracture is to be operated on, it must be done through atraumatic techniques which do not interfere with the blood supply (see Fig. 4.13)

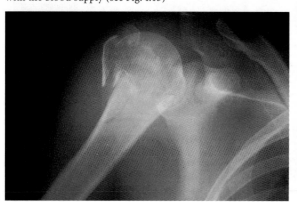

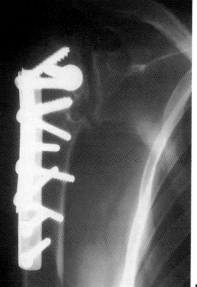

Fig. 4.15 a–c. Two-part fracture-dislocations. **a** Two-part anterior fracture-dislocation associated with an avulsed greater tuberosity. **b** Anterior dislocation of the shoulder associated with an avulsion of the rotator cuff. **c** Anterior dislocation of the shoulder with an interposed long head of biceps tendon preventing reduction of the dislocation

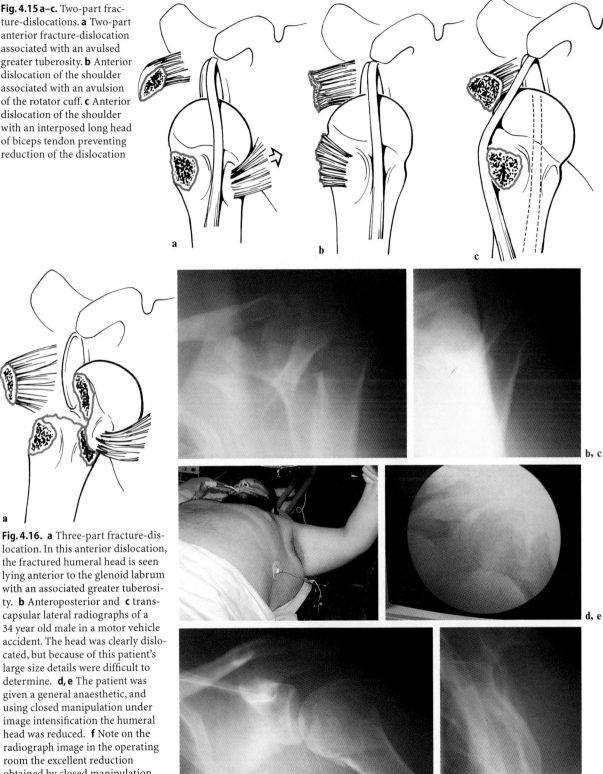

Fig. 4.16. a Three-part fracture-dislocation. In this anterior dislocation, the fractured humeral head is seen lying anterior to the glenoid labrum with an associated greater tuberosity. **b** Anteroposterior and **c** transcapsular lateral radiographs of a 34 year old male in a motor vehicle accident. The head was clearly dislocated, but because of this patient's large size details were difficult to determine. **d, e** The patient was given a general anaesthetic, and using closed manipulation under image intensification the humeral head was reduced. **f** Note on the radiograph image in the operating room the excellent reduction obtained by closed manipulation. **g** The patient was treated with an abduction splint until the fracture healed with an excellent end result and no avascular necrosis

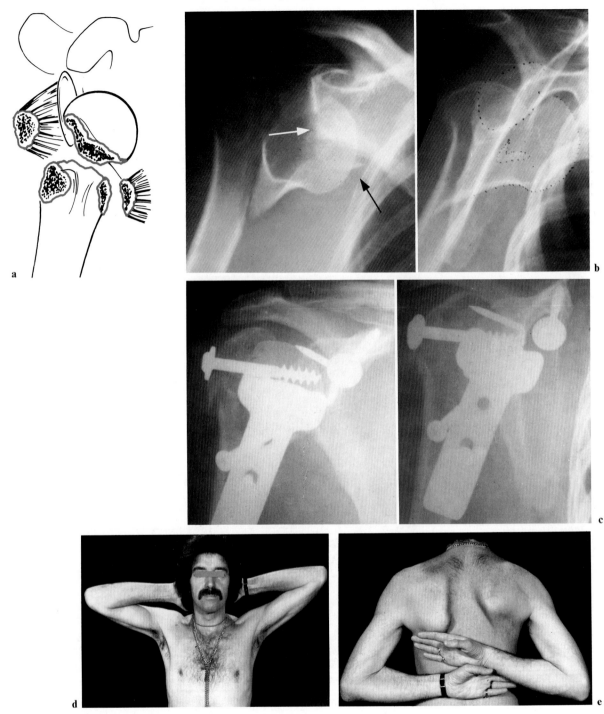

Fig. 4.17 a–e. Four-part fracture-dislocations. **a** The head is anteriorly dislocated. Both the lesser and greater tuberosities are avulsed. The humeral head may be attached by a small amount of capsule inferiorly or may be completely devoid of soft tissue attachment. The presence of the inferior triangle of bone is a good prognostic sign and may indicate that the blood supply is intact. **b** Anteroposterior and lateral radiographs of a four-part anterior fracture-dislocation. The *lower arrow* points to an avulsion from the glenoid labrum, the *upper arrow* to that portion of the glenoid from which the bone was avulsed. Open reduction and internal fixation were performed through an anterior deltopectoral approach. **c** The greater tuberosity was replaced with a lag screw, the major fracture with a lag screw plus T plate, and the glenoid fracture with a screw and staple. **d, e** The result at 18 months, with full movement and no avascular necrosis.

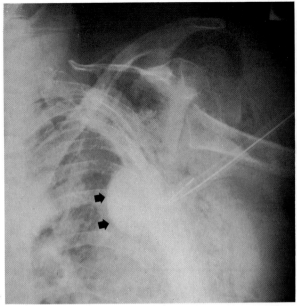

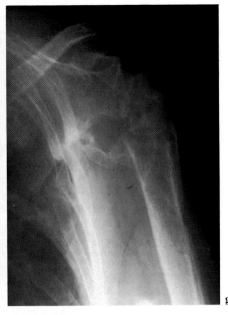

f

g

Fig. 4.17 f, g. Intrathoracic fracture-dislocation of the humeral head. **f** Humeral head in the left pleural cavity outlined by the *arrows*; chest drain in place. **g** Appearance after removal of the humeral head, 12 months after trauma

and internal fixation are desirable. The surgeon must respect the soft tissue attached to the head fragment envelope in order not to destroy the attached soft tissue.

Four-Part. Fracture-dislocations involving the anatomical neck of the humerus propel the small crescentic head fragment inferiorly, anteriorly (Fig. 4.17 a–e), posteriorly, or occasionally intrathoracically (Fig. 4.17 f, g). In almost all cases, this small head fragment has no attached soft tissue and will be avascular; therefore, the prognosis must be guarded. Closed manipulation under general anesthesia may restore the head fragment to its normal position. However, in our experience, this is extremely difficult, and anatomical reduction is rarely

achieved. Open reduction is usually indicated, but the patient must be informed that avascular necrosis of the humeral head is likely. In young patients, every effort should be made to retain the head fragment; in older patients it should be discarded in favor of a prosthesis (Hawkins and Switlyk 1993).

4.3.3 Articular Fractures

4.3.3.1 Impacted (Hill-Sachs)

Impaction of the articular surface, the so-called Hill-Sachs lesion, may occur with any type of fracture-dislocation. In anterior dislocations the impaction of the articular surface occurs posteriorly, the reverse being true for the posterior dislocation (Fig. 4.18). Very little can be done surgically to restore the normal anatomy,

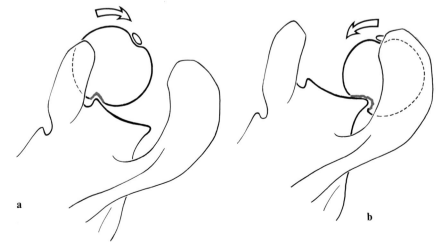

a

b

Fig. 4.18 a, b. Impacted articular fractures. Impaction of the articular surface may occur with any type of fracture-dislocation. **a** In anterior dislocations, the impaction of the articular surface occurs posteriorly. **b** In posterior dislocations, the impaction occurs anteriorly

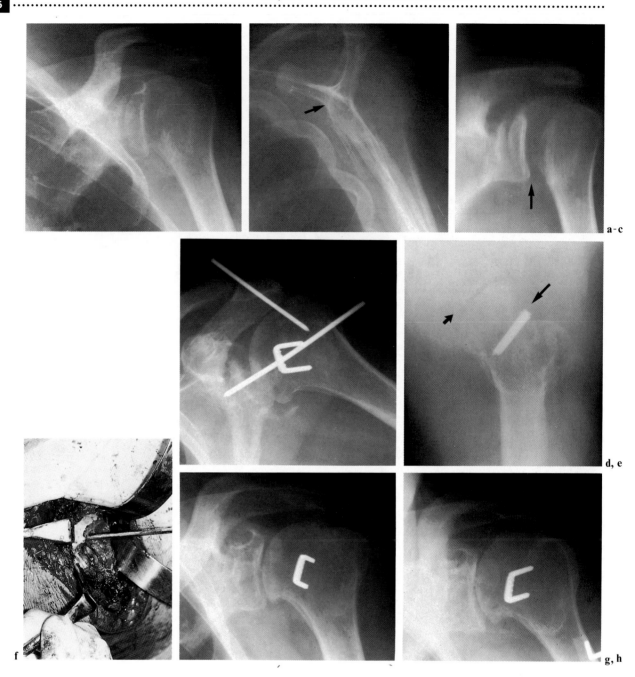

Fig. 4.19 a–h. Late posterior dislocation of the shoulder. **a, b** Anteroposterior and lateral radiographs of a 48-year-old epileptic who had sustained a posterior dislocation of the left shoulder 4 months previously. **c** Tomogram showing large anterior humeral head defect. **d** Surgery through an anterior approach reduced the head; it was maintained with Kirschner wires and the subscapularis tendon was inserted into the defect. **e** The Kirschner wires were removed with stability maintained. **f** Intraoperative photograph showing the massive defect. **g, h** The final result: joint narrowing is apparent but function is satisfactory

and recurrent dislocation may ensue, to be dealt with secondarily by standard means. In late, unreduced fracture-dislocation the defect may be so large that specialized techniques such as insertion of the subscapularis tendon into the anterior defect (McLaughlin 1960) or osteotomy of the humerus or scapular neck for the posterior defect (Müller et al. 1979) may be required to restore stability to the shoulder (Fig. 4.19).

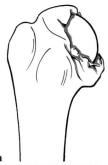

a

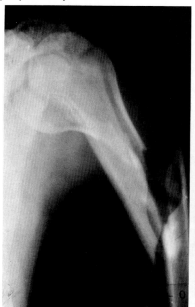

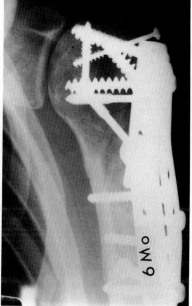

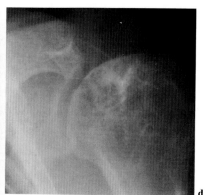

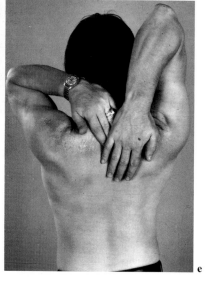

b,
c

d

e

Fig. 4.20 a–e. Articular fractures of the humeral head. **a** Impaction of the articular cartilage. **b** Anteroposterior radiograph of a 19-year-old motorcyclist with an injury to the proximal humerus. Note the articular impaction, the marked comminution, and the fracture of the proximal shaft. **c** Open reduction and internal fixation included elevation of the articular surface and bone grafting, as well as stable internal fixation using interfragmental screws and T plates. **d** After removal of the fixation 3 years after injury, the anteroposterior radiograph shows no evidence of avascular necrosis and a good cartilage space. **e** Function at that time was satisfactory, although definite restriction of external rotation was noted

4.3.3.2 Humeral Head

As in any other joint, major shearing forces applied to the joint surface may shatter the articular cartilage. The degree of articular damage may vary from small osteochondral fractures to major splits in the humeral head. In this situation, we must revert to basic principles in the management of any joint fracture, i.e., open anatomical reduction and stable fixation, followed by early motion if technically possible (Fig. 4.20). The upper extremity, however, is much more forgiving than the lower extremity; hence, closed methods may be more prudent than

open methods, which could jeopardize the blood supply to the small fragments. These fractures present extremely difficult management problems and require careful analysis before a definitive decision is made.

4.3.3.3 Glenoid Labrum

The usual pathological lesion associated with an anterior dislocation of the shoulder is an avulsion of the glenoid labrum (Bankart lesion) and a posterior impaction fracture of the humeral head (Hill-Sachs lesion). On

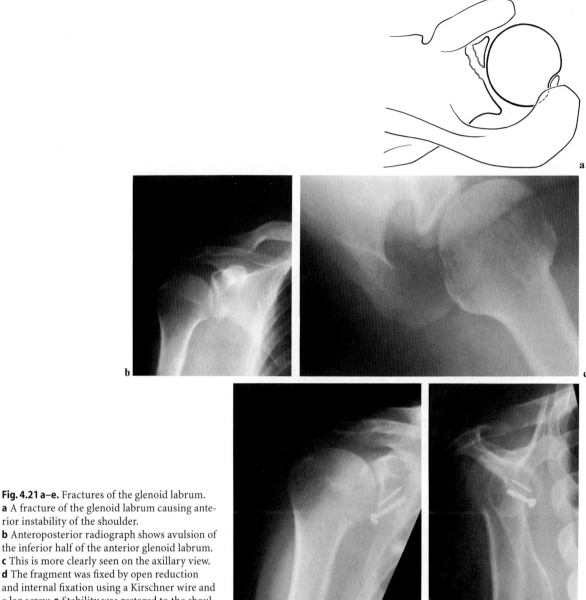

Fig. 4.21 a–e. Fractures of the glenoid labrum.
a A fracture of the glenoid labrum causing anterior instability of the shoulder.
b Anteroposterior radiograph shows avulsion of
the inferior half of the anterior glenoid labrum.
c This is more clearly seen on the axillary view.
d The fragment was fixed by open reduction
and internal fixation using a Kirschner wire and
a lag screw. **e** Stability was restored to the shoulder and function was good

occasion, the glenoid labrum is avulsed with a small segment of bone which, upon reduction, does not affect the
acute stability of the shoulder, but may be associated
with recurrent dislocation. Rarely, with anterior dislocation, a large anterior segment of the glenoid is fractured
and displaced, rendering the shoulder unstable
(Fig. 4.21). This fracture may occur with simple dislocations or with the more complex fracture-dislocations.

If displaced, open reduction and internal fixation are
desirable for the following reasons: (a) redisplacement
of the shoulder will readily occur with external rotation
because of the loss of the anterior portion of the glenoid

labrum; (b) since the fragment contains a major portion
of the articular surface of the joint, it requires anatomical reduction for optimal results. Closed treatment cannot accomplish this; therefore, operative fixation is *mandatory* when the fragment is large enough to affect the
stability of the joint. The opposite lesion may occur with
a posterior dislocation, i.e., a large posterior fragment of
the glenoid labrum may be fractured and will require
operative reduction.

4.4 Management

4.4.1 Assessment

4.4.1.1 Clinical

The first step in logical decision making is a careful clinical and radiological assessment. A painstaking history may indicate the physiological state of the patient, his or her expectations, and the degree of violence involved in the injury. For example, a markedly displaced fracture-dislocation through the proximal humerus of a young patient with normal cancellous bone has a vastly different outlook from that of a fracture-dislocation of similar appearance caused by a simple fall in an elderly individual. Physical examination will determine both the general state of the patient and the local condition of the limb. Complicating factors such as severe soft tissue injury, whether open or closed, and the presence of neurovascular injury will affect the decision to operate and its timing.

Careful manipulation of the limb will often reveal more information about the stability of the fracture than the radiograph. In grossly unstable fractures, the humeral shaft may be easily palpated in the deltoid muscle mass, moving independently of the proximal fragment.

4.4.1.2 Radiological

Careful radiological assessment is required prior to choosing a definitive treatment method. Standard roentgenograms of this area are often confusing and may be supplemented with tomograms or computed tomography (CT) scans (see Fig. 4.12 b). Tomographic investigation will reveal the position and size of the humeral head fragment, the number of segments, and the degree of instability.

Through a careful combination of the clinical and radiological assessments, a proper management scheme for the individual patient will evolve.

4.4.1.3 Examination Under Anesthesia

In most patients, a careful clinical assessment will indicate the degree of instability without the need for a general anesthetic. These individuals may be examined with adequate sedation, their fracture viewed on the image intensifier, and the degree of instability ascertained. With those patients in whom stability cannot be assessed because of severe pain, examination under anesthesia with image intensification will be helpful. Also, in some fracture-dislocations, the radiographs may be confusing; therefore, examination under anaesthesia may serve two purposes: first, giving more information about the injury and second, affording the surgeon the possibility of treatment by closed reduction (see Fig. 4.16). The surgeon should be prepared to proceed with immediate definitive surgical management if indicated.

4.4.2 Decision Making

The natural outcome of most stable and minimally displaced unstable proximal humeral fractures is a healed fracture and a satisfactorily functioning extremity. However, unstable fractures or fracture-dislocations have a high probability of delayed union or nonunion, avascular necrosis, irreducibility of the dislocation, and articular cartilage damage. Surgery is indicated where the probability of such complications with closed treatment is high, as previously discussed. The surgeon should assess the *personality* of the injury: this includes the fracture pattern, the condition of the limb, and the patient, as well as his or her own expertise. [The term "personality of the fracture" was first coined by Nicoll (1964) in connection with fractures of the tibia; see Sect. 17.2]. These factors are considered in the decision-making algorithm (Fig. 4.22).

4.4.2.1 Stable Fractures

If the clinical and radiological assessment indicates a stable fracture, i.e., the patient can actively move the extremity without pain, and the limb can be moved passively with little pain and no abnormal motion between the shaft and head fragments, the patient should be treated *nonoperatively*. The blood supply to a fractured proximal fragment is often so fragile that ill-advised open reduction will threaten the viability of the humeral head and must be avoided at all costs in stable situations (see Figs. 4.10 and 4.14). The arm may be immobilized in a sling and early motion started immediately. An excellent functional result may be expected in this situation (Rasmussen et al. 1992). The only exception to this rule would be a stable fracture with such gross displacement that the function of the extremity would be adversely affected. We agree with Neer that an impacted humeral neck with an adduction deformity of more than 50° would certainly affect the end result, and in rare circumstances this would constitute an indication for open reduction.

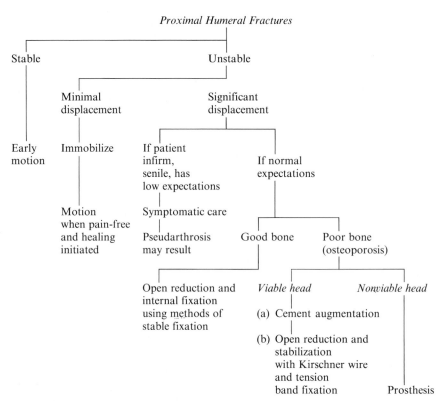

Fig. 4.22. Decision-making algorithm for proximal humeral fracture

Proximal Humeral Fractures

Stable — Unstable

Minimal displacement — Significant displacement

Early motion

Immobilize

If patient infirm, senile, has low expectations — If normal expectations

Motion when pain-free and healing initiated

Symptomatic care

Pseudarthrosis may result — Good bone — Poor bone (osteoporosis)

Open reduction and internal fixation using methods of stable fixation

Viable head — *Nonviable head*

(a) Cement augmentation

(b) Open reduction and stabilization with Kirschner wire and tension band fixation — Prosthesis

4.4.2.2 Unstable Fractures

If the clinical and radiological assessment indicates an unstable fracture, i.e., independent motion is present between the shaft and head fragments, further decision-making will depend upon the degree of displacement and instability present.

a) Minimally Displaced

If the fracture is minimally displaced (Fig. 4.5 a, b), no matter how many segments are involved, one might reasonably expect the presence of an intact soft tissue envelope in some portion of the fracture. Examination under image intensification may indicate lack of independent motion between the shaft and the proximal fragment at various degrees of rotation and abduction, confirming the presence of an intact soft tissue envelope. Patients with these fractures have more pain than do patients with a firmly impacted stable fracture; therefore, immobilization is required until sufficient fracture healing has taken place to render the patient pain-free. This is followed by a period of active rehabilitation of the injured limb; this period may vary from 2 to 6 weeks, depending upon the specific fracture. Since most fractures of the proximal humerus fall into the above two types, either the stable or the minimally displaced unstable fracture, it follows that most fractures of the proximal humerus may be managed by closed means.

b) Displaced

If a careful assessment indicates an unstable fracture or fracture-dislocation, the situation changes markedly. In Sect. 4.3 we discussed in some detail those injuries requiring open reduction. Having determined that the fracture at hand would best be treated by open reduction and stable internal fixation, other factors must now be considered.

Even in the best of circumstances surgery may be difficult; therefore, the stated goal of open reduction – stable fixation allowing early motion – may not be realized because of the many technical problems inherent in this area. Therefore, surgery should only be performed in cases where the surgeon is confident of overcoming these difficulties and experienced enough to achieve the stated goal. Of prime importance is the *general state of the patient*.

Poor Patient Expectations. If the patient is infirm, senile, and with low functional expectations, the surgeon should consider nonoperative symptomatic treatment, i.e., judicious neglect. Such patients are immobilized in any type of binder or sling for comfort. Between the fourth and sixth week their pain usually subsides. Delayed union and eventually nonunion become apparent in many cases of three- and four-part fractures. With persistence of this nontreatment, the surgeon may be pleasantly surprised at the degree of shoulder function

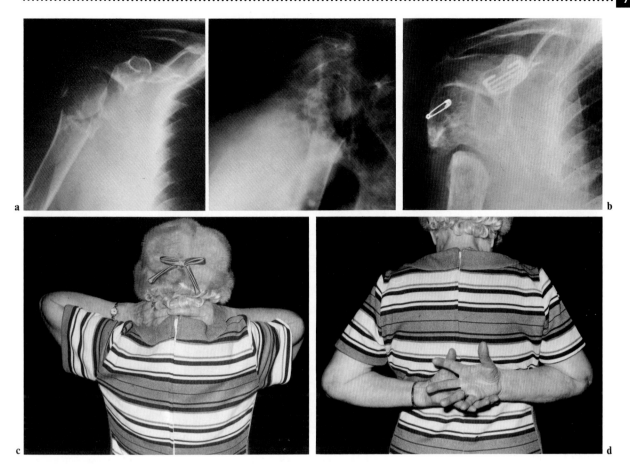

Fig. 4.23 a–d. An 82-year-old woman fell and sustained a three-part fracture of the right proximal humerus, seen on the anteroposterior and lateral radiographs (**a**). The patient was treated with a short period of immobilization followed by rehabilitation. **b** At 2 years, a clear pseudoarthrosis is seen on the anteroposterior radiograph. **c,d** The patient's function, however, was excellent, with a full range of motion and minimal discomfort. Her major disability was weakness in the right arm

regained by these patients. By 6 months, many patients have little pain and a surprisingly good range of motion (Fig. 4.23). They complain of weakness in their extremity and inability to lift heavy objects, but usually carry out their normal daily routine without difficulty. We recommend this pseudoarthrosis treatment only in exceptional circumstances, such as for patients with severe physical or mental disease.

Normal Expectations. If our assessment reveals that the patient has expectations for a normally functioning upper extremity, it then becomes necessary to carefully appraise not only the type of fracture present, but also the physiological state of the bone. It is obvious that this state is not an absolute, i.e., either good or bad, but a spectrum. Assessment of the bone may be difficult; nevertheless, it is extremely important if major errors in technique are to be avoided. Many of these fractures occur in elderly individuals with osteoporotic bone. Standard AO/ASIF techniques will fail because of the poor holding power of the screws in such bone. Therefore, the surgeon might achieve an excellent-looking postoperative radiograph, but will find that with early motion the screws will often pull out, with disastrous results (Fig. 4.24). Other techniques to be described are preferable in that situation (Figs. 4.25, 4.26).

If the bone is *normal,* i.e., if the state of the skeleton is good enough to ensure the holding power of the screws, anatomical open reduction followed by stable internal fixation is indicated. This may be readily achieved in the two- and three-part configurations, unless comminution or destruction of the articular cartilage is great. Early motion may be instituted and a good result can be expected (see Fig. 4.17 a-e) (Esser 1994).

In the four-part fracture, the result is more dependent on the state of vascularity of the head fragment, which may compromise the end result. In the young individual, however, we feel that every effort should be made to retain the crescentic head and to institute early rehabilitation. If the ensuing avascular necrosis becomes a

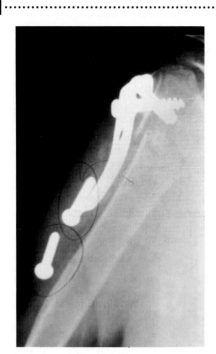

◀ **Fig. 4.24.** Anteroposterior radiograph taken 4 days following an excellent internal fixation of a four-part proximal humerus fracture in a 79-year-old woman, showing failure of the fixation because of osteoporotic bone, so common in proximal humeral fractures in the elderly

Fig. 4.25 a–d. Impaction tension band technique of internal fixation. If open reduction is indicated in elderly patients with osteoporosis, the technique will afford good stability. **a** After exposing the fracture, a small portion of soft osteoporotic bone should be curetted from the femoral head and neck. **b** This will allow impaction of the shaft into the defect so created. This impaction will restore some stability to the unstable fracture, and the head and shaft can move as a unit. **c** Fixation is achieved with multiple Kirschner wires into the head and shaft, crossing the tuberosities as necessary. **d** A tension band wire is then inserted around the Kirschner wires over the inferior portion of the rotator cuff

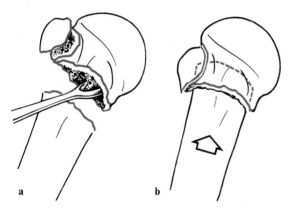

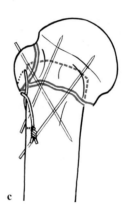

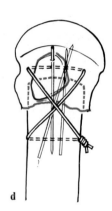

a   b   c   d

major symptomatic problem, secondary prosthetic replacement or shoulder arthrodesis may be performed if necessary.

If the pre- or intraoperative assessment indicates the presence of bone so poor that the holding power of screws would be negligible, other measures must be taken to achieve stability. The surgeon must first determine whether the proximal fragment is viable or not viable. In two- and three-part fractures the head is usually viable, unless the soft tissue is indiscriminately removed by the surgeon. A small crescentic head segment in the four-part fracture is almost always avascular.

If the head fragment is viable, i.e., if the proximal segment is vascular as in the two- and three-part fractures, but the bone is so poor that it is unlikely that a screw will hold, other options are available. Because the viability of the proximal fragment is not in question, it should

always be retained and the use of a prosthesis should not be considered. The other options are:

1. *Impaction tension band technique.* By curettage of some cancellous bone from the proximal fragment and impaction of the shaft into that area, stability may be restored to the fracture (Fig. 4.25 a, b). Multiple Kirschner wires through the fracture fragments surrounded by a tension band wire will maintain this stable situation (Fig. 4.25 c, d; H. Rosen, personal communication). Screws are not used; fixation is dependent upon the multiple Kirschner and tension band wires (Fig. 4.26; Kocialkowski and Wallace 1990; Flatow et al. 1991; Jaberg and et al. 1992; Cornell and Levine 1994).

2. *Cement composite fixation.* A second alternative is to use cement in the intramedullary portion of the fracture to improve its stability or in the predrilled screw holes to improve the holding power of the screws.

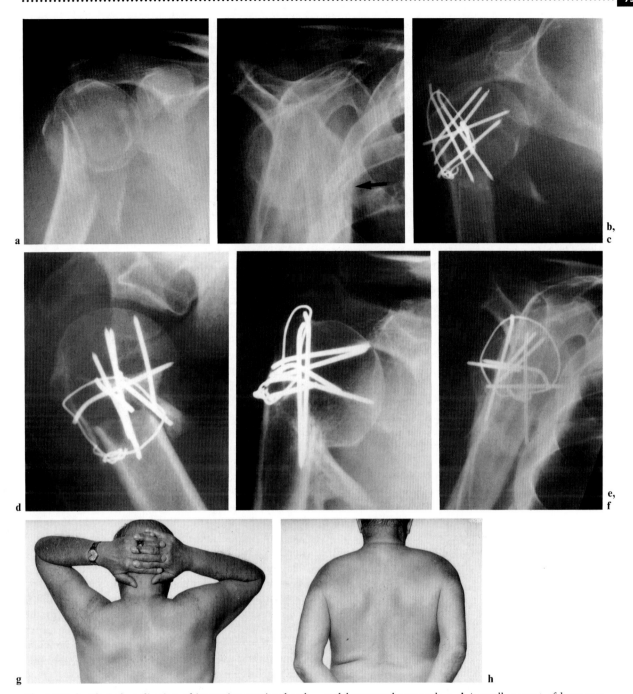

Fig. 4.26 a–h. Clinical application of impaction tension band technique. **a, b** The anteroposterior and lateral radiographs of this 73-year-old man show the typical moon-shaped head of a three-part unstable fracture of the right proximal humerus. The *arrow* points to the anterior location of the shaft with no contact to the humeral head. The fracture was exposed through a deltopectoral approach. **c, d** A small amount of bone was curetted and the shaft was impacted and fixed with multiple Kirschner wires and a tension band wire, as seen on the post-operative radiographs. **e, f** At 8 months the radiographs show sound union. **g, h** The clinical photographs show excellent function

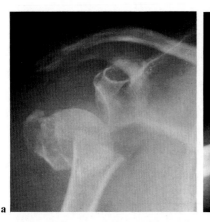
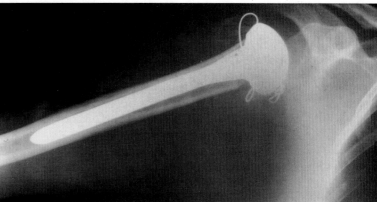

a   b

Fig. 4.27 a, b. Four-part fracture; treatment by unipolar prosthesis. **a** Anteroposterior radiograph indicating an unstable
four-part proximal humerus fracture. A small crescentic head
is nonviable. **b** It was replaced with a unipolar Neer-type prosthesis. Note the rotator cuff reposition with a wire suture

If the surgeon has begun a traditional type of open
reduction and finds that the screws are not holding in
the metaphysis, nuts may be affixed to the cortical
screws to increase their holding power. However, in the
upper humerus, the major problem is usually poor fixation of the screws in the proximal fragment, for which
this technique is obviously unsuitable. The above two
alternatives are more suitable for that particular problem.

If the head is nonviable – as in a four-part fracture –
i.e., if the crescentic fragment is totally avascular and the
bone is poor, a unipolar prosthetic replacement should
be inserted primarily, great care being taken to restore
the function of the rotator cuff by carefully reattaching
the rotator cuff or the avulsed tuberosities (Fig. 4.27;
Hawkins and Switlyk 1993; Moeckel et al. 1992).

4.4.3 Surgical Technique

4.4.3.1 Timing

Since fractures of the proximal humerus are articular or
periarticular injuries, we prefer to operate as soon as possible, once the decision has been made that surgery is
necessary. This will, of course, depend upon the state of
the soft tissues and the precise time that the patient is
seen following the accident. Surgery should *never* be performed through compromised soft tissues. Delayed surgery, especially between the third and seventh day after
injury, may result in excessive heterotopic ossification
however, there is no definite clinical proof at this time.

4.4.3.2 Approaches

Where an extensile approach is indicated, the standard
anterior deltopectoral approach will suffice (Henry
1927). Since it is extensile, the incision may be continued
distally to expose the entire humeral shaft on its anterolateral surface. The *posterior approach* may be used for
irreducible posterior fracture-dislocations, but is not
indicated for other reconstructive procedures in the area
of the shoulder.

However, the trend at this time is for more limited
approaches for fracture care, in order to preserve the
blood supply to the bony fragments *(biological internal
fixation)*. In the shoulder, a limited approach to fixation
by tension band techniques and intramedullary devices
is the deltoid split with or without acromion osteotomy.

a) Anterior Deltopectoral Approach

The anterior incision should be made along the medial
border of the deltoid muscle extending laterally to the
humeral shaft (Fig. 4.28 a). The deltopectoral triangle is
identified and the cephalic vein protected. Proximal
exposure will depend upon the fracture configuration. If
the surgical neck is fractured without extension into the
tuberosities, very little deltoid reflection is necessary
(Fig. 4.28 b), whereas if greater access to the proximal
humerus is required, a more radical removal of the deltoid will be necessary.

The deltoid muscle should be removed from the clavicle by raising an osteoperiosteal flap laterally to the
acromion. In the three- and four-part configurations, an
osteotomy of the acromion, which can be readily reattached with internal fixation, will allow wide access to
the proximal humerus. In our opinion, the advantage
gained by this increased exposure far outweighs the
potential disadvantage of the deltoid removal and its
possible avulsion in the postoperative period. It will also
allow the surgeon to work with relative ease on the proximal fragment, so that the vascular soft tissue attachments to that fragment are not further damaged.

Fig. 4.28 a–d. Anterior approach to the proximal humerus. **a** Anterior incision. **b** Deep dissection in the deltopectoral triangle. Note position of the long head of the biceps muscle. **c** Line of resection of deltoid from clavicle *(heavy dotted line)* and level of acromion osteotomy *(small dotted line)*. **d** Increased exposure of the proximal humerus by acromion osteotomy

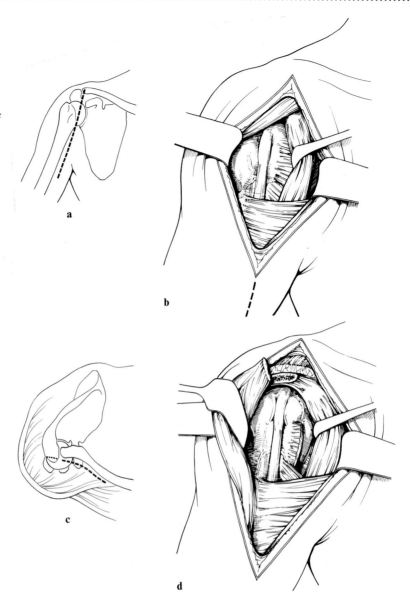

b) Deltoid Muscle Splitting With or Without Acromion Osteotomy

This approach may suffice for limited access to the greater trochanter and some two-part fractures for intrameduallary devices. If greater access is required, the acromion may be osteotomized (Fig. 4.29 a). This allows access to impacted four-part fractures, leaving the shoulder capsule and blood supply to the head intact by operating through the fracture.

The incision extends across the acromion and laterally over the deltoid muscle mass 4–5 cm. The deltoid fibers are split longitudinally (Fig. 4.29 b). If necessary, the acromion is osteotomized (Fig. 4.29 c), allowing greater access to the rotator cuff and fracture. Distally, the deltoid split must be not more than 3–5 cm to avoid damage to the axillary nerve.

The acromion is usually restored by a tension band wire, with or without screw fixation.

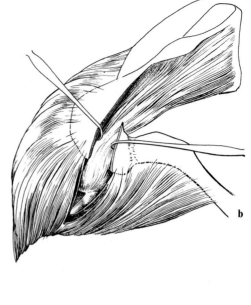

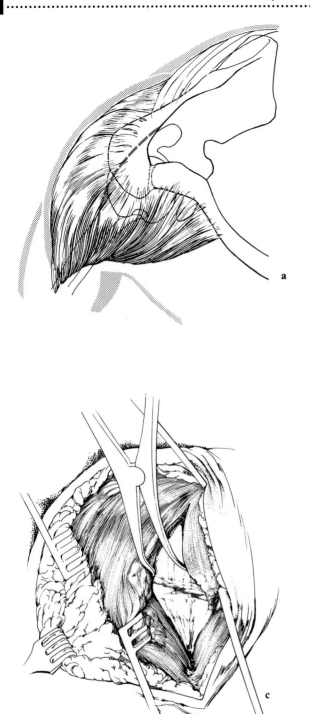

Fig. 4.29 a–c. Transacromial approach. The distal end of this approach is deltoid splitting, therefore it is of limited value only without an osteotomy of the acromion. The incision is made across the acromion and to the mid portion of the deltoid, but the deltoid split should not be performed further than 3 cm distal to the acromion because of the presence of the axial nerve. If further exposure is needed the acromion is osteotomized as shown in the drawing (**b**). Insertion of a laminar spreader will allow visualization of the rotator cuff. In the four-part impacted fracture in elderly patients this will allow the surgeon to reduce the fracture without division of the capsule, and makes fixation with a tension band figure of 8 wire relatively easy (**c**).

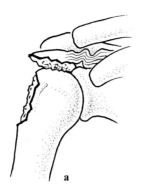
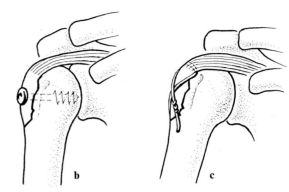

Fig. 4.30. a Avulsion fracture of the greater tuberosity with sub-acromial impingement.
b, c Reduction and internal fixation with either cancellous screw (**b**) or a tension band wire (**c**). (From Müller et al. 1979)

4.4.3.3 Reduction

Once easy access has been obtained by reflecting the deltoid, with or without a portion of the acromion, the fracture must be exposed through the disrupted soft tissues. No incisions should be made through intact soft tissues, no soft tissue should be removed from any of the bony fragments, and only minimal dissection should be performed along the fracture itself. In the upper humerus, anatomical reduction of the surgical neck and the comminuted fragments is not essential; therefore reduction should be obtained by applying traction, without disturbing the blood supply to the fragments. Once adequate reduction has been obtained, impaction of the fragments by applying a blow to the elbow will restore some stability to the fracture. Reduction of the head fragment should be performed atraumatically, especially if the fragment is small (see Fig. 4.13). The lesser tuberosity will be found attached to the subscapularis and the rotator cuff to the greater tuberosity. Often, the two are combined as a single fragment, with the long head of the biceps tendon running through it.

If the head fragment in the four-part fracture or fracture-dislocation is completely devoid of soft tissue, avascularity, of necessity, must be present; therefore, a decision must be made to retain or discard this avascular humeral head, depending upon the physiological age of the patient.

4.4.3.4 Methods of Internal Fixation

a) Good Bone

If the bone is of normal consistency and will hold a screw, the surgeon may proceed with standard techniques of internal fixation, using lag screws and plates where required.

Tuberosity Fractures. Fractures of the tuberosities are true avulsion fractures; therefore, they require dynamic compression techniques for stabilization, either by ten-sion band wiring or – in complex fractures – by incorporation of the tuberosity fracture in a tension band plate fixation. Occasionally, cancellous lag screws with washers may be used to achieve stable fixation (Fig. 4.30).

Humeral Neck Fractures. The choice of implant will depend upon the fracture pattern. The implants available for the upper humerus are the T plate, the L plate, standard 4.5-mm dynamic compression (DC) plates, the 6.5-mm cancellous screws, both lag and fully threaded, and 4.5-mm cortical screws. In the two-part surgical neck fractures a standard, laterally placed DC plate may be used if there is ample room for two screws proximal to the fracture (Fig. 4.31; see also Fig. 4.7). In the three-part fracture, the DC plate may be supplemented by a tension-band wire, fixing the tuberosity fragments. Two 6.5-mm cancellous screws inserted well into the subchondral area must be used to fix the proximal portion of the plate. These screws should be *fully threaded* to increase their holding power. The use of the DC plate will obviate the need for a T plate placed across the long head of biceps.

If the obliquity of the surgical neck fracture allows, a lag screw should be placed through the plate across the fracture line. This will greatly enhance the stability of the system (see Fig. 4.7).

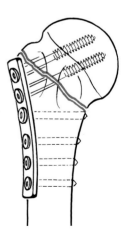

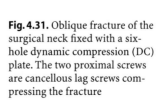

Fig. 4.31. Oblique fracture of the surgical neck fixed with a six-hole dynamic compression (DC) plate. The two proximal screws are cancellous lag screws compressing the fracture

78 ·

Chapter 4 **Fractures of the Proximal Humerus**

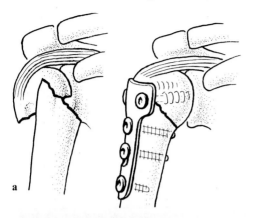

Fig. 4.32. a Reduction and fixation of a fracture with a T plate. (From Müller et al. 1979). **b, c** Clinical example of a three-part fracture treated with an interfragmental screw and a long T plate

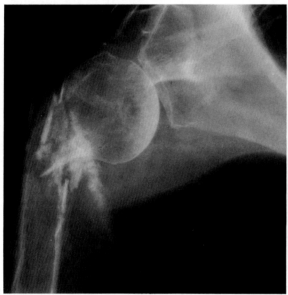

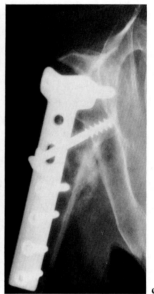

In the three- and four-part fracture types, the T or L plates are the implants of choice (Fig. 4.32). If the T plate is chosen, the anterior limb of the T usually crosses the long head of biceps. This can be prevented by the use of the L plate, which allows fixation of the proximal fragment with two large cancellous screws into the proximal fragment and cortical screws into the shaft. The greater tuberosity should be incorporated into the fixation device or, alternatively, may be fixed with tension band wiring.

Either the DC, the T, or the L plate may be applied as a neutralization, buttress, or tension band plate.

The various fracture types require different techniques:

1. *Transverse or short oblique fractures*
   - Surgical neck: since these unstable fractures occur in cancellous bone as a result of shearing forces, ideally, the major fragments should be compressed. Transverse or short oblique fractures of the surgical neck are suitable for compression techniques using plates with lag screws across the fracture where possible (Fig. 4.29).
   - Anatomical Neck: oblique fractures through the anatomical neck may be compressed by using large cancellous lag screws alone with washers or through a plate (Fig. 4.33).

2. *Comminuted or spiral fractures.* Grossly comminuted or spiral fractures require provisional fixation with Kirschner wires supplanted by permanent interfragmental screws. If the fragments are so small that a screw cannot be used, the Kirschner wire should remain as part of the definitive fixation. The fracture must then be stabilized by a neutralization or buttress plate, care being taken to incorporate the avulsed tuberosities, if present, into the system. All soft tissue should be retained, if possible.

3. *Articular Fractures.* Displaced fractures of the articular surface of the humeral head (Fig. 4.20 a) should be managed by open anatomical reduction and stable

Fig. 4.33 a–d. Fixation of anatomical neck fractures. **a** Anatomical neck fractures may be fixed with two screws using washers or through a plate used as a washer. These screws must be lag screws, as depicted. In osteoporotic bone, these screws may not hold and may pull out of the distal fixation. **b** Anteroposterior radiograph of a four-part fracture of the proximal humerus in a 74-year-old woman. **c, d** The fixation failed, as shown by the radiographs taken 4 months later. The patient's end result was poor

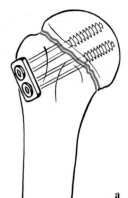
a

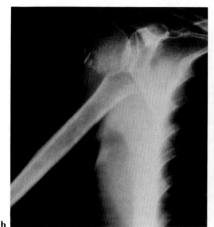
b

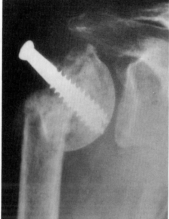

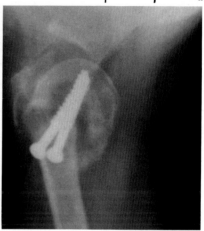
c,
d

fixation (Fig. 4.20 b–e). If the fracture has been impacted, elevation of the fragments will create a gap which must be filled with cancellous bone. Fixation of the joint fragments may be done with lag screws or occasionally, if they are small, with Kirschner wires. Small avascular fragments should be discarded, as they will usually displace into the joint during rehabilitation and act as loose bodies in the shoulder.

A large anterior or posterior glenoid rim fracture affecting joint stability *must* be internally fixed. If the fragment is large enough, it is best fixed with one or two 4.0-mm cancellous lag screws. Occasionally, if the fragment is small, it may be fixed with a staple or with Kirschner wires. Care must be taken that the metal does not penetrate the articular surface – direct visualization of the joint surface is the best way to avoid this complication (see Fig. 4.21).

In cases of complex two-, three-, and four-part fracture-dislocations, this glenoid rim fracture should be fixed last, after reconstruction of the other injuries.

b) Poor Bone

Viable Head; Cement Augmentation. Most surgeons develop a rather uneasy feeling during surgery if the cancellous screws in the proximal fragment just keep turning and turning and turning! If only one screw is not holding but the remainder of the fixation is good, then that screw should be removed, low-viscosity cement injected into the screw hole, and the screw replaced. This composite type of fixation may reverse a difficult situation. If the entire purchase on the proximal fragment is poor, then low-viscosity cement should be injected into the fracture site as well as into the proximal screw holes to ensure adequate fixation. We have also used this method in other situations where excessive movement may be expected in the postoperative period, for example, in patients with severe tremor due to parkinsonism. On the rare occasion where the proximal fixation is good but the distal fixation poor, nuts may be used on the cortical screws to enhance their fixation.

Impaction and Tension Band Techniques. If the surgeon recognizes preoperatively that the bone is poor and that screws will not hold, a completely different approach is indicated. Under these circumstances, anatomical reduc-

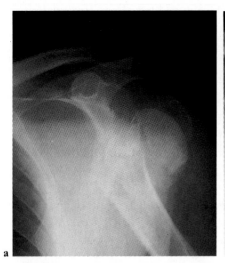 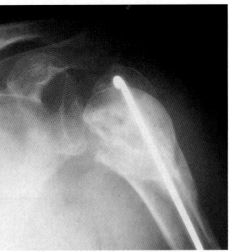

a   b

Fig. 4.34 a, b. Four part fracture of the proximal humerus with the articular surface rotated 90 degrees posterolateral, as noted in the radiograph **a**. The fracture was fixed with a percutaneous Rush pin. Unfortunately, the fracture was not reduced and healed with the humeral head facing laterally causing major symptoms for the patient (**b**)

tion is not attempted; stability is restored to the fracture by scooping out a portion of the very soft bone in the proximal fragment with a curet and impacting the humeral shaft into the hole so created (Fig. 4.25 a,b). This impaction can be done manually by placing the distal fragment into the hole and striking the elbow until impaction occurs. The shaft and head fragments should then move together as one unit, which can be fixed with Kirschner wires (Fig. 4.25 c,d). Fine 1.6-mm or 2-mm Kirschner wires are driven across the main fragments with a power drill; other fragments of bone are similarly fixed. The tuberosity fragments with the attached rotator cuff can also be provisionally fixed with Kirschner wires. A large tension band wire is then inserted around the Kirschner wires in the tuberosities and inserted in the shaft, thereby imparting further stability to the fracture. Stability depends upon the degree of impaction achieved between the shaft and head fragments and upon the tension band wire. Usually, enough stability is obtained to allow early protected motion without fear of the fixation falling apart (see Fig. 4.26). Occasionally, cement may be used at the fracture to ensure maintenance of the reduction and to aid in stability.

Percutaneous Techniques. For osteoporotic bone, many percutaneous techniques have been attempted, especially Rush pins through the tuberosity into the shaft. This technique has given variable and inconsistent results

and cannot be recommended except where the patient is in poor medical condition. The pin tended to displace into the proximal fragment, allowing loss of reduction (Fig. 4.34). However, Robinson and Christie (1993) compared this technique with open reduction and internal fixation (ORIF) (AO) in older osteoporotic patients and found the results to be more favorable. Retrograde pins have also been used (Zifko et al. 1991) with reasonable results in these difficult patients.

Nonviable Head. In a four-part fracture or fracture-dislocation through osteoporotic bone, the head fragment is usually free and avascular. Often, the bone is so soft that fixation is impossible. Even if fixation were possible, avascular necrosis would certainly ensue, compromising the final result. Under these circumstances, especially in elderly individuals, we suggest a *unipolar prosthetic replacement* (Fig. 4.27). Precise attention to detail, including the correct retroverted position of the prosthetic head and careful restoration of the tuberosity fragments containing the rotator cuff, will give satisfactory results (Neer 1955). We feel that a four-part fracture or fracture-dislocation in an older patient with a totally avascular crescentic head fragment, devoid of all soft tissue, is the *only* indication for primary prosthetic replacement of the humeral head. The results of this procedure, if strict attention to technical detail is followed, are good (Hawkins and Switlyk 1993). However, many reports to the contrary make this a controversial issue at this time. In younger patients with a nonviable humeral head, shoulder arthrodesis may be indicated (Fig. 4.35). This should rarely be done as a primary procedure, since avascular necrosis of the humeral head may be tolerated by the patient.

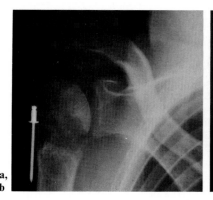
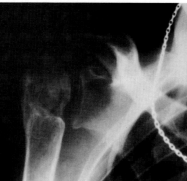
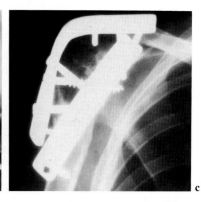

a,
b

c

Fig. 4.35. a Avascular necrosis of a small crescentic head fragment following fracture-dislocation. **b** Seven months later, the
fracture had healed, but the humeral head had collapsed.
c Managment of this 22-year-old man was by arthrodesis

4.4.3.5 Wound Closure

The deltoid muscle should be reattached with nonabsorbable sutures through the attached osteoperiosteal
flaps into the clavicle. If the acromion has been osteotomized, nonabsorbable sutures or wire may be used to
reattach it. Occasionally, a screw through a predrilled
hole may be inserted. The deltoid muscle will then cover
the entire fracture complex and the implant. The skin
should be closed primarily over suction drains. If the
fracture was open, that portion of the skin previously
open should be left so and can be dealt with by closure
on the fifth day, if clean granulation has appeared.

4.4.3.6 Postoperative Care

a) Early

The early postoperative care will depend upon the
surgeon's assessment of the degree of stability present.
In the immediate postoperative period, we prefer to
immobilize the patient in abduction, either with the use
of pillows or with skin traction. If the stability of the
fracture is sound, the patient may be taken out of the
abducted position on the second postoperative day and
allowed pendulum exercises. Active contractions of the
deltoid muscle are encouraged if there is no concern
about the deltoid resuture. Young patients with anatomical reduction and rigid fixation will rapidly regain full
shoulder motion, often to a surprising degree within the
first 2 weeks following surgery. If there is concern about
the deltoid suture, an abduction splint is applied, the
patient being allowed out of the splint for pendulum
exercises only. In these circumstances we do not allow
active deltoid contraction against resistance until bio-

logical healing of the deltoid muscle insertion has
occurred, usually within 4–6 weeks.

If the stability of the fracture is in question, the surgeon must use his or her own judgment as to the best
method and timing of the rehabilitation process.
Pendulum exercises without resistance can usually be
carried out with any stable internal fixation, but if the
bone is so poor that the fixation is in jeopardy, the
patient should be immobilized in an abduction splint
until some sign of bone union is noted, usually by the
sixth week.

If a prosthetic replacement has been used, the patient
is immobilized in abduction in the immediate postoperative period and the abduction splint is used for
4–6 weeks; pendulum and resisted deltoid exercises are
allowed during this period.

b) Late

The patient should be followed up carefully for clinical
and radiological signs of implant failure, such as lucency around the screws, loss of plate fixation, or movement
at the fracture site. If any of these are noticed, it is far better to immobilize the patient in an abduction splint until
union has occurred than to persist with early motion,
which may result in total loss of the fixation.
Reoperation would be more hazardous, because the
already porotic bone would be even worse a few weeks
after the injury.

References

Burstein AH (1993) Fracture classification systems: do they work and are they useful? J Bone Joint Surg 75A/12:1743

Codman EA (1934) The shoulder. Rupture of the supraspinatus tendon and other lesions in or about the subacromial bursa. Todd, Boston

Cornell CN, Levine D, Pagnani MJ (1994) Internal fixation of proximal humerus fractures using the screw-tension band techniques. J Ortho Trauma 8/1:23–27

Esser RD (1994) Treatment of three and four-part fractures of the proximal humerus with a modified cloverleaf plate. J Ortho Trauma 8/1:15–22

Flatow EL, Cuomo F, Maday M et al (1991) Open reduction and internal fixation of two-part displaced fractures of the greater tuberosity of the proximal part of the humerus. J Bone Joint Surt 73A/8

Hawkings RJ, Switlyk P (1993) Acute prosthetic replacement for severe fractures of the proximal humerus. Clin Ortho Relat Res 289:156–160

Henry AK (1927) Exposure of the long bones and other surgical methods. Wright, Bristol

Jaberg H, Warner J, Jakob RP (1992) Percutaneous stabilization of unstable fractures of the humerus. J Bone Joint Surg 74A/4

Jakob RP, Miniaci A, Anson PS et al (1991) Four-part valgus impacted fractures of the proximal humerus. J Bone Joint Surt 73B/2

Kocialkowski A, Wallace WA (1990) Closed percutaneous K-wire stabilization for displaced fractures of the surgical neck of the humerus. Injury 21:209–212

McLaughlin HL (1960) Recurrent anterior dislocated shoulder. Morbid anatomy. Am J Surg 99:628–632

Moeckel BH, Dines DM, Warren RJ et al (1992) Modular hemiarthroplasty for fractures of the proximal part of the humerus. J Bone Joint Surg 74A/6

Müller ME, Allgöwer M, Willenegger H (1979) Manual of internal fixation, 2nd edn. Springer, Berlin Heidelberg New York

Müller ME, Allgöwer M, Schneider R, Willenegger H (1991) Manual of internal fixation, 3rd edn. Springer, Berlin Heidelberg New York

Neer CS (1955) Articular replacement for the humeral head. J Bone Joint Surg 37A:215–228

Neer CS (1970) Displaced proximal humeral fractures. I. Classification and evaluation. J Bone Joint Surg 52A: 1077–1089

Nicoll E (1964) Fractures of the tibial shaft. A survey of 105 cases. J Bone Joint Surg [Br] 46B:313–381

Rasmussen IH, Dalsgaard J, Christensen BS, Holstad E (1992) Displaced proximal fractures: results of conservative treatment. Injury 23/1:41–43

Robinson CM, Christie J (1993) The two-part proximal humeral fracture: a review of operative treatment using two techniques. Injury 24/2:123–125

Sidor ML, Zucherman JD, Lyon T et al (1993) The Neer classification system for proximal humeral fractures. J Bone Joint Surg 75A/12

Siebenrock K, Gerber C (1993) The reproducibility of classification of fractures of the proximal end of the humerus. J Bone Joint Surg 75A/12

Szyszkowitz R, Seggl W, Schleifer P, Cundy P (1993) Proximal humeral fractures. Management techniques and expected results. Clin Orth Relat Res 292:13–25

Zifko B, Poigenfurst J, Pezzei C, Stockley I (1991) Flexible intramedullary pins in the treatment of unstable proximal humeral fractures. Butterworth-Heinemann, London

5 Fractures of the Humerus (12-A, B, and C)

J. Schatzker

5.1 Introduction

Most fractures of the humerus can be treated successfully by closed means. They unite rapidly. Minor angular and rotational deformities do not result in loss of function, and shoulder and elbow stiffness does not occur. There are circumstances, however, when an open reduction and internal fixation is indicated.

Fig. 5.1. a A long spiral fracture of the humerus. The gap did not close when rotational alignment was restored because of soft tissue interposition. **b** Complete failure of healing at 3 months

5.2 Indications for Surgery

5.2.1 Failure to Obtain a Satisfactory Reduction

a) Long Spiral Fractures

If displaced with a gap which does not close when rotational alignment is restored (Fig. 5.1), long spiral fractures are almost impossible to reduce because of muscle interposition. If left in good alignment, but with a significant gap between the fracture fragments, the outcome of these fractures is always an atrophic nonunion.

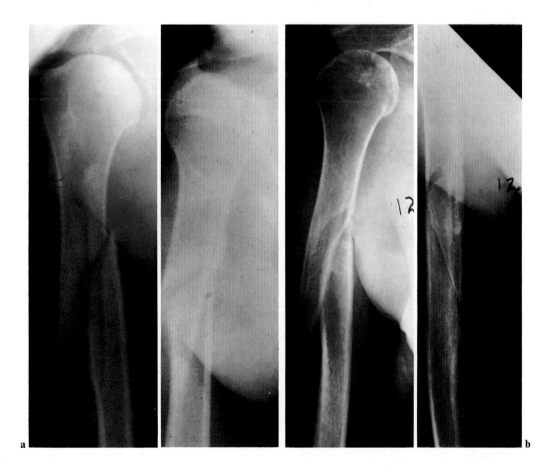

a   b

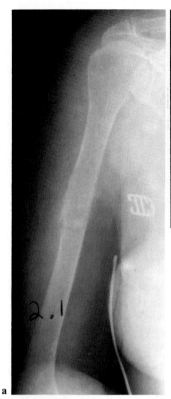

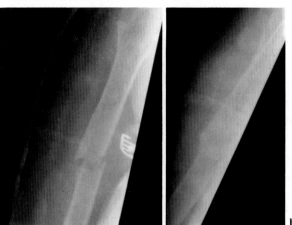

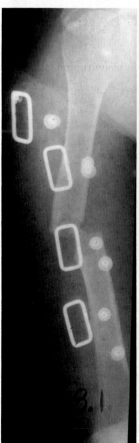

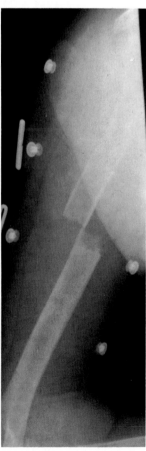

Fig. 5.2. a A transverse fracture of the humerus. Note the slight distraction at the time of the initial X-ray. **b** The same fracture after the application of a sugar-tong plaster splint and a sling. The distraction is more marked. **c** The arm was transferred into a cast brace in the hope that active muscle contraction would bring the fracture ends together. The fracture brace could not control the instability of the fracture, and it displaced

b) Transverse Fractures

Similarly, a transverse fracture which is overdistracted, either as a result of the initial trauma or closed treatment (traction or hanging cast), should be operated upon (Fig. 5.2). Attempts to treat such fractures closed are frustrating to both the patient and the surgeon, first, because the fracture gap cannot be closed by nonoperative means, and second, because alignment is difficult to control. Prolonged immobilization, although frequently employed, is in vain. By the time the clinician finally accepts that nonunion has occurred, some permanent shoulder and elbow stiffness will have become established.

c) Short Oblique Fractures

Short oblique fractures through the distal portion of the shaft just above the olecranon fossa, if displaced, are difficult to reduce and very difficult to maintain in the reduced position. Furthermore, because they are periarticular, prolonged immobilization leads to irreversible elbow stiffness. For these reasons, an open reduction and internal fixation is frequently the best form of treatment.

5.2.2 Failure to Maintain Reduction

The "sugar-tong" plaster of Paris splint, combined with a Velpeau bandage, is the most effective and most commonly employed method of immobilization of humeral

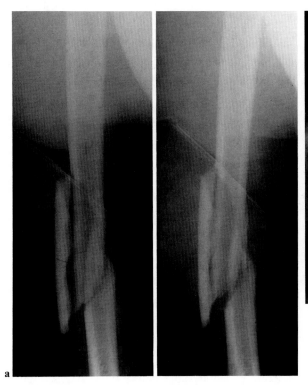

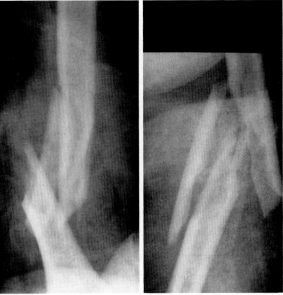

Fig. 5.3. a A comminuted fracture of the humerus in an obese woman with large breasts. Note the initial satisfactory alignment. **b** An attempt to brace the humeral shaft against the bulging breast and chest wall resulted in unacceptable displacement

fractures. Very occasionally, we have used a thoracobrachial spica to prevent excessive internal rotation of the fracture. We have found the hanging cast a somewhat illogical and unsuccessful method. In order for the hanging cast to exert any degree of traction to effect alignment, the patient must remain upright at all times. As soon as the patient lies down, all traction is lost and the cast acts like a lever, causing displacement, since frequently its upper end is at or just above the fracture. Whenever the patient moves while upright, despite the collar and cuff, the cast tends to swing. This not only causes a great deal of pain, but also excessive movement at the fracture. Therefore, we feel that if a fracture cannot be controlled in a sugar-tong cast, the hanging long arm cast is not a logical solution.

In the majority of patients, if the arm in the sugartong cast is bound to the chest wall, the fracture remains reduced, the patient is comfortable, and the fracture unites. However, if a satisfactory position cannot be maintained, then an open reduction and internal fixation is indicated. Sometimes reduction is lost because of the deformity of the chest wall. This is true in very obese patients and in women with very large breasts (Fig. 5.3). Further manipulative attempts are futile and open reduction and internal fixation should be carried out.

5.2.3 Injuries to the Chest Wall

Patients with coexistent injuries to the chest wall (e.g., rib fractures, flail chest, sucking wound) cannot have the arm bound to the chest wall because it would interfere with ventilation and with care of the chest wall injury.

5.2.4 Bilateral Humeral Fractures

In patients with bilateral fractures, at least one humerus should be stabilized to facilitate self-care. Otherwise, the immobilization results in total disability.

5.2.5 Multiple Injuries

Occasionally, in patients with multiple injuries, open reduction and internal fixation of the humerus are required to facilitate the care and rehabilitation of the patient.

5.2.6 Vascular Lesions

In fractures associated with vascular lesions, the fracture should be stabilized before the vascular repair is carried out.

5.2.7 Neurological Lesions

Fractures of the humeral shaft are at times associated with injury to the radial nerve. The management of the fracture associated with a radial nerve lesion continues to be a controversial issue, with some favoring a delay to see whether the radial nerve will recover and others favoring a policy of immediate exploration, reduction, stabilization of the fracture, and primary nerve repair if the nerve is torn.

The radial nerve is commonly at risk if the fracture is at the junction of the middle and distal thirds of the humeral shaft and particularly if the fracture is associated with lateral displacement of the distal fragment (Fig. 5.4). At this point, the radial nerve emerges from the spiral groove and is tethered as it pierces the intermuscular septum. It cannot yield to the lateral displacement of the distal fragment and is therefore frequently seriously damaged. We feel, therefore, that in the presence of this fracture pattern, immediate exploration is indicated.

If radial nerve function disappears as a fracture is manipulated and reduced, the nerve is caught in the fracture. Spontaneous recovery will not occur if the nerve is not freed and, if the nerve is not explored immediately, the nerve becomes even more enveloped in the callus of fracture repair. This makes its ultimate exploration very difficult. Therefore, we feel immediate explora-

tion with freeing of the nerve and surgical repair of the fracture is indicated in all instances where radial nerve function is lost as a consequence of closed reduction. In all other closed fractures of the humerus associated with radial nerve lesions, if there are no other indications for surgery, a delay of 3–4 months is justifiable. By then the fracture should have united and rehabilitation begun. If the nerve has not recovered, electromyography (EMG) of the most proximal muscles supplied by the radial nerve distal to the fracture should be performed. If there is no sign of recovery, the lesion was a neurotmesis and the patient will require either a free nerve graft or multiple tendon transfers.

5.2.8 Fractures of the Shaft Associated with Intra-articular Fractures or Articular Extensions of the Fracture

The successful outcome of all intra-articular fractures depends on the anatomical reduction and stable fixation of the fragments and early motion. Therefore, if a fracture of the humerus either extends into a neighboring joint or is associated with a separate intra-articular fracture of the shoulder or the elbow (Fig. 5.5), then both the shaft and the intra-articular fracture are best managed by an open reduction and internal fixation. This will ensure that the outcome of the intra-articular fracture is not prejudiced by the desire to treat the shaft

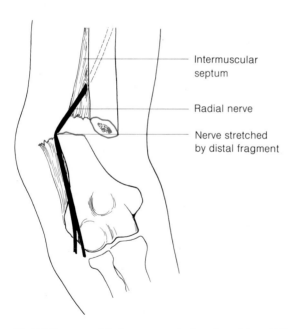

Intermuscular septum

Radial nerve

Nerve stretched by distal fragment

Fig. 5.4. Fracture of the humerus at the junction of the middle and distal thirds (Holstein fracture). Note the lateral displacement of the shaft and the tethering of the nerve by the intermuscular septum

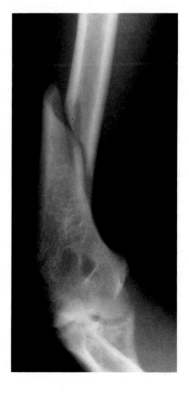

Fig. 5.5. a Association of a midshaft fracture of the humerus with a fracture of the olecranon. **b** Internal fixation of both fractures

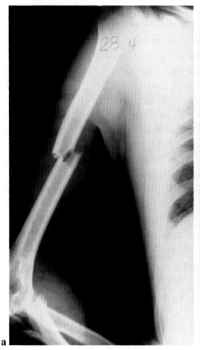
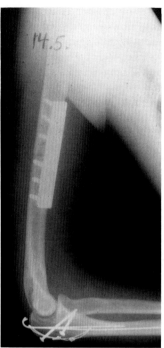

fracture nonoperatively. There is no adequate method of splinting the shaft and permitting full mobilization of the shoulder and elbow. If the joint were to be kept immobilized after an open reduction and internal fixation, then serious stiffness of the joint would be certain.

5.2.9 Open Fractures of the Humerus

All open fractures, after thorough débridement, require skeletal stability (see Chap. 3).

5.2.10 Pathological Fractures of the Humerus

Many pathological fractures of the humerus will unite if splinted and treated with radiation. In some patients such immobilization may be impractical because of other considerations such as loss of use of the other upper extremity or inability to splint the humerus to the chest wall. Locked intramedullary nailing is an excellent method of securing stability and function (see Fig. 5.12). Composite fixation is another useful method but one which requires more surgery (see Fig. 5.14). Regardless of the method chosen, the fractures can then be radiated if the tumor is radiosensitive. The indications for internal fixation of pathological fractures will depend, of course, not only on the factors mentioned but also on the extent of pathological involvement. Some bones are so

extensively involved that surgical stabilization is not possible.

5.3 Surgical Approaches

We feel that the best approach to the proximal third of the shaft is the standard deltopectoral approach. The more proximal the fracture, the more likely it will be necessary in order to gain exposure to release the deltoid distally from its insertion into the deltoid tuberosity. Reattachment of the deltoid is not necessary, as the muscle reattaches to bone spontaneously without any subsequent functional deficit. Occasionally it may become necessary to detach the anterior third of the deltoid muscle from the clavicle. In doing this, it is important to preserve both the superficial and deep fascia which invests the deltoid muscle. We no longer leave a cuff of muscle attached to the clavicle to effect a closure, because we have found the following method to be more effective. We pass our sutures carefully through both the deep and superficial fascia of the deltoid and then through the fascia of the trapezius muscle at its insertion into the clavicle. As the sutures are tied, the deltoid is drawn snugly up to and over the edge of the clavicle, effecting a strong muscle closure.

In order to protect the resutured portion of the deltoid from avulsion during early mobilization, we insist on passive elevation and abduction for the first 4 weeks. With this method, we have not had a single deltoid avulsion. As we extend the incision distally, we approach the insertion of the deltoid. At this point it is important to identify the origin of the brachialis muscle, which merges here with the insertion of the deltoid, because the radial nerve lies a fingerbreadth below and behind the deltoid insertion as it comes forward around the humerus. This is invariably an area where brisk bleeding is encountered as the planes are developed, and the surgeon should be ready to coagulate the bleeding vessels. Further exposure distally is gained by splitting the brachialis muscle down its middle. The lateral half of the muscle is used to protect the radial nerve. By splitting the brachial muscle, exposure can be extended as far as the elbow joint.

For this part of the approach, we like to have the patient positioned supine with a folded sheet under the scapula to lift the shoulder off the table. This facilitates cleansing of the skin posteriorly and subsequent draping of the shoulder to leave the arm free and fully exposed. The arm is positioned at the patient's side and is supported on an arm board.

It is best to approach the distal third of the humerus posteriorly. For this exposure, the patient is positioned lying on the uninjured side. After draping, which should leave the shoulder and elbow fully exposed, the arm is supported on a rolled sheet and the elbow is flexed. It is extremely advantageous to support the humerus while it is being exposed, because it obviates the need for an assistant and makes the handling of the fracture fragments much simpler. The triceps aponeurosis is split down the middle or is reflected down as a tongue. The underlying triceps is then split in line with its fibers. If the approach has to be extended more proximally or if the humerus has to be approached from the back, as might occur in the case of an open fracture which has penetrated muscle and skin posteriorly, then a formal posterior approach to the bone has to be used. This is done by developing the interval between the long head of the triceps medially and the lateral head laterally. The radial nerve is encountered in the more proximal portion of the exposure coursing from high medial to low lateral. It is important to realize that, although described as running along the radial grove of the humerus, the nerve does not lie on bone but on the medial head of the triceps.

5.4 Surgical Methods of Stable Fixation

5.4.1 Biomechanical Considerations

The cortex of the humerus splinters very easily. Therefore, even long spiral fractures must be protected after lag screw fixation with a neutralization plate, and it is imperative never to rely on screw fixation alone.

Furthermore, to prevent longitudinal fissuring whenever the humerus is plated, a broad plate should be used. The screw holes in these broad plates are staggered, which increases the distance between successive screws and decreases the likelihood of fissuring the bone longitudinally.

In patients with a normal elbow, the posterior cortex is under tension (Müller et al. 1970). If the patient has a stiff elbow, the anterior cortex becomes the one under tension (Weber and Cech 1976). This would mean that in patients with a mobile elbow, the "compression" or tension band plates should be applied posteriorly, and in patients with a stiff elbow, anteriorly.

Because the radial nerve lies in the spiral groove posteriorly, the posterior surgical approach to the mid-diaphysis is more difficult and the radial nerve is at great risk of injury. For this reason, we prefer Henry's anterior approach to the upper and mid-diaphysis (Henry 1959) and apply the plates most commonly to the anterolateral surface of the bone. Because the humerus is not a weight-bearing bone and is not subjected to forces as great as those acting on the femur or the tibia, this biomechanical infringement has not resulted in any failures of fixation.

Fractures of the distal third should be plated posteriorly. There are four reasons for this. The humerus is flat posteriorly and it is easier to apply the broad plate to that surface. It is much easier to insert the most distal screws from the posterior approach because the surgeon is not close to the cubital fossa with all its converging soft tissue structures, which create a very tight envelope and make anterolateral or anterior screw insertion difficult and hazardous. If applied posteriorly, the plate can also reach further distally without compromising elbow flexion. Furthermore, a distal diaphyseal fracture of the humerus sometimes lends itself to stabilization with two semitubular plates (Fig. 5.6) or two 3.5-mm dynamic compression (DC) plates. This greatly increases the stability of fixation in this difficult transition zone of the humeral shaft.

When exposing the distal third of the humerus posteriorly, the surgeon must remember that the radial nerve will be close to the upper end of the exposure. It may have to be isolated and protected. If the exposure approaches the elbow, then the ulnar nerve has to be isolated and protected as it passes behind the medial epicondyle.

With the exception of the supracondylar area, where the small-fragment 3.5-mm cortex screws, 4.0-mm cancellous screws, and the corresponding plates are used, the 4.5-mm large fragment screws and the corresponding plates should be used for fixation of the humeral shaft. As already emphasized, the broad plates should be used on the diaphysis to prevent longitudinal fissuring of the bone. An exception might be made in an extreme-

Fig. 5.6. a A single plate failed to provide adequate stability and the outcome of the fracture was nonunion. **b** In the metaphysis, we can use two plates without running the risk of stress shielding. Thus, two shorter and thinner plates (semitubular) applied to the rounded posteromedial and posterolateral edge have provided significant stability

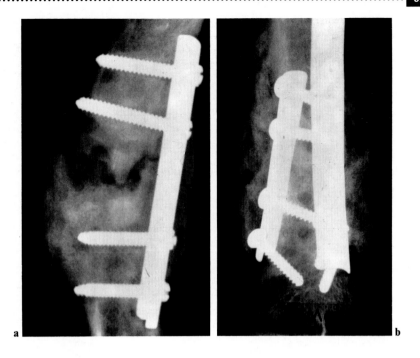

ly small individual with very slender bones; in such cases, the narrow 4.5-mm DC plate can be used. The 3.5-mm DC plates should be used only in the supracondylar area (Fig. 5.7). In the proximal portion of the shaft, where the bone flares to meet the metaphysis, the cortex is very thin and very difficult to tap. If the tap is inadvertently allowed to wander, it can easily miss the hole in the far cortex and then either strip the thread in the near cortex or break out a segment of bone from the opposite cortex. Great care must be exercised to prevent this complication.

As already emphasized, even in long oblique or spiral fractures, lag screws must not be used alone to secure internal fixation (Fig. 5.8). The lag screw is the most efficient means of securing interfragmental compression, and as such it is the principal means of securing a stable fracture interface and structural continuity of fragments. However, mechanically, such fixation is not sufficiently strong to withstand the forces of bending shear and torque. Therefore, the lag screw fixation must be protected with a neutralization plate (Fig. 5.9).

Transverse or short oblique fractures are stabilized by means of axial compression. The stability of the fixation is greatly enhanced if a lag screw is passed through the

Fig. 5.7. The different plates and their place on the humerus: ▶ *A*, T plate; *B*, narrow 4.5-mm dynamic compression (DC) plate; *C*, broad 4.5-mm DC plate; *D*, 3.5-mm DC plate; *E*, one third tubular plate (3.5-mm screws); *F*, semitubular plate (4.5-mm screws)

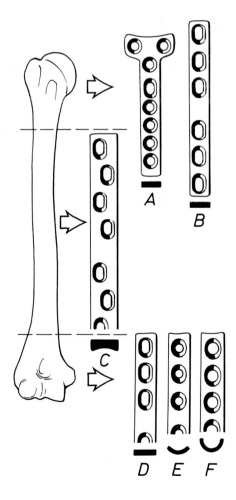

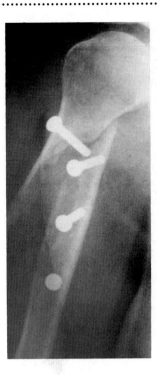

Fig. 5.8. Even in a long spiral fracture, lag screws alone cannot provide adequate stability

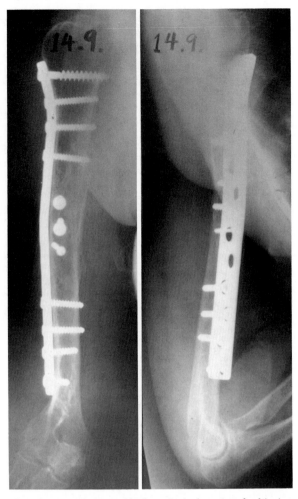

Fig. 5.9. Lag screws provide the principal means of achieving interfragmental compression and, in this way, structural continuity. The neutralization plate protects the stability achieved by means of lag screws

plate and across the fractures. If technically, because of the configuration of the fracture, the lag screw cannot be passed through the plate, it should still be inserted across the fracture to improve the stability of the fixation (Fig. 5.10). In the distal third of the humerus, there is only a small portion of the brachialis muscle which separates the radial nerve from the plate applied to the anterolateral surface of the bone. In some patients, the nerve has been left in direct contact with the plate. We have not observed any damage to the nerve, either early or late, as a result of this. The relationship of the nerve to the plate and, in particular, where it crosses the plate in relationship to the screw holes, should be carefully recorded in the operative report. This will protect the nerve from damage at the time of plate removal if this becomes necessary.

For stable fixation of the humerus, screw purchase is necessary in the cortex in six places on each side of the fracture. This means that the shortest plate that can safely be used on the humerus is a six- to seven-hole plate. With osteoporosis, the number of screws on each side of the fracture must be increased and a longer plate used. The fixation on each side of the fracture must be equally strong. Therefore, as we approach the metaphysis, we use either two plates or specially shaped buttress plates which permit the insertion of a greater number of screws through a shorter segment of the plate are used.

Unlocked intramedullary nailing has had little place in the treatment of acute fractures. We have used Hackethal retrograde stacked pinning with success in

the treatment of undisplaced pathological fractures of the humerus (see Fig. 5.11). This type of fixation does not provide sufficient stability for the treatment of displaced acute fractures. In recent years, surgeons have developed locked intramedullary nailing for the humerus. The Seidel nail, developed by Dr. Seidel of Hamburg, Germany, was the first one we used. This nail was locked proximally by a screw. For distal locking the Seidel nail depended on deployment of intramedullary fins. This nail provided reasonable axial stability but very poor rotational stability. It was also extremely difficult to remove because bone blocked the intramedullary fins from retraction. We have now abandoned its use. More recently, the Smith Nephew Richards company has marketed a nail which locks with screws both proximally and distally. We have used this nail with success, but it is not without its problems. We feel that it should be used preferably in the treatment of complex fractures of the

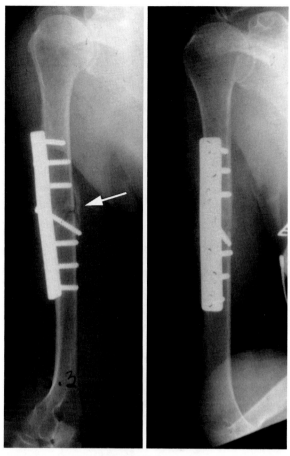

Fig. 5.10. Lag screw used to increase the stability achieved by means of a tension band plate

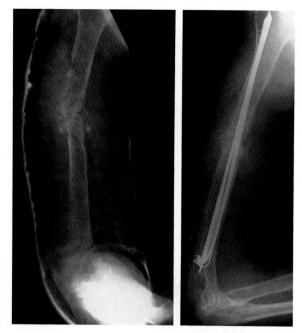

Fig. 5.11. Hackethal stacked intramedullary pinning of the humerus

shaft which are difficult to stabilize with plates and screws because of their fracture morphology. Proximal insertion of the nail carries the risks of damage to the rotator cuff and of stiffness of the shoulder. This can be avoided to some degree if the nail is inserted through a minimal split in the deltoid just below the rotator cuff insertion between the superior facet and the lesser tuberosity (Fig. 5.12). Distal retrograde insertion carries the risk of fracturing of the humerus and of myositis ossificans of the triceps and subsequent elbow stiffness. Whenever we have used an intramedullary nail in acute fractures, we have always carried out a limited exposure of the displaced portion of the fracture to make certain that the radial nerve was not interposed. Locked intramedullary nailing has also proven very useful in the treatment of pathological fractures of the humerus (Fig. 5.13).

In displaced pathological fractures, we have found the so-called composite type of fixation of methyl methacrylate and plating to be most reliable (Fig. 5.14). The fracture is reduced before any attempt is made to evacu-

ate the tumor mass. A plate is then contoured, applied to the anterolateral surface of the bone, and fixed with one or two screws proximally and distally. In pathological fractures, because of the frequent destruction of cortex and osteoporosis, longer plates must be used than in nonpathological fractures. Care should also be taken that the plate does not stop at or near a metastatic deposit. Once the bone is provisionally stabilized, a window is cut to permit the introduction of a curette and methyl methacrylate. This window should bridge both fragments and encompass at least three or four screw holes on each side of the metastatic deposit, but it should not extend to the end of the plate. Once the window is cut, all of the tumor is removed with curettage and suction. The screw holes are then predrilled, measured, and tapped, and the screws prepared in the order of insertion. Methyl methacrylate bone cement is then mixed and, while in the early doughy stage, rapidly pushed into the prepared trough and defect. Before the cement sets, the screws are rapidly screwed in and finally tightened once the methyl methacrylate has polymerized.

5.5 Postoperative Regimen

Following surgery, it is best to immobilize the arm on a posterior plaster splint with the elbow in almost full extension and to suspend it for 24–48 h from an intravenous drip pole to minimize postoperative edema. The

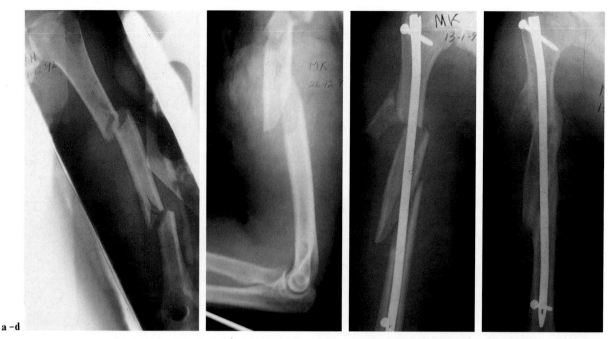

a –d

Fig. 5.12 a–d. Note the insertion point of the nail as well as the two locking screws. Note also that the displacement between the fragments did not prevent union. Postoperatively the patient was allowed to mobilize the limb but was advised to avoid torsion and lifting. Union is by callus

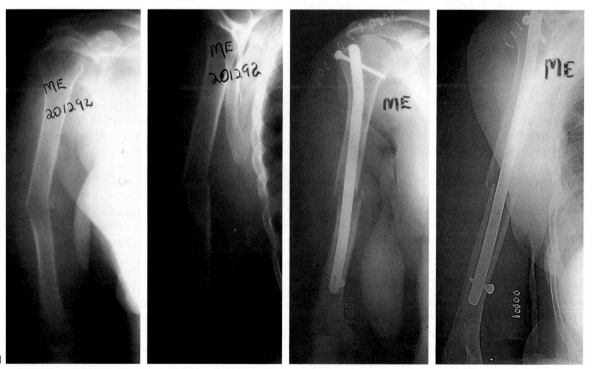

a – d

Fig. 5.13 a–d. This pathological fracture was stabilized with the locked intramedullary nail without the adjunct of methyl methacrylate. Some shortening resulted, but this was of no functional significance

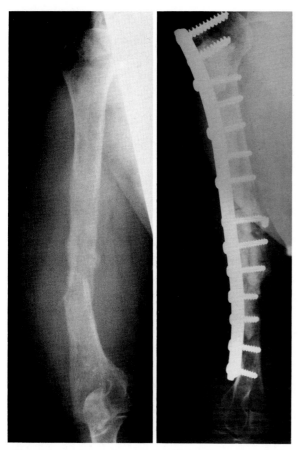

Fig. 5.14. Composite fixation (plate and methyl methacrylate cement) of a pathological fracture of the humerus

patient is allowed up for meals and to go to the toilet. Suction drains are removed after 24–36 h, depending on the amount of drainage. The wound is inspected daily. If healing is progressing satisfactorily without any complicating features such as hematoma or sepsis, active mobilization is started on the second or third postoperative day.

If the fixation is stable, apart from minor wound discomfort, mobilization is painless. A cooperative patient will carry out active mobilization exercises as instructed and will not require a formal program of rehabilitation. An anxious or less well motivated individual requires supervision, but strict instructions must be issued to the physiotherapist not to carry out joint manipulations or resisted exercises lest the fixation be lost from mechanical overload.

The surgeon is the only individual able to judge accurately the stability of any fixation because only the surgeon knows how well each screw held as it was tightened in bone. If the fixation is judged to be unstable, then of course this program of early mobilization has to be modified and the extremity protected.

In cases of early failure of the fixation, either in the early postoperative period or during the phase of fracture healing, a surgical revision of the fixation should be undertaken if it is technically feasible. It is important to recognize modes of failure.

Early failure, the result of mechanical overload, either because of inadequate primary fixation or because of the patient overloading the fixation, should be revised surgically to a stable internal fixation.

If failure of fixation is recognized at, say, 6 weeks or later, it is important to differentiate between instability in the presence of an irritation callus and instability without an irritation callus, which displays a widening fracture gap, a halo around the screws, periosteal reaction at the plate ends, and resorption of cortex deep to the plate. In the former, with an evident irritation callus, protection of the extremity from load by immobilizing it in a cast will usually result in the irritation callus changing to a fixation callus with healing of the fracture. In the latter, with evidence of failure but no callus, further immobilization and protection are of no avail. Surgical revision must be performed. Stable fixation has to be achieved by revising the existing internal fixation. Usually it is also necessary to perform bone-grafting to promote union.

The above applies only if absolutely stable fixation has been attempted. If a complex or wedge fracture has been stabilized with a bridge plate following an indirect reduction with attention paid to the preservation of the blood supply of all the intervening fragments, then union will be by callus. This fixation callus, which characterizes the union of viable fragments of bone in the presence of motion, is characteristically seen in fractures which have been splinted, such as those fixed with a bridge plate or an intramedullary nail. It is smooth and rounded in outline, homogeneous in consistency, and continuous and it bridges the fragments. Irritation callus is ill defined, nonhomogeneous, and not smooth in outline, and it does not bridge the fragments.

Fractures of the humerus are usually solidly united in 3 months. If union should be delayed but the fixation remain stable, unlike in the lower weight-bearing extremity, where failure of the plate would be almost certain, in the upper extremity we can afford to wait for consolidation to occur. Clearly the patient would be completely symptom free and the only clue to the delayed union would be radiological.

5.6 Removal of Internal Fixation

Plates should be removed only if they give rise to symptoms. In removing plates from the humerus, the proximity of the radial nerve to the plate and the danger of leaving the patient with a radial nerve palsy should always be borne in mind. Following plate removal, the patient should abstain from heavy lifting for a period of 6–8 weeks.

References

Henry K (1959) Extensile exposure. Livingstone, Edinburgh, p 25

Müller ME, Allgöwer M, Willenegger H (1970) Manual of internal fixation, 1 st edn. Springer, Berlin Heidelberg New York, p 121

Weber BG, Cech O (1976) Pseudoarthrosis. Huber, Bern, p 109

6 Fractures of the Distal End of the Humerus (13-A, B, and C)

J. SCHATZKER

6.1 Introduction

Fractures of the distal end of the humerus fall into two categories: the simple metaphyseal type A and the partial articular type B condylar fractures, and the difficult complete articular type C fractures. The former, although sometimes part of a more complex injury, such as dislocation of the elbow, are relatively easy to treat and usually have a good prognosis. They will be discussed first. In the remaining part of the chapter we will discuss supracondylar fractures, which continue to be a difficult and controversial problem. Although we will indicate, for the benefit of those who wish to refer to the *Manual of Internal Fixation* (Müller et al. 1979), the designation of each fracture in accordance with the comprehensive classification (Fig. 6.1), we do not entirely agree with this classification of fractures around the elbow. We feel that a classification of fractures should group fractures which have similar problems in treatment and a similar prognosis. The fate of fractures around the elbow is determined by the anatomical part involved, by the degree of displacement, and by the degree of comminution. Thus the problem lies in grouping the extra-articular epicondylar fracture (A1) together with the difficult supracondylar A2 and A3 fractures or the grouping of the condylar B1 and B2 fractures with the coronal osteochondral B3 fractures, of which a capitellar fracture is a good example. All three are intra-articular, but that is the only feature which B3 shares with B1 and B2. B3 differs in the mechanism of injury, in the treatment, and in the prognosis. We feel, therefore, that from a prognostic point of view, it is more prudent to group fractures around the elbow into those with a good prognosis and those with a poor prognosis and to discuss each type separately, since each has its distinguishing features worthy of mention. Similarly, the supracondylar fractures and those with extension into the joint will be grouped together, because they share the mechanism of injury, anatomical features, surgical exposures, methods of internal fixation, and prognosis. The individual differences in this group may be expressed by isolating these fractures into subtypes.

6.2 Fractures with a Good Prognosis

6.2.1 Fractures of the Epicondyles

6.2.1.1 Fractures of the Lateral Epicondyle (13-A1.1)

An avulsion fracture of the lateral epicondyle is an extremely rare injury in adults. It may occur as part of a posterolateral or posterior dislocation of the elbow. In the latter case, it is frequently associated with a fracture of the medial epicondyle. In children where the lateral epicondyle is avulsed with varying portions of the capitellum, it may turn on itself through 180° and turn the fracture surface outward, and the outcome may be a nonunion and deformity. This complication is not seen in adults. When the elbow is reduced, the epicondylar fragment reduces and heals in place, usually by bone, although occasionally by fibrous tissue.

6.2.1.2 Fractures of the Medial Epicondyle (13-A1.2)

Fractures of the medial epicondyle are most common in children, but may be seen in adults either as a result of a direct injury or as an avulsion. The fragment may vary in size, displacement, and degree of comminution. If small and undisplaced, it does not require surgical treatment. If displaced and caught in the joint, as may occur in the reduction of a lateral dislocation of the elbow, it has to be reduced surgically and fixed in place. This is best done with a small, 4.0-mm cancellous screw. If the fragment is comminuted, only suture to the adjacent soft tissues may be possible. Occasionally, the fragment may be quite large and displaced. Whenever displaced or comminuted, it should be openly reduced and stabilized by internal fixation to prevent the onset of ulnar palsy. The approach is medial. The ulnar nerve must be identified and protected before the reduction is attempted. Anterior transposition of the nerve may be necessary if the nerve comes to rest on bony irregularities or the internal fixation.

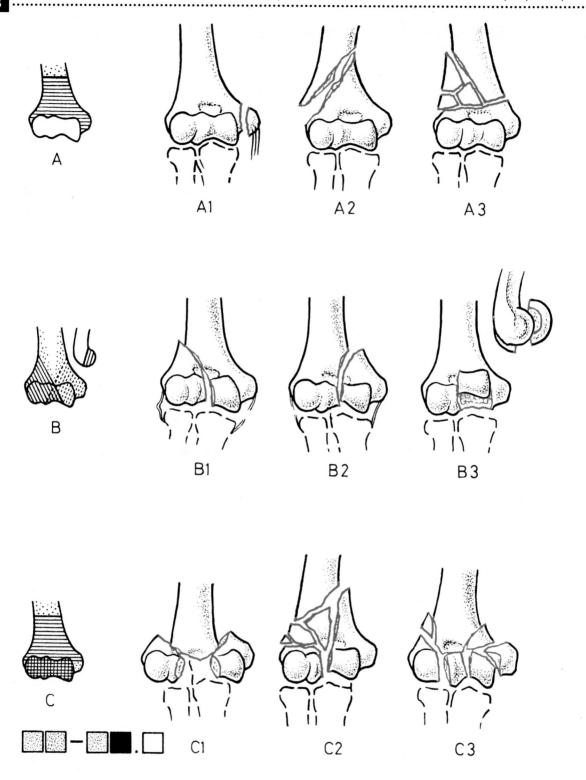

Fig. 6.1. Distal humerus: the groups. *A1*, extra-articular fracture, apophyseal avulsion; *A2*, extra-articular fracture, metaphyseal simple; *A3*, extra-articular fracture, metaphyseal multifragmentary; *B1*, partial articular fracture, lateral sagittal; *B2*, partial articular fracture, medial sagittal; *B3*, partial articular fracture, frontal; *C1*, complete articular fracture, articular simple, metaphyseal simple; *C2*, complete articular fracture, articular simple, metaphyseal multifragmentary; *C3*, complete articular fracture, multifragmentary

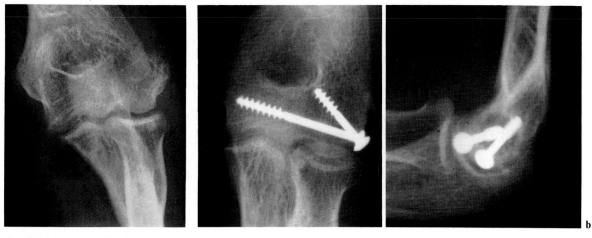

Fig. 6.2 a, b. Fracture of the lateral condyle extending medially to involve the trochlea. Secure fixation is accomplished with two lag screws

6.2.1.3 Fractures of the Lateral Condyle (B1)

In adults this fracture is comparable to the fracture of the lateral condyle in children. It is always larger than it appears on X-ray. In our experience, it always extends medially and involves part of the trochlea (13-B1.3). It is a major intra-articular fracture and must be accurately reduced and fixed to ensure preservation of normal joint function (Fig. 6.2).

The approach is lateral. We prefer two small, 3.5-mm cancellous screws for fixation. We favor internal fixation, even if the initial displacement is minimal, because we feel that early motion is essential to prevent stiffness. If the fracture is not stabilized, early motion could lead to displacement, with dire consequences.

6.2.1.4 Fractures of the Capitellum (13-B3.1)

The capitellum is the smooth, rounded, knob-like portion of the lateral condyle, covered with articular cartilage only on its anterior and inferior surfaces. The head of the radius rotates on its anterior surface when the elbow is in flexion and on its inferior surface when the elbow is in extension.

We have seen fractures of the capitellum more commonly as part of comminuted supracondylar fractures (13-C) than as isolated injuries. As an isolated injury, the fracture occurs as a result of the head of the radius being forcibly driven against the capitellum with the elbow in some degree of flexion or from a direct blow to the elbow when it is fully flexed (Alvarez et al. 1975). When fractured, the capitellum becomes a free intra-articular osteochondral body and is always displaced anterosuperiorly into the radial fossa. We feel that this fracture requires

special mention because closed manipulation always fails (Keon-Cohen 1966; Alvarez et al. 1975) and because attempts at internal fixation of the isolated fragment have given poor results. The recommended treatment of an isolated fracture of the capitellum is excision of the fragment (Alvarez et al. 1975).

When we have encountered this fracture as part of a supracondylar fracture, we have visualized it in every instance through a posterior approach combined with an osteotomy of the olecranon. Reduction is difficult to maintain because the fragment tends to slide upward out of view. It has to be held in place with a small hook while it is provisionally fixed with a small Kirschner wire (Fig. 6.3). Definitive fixation is then carried out with small, 3.5-mm cancellous screws introduced from back to front. The fixation is always difficult because the frag-

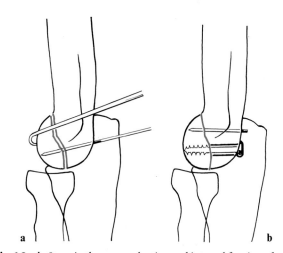

Fig. 6.3 a, b. Steps in the open reduction and internal fixation of a fracture of the capitellum

ment is small and is subjected to considerable shearing forces which tend to displace it. In isolated fractures of the capitellum, if the fragment is small it should be excised. If it is sufficiently large to allow for stable fixation as described previously, then we prefer to fix it. The exposure is lateral with the fixation from the posterior aspect. Another option is to fix the capitellum transarticularly. If such an approach is used, the head of the screw must be countersunk below the level of the articular cartilage.

6.3 Fractures with a Poor Prognosis: The Extra-Articular Group A2 and A3 and Complete Articular Type C

6.3.1 Supracondylar Fractures

6.3.1.1 Natural History

Stiffness and pain in the elbow are the results of failure of treatment. Varus or valgus deformity, frequently seen following improperly treated supracondylar fractures in children, is not as significant a problem in adults as is stiffness.

In order to prevent stiffness, all periarticular and intra-articular fractures require early active motion. Prolonged plaster immobilization leads to irreversible

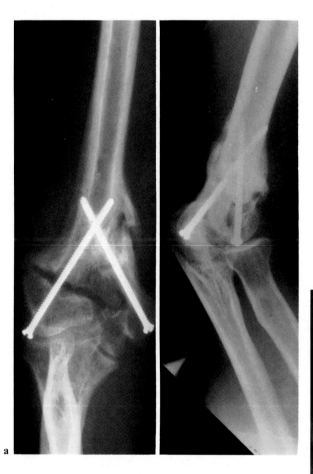

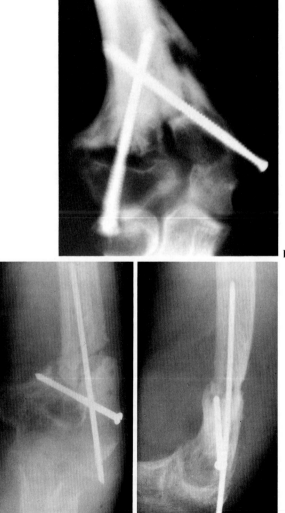

Fig. 6.4. a Screw fixation of a supracondylar fracture of the humerus. **b** Note, in this tomograph of this fracture, the malreduction of the joint and the nonunion of all fracture lines. **c** In another patient, the threaded Compere wire failed to provide adequate stability and the outcome of the supracondylar fracture was nonunion

joint stiffness. Traction, although it affords some degree of immobilization and pain relief, and although it permits early active motion, does so only within a limited arc of movement. Furthermore, although traction may improve the position of displaced intra-articular fragments, it almost never leads to the accurate joint reduction required for the return of normal function.

Early attempts at open reduction and internal fixation relied on screws, Kirschner wires, and occasionally on plates for stability (Fig. 6.4). Although the radiological appearance of the fracture was frequently improved, the need for postoperative plaster immobilization, which was carried out for 3–6 weeks or longer, resulted in a considerable degree of elbow stiffness. Internal fixation without the use of compression was not stable. Attempts at early active movement resulted not only in an increased incidence of malunion or nonunion, but also in stiffness. The patients felt severe pain because of instability and were unable to execute the required range of movement.

Passive manipulation of these fractures rarely improved the result and was sometimes disastrous because it led to myositis ossificans which permanently marred the result. Controversy continued and, whereas most surgeons were opposed to any form of surgical intervention (Keon-Cohen 1966; Riseborough and Radin 1969), others championed the operative approach (Bickel and Perry 1963; Miller 1964). The opponents of surgical intervention felt that the results of internal fixation were extremely bad (Keon-Cohen 1966) and that stiffness was the result of surgical dissection, necessary for the exposure of all components of the fracture and insertion of the internal fixation. Inability to achieve a reasonable reduction by manipulation and traction was considered to be the only indication for an open reduction and internal fixation.

The champions of the surgical approach have clearly outlined the disadvantages of closed treatment. Manipulation and traction often fail to restore perfect joint alignment. Thus the patient not only faces stiffness, but pain from joint incongruity and post-traumatic osteoarthritis. Traction is often required for 4–6 weeks before sufficient stability is gained to permit guarded mobilization. Traction may not be possible because (a) the patient may not tolerate the imposed supine position because of age or temperament; or (b) because of associated injuries which demand mobilization. Furthermore, traction may have to be discontinued because the anticipated satisfactory reduction is not obtained. Unfortunately, this decision is often reached at an inopportune time for an open reduction. Because of delay, the fragments will have usually become matted together by callus, softened by disuse and hyperemia, and the joint will have become stiff because of the trauma and inactivity.

The advocates of surgical treatment (Bickel and Perry 1963; Miller 1964) have further pointed out the following. In the displaced fracture, an anatomical reduction of the joint can be obtained only by operative means. Furthermore, in the absence of any inherent stability of the bony fragments, the reduction can only be maintained by internal fixation. Open reduction and internal fixation hasten ambulation of the patient and active motion of the elbow.

The development by the AO group of stable internal fixation, utilizing compression as the keystone of stability, and the development of new implants and operative techniques have greatly increased the scope of surgery for the supracondylar fracture. Of particular help in the treatment have been the small cortex and cancellous screws, the one-third tubular plates, the small dynamic compression (DC) plates and more recently the low contact DC (LCDC) plates, and the small reconstruction plates. They have made it possible to achieve the goals of internal fixation, namely, stable fixation and early motion.

6.3.1.2 Factors Influencing Decisions in Treatment

Our own experience strongly supports the view of those who have championed surgery as the method of treatment of this fracture. We are of the opinion that accurate anatomical reconstruction of the joint surfaces, stable internal fixation, and early active motion are the only means available to ensure a patient with this fracture a return of function as close to normal as possible. Surgery, however, is not always possible nor advisable. Surgeons must carefully evaluate all factors before deciding on a course of treatment. Technique must not triumph over reason. We stress repeatedly throughout this book the concept of the "personality" of the fracture as a guide in decision making. This is perhaps nowhere as important as in the evaluation of an intra-articular fracture. The factors which limit success are the degree of comminution, the degree of joint involvement, and osteoporosis.

Age and Osteoporosis

The typical mechanism which leads to the so-called Y or T supracondylar fracture is a fall on the point of the elbow. But how different these injuries are in a young, healthy man (Fig. 6.5) and in an elderly, frail, and osteoorotic woman (Fig. 6.6)! The weakest link in any correctly executed internal fixation is the bone. If the bone is fragile and osteoporotic, the surgeon may have difficulty in securing a satisfactory purchase for any screws. Thus the first factor to be determined is the patient's age. This

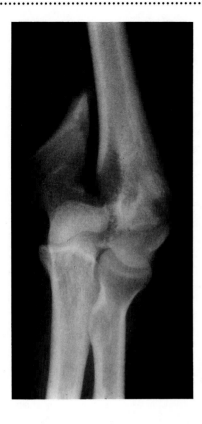

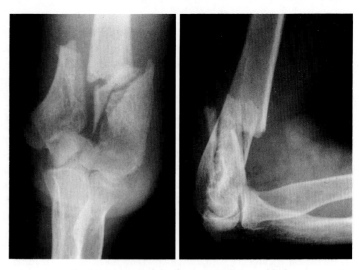

Fig. 6.6. Supracondylar fracture (C3) in an elderly osteoporotic woman. Note the severe degree of comminution

◀ **Fig. 6.5.** Supracondylar fracture in a young man (C1). There is no comminution

will not only shed some light on the expected degree of osteoporosis, but may modify the goals of treatment. Clearly, the goals will be different for a young, athletic man person than for a retired octogenarian.

Type of Fracture

The next factor to be determined is the type of fracture. The metaphyseal extra-articular supracondylar fractures A2 and A3 (see Fig. 6.1) may pose difficulties, particularly if the distal fragment is small or if the metaphysis is badly comminuted. These difficulties, however, are greatly overshadowed by the difficulties posed by a comminuted articular surface.

Degree of Displacement

An undisplaced fracture may not require surgery. Displacement, particularly of the joint fragments, is clearly an indication for an open reduction. Displacement is also an index of the ease of reduction and the degree of devitalization. Considerable displacement is usually the result of high-velocity force, which not only drives the fragments apart in an explosive fashion, but strips them of their soft tissue attachment and blood

supply. Devitalization prolongs the healing process. Therefore, such a fracture would be more prone to failure of its internal fixation, yet the displacement makes open reduction almost mandatory.

Degree of Comminution and Joint Involvement

The extra-articular supracondylar fractures A2 and A3 (see Fig. 6.1) may pose difficulties with internal fixation, particularly if the distal fragment is small or if the metaphysis is badly comminuted. These difficulties, however, are greatly overshadowed by the almost insurmountable problems of the severely compressed and comminuted articular surface of a C3 fracture (Riseborough and Radin 1969).

It is most important to evaluate the degree of joint comminution before embarking on surgery. The displacement of the fragments may be such that it is impossible to interpret the radiograph. In these cases, we have found it very useful to obtain our radiograph while the patient is under anesthesia and traction is applied to the elbow (Fig. 6.7). This may restore sufficient alignment to make an analysis possible.

In our experience, the only major contraindications to surgery have been severe osteoporosis and advanced age. We have found all too frequently at the time of sur-

Fig. 6.7. a Before application of traction.
b After application of traction: the pattern of the fracture becomes discernible. The screw in the ulna served to provide temporary pre-operative overhead traction

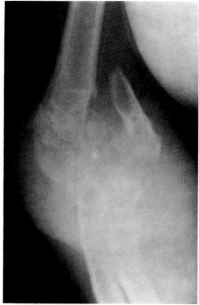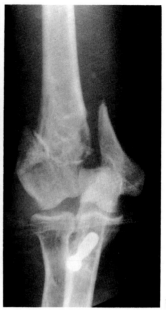

a   b

gery that a radiograph of an osteoporotic humerus with an intra-articular fracture did not give an accurate indication of the degree of comminution, particularly of the joint. The multiplicity of the fragments, their small size, and the poor holding power of the bone have been the chief causes of less than satisfactory results. In younger patients, we have achieved our treatment goals, but we would like to offer a word of caution about the C3 fracture. The tremendous comminution and compression of the articular surface and of the subjacent bone leads at times to irreconstructible conditions of the articulation. These fractures are examples of extremes of violence and extremes of intra-articular injury where the return of any degree of useful function can be judged as satisfactory because the results are usually poor. In dealing with these fractures, it is particularly important to evaluate carefully whether the trochlea can be reconstructed.

If the trochlea can be reconstructed, then a useful degree of function can be anticipated, which is better than what can be achieved by closed treatment. If the trochlea is beyond the scope of surgical reconstruction, then traction with early motion is preferable to the failure of an ill-advised surgical attempt. The recent reports of excellent outcomes achieved with total elbow replacements performed as primary treatment for the irreconstructible type C fractures suggests strongly that a primary elbow arthroplasty should be considered for the active elderly patient with an irreconstructible injury.

There are certain situations where the decision to operate must be made on considerations other than the fracture.

6.3.1.3 Indications for Surgery

Open Fracture

We feel that, in addition to débridement, the single most important prophylactic measure in preventing sepsis is stable internal fixation. The surgeon who carries out a débridement and then secures immobilization, either in a cast or traction, in order to execute a delayed open reduction should sepsis have been prevented, compromises the only chance the patient may have to regain good function. We are not advocating extremes of exposure with further devitalization of fragments, nor are we advocating massive internal fixation, but we do feel that a successful joint reconstruction can only be achieved early. The amount of internal fixation used should be sufficient to provide initial stability. Mechanical overload and failure as a result of movement may destroy such marginal fixation, but we would rather revise a failed internal fixation in a patient with mobile soft tissues and a mobile joint free of sepsis than face a stiff joint and a scarred soft tissue envelope or an unstable joint which has become infected. Recent evidence has destroyed the notion that the presence of metal raises the incidence of sepsis. That was true if fixation was unstable. Even if disaster should strike and sepsis develops, we are in a far better position to treat this complication in the presence of stable internal fixation. These techniques apply, of course, only if there is a soft tissue envelope and a joint which has not been totally deformed and destroyed. If the soft tissue injury is severe, we advocate reduction and fixation of the articular component and then bridging of the elbow with an external fixator to provide immobilization and allow for easy access and care of the soft tissue. Once the soft tissues have healed, an evaluation can be made of what further reconstruction is possible.

Vascular Injury

The fibers of the brachialis muscle are the only protection afforded the brachial artery from the jagged and sharp ends of the thin and flared portion of the distal humerus. Thus it is not surprising that vascular injuries, particularly in children, are not rare. We feel that if a vascular injury is present, surgical stabilization of the skeleton is required in order to safeguard the surgical repair of the vascular lesion.

Associated Fractures

An associated fracture of the humerus or radius and ulna requires surgical stabilization of all fractures to safeguard the function of the elbow (see Chap. 9).

Associated Injuries

The care of associated injuries such as chest injuries or other fractures (e.g., femur, pelvis) may require an upright and mobile patient and may make surgical stabilization of the supracondylar fracture advisable.

6.3.1.4 Surgical Treatment

Timing of Surgery

The supracondylar fracture is a complex intra-articular injury which requires very careful evaluation, preparation for surgery, and surgical execution. Unfortunately, time is a luxury rarely available. Supracondylar fractures frequently require emergency surgery because of an associated vascular lesion or an open fracture. Even if not faced with an emergency, we do not like to delay unduly because the elbow tends to swell rapidly, which may severely compromise the soft tissue closure following an internal fixation. Furthermore, a delay of even 5 days has been associated with a disturbingly high incidence of myositis ossificans. Therefore, we favor carrying out open reduction and internal fixation as soon as possible, but not before a careful radiological evaluation of the fracture, which may require a computed tomography (CT) scan for proper definition of the fracture pattern. If the elbow is too swollen to permit closure of the soft tissues without tension, we insert a few approximat-

ing sutures and leave the wound open to carry out a secondary closure once the swelling has subsided.

In patients who are to be treated by closed means, we insert a cancellous screw into the dorsal aspect of the olecranon at the level of the coronoid process and suspend the patient's arm in overhead traction (Fig. 6.8). The advantage of the cancellous screw is the great ease of insertion and the avoidance of all danger to the ulnar nerve, which can be pierced by a Kirschner wire inserted into the olecranon for traction. Mobilization of the elbow can be started while it is still in traction. Once the fracture becomes "sticky" (i.e., deformable, but not displaceable), we transfer the extremity into a cast brace.

Diagnosis

The case history is important because it sheds light on the mechanism of injury and on the forces involved. It also informs the surgeon about associated vascular or neurological injuries, which so commonly accompany this fracture. The physical examination discloses a swollen, painful elbow which the patient holds protectively and refuses to move. Physical examination will serve little in delineating the exact pattern of the fracture, but it is invaluable in the evaluation of an associated vascular injury, compartment syndrome, or an associated neurological complication.

The radiological examination is the only method available which will give a detailed picture of the fracture. It is important to remember that, despite this, a patient with a vascular compromise must not be sent off to the radiology department. If a pulse does not return

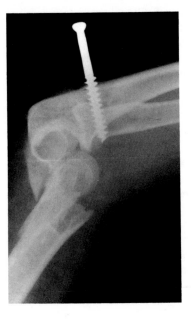

Fig. 6.8. Olecranon screw used for overhead traction

following gentle realignment, the patient must be taken to the operating room as an emergency and any radiological assessment, including angiography, should be carried out while the patient is being prepared for surgery.

At times, the elbow is so distorted that it is impossible to make out the definition of the fracture fragments. Tomography can be very helpful in such cases. In complex fractures we prefer a CT scan, which allows a precise evaluation of the fragmentation and of the three-dimensional pattern of the fracture. If the distortion is great, we have found it very useful to obtain an X-ray with the patient under anesthesia while traction is applied to the forearm with the elbow in extension. This often results in sufficient reduction to make possible the identification of the fragments and of the fracture pattern (see Fig. 6.7).

Classification

Although we continue to use the comprehensive classification of these fractures (see Fig. 6.1), we do so with the reservations we have already mentioned. We would like to reiterate that epicondylar and condylar fractures are sustained by a different mechanism to supracondylar fractures, are relatively simple to treat, and have a good prognosis. The supracondylar A2 and A3 fractures and the supracondylar intra-articular fractures C1, C2, and C3 pose common problems which relate to the fracture and to the anatomical region. They share methods of treatment and prognosis and therefore should be considered together.

Surgical Anatomy of the Distal Humerus

The distal end of the humerus is flattened, expanded transversely, and rounded at the end (Fig. 6.9). The rounded end of the condyle presents articular and nonarticular surfaces. The articular portion forms the elbow joint and articulates with the radius and ulna. The lateral convex surface of the condyle is the capitellum, which is covered on its anterior and inferior surfaces with articular cartilage. It articulates with the head of the radius. The fact that the posterior surface is nonarticular is important in the fixation of the fractures of the capitellum, since lag screws can be inserted from back to front through the nonarticular surface without interfering with the joint (see Fig. 6.3).

The trochlea is medial, larger, pulley-shaped, and completely covered with articular cartilage. It articulates with the trochlear notch of the ulna. When the elbow is extended (Fig. 6.9 c), the inferior and posterior aspects of the trochlea are in contact with the ulna and the tip of

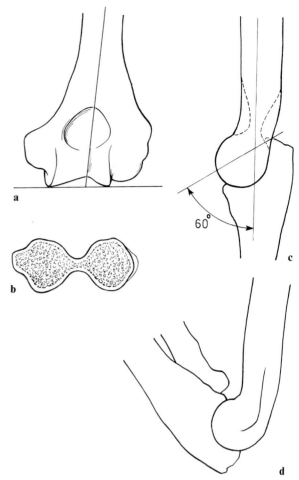

Fig. 6.9 a–d. The distal end of the humerus. **a** Note the distribution of the articular cartilage. The posterior aspect of the capitellum has no articular cartilage. Note also the downward projection of the trochlea, responsible for the carrying angle. **b** The distal humerus in cross-section at the level of the fossa olecrani. The two columns of bone on either side of the fossa are dense and strong and offer a good hold for screws. **c** With the elbow in extension, the tip of the olecranon lodges in the olecranon fossa. If the fossa is blocked by a screw or plate, extension of the elbow is impossible. **d** Note also the 60° anterior angulation of the articular portion of the humerus. This forward angulation makes it difficult to apply a plate to the radial aspect of the distal end of the humerus

the olecranon lodges within the olecranon fossa. When the elbow is flexed, the trochlear notch of the ulna rolls on to the anterior aspect of the trochlea and the coronoid process rests in the coronoid fossa and the radial head in the radial fossa. The downward projection on the medial side of the trochlea is responsible for the physiological valgus tendency of the elbow in full extension. This valgus tendency is referred to as the carrying angle and is approximately 170° (Fig. 6.9 a).

104 ·

Chapter 6 **Fractures of the Distal End of the Humerus (13-A, B and C)**

The portion of the humerus immediately above the trochlea is hollowed out and, as indicated, anteriorly forms the coronoid fossa and posteriorly the olecranon fossa. The two fossae share a common floor, which in some individuals may be absent and be represented by a hole. The two columns of bone on either side of the fossa (Fig. 6.9 b) are dense and strong and very important in the internal fixation of a supracondylar fracture (Müller et al. 1965); they are the only portions of bone in this region into which screws can be inserted, since the olecranon and coronoid fossa must not be obstructed in any way. The medial epicondyle forms an extension of the medial column medially. It is grooved on the posterior aspect by the ulnar nerve. When the ulnar nerve is lifted out of its groove and transposed to the front, the medial epicondyle becomes a very useful portion of bone for the insertion of screws.

Planning the Surgical Procedure

A simple fracture requires little planning. By contrast, a complex fracture requires a very careful fracture analysis and careful planning of the internal fixation (Fig. 6.10). It is extremely helpful to obtain an anteropos-terior radiograph of the normal elbow, to serve as a template of the distal humerus (Fig. 6.10 a). We turn the radiograph over and trace the outline of the normal distal humerus on tracing paper. Since both the fractured elbow and the normal elbow are radiographed at the same distance from the X-ray tube, the magnification is the same. It is now possible, with the aid of the antero-posterior radiograph of the fractured elbow, to mark in the fracture lines on the tracing (Fig. 6.10 b). It is important to draw in the comminution as well as any bone defects which exist. We are now in a position to plan the internal fixation.

The reconstruction of an intra-articular fracture always begins with the reconstruction of the joint. It needs to be decided whether the trochlear and capitellar fragments will be lagged together with one or two small, 3.5-mm cancellous screws. If a defect exists in the articular surface, it is wrong to lag the fragments together because this narrows the hinge and makes the elbow joint incongruous. In such a case, one should plan to fix the condylar fragments with a 4.5-mm cortical screw. Both fragments are tapped. The cortical screw then acts as a fixation screw rather than as a lag screw and maintains the fragments the correct distance apart.

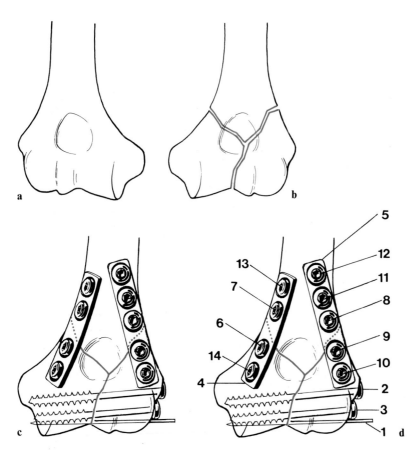

Fig. 6.10 a–d. The preoperative plan. **a** The outline of the radiograph of the normal side. This serves as a template for the reduction and internal fixation. **b** The radiograph is turned over, traced, and the fracture lines are marked in, as well as any comminution. **c** The planned internal fixation. It should correspond to the final radiograph. **d** Working drawing. The implants, their function, and the steps are labeled. *1*, Kirschner wire – provisional fixation; *2, 3*, 3.5-mm cancellous screws; *4, 5*, 3.5-mm dynamic compression (DC) plates; *6, 7*, first two screws – achieve interfragmental compression; *8, 9*, next two screws – achieve interfragmental compression. Note: screws *7* and *9* are "load screws." The remaining screws are inserted to complete the fixation. Their exact order is not as important

Once the joint is reconstructed, the fixation of the supracondylar fracture should be planned. The first rule to be kept in mind is that no piece of internal fixation must encroach on the olecranon fossa, because this would permanently block extension. The second is that screws alone cannot achieve stable fixation of the supracondylar fracture. The diaphyseal segment should be assessed to see whether there are fragments which should be reduced and lagged together. This is an important step because it increases the stability of the fixation and reduces the number of fragments to deal with, which makes reduction easier. It is important to mark on

the drawing the exact position and direction of the lag screws. Frequently, it is advantageous to predrill a gliding hole or a thread hole before the reduction is carried out. If possible, the supracondylar fracture is fixed with two one-third tubular or two 3.5-mm DC plates. If this appears impossible, then we try to apply a plate along the lateral border of the shaft with the last screw of the plate opposite the condylar fragment (Fig. 6.11). We use the 3.5-mm reconstruction plate for this purpose because it is easier to contour in order to accommodate the anterior angulation of the distal epiphysis. The last screw through the plate must go into the condyles and may

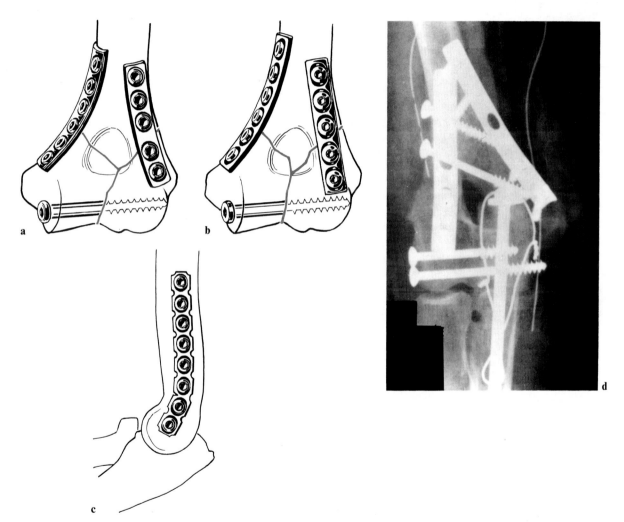

Fig. 6.11 a–d. Internal fixation of the distal humerus. **a** Two one-third tubular plates. The medial one can be contoured to lie along the posteromedial border and extend to the epicondyle. The lateral one lies at almost 90° to the medial and reaches to the posterior aspect of the capitellum. **b** Two 3.5-mm dynamic compression (DC) plates are applied, one medially and one laterally. Because the DC plates are flatter, the medial one comes to lie more posteriorly in the plane of the medial epicondyle. **c** The 3.5-mm reconstruction plate, because of its

notching, can be bent forward; thus it is best suited if a plate is to be applied laterally and reach as far as the lateral condyle. **d** Note in this postoperative X-ray the two lag screws used to stabilize the oblique fracture line between the medial epicondylar and condylar fragment and the shaft. Whenever possible, lag screws should be used to achieve primary stability. The plates then function in addition to their tension band effect as neutralization plates

even be used to lag them together. It must be remembered, however, that the longitudinal axis of the lateral condyle makes a 60° angle with the longitudinal axis of the shaft. The plate must, therefore, be angled forward or an extension deformity of the distal fragment will result (see Fig. 6.9 c).

Thus, the final working drawing (Fig. 6.10 d) will have marked on it all the screws and plates, their function, and the order of insertion. The time spent on preoperative planning gives the surgeon that much more time to spend on the internal fixation, ensures thorough familiarity with the individual fracture, and will vastly improve the quality of the internal fixation and thus the final result.

Positioning and Draping the Patient

The positioning of the patient will be determined by the habitus of the patient and any associated injuries. We prefer to position the patient lying on the side opposite the involved extremity (Fig. 6.12). This position automatically exposes the posterior aspect of the elbow and allows a direct, unobstructed surgical approach. The elbow must be free to be flexed through a full range, which is extremely important in the surgical exposure and reduction of the fracture. With the patient lying on the uninjured side, the force of gravity maintains traction on the forearm and keeps it in the correct position throughout surgery. This obviates the need for an assistant, who would otherwise be required to hold the forearm in a position indicated by the surgeon. As the assistant tires, the arm begins to wander and the exposure (and sometimes even the reduction) can be lost. This can lead to a great deal of unnecessary tension and frustration and may adversely affect the outcome of surgery. With the patient in the lateral decubitus position, the position of the elbow and forearm is adjusted simply by placing a rolled-up sheet under the forearm and elbow and shifting it as required.

We wish to stress that particularly patients with an associated vascular lesion must not be positioned prone. This obstructs the access to the anterior arm and cubital fossa and makes vascular repair impossible. With the patient lying on the uninjured side, the surgeon has easy access to the front and back of the elbow. Two surgical incisions are necessary if a vascular repair has to be performed. It is impossible to deal adequately with a supracondylar fracture from in front or through one or two side incisions.

Draping

An assistant should apply traction to the upper extremity and hold it with the elbow in extension while the surgeon scrubs it from the axilla to the wrist. The upper extremity is then draped free to allow for free manipulation and full unobstructed flexion and extension of the elbow.

Tourniquet

Where feasible, we prefer to use a tourniquet on all intra-articular fractures. This decreases bleeding, allows better visualization of the intra-articular components, and leads to a more accurate reconstruction of the joint.

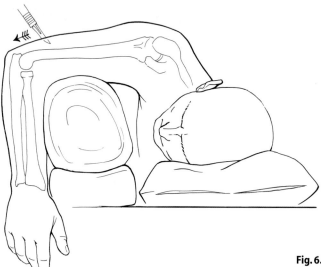

Fig. 6.12. The lateral position of the patient. The elbow is flexed. The weight of the forearm applies traction

Surgical Exposure of the Distal Humerus

The surgical exposures for simple fractures of the distal humerus have already been discussed (see p. 88). We shall concern ourselves now with the surgical exposure of complex supracondylar fractures. As suggested by our preferred positioning of the patient, we favor the posterior approach. Fractures which do not involve the joint are approached through the tongue-of-triceps approach, as described by Van Gorder (1940). Fractures which involve the joint are approached through a transverse osteotomy of the olecranon, as described by Cassebaum (1952).

The skin incision is begun posteriorly in the center of the distal arm and is extended distally on the medial side of the olecranon to a point four to five fingerbreadths distal to the point of the olecranon. The incision should not cross the tip of the olecranon, as this might lead to a

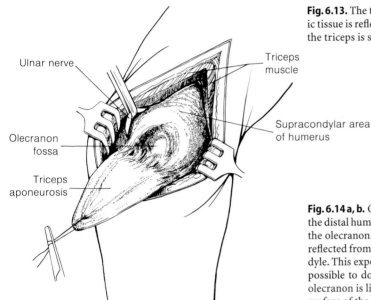

Ulnar nerve

Triceps muscle

Supracondylar area of humerus

Olecranon fossa

Triceps aponeurosis

Fig. 6.13. The tongue-of-triceps approach. Only the aponeurotic tissue is reflected as a tongue. The underlying muscle mass of the triceps is split in line with its fibers

Fig. 6.14 a, b. Olecranon osteotomy in the surgical approach to the distal humerus. **a** Note the sawcut is only four fifths through the olecranon. The anconeus muscle is identified and partially reflected from the radial side of the ulna and the lateral epicondyle. This exposes the trochlear notch of the ulna and makes it possible to do the osteotomy under direct vision. **b** Once the olecranon is lifted up and the elbow flexed, the whole articular surface of the distal humerus comes into view

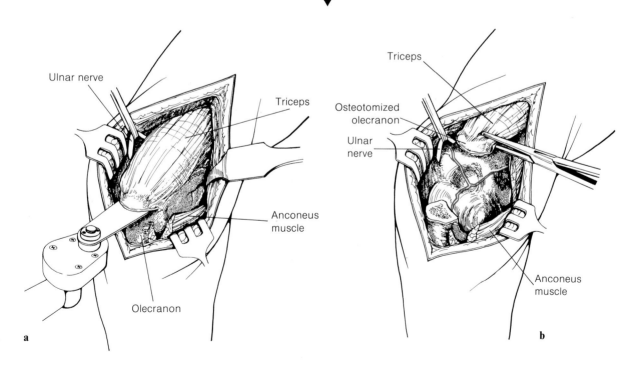

Ulnar nerve

Triceps

Anconeus muscle

Olecranon

Triceps

Osteotomized olecranon

Ulnar nerve

Anconeus muscle

a

b

painful scar. We prefer the incision on the medial side for two reasons. First, it is cosmetically less apparent, and second, it allows ready exposure of the ulnar nerve. If the olecranon is not osteotomized, we make an effort to preserve the olecranon bursa.

The first step in the posterior approach is the isolation and protection of the ulnar nerve. Normally, it is readily found and easily palpated in the groove posterior to the medial epicondyle. The distorted skeleton and swollen ecchymotic soft tissues can make isolation of the ulnar nerve difficult. However, it must be found and protected, for it is easily injured. Sometimes it is easier to isolate it more proximally and trace it distally through the distorted tissues.

In the tongue-of-triceps approach (Fig. 6.13) a tongue of the triceps aponeurosis is developed with the apex proximally and the base at the olecranon. It is then turned down and the remaining fibers of the triceps are split and elevated with a periostial elevator. The muscle masses are retracted medially and laterally and held with Hohmann retractors. Great care must be taken on the lateral side in positioning the tip of the retractor, because it can easily be placed around the radial nerve anteriorly and inadvertently damage the nerve.

If the fracture extends into the joint, we favor the transolecranon approach (Fig. 6.14). The olecranon is exposed, and the anconeus muscle is partially lifted from the radial side of the ulna to expose the lateral edge of the trochlear fossa. A 3.2-mm drill hole is made in the center of the olecranon and is directed along the long axis of the ulna. This hole is tapped with the large cancellous tap for subsequent insertion of a cancellous screw. With the articular margin in sight medially and laterally, a transverse cut is made with an oscillating saw in the olecranon opposite the deepest point of the trochlear fossa. The cut is extended through four fifths of the olecranon. A broad osteotome is then inserted into the cut and the olecranon is pried apart. Thus, the osteotomy is completed by fracturing through the subchondral bone. This leads to irregular bony spicules in the subchondral bone which are used at the end of the procedure as a guide to reduction. The sawing also results in about 1 mm loss of bone. If we were to cut right through, the articular cartilage might be damaged and a 1-mm loss of the articular surface might result.

The olecranon is separated medially and laterally and is lifted proximally, together with the triceps muscle, which is dissected free from the underlying bone. Hohmann retractors aid in the exposure. The same care must be exercised on the lateral side in inserting the Hohmann retractor. On the medial side, care must be taken, of course, not to injure the ulnar nerve. The exposure of the joint can be further increased by flexion of the elbow. This gives a full and unobstructed view of the joint and allows reduction and fixation of all the fragments.

At the end of the procedure, the olecranon is lagged in place with a large cancellous screw. The predrilling and tapping of the hole ensures an anatomical reduction. The lag screw fixation alone is not adequate and must be protected with a tension band wire which is passed deep to the triceps tendon (see p. 117).

Technique of Reduction and Internal Fixation of a Supracondylar Fracture

In dealing with an intra-articular fracture, the surgeon should always begin with the reconstruction of the joint. It is important to expose the joint, evaluate the comminution, and decide which is the major and best-preserved fragment. The small articular fragments should not be discarded, and care should be taken in the exposure not to allow any significant fragment to fall out. The only time a segment of the articulation might be discarded and replaced by a cancellous graft is when that portion is completely crushed and comminuted. Once all the fragments are identified, it is important to compare the findings with the sketched plan of the operation. The fragments should be carefully manipulated, rotated, and aligned until the surgeon is certain of their exact fit and of the steps in the reduction. The most important step in the procedure is a meticulous reconstruction of the trochlea. The trochlea forms the hinge of the elbow, and if it is not anatomically reconstructed, the elbow will be incongruous and the result correspondingly poor.

The fragments should be provisionally fixed with Kirschner wires. Depending on the size of the fragments involved, we use either 0.5-mm or 1.0-mm Kirschner wires for the provisional fixation. These wires must be inserted with a power drill. A hand drill wobbles too much and can frequently result in the loss of a difficult reduction.

The insertion of the first 1.0-mm Kirschner wire is crucial because it will serve as a guide to the internal fixation of the condylar fragments. The surgeon must decide which is the major articular fragment. Preferably, the radial fragment should be selected, because it is better to insert the lag screws in a radioulnar direction since this offers less chance of damage to the ulnar nerve later when the metal is removed. However, if the radial fragment is too small or comminuted, the surgeon begins with the ulnar fragment. The first Kirschner wire must be drilled through the center of the fragment, equidistant from the anterior and posterior articular cartilage but low enough to permit the insertion of a screw above it (Fig. 6.15).

Once the first wire is drilled through, the articular fragments are carefully reduced and, if necessary, kept in place with fine 0.5-mm Kirschner wires. The first

Fig. 6.15. The technique of open reduction and internal fixation of the supracondylar fracture. (Modified from Heim and Pfeiffer 1972)

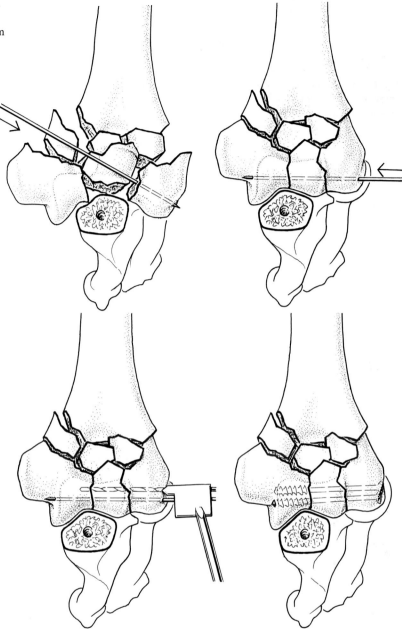

Kirschner wire is then drilled in a retrograde fashion into the other major condylar fragment and, if possible, through any other major intervening articular fragments. The pointed 2.0-mm three-hole drill guide is then slipped over the Kirschner wire, which serves not only as the major provisional fixation of the articular fragments, but also as a guide for the drilling of the hole for the first lag screw. After the 2.0-mm hole has been drilled and tapped, the 3.5-mm small cancellous screw is inserted as a lag screw for fixation of the fragments. Extreme care must be taken to preserve the width of the trochlea.

If a defect is present, the condylar fragments must be fixed with a 4.5-mm cortical screw, which is inserted as a fixation screw. This means that all the fragments are tapped. When the screw is inserted, no compression results and the trochlea is not narrowed. The gap between the condylar fragments is filled with a cancellous bone graft. The recent development of cannulated screws has further simplified the fixation of the articular fragments. Instead of a regular K-wire, the guide wire for a cannulated screw should be drilled in a prograde fashion through the larger fragment. This is necessary because the tip of the guide wire is threaded. The fracture is then reduced and the guide wire advanced into the second fragment until it engages the opposite cortex. The depth is then measured, the hole is drilled with the cannulated drill, the thread is cut with the cannulated tap, and the cannulated screw is inserted. One 3.5-mm screw is usually enough, but if the patient is large two may be necessary.

Once the joint is reconstructed, the surgeon proceeds to the fixation of the supracondylar fracture. As already described on p. 105, the diaphyseal segment should be assessed, and if any major fragments can be lagged to the shaft, this should be done before attempting to fix the supracondylar fracture itself. This is an important step in the procedure. The lag screw fixation of comminuted fragments will increase the stability of the fixation and will reduce the number of fragments to deal with. This makes the reduction easier. In doing this great care must be taken not to strip the fragments of their soft tissue attachments and render them avascular.

The first rule to be kept in mind is that no piece of internal fixation may encroach on the olecranon fossa or coronoid fossa, because it would block extension or flexion, respectively. The second rule is that crossed lag screws or threaded pins cannot achieve stable fixation of the supracondylar fracture. The supracondylar fracture should be reduced and held provisionally with Kirschner wires while the reduction is checked, the situation again compared with the preoperative plan, and the final fixation decided upon.

If possible, we prefer to fix the supracondylar fracture with two 3.5-mm low contact dynamic compression (LCDC) plates or occasionally, in very small bones, with one-third tubular plates, which must be carefully positioned and contoured to fit the medial and lateral ridges on either side of the olecranon fossa (see Fig. 6.11). Clearly, in a simple fracture without comminution, these two plates should be inserted as compression plates, which will greatly enhance the stability of the fixation. If comminution exists, these plates will function as buttress plates or neutralization plates where they protect a lag screw fixation. The plates have to reach the diaphysis; however, if the fracture pattern is such that it is impossible to fix it with two plates, then we resort to one plate, which is best carefully contoured and applied along the lateral border of the humerus (see Fig. 6.11 c) in such a way that the lowermost one or two screw holes will permit insertion of one or two screws into the condylar fragment. This plate should be either a 3.5-mm reconstruction plate or a regular dynamic compression (DC) plate. The choice will clearly depend on the length of plate required as well as on the segment of humerus involved. If the plate is designed to fix the lower diaphysis, then it should be stronger and we would favor the 4.5-mm DC plate. The choice of plate must, of course,

also be governed by the size of the patient. In applying this side plate, the anterior angulation of the lateral condyle must be borne in mind. This is best accommodated for with the reconstruction plate. If difficulty is encountered with the lateral plate, then it can be applied medially and extended over the epicondyle (see Fig. 6.11 b, c).

Postoperative Care

The elbow is splinted in approximately 120°–130° extension on a well-padded posterior plaster slab and suspended for elevation for the first 24–36 h from an overhead bar or pole. On the second day we remove the suction drain, and on the third day we remove the splint and the dressing and examine the wound. If no complications are found, active flexion–extension exercises are begun.

Early active movement is essential if function is to be regained. If the internal fixation is such that external protection and immobilization are required, then all the advantages of surgery will be lost. The only person who can accurately assess the stability of the internal fixation is the surgeon. A radiograph projects the configuration of the internal fixation, but only the surgeon can attest to the quality of the bone and to the holding power of the screws. Sometimes, despite proper judgement and care, we are left with an internal fixation which must be protected or mechanical overload with failure is certain. Under these circumstances, we have made use of cast bracing. This has permitted early, active mobilization with a certain degree of protection of an otherwise tenuous fixation. We feel that plaster of Paris fixation, recommended for 3 weeks or longer by some, is almost certain to become associated with a serious degree of stiffness.

We have found hydrotherapy a useful adjunct in the active mobilization of joints. Under no circumstances should passive manipulation be employed. It robs the patient of the protective sensory feedback and may lead to a ripping apart of the internal fixation. It may also lead to a rapid onset of myositis ossificans which can lead to irreversible stiffness. If, in the course of active mobilization, the patient develops local pain, redness, and swelling, and one can be certain that these are manifestations of instability rather than sepsis, then immobilization must be instituted until some degree of biological stability has been achieved. We have made use of continuous passive motion machines (CPM) in the postoperative treatment of supracondylar fractures and have found the recovery period to be shorter, the mobilization less painful, and the recovery of movement more rapid. Use of the machine is started as early as possible and motion continued without any lengthy interruptions for the first week. We have found the Mobilimb (Toronto Medical

Corporation) particularly useful because it is portable and allows patient mobilization. After the first week, the patient is treated in the same manner as patients who began with early active mobilization. In comparing the two groups of patients, we feel that postoperative mobilization with the aid of a CPM is preferable. The patients are more comfortable, the edema subsides more rapidly, and the range of motion in the joint returns more quickly. In addition, there is the beneficial effect of continuous passive motion on the healing of articular cartilage (Salter et al. 1980). If a CPM is not readily available, almost equally good results can be achieved with early active mobilization. This, however, is not true if a late reconstruction is being carried out, such as an intra-articular osteotomy or nonunion, or a stiff elbow is being mobilized. Under these circumstances a CPM is essential.

References

Alvarez E, Patel MR, Nimberg G, Pearlman HS (1975) Fractures of the capitelum humeri. J Bone Joint Surg 57A:1093–1096

Bickel WE, Perry RE (1963) Comminuted fracture of the distal humerus. JAMA 184:553–557

Cassebaum WH (1952) Operative treatment of T and Y fractures of the lower end of the humerus. Am J Surg 83:265–270

Heim U, Pfeiffer KM (1972) Periphere Osteosynthesen. Springer, Berlin Heidelberg New York

Keon-Cohen BT (1966) Fractures of the elbow. J Bone Joint Surg 48A:1623–1639

Miller WE (1964) Comminuted fractures of the distal end of the humerus in the adult. J Bone Joint Surg 46A:644–657

Müller ME, Allgöwer M, Willenegger H (1965) Technique of internal fixation of fractures (Fig. 210). Springer, Berlin Heidelberg New York, p 196

Müller ME, Allgöwer M, Schneider R, Willenegger H (1979) Manual of internal fixation, 2nd edn. Springer, Berlin Heidelberg New York

Riseborough EJ, Radin EL (1969) Intercondylar fractures of the humerus in the adult. J Bone Joint Surg 51A:130–141

Salter RB, Simmonds DF, Malcolm BW, Rumble EJ, MacMichael D (1980) The biological effects of continuous passive motion on the healing of full thickness defects in articular cartilage: an experimental investigation in the rabbit. J Bone Joint Surg 62A:1232–1251

Van Gorder GW (1940) Surgical approach in supracondylar "T" fractures of the humerus requiring open reduction. J Bone Joint Surg 22:278–292

7 Fractures of the Olecranon (12-B1)

J. SCHATZKER

··

7.1 Introduction

A fracture of the olecranon with displacement represents a disruption of the triceps mechanism and, as a consequence, the loss of active extension of the elbow. The necessity for surgical repair has been appreciated ever since Lord Lister attempted an open reduction and suture of the olecranon (Keon-Cohen 1966). The methods of surgical repair have varied. Some authors have advocated excision of the fragment or fragments with repair of the triceps aponeurosis (Keon-Cohen 1966). Others have advocated the fixation of the fragment with intramedullary nails, screws, or plates (Weseley et al. 1976). As indications became more clearly defined, resection of the proximal fragment and reattachment of the triceps tendon to the distal fragment was reserved for elderly patients in whom the fracture was proximal to the middle of the trochlear notch (Rowe 1965). Younger patients were subjected to an open reduction and an attempt was made to stabilize the fragments, either with a through-and-through loop of wire (Fig. 7.1) or with a long intramedullary lag screw (Fig. 7.2).

If the olecranon fragment was small, excision usually resulted in a stable elbow with a satisfactory range of motion. If the fragment was large, it became increasingly more difficult to preserve an adequate cuff of the triceps aponeurosis to effect a repair. If the fragment involved more than 50% of the articular surface,

instability of the elbow followed resection. Instability was a serious problem because it compromised function, and therefore excision was abandoned as a form of treatment for any but the smallest of fragments.

The methods of internal fixation with either the wire loop, intramedullary Rush rod, or an intramedullary lag screw did not provide sufficient stability to allow early motion. The joint had to be immobilized until union occurred. Despite plaster of Paris immobilization, the triceps pull was frequently sufficient to cause displacement (Fig. 7.2). Typically, the fracture gaped dorsally, and frequently some separation of the fragments occurred, which led to gaps in the articular surface and to joint incongruity.

The duration of immobilization and the associated joint disorganization frequently led to varying losses in the range of flexion and extension. The dorsal gaping with displacement of the proximal fragment hindered full extension. Therefore, the loss of extension was often more severe than the loss of flexion. Because the elbow is not a weight-bearing joint and does not transmit such great forces as the knee joint, incongruity does not result rapidly in post-traumatic osteoarthritis. However, if the patient is called upon to perform heavy work requiring elbow flexion and extension against resistance, then progression of the osteoarthritis and an increase in pain and disability are to be expected.

In 1965, the AO group published the *Technique of Internal Fixation of Fractures* (Müller et al. 1965), which

Fig. 7.1. A wire loop inserted through the substance of the olecranon **(a)** is unable to resist the pull of the triceps and brachial muscles against the intact trochlea **(b)**. Gaping of the fracture with varying degrees of displacement, despite protection in a cast, is the usual outcome

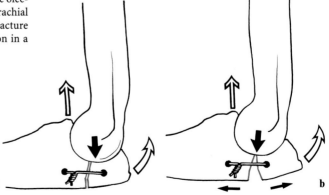

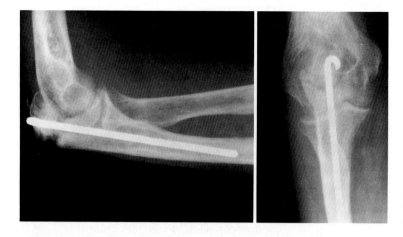

Fig. 7.2. A Rush rod or an intramedullary screw is also unable to resist the pull of the triceps and brachial muscles. Note the displacement of the olecranon

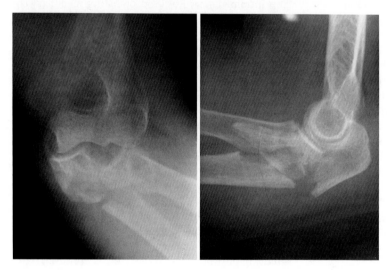

Fig. 7.3. A fracture of the olecranon with displacement. Note in this example the associated disruption of the elbow joint with subluxation

introduced tension band wiring as the most effective method of internal fixation of olecranon fractures. Their experiments showed tension band wiring to be six times stronger than any other fixation technique. By using this technique, it was therefore possible to forego the application of a plaster fixation and to begin active movement soon after surgery. At 4–6 weeks, the olecranon fracture was usually sufficiently healed to allow the patient full function. The rate of malunion or nonunion was extremely low, as was the degree of residual disability.

7.2 Methods of Evaluation and Guides to Treatment

The indication for surgery is an olecranon fracture with displacement, which represents a disruption of the triceps mechanism and loss of active extension of the elbow. If the fracture is undisplaced, the surgeon must determine whether the triceps aponeurosis is intact or not. With an intact triceps aponeurosis, a patient is able to extend the elbow against gravity without causing any displacement of the fragments. Such a fracture is stable, will not displace under the influence of physiological forces, and requires only symptomatic treatment. If any doubt exists as to the continuity of the triceps aponeurosis, the elbow should be examined with the aid of an X-ray image intensifier. Any degree of displacement on full flexion signifies damage to the triceps aponeurosis.

The diagnosis is simple. Typically, the patient gives a history of having fallen and of not being able to use the elbow. The olecranon is very painful, swollen, and bruised. The exact diagnosis is established on an appropriate anteroposterior and lateral radiograph (Fig. 7.3). The anteroposterior view is more useful for an overall examination of the elbow to exclude other injuries, but the olecranon itself is obscured in this view. The lateral projection gives a clear view of the olecranon. If there are any doubts as to the degree of comminution or articular surface depression, lateral tomograms should be requested in order to obtain an accurate definition of the fracture.

7.3 Classification

7.3.1 Intra-articular Fractures

7.3.1.1 Transverse (21–B1.1)

The simple fracture occurs at the deepest point of the trochlear notch (Fig. 7.4). It is an avulsion fracture and results from a sudden pull of both the triceps and brachialis muscles. It may also result from a direct fall on the olecranon itself.

Complex fractures which result from a direct force, such as a fall, frequently have comminution and depression of the articular surface (Fig. 7.5).

7.3.1.2 Oblique (21–B1.1)

An oblique fracture usually result from a hyperextension injury of the elbow. It begins at the midpoint of the trochlear notch and runs distally (Fig. 7.6).

7.3.1.3 Comminuted Fractures and Associated Injuries

Comminuted fractures and associated injuries are the result of a high-velocity direct injury to the elbow, such as might result from a considerable fall directly on the elbow. The fracture lines are variable, but certain features must be distinguished.

1. *Fractures of the coronoid process.* Small fractures of the coronoid process itself are unimportant. If the fragment is large, it represents the distal articular surface of the trochlear notch and cannot be neglected, because of resultant instability of the elbow in extension (Fig. 7.7).
2. *Distal extent of the fracture.* If the fracture extends distally past the midpoint of the trochlear notch (Fig. 7.8), it is no longer merely a disruption of the triceps mechanism. It compromises the stability of the elbow in withstanding varus or valgus forces.
3. *Fracture or dislocation of the radial head.* An associated fracture of the radial head comprises a dislocation of the elbow and is usually associated with a disruption of the medial collateral ligament (Fig. 7.9). It implies ligamentous instability of the elbow which may not be corrected by reduction of the fracture and repair of the ligament. The radial head has to be reduced and fixed or replaced by a prosthesis.

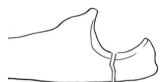

Fig. 7.4. A transverse fracture of the olecranon

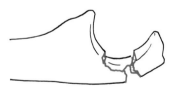

Fig. 7.5. A complex transverse fracture. Note the impaction of the central portion of the articular surface. This fragment is frequently difficult to reduce and, because of its position, difficult to fix. Once the fragment is disimpacted, a hole is left which may occasionally have to be bone-grafted

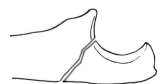

Fig. 7.6. An oblique fracture of the olecranon – the result of hyperextension

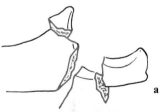

a

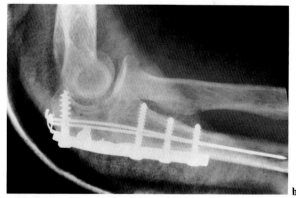

b

Fig. 7.7. a Severe comminution. Note also the fracture of the coronoid process. Such a comminuted fracture requires a neutralization plate, which can also act as a tension band. **b** A comminuted fracture of the olecranon fixed with a plate, Kirschner wires, and a tension band wire

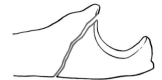

Fig. 7.8. A fracture of the olecranon which is distal to the mid-point of the trochlear notch. If not comminuted, such an oblique fracture should be first stabilized with one or two lag screws. Kirschner wires are not enough for lateral support. To overcome varus/valgus instability and resistance to torque, these distal fractures, even if fixed with lag screws, should be fixed with a plate. Semitubular plates are not strong enough to resist torsional forces. The 3.5-mm dynamic compression (DC) plates should be used to stabilize these fractures

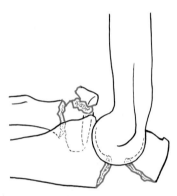

Fig. 7.9. A fracture of the olecranon associated with a fracture of the radial head (21–B3.3). These fractures are frequently associated with a rupture of the medial collateral ligament of the elbow. The elbow remains unstable until the olecranon fracture is fixed, the medial collateral ligament repaired, and the radial head either reduced and fixed with screws or replaced with a prosthesis. Resection of the radial head will result in valgus subluxation of the elbow

···········

7.3.2 Extra-articular Fractures

Avulsion fractures of a small part of the tip of the olecranon with the attached triceps tendon result in the same loss of function as a transverse fracture of the olecranon. The mechanism of injury is probably the same.

··········

7.4 Surgical Treatment

7.4.1 Positioning the Patient

The patient should be positioned either prone or lying on the uninjured side. This position automatically exposes the posterior aspect of the elbow and allows a direct unobstructed surgical approach. The elbow is free to be flexed or extended. The force of gravity maintains traction on the forearm and keeps it in the correct position throughout surgery. This obviates the need for an assistant, who would otherwise be required to hold the forearm of a supine patient in a position indicated by the surgeon. With the patient lying on the uninjured side or prone, the position of the forearm is adjusted simply by placing a rolled-up sheet under the forearm as required (see p.106).

··········

7.4.2 Draping

The surgical scrub should extend from the level of the tourniquet, which is applied as high as possible on the arm, to the wrist. The extremity must be draped free to allow for unobstructed flexion and extension of the elbow.

··········

7.4.3 Tourniquet

We prefer to use a tourniquet on all intra-articular fractures. It reduces bleeding, allows better visualization of the intra-articular components, and leads to a more accurate reconstruction of the joint.

··········

7.4.4 Surgical Exposure

The incision is begun posteriorly in the middle of the supracondylar area of the humerus and is extended distally on the medial side of the olecranon to a point three or four fingerbreadths distal to the fracture. The incision should not cross the point of the olecranon, as it might lead to a painful scar. We prefer to use an incision on the medial side of the olecranon for two reasons. First, it is cosmetically more pleasing because it is less apparent. Second, we feel that the ulnar nerve should be identified and protected during the surgical exposure and reduction (Fig. 7.10). If the incision is radial, it is more difficult to expose the ulnar nerve and follow it distally without undermining a considerable flap. The olecranon bursa is incised and no effort is made to protect it. If the fracture is exposed with the elbow flexed it usually gapes, which facilitates the identification of the fracture lines without undue stripping of the flexor carpi ulnaris muscle from the medial side of the olecranon. The fracture and the articular surface should be exposed through the fracture by increasing the deformity of the proximal fragment. If the fracture is comminuted, but particularly if the joint surface is depressed, it is necessary to visualize the articular surface to check the accuracy of the reduction. This cannot be done safely from the medial side because of the ulnar nerve and because of the attachment of the deltoid ligament. Good exposure of the joint can be

Fig. 7.10. Surgical exposure of the olecranon. Note the isolated and protected ulnar nerve which dips into the tunnel of the ulnar flexor muscle of the wrist next to the fracture. To visualize the joint, the fibers of the ulnar flexor muscle of the wrist and anconeus muscle must be reflected

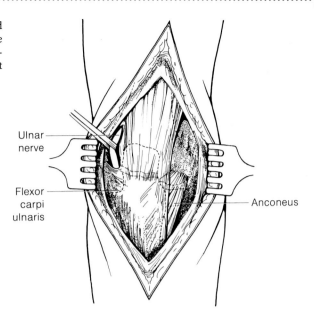

Ulnar nerve

Flexor carpi ulnaris

Anconeus

obtained from the lateral side by detaching some of the fibers of the anconeus muscle from the radial side of the ulna (Fig. 7.10).

7.4.5 Techniques of Reduction and Internal Fixation

7.4.5.1 Transverse Fractures

The reduction of the olecranon fracture is easiest with the elbow in extension, which relaxes the pull of the triceps muscle. Once carefully reduced, the fracture should be held reduced with a pointed reduction clamp. Two Kirschner wires are then inserted. These must be parallel to one another in the direction of the long axis of the ulna. A common error is to cross them. This holds the fracture apart and prevents compression. Another common error is to angle them anteriorly and exit them through the anterior cortex near the coronoid process, where they may damage vital structures. If they are angled too far anteriorly, they may enter the joint. Correct insertion of the wires is greatly eased if the elbow is slightly flexed and if the cortex of the olecranon is predrilled with a 2.0-mm drill bit. The Kirschner wires should be 1.6 mm in diameter. If they are any thicker, they are too difficult to bend. They should be inserted with a power drill with the help of a telescoping wire guide. The surgeon should aim parallel to the subcutaneous border of the ulna. These wires are important because they are an internal splint which prevents rotation and lateral displacement.

The wire for the tension band is inserted through a 2.0-mm drill hole which is drilled distally, approximate-

ly the same distance from the fracture as the tip of the olecranon. The drill hole must be deep to the subcutaneous cortex of the ulna. If it is too superficial, the wire will cut out. The wire for the tension band should be 1.0–1.2 mm in diameter and should be made of stainless steel, which is sufficiently ductile to permit twisting.

The tension band wire must pass deep to the triceps tendon and be just proximal to the two Kirschner wires. We have found a gauge 14 or 16 needle a great help in passing the wire correctly deep to the triceps tendon. If the wire is passed only arround the two Kirschner wires, there is a risk of the Kirschner wires backing out and perforating the skin.

B.G. Weber (circa 1972, personal communication) suggested that before the figure-of-eight tension band is tightened, two loops should be made to allow simultaneous twisting and tightening of both limbs of the figure-of-eight, to ensure uniform compression on both sides of the fracture. The two loops are not absolutely essential as long as the surgeon ensures that the wire is straightened out and pulled very tight before it is placed under tension by twisting. Once tension is applied, the wire binds and will not slide in bone. If the wire is not pulled tight and straightened before it is tightened, it may straighten after the internal fixation is completed and thus lengthen, which loosens the tension band and leads to failure of the fixation. The tension band should be tightened in full extension to effect a slight overreduction of the fracture, which will disappear as the elbow is flexed. This ensures dynamic compression on the whole fracture surface.

As the tension band is tightened, a slight gap in the articular surface is created, and the only part of the bone under constant axial compression is the posterior cortex and some adjacent cancellous bone. This is the only part which heals by primary bone healing. The remainder of the fracture is subjected to changing degrees of compression because the compression increases when the elbow is flexed and decreases when it is extended. This flux in the degree of compression was seen in an experimental investigation to result in the central and subchondral areas of the fracture healing by endochondral ossification. The articular defect heals by the formation of fibrocartilage (Schatzker 1971).

With tension band fixation, flexion of the elbow increases the axial compression. This is fortunate because it increases the stability of the reduction and fixation, while with lag screw fixation or loop cerclage wiring, flexion causes displacement because of the unopposed pull of the triceps. Fractures of the olecranon fixed with a tension band wire should not be splinted in extension, therefore, but should be allowed early active flexion, since this actually increases compression and stability. A further advantage of tension band fixation is that it can be employed successfully in osteoporotic bone, since its strength does not depend on the holding power of a screw in the bone. Its strength is determined by the resistance of the bone to the cutting out of the wire where it traverses the ulnar cortex and by the stability and resistance of the two parallel Kirschner wires which support the tension band wire deep to the triceps tendon.

7.4.5.2 Transverse Fractures with Joint Depression

The transverse fracture with comminution and joint depression requires special attention (see Fig. 7.5). The articular fragment which is depressed and driven into the underlying cancellous bone represents a separate piece of bone with a disrupted blood supply. If it is large and left unreduced, joint incongruity and instability result. Therefore, it must be elevated in a manner similar to that described for the tibial plateau (see Sect. 16.4.5). The resultant defect must be bone-grafted. The graft, together with the axial compression, will aid in preventing redisplacement. Occasionally, it may also be possible to splint it in position with one of the two axial Kirschner wires. At the end of the procedure, the Kirschner wires are bent and cut to length and the free ends are driven into the bone, which further increases the stability of the fixation and hinders the wires from backing out.

7.4.5.3 Oblique Fractures

The oblique fracture is reduced in the same way as a transverse fracture. The stability of the fixation can be greatly increased if a lag screw is inserted at right angles to the fracture line. The internal fixation then follows, as described previously, with the two Kirschner wires and a tension band wire. In this instance, the tension band wire can be viewed as a neutralization wire, protecting the compression and fixation achieved with the lag screw. If the fixation with the lag screw is secure, the Kirschner wires can be omitted. The tension band wire alone will be enough. If the fracture is distal, a plate should be used for fixation instead of a wire (see Fig. 7.7 b).

7.4.5.4 Comminuted Fractures

Comminuted fractures, the result of high-velocity injury, are frequently complex and may pose great difficulties when reduction and fixation are attempted. Reduction may be made easier if indirect reduction techniques are used. However, this must not be at the expense of an anatomical reduction of the articular surface. If the surgeon decides to use direct reduction techniques, then the reduction should commence distally and proceed toward the joint. Thus, if there is an extension wedge fragment distal to the coronoid process, an attempt should be made to reduce it and fix it with a lag screw before proceeding with the reduction of the joint surface. The articular surface of the distal fragment must be clearly visualized. Frequently, this can only be achieved if the proximal and distal fragments are widely separated.

The fracture of the coronoid, if significant in size, should be reduced first and held provisionally with small bone-holding forceps or a Kirschner wire while it is fixed with a lag screw passed up through the posterior cortex of the ulna. The reduction and fixation of this fragment is important if stability of the elbow in extension is to be restored. The remaining fragments are then reduced and fixed to each other by whatever means is most suitable. Once reduced, the olecranon is then splinted by the insertion of the two axial Kirschner wires.

If the fracture extends past the coronoid process, it can no longer be viewed as an isolated fracture of the olecranon subjected only to the pull of the triceps. Once the fracture involves the whole trochlear notch of the ulna and extends distal to the coronoid process, it becomes subjected to considerable torque and valgus/varus stress, and the simple Kirschner wires and tension band fixation are no longer enough. For such fractures, we like to combine the Kirschner wire and tension band fixation with a plate which is applied along the posterior cortex of the ulna and olecranon (see Fig. 7.1 b). This plate protects the fracture from the varus/valgus and torsional stresses. Occasionally, we resort to the use of a plate even if the fracture does not extend distal to the coronoid process, but is very comminuted so that no continuity exists in the posterior cortex. In such a case, as a tension band is tightened, the fragments tend to telescope, and the reduction might be lost and the joint become deformed. For such fractures, we use a plate, which buttresses the fragments and helps maintain their relative position. We have found the small, 3.5-mm dynamic compression (DC) plate very useful for this purpose. A semitubular plate should not be used because it is too weak and tends to break.

7.5 Postoperative Care

Suction drains are used to prevent hematoma formation. These are removed after the first 24–36 h. The olecranon is held at 90° flexion on a padded posterior plaster splint for the first 2–3 days. The splint is then removed and the wound carefully inspected. If no complications exist, the patient is encouraged to begin active flexion–extension exercises, which continue until a full range of movement is regained. The fractures, if uncomplicated, are usually healed in 6 weeks. At this point, full unprotected use of the extremity can be resumed. Comminuted fractures, particularly those with extension into the diaphysis of the ulna and those with devitalized bone fragments, require a longer time for consolidation and must be protected from overload to prevent implant failure with malunion or nonunion. Initially, we were very enthusiastic about the use of continuous passive motion machines (CPM) in elbow fractures. Although we still feel that they have a major role to play in the complex reconstructive procedures, simpler olecranon fractures do equally well with well-supervised early active mobilization.

References

Keon-Cohen BT (1966) Fractures of the elbow. J Bone Joint Surg 48A:1623–1639

Müller ME, Allgöwer M, Willenegger H (1965) Technique of internal fixation of fractures. Springer, Berlin Heidelberg New York

Rowe CR (1965) Management of fractures in elderly patients. J Bone Joint Surg 47A:1043–1059

Schatzker J (1971) Fixation of olecranon fractures in dogs. J Bone Joint Surg 53B:158

Weseley MS, Barenfeld PA, Risenstein AL (1976) The use of the Zuelzer hook plate in fixation of olecranon fractures. J Bone Joint Surg 58A:859–862

8 Fractures of the Radial Head (21-A2.2, 21-B2.1, 21-B2.2, and 21-B2.3)

J. Schatzker

8.1 Introduction

The goal of treatment of fractures of the radial head is the preservation of elbow flexion and extension as well as pronation and supination of the forearm.

8.2 Mechanism of Injury

The vast majority of fractures of the radial head are sustained in a fall onto the outstretched hand. The force of the fall is transmitted through the radius to the elbow, where the head of the radius is driven against the capitellum. Thus, the damage may not only be to the radial head, but also to the capitellum. Occasionally, the radial head may fracture as a result of a valgus force to the elbow, when the injury may also become complicated by a fracture of the olecranon. In these complex injuries, it should be remembered that the medial collateral ligament of the elbow is frequently torn. The rupture of the collateral ligament on one side and the fracture of the radial head on the other render the elbow joint completely unstable.

8.3 Guides to Treatment

Considerable confusion continues to exist on how best to treat fractures of the radial head. Much of the confusion has been caused by an attempt to treat the radiograph rather than the patient. Some have advocated excision of the radial head if the fracture involved more than one ninth of the circumference, while others have asserted with equal dogmatism that it should be one sixth and some that it should be one third. Some surgeons, guided by the experience that not only is the fragment always bigger than suggested by the radiograph but also that the damage to the radial head, in the form of comminution and articular depression, is always greater than anticipated, have gone so far as to advocate the following: "When in doubt, operate" and excise (Keon-Cohen 1966).

Since the goal of treatment is the preservation of function, the treatment must be directed to preserving motion at the elbow. Permanent loss of motion occurs either as a result of a bony block caused by a displaced piece or pieces of bone or by capsular and pericapsular scarring. Early movement is the only measure available to prevent capsular and pericapsular scarring. Loss of movement due to a bony block can be corrected only by removal of the block. Thus, we feel that once the diagnosis of a displaced fracture of the radial head has been established radiologically, the surgeon must establish beyond doubt whether a bony block to movement exists or not.

An intra-articular fracture is invariably associated with varying degrees of hemarthrosis. The distended joint is painful and the patient is reluctant to attempt any active movement or permit any passive manipulation. Considerable relief of pain is gained by aspiration of the hemarthrosis and infiltration of the joint with a local anesthetic, such as 2% Xylocaine (lidocaine). The advantage of local anesthesia is that once the joint becomes relatively painless, it is possible to determine whether or not there is a bony block to motion. If no block to motion is present, then early active motion is to be encouraged. We have treated displaced fractures in this fashion, regardless of their radiological appearance. The results have been gratifying, and despite incongruity of the articulation between the radial head and the capitellum, post-traumatic osteoarthritis has not developed. Loose intra-articular fragments and fractures with a block to motion under anesthesia, however, constitute an indication for surgery.

Excision of the radial head is not advisable. Studies by Pennal and Barrington (T. Barrington, personal communication) have demonstrated that in those who make heavy demands on their wrist and elbow, such as manual workers, excision of the radial head is followed by proximal migration of the radius. This leads to inferior radioulnar joint disturbance with pain and weakness of the wrist.

Radiographs of a fractured radial head are difficult to interpret and are often misleading. An accurate assessment of the fracture is only possible at the time of surgery. It is then possible to determine whether open reduction and internal fixation of the radial head are feasible or whether the radial head should be excised. We do not believe in partial excision of the head, because the results have been uniformly less satisfactory than after excision of the whole head.

8.4 Surgical Treatment

We consider the following to be indications for surgery:
- Major loose intra-articular fragments
- Displaced fractures which under anesthesia can be demonstrated to constitute a block to motion
- Displaced fractures of the radial head associated with fractures of the olecranon or with rupture of the ulnar collateral ligament, or with both

Although excision of the radial head might be contemplated as definitive treatment for a comminuted fracture if such a fracture is in isolation, it cannot be considered as an option if the fracture of the radial head is associated with rupture of the ulnar collateral ligament. A repair of the ulnar collateral ligament will not render the elbow stable if the radial head is missing. Therefore, under these circumstances, either an open reduction and internal fixation of the radial head fracture can be performed or the radial head can be excised and replaced with a prosthesis, which will act as a spacer and will stabilize the joint. We feel that preservation of the radial head is preferable to excision. The decision whether an open reduction and fixation is feasible has to be based, as in all other fractures, on the personality of the fracture.

8.4.1 Classification

In evaluating radial head fractures, we recognize three types:
- *Type I: split-wedge fracture.* The fracture consists of a simple split-wedge fragment which may be displaced or undisplaced (Fig. 8.1 a).

- *Type II: impaction fracture.* In this fracture pattern, part of the head and neck remain intact. The portion involved in the fracture is tilted and impacted, with the amount of comminution being variable (Fig. 8.1 b).
- *Type III: severely comminuted fracture.* The hallmark of this fracture is that no portion of the head or neck remains in continuity and that the comminution is very severe (Fig. 8.1 c).

The *Comprehensive Classification of Fractures* (Müller et al. 1990) is not very helpful in distinguishing the different fracture patterns. The isolated fracture of the radial neck is a type A and therefore would be coded as 21-A2.2 and 21-A2.3. The split wedge type I and the impaction types II and the multifragmentary types III are all partial articular fractures and are coded as B, which does not indicate the severity of the articular head fracture. The split wedge type I would be 21-B2.1. The impaction type II would be either 21-B2.2 or 21-B2.3 depending on the degree of fragmentation and depression. The severely comminuted fracture type III could be either 21-B2.2 or more likely 21-B2.3. Thus we feel that for coding puposes and for documentation the comprehensive classification is useful, but not for daily practice, where we feel the simple terms split wedge, impaction, or multifragmentary is more useful. Articular fractures of the radial head associated with olecranon fractures are classified as type C.

Severely comminuted fractures are irreconstructible. If a block to motion exists, the surgeon must decide between simple excision or excision and prosthetic replacement. If the fracture of the head is part of a fracture dislocation of the elbow one must either reconstruct or replace the head with a prosthesis. In the other two fracture patterns, if there is an indication for surgery because of a block to motion, the decision between excision on the one hand and reduction and fixation on

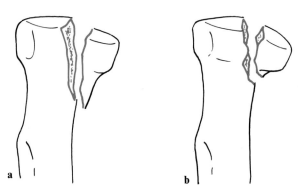
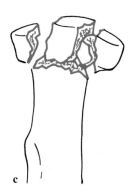

Fig. 8.1. a A split-wedge fracture. In this fracture, a part of the head remains intact. Fixation is simple with two 2.7-mm cortical screws used here as lag screws. The heads are recessed below the level of the articular cartilage. **b** An impaction fracture. Here again, a part of the head remains intact. The fracture fragments may be single, but more often there is some comminution. The fragments are tilted and the bone beneath them crushed or impacted. There may also be a transverse fracture across the neck. **c** A severely comminuted fracture. There are many fracture fragments, usually with significant displacement

the other has to be made on the basis of the personality of the fracture. As already stated, in younger patients we prefer reduction and fixation to excision.

8.4.2 Positioning and Draping the Patient

The patient is placed in a supine position. The limb is prepared from the axilla to the wrist and is draped free to permit pronation and supination of the forearm. The procedure is performed under tourniquet control.

8.4.3 Surgical Exposure

The approach is lateral. The incision begins at the lateral epicondyle and is extended just distal to the radial head. The common extensor muscle is split along the line of its fibers in line with the skin incision. Care must be taken to stay posterior to the radial nerve, which crosses just in front to enter the substance of the supinator muscle, approximately 2 cm distal to the radial head. The incision must therefore not extend distally below the annular ligament. Furthermore, if damage to the nerve is to be avoided, retraction must be gentle; if difficulty in visualization of the joint is encountered, it is best to release the lateral collateral ligament with an attached piece of the lateral epicondyle. At the close of the procedure the continuity of the collateral ligament is reestablished by screwing the osteotomized piece of bone back into place. The capsule is opened laterally and the radial head is visualized. Pronation and supination permit different portions of the head to be brought into direct vision. Another useful approach is the dorsal one. Exposure of the radial head and neck is achieved by detachment of the anconeus muscle from the ulna and the lateral epicondyle. This gives a better exposure of the medial portion of the head and of the radioulnar articulation.

8.4.4 Techniques of Reduction and Internal Fixation

8.4.4.1 Comminuted Fractures

The type III severely comminuted fracture in which there is no continuity of the head and neck cannot be reduced and fixed. The head is therefore excised. The decision as to whether a prosthetic replacement should be carried out must be made in each individual case. We feel that the only absolute indication for prosthetic replacement of the radial head is a dislocation of the elbow with rupture of the medial collateral ligament, with or without an associated fracture of the olecranon. The prosthesis is required to act as a spacer and prevent

valgus displacement and possible redislocation, even if a direct repair of the medial collateral ligament is carried out.

8.4.4.2 Split-Wedge Fractures

Type I split-wedge fractures are easily reduced and fixed with a lag screw. We have found the mini or small cortical screws best for fixation of these fractures. If the screw is inserted through the articular cartilage of the head, it should be recessed below the articular surface (Fig. 8.2).

8.4.4.3 Impaction Fractures

Type II impaction fractures are the most common type. They fall in complexity between type I and type III. The fragments are tilted, depressed, and impacted. Whether reduction and fixation is possible depends on the degree of comminution. If only one or two fragments are present, reduction is usually possible. The fragments should be elevated, provisionally fixed with a Kirschner wire, and then lagged to the remaining portion of the head and neck with one or two 2.7-mm screws as in type I. Since the injury is usually the result of a valgus force with the forearm in supination, the medial portion of the head and neck is usually intact (Figs. 8.3–8.5). Occasionally, the central comminution may be such that compression with a lag screw would narrow and distort the head. In such cases, this will prevent the screw from acting as a lag screw. All fragments should be drilled with the 2.0-mm drill bit and tapped with the 2.7-mm tap. We have indicated the use of the 2.7-mm cortex screws. If the fragments are smaller, the surgeon should resort to using the 2.0-mm or even the 1.5-mm cortex screws, as indicated.

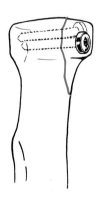

Fig. 8.2. The fixation of a wedge fracture is simple. Two 2.7-mm cortical screws are used as lag screws. The heads of the screws are recessed below the level of the articular cartilage

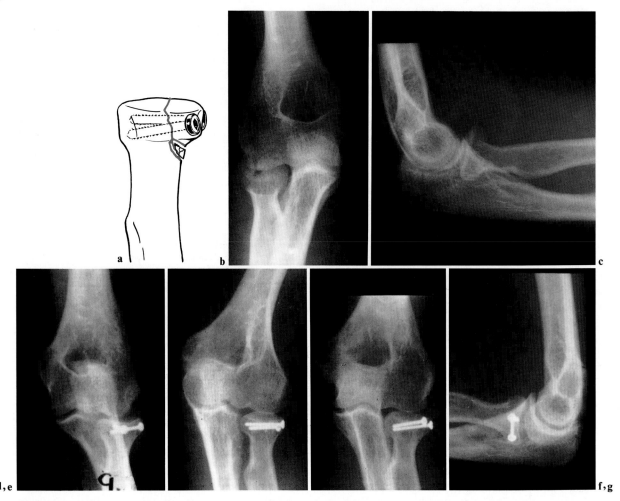

Fig. 8.3. a In an impaction fracture, if a portion of the head remains intact, fixation is relatively simple. The fragments are lagged to the intact portion of the head. Again, 2.7-mm screws are used for fixation. **b–g** A preoperative radiograph, 4 months after surgery

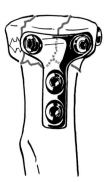

Fig. 8.4. If there is a transverse fracture of the neck, fixation of the head must be supplemented with a plate. The mini T plate must be carefully contoured and positioned in such a way as not to interfere with the radioulnar articulation in pronation or supination

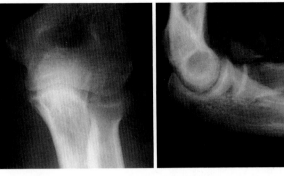 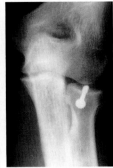 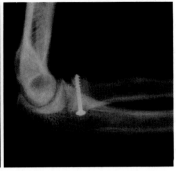

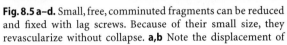

a, b   **c, d**

Fig. 8.5 a–d. Small, free, comminuted fragments can be reduced and fixed with lag screws. Because of their small size, they revascularize without collapse. **a,b** Note the displacement of the fragment. It blocked flexion of the elbow. **b,c** Six months after reduction and fixatio

8.4.5 Postoperative Care

Suction drainage is used for the first 24 h. Stable fixation eliminates bone pain and makes it safe and possible to begin early active flexion–extension and pronation–supination exercises. We immobilize the elbow at 90° in a padded posterior splint. On the second or third day, the dressings are removed and, if no complications exist, active mobilization exercises are started. We discourage the use of a sling because it maintains the elbow in flexion. Pronation, supination, and flexion usually return almost to normal without much difficulty. The last 10°–15° of extension are very difficult to regain, no matter what form of treatment is used. We have concluded from a trial that continuous passive motion machines (CPM) are not useful in fractures of the radial head.

References

Keon-Cohen BT (1966) Fractures of the elbow. J Bone Joint Surg 48A:1623–1639

Müller ME, Nazarian S, Koch P, Schatzker J (1990) The comprehensive classification of fractures of long bones. Springer, Berlin Heidelberg New York

9 Fractures of the Radius and Ulna

M. TILE

9.1 Introduction

Fractures of the forearm present unique management problems. In these particular diaphyseal fractures, perhaps more than any others, the combination of anatomical reduction and skeletal stability with mobility of the extremity is necessary to produce excellent functional results. The ASIF system of stable internal fixation is admirably suited to this end; therefore, it is not surprising that the use of this system in diaphyseal fractures of the radius and ulna has revolutionized their management and improved the end results.

9.2 Natural History

9.2.1 Closed Treatment

For many years, surgeons have grappled with the difficulty of restoring early function to the fractured forearm. Early authors recommended closed reduction followed by lengthy plaster immobilization, but the deficiencies of this method were soon recognized. Malunion and nonunion were frequent complications with resultant poor functional results.

Böhler (1936) recognized that to maintain skeletal length, continuous traction was often required. He recommended Kirschner wires inserted above and below the fracture and held by a plaster cast to achieve this goal; however, the results were not significantly improved. Perhaps the most severe indictment of the closed method was made by Hughston (1957), reporting 92 % unsatisfactory functional results in the treatment of 41 isolated, displaced radial shaft fractures (Galeazzi type). Therefore, even Charnley (1961), in his classic treatise *Closed Treatment of Common Fractures*, strongly recommended operative treatment of forearm fractures.

9.2.2 Open Treatment

Early attempts at enhancing the functional results by open reduction and internal fixation did little to improve the situation, but they represented pioneering efforts. Unstable fixation with inadequate and poorly applied plates required long-term plaster immobilization, again compromising the final results. In spite of the necessary cast immobilization, which resulted in some stiffness of the injured extremity, the nonunion rate remained significantly high. This was particularly evident in the report of Knight and Purvis (1949).

Smith and Sage (1957) attempted to change this outlook by the development of specialized intramedullary devices, with improved results, but their nonunion rate was unacceptably high. Intramedullary devices cannot restore the most important rotatory stability to the injured forearm. Also, they tend to straighten the normal dorsoradial bow of the radius and are therefore not well suited to the radius; however, locked intramedullary nails have been developed (De Pedro et al. 1990).

9.2.3 AO/ASIF Techniques

Major improvements in the results of this injury awaited the development of advanced techniques. Danis (1947) is generally credited with initiating the era of compression plates. The introduction of AO implants and the strict adherence to AO principles have changed the outlook dramatically. Stable internal fixation using these proven techniques has eliminated most external casts and splints; this, in turn, has led to markedly improved functional results for the patient, depending on the degree of soft tissue injury. Malunion should be eliminated with use of the proper technique and nonunion should almost disappear, further enhancing the results. Most recent surveys have indicated a nonunion rate of less than 5 %. Even if nonunion does develop, the final result should not be compromised, since these patients, free of all external casts and splints, can maintain full function of the extremity during this period.

Lack of recognition of the important biological and biomechanical principles of modern techniques of internal fixation is the most common cause of failure. In our first 60 consecutive cases in which this method was used prior to obtaining the sophisticated skills later possessed, we achieved 90 % excellent functional results (Tile and Petrie 1969). All our failures were technical, as were those of Anderson et al. (1975), who achieved union rates of 97.9 % for the radius and 96.3 % for the ulna, with excellent functional results. These results and those of others are a far cry from those reported only a decade earlier, when the usual scenario for the fractured forearm was an open reduction with imperfect fixation, requiring the use of a plaster cast for a minimum of 8–12 weeks. Even then, a nonunion rate for one or the other bone of 20 % or more was expected.

More recent reports have continued to show excellent functional results with anatomical reduction, stable fixation with plates and early motion (Chapman et al. 1989; Schemitsch and Richards 1992; Duncan et al. 1992).

9.3 Management

9.3.1 Principles

To achieve excellent results, anatomical reduction and stable fixation are required. The forearm fracture requires anatomical reduction for the following reasons: (a) restoration of normal radial and ulnar length will prevent subluxation of either the proximal or distal radioulnar joint and will reestablish length to the muscles controlling that most beautiful tactile instrument of the body, the hand; and (b) restoration of rotational alignment is essential for normal pronation–supination function of the forearm. The restoration of the normal dorsoradial bow of the radius is essential to maintain this rotatory function – again, difficult to achieve with intramedullary devices. Therefore, intramedullary devices are not suited for the treatment of forearm fractures, especially the radius. If locked intramedullary devices are used in the ulna, it is essential that ulnar length and rotation are anatomical.

The principle of anatomical reduction in forearm fractures must be upheld in this era of *biological reduction. While it is important to maintain bone viability by improved techniques, in the forearm it is more important to achieve anatomical reduction.*

Anatomical reduction and stable internal fixation with plates will reduce pain and allow early soft tissue rehabilitation, without the use of external splints or casts. Rapid restoration of both hand and forearm function is assured by the use of plates, either as a tension band, axially compressing the fracture, or as a neutralization plate with prior interfragmental compression.

In summary, the forearm fracture, whether of one or both bones, more than any other diaphyseal fracture in the body, requires open anatomical reduction with stable fixation, preferably with plates, for optimal functional results.

9.3.2 Indications for Surgery

As stressed in other chapters in this book, the indications for surgery in this type of fracture are dependent upon a knowledge of the natural history of the fracture combined with an assessment of its personality. The natural history of the forearm fracture, under almost all circumstances, is so uncertain when treated by means other than anatomical open reduction, stable fixation with plates, and early motion of the extremity that this treatment alone can be recommended in almost all of the cases described below.

9.3.2.1 Fractures of Both Bones

For reasons previously discussed, displaced fractures of both radius and ulna should be treated by open reduction, stable internal fixation, and early motion.

9.3.2.2 Fracture of One Bone

a) Fractures of the Shaft of the Radius or the Ulna with Radioulnar Subluxation (Galeazzi or Monteggia Fractures)

Displaced single-bone fractures of the radius or ulna, if treated nonoperatively, have a notoriously poor outcome. Displacement at the fracture site is always accompanied by displacement at the corresponding radioulnar joint, whether proximal or distal. Reduction must be absolutely anatomical or subluxation of that radioulnar joint will remain, with significant functional loss. Therefore, the displaced fracture of the radial shaft with distal radioulnar subluxation (Galeazzi fracture; see Fig. 9.11 b–e) and the displaced fracture of the ulnar shaft with proximal radioulnar subluxation (Monteggia fracture) constitute *absolute* indications for surgery.

b) Isolated Fracture of the Ulna

The management of this fracture, usually caused by a direct blow and not associated with a proximal radial head dislocation, has been a subject of controversy. Even with minimal displacement and prolonged immobilization in a plaster cast, union may be delayed (Fig. 9.1).

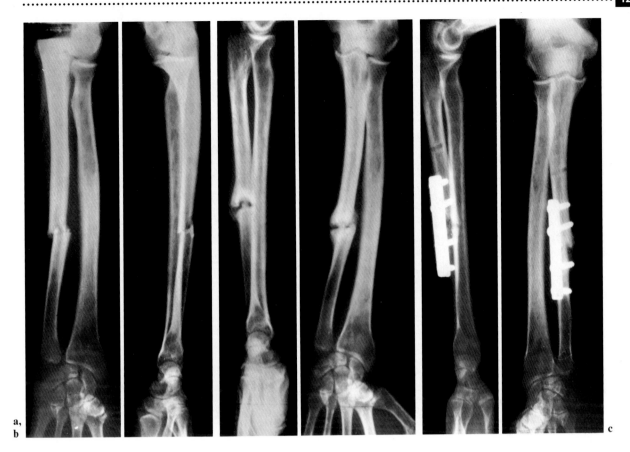

Fig. 9.1 a–c. Isolated fracture of the ulna – nonoperative management. **a** Anteroposterior and lateral radiographs of an isolated fracture of the ulna caused by a direct blow. No injury to the elbow or wrist is apparent. **b, c** After 24 weeks of immobilization in plaster, the radiograph shows nonunion requiring internal fixation

Proximal ulnar fractures are the most dangerous, as they are subjected to a greater torque and may bow. Therefore, to obviate these problems, surgery may be indicated for this seemingly innocuous fracture.

Reports by Sarmiento et al. (1975) Goel et al. (1991), and Gebuhr et al. (1992), and others, dispute this, indicating universally good functional results with a simple below-elbow splint. We feel that most of these fractures, if relatively undisplaced, may be treated with casts or splints with the expectation of a good result (Fig. 9.2). However, in certain instances, open reduction and internal fixation may be preferable to prolonged splinting for the patient. In these cases, the patient should share in the decision-making process, after being informed of the advantages and disadvantages of each method (Fig. 9.3).

9.3.2.3 Open Fracture of the Forearm

Open fractures of the forearm require open reduction and internal fixation, for the same reasons as closed fractures do. Early restoration of mobility and function is even more important in these cases, so stability must be restored early. Some surgeons delay internal fixation for several days, but we prefer to fix the fracture at the time of the original cleansing and débridement, having noted no difference in the rate of sepsis or the complications in those so treated, where careful open wound management was maintained (Moed et al. 1986; Duncan et al. 1992).

9.3.3 Timing of Surgery

Since surgery is usually indicated for all displaced forearm fractures, we prefer to proceed with it as soon as possible following injury.

Early surgery is desirable but not essential. The advantages of early surgery are both technical and functional. One of the technical advantages is ease of reduction prior to shortening of the bone ends, which ensures the anatomical reduction so necessary in this fracture.

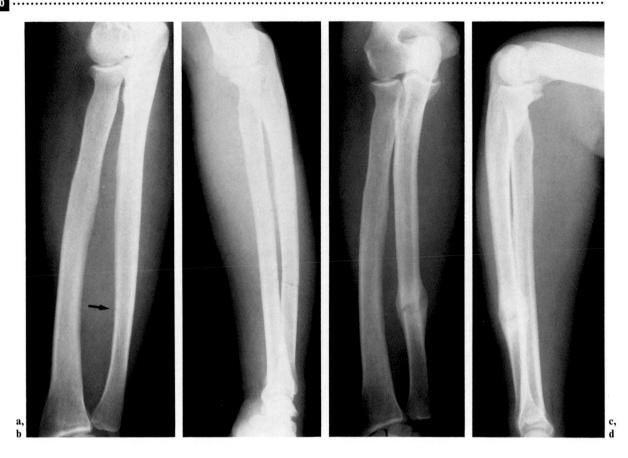

a,
b

c,
d

Fig. 9.2. a, b Anteroposterior and lateral radiographs of a 45-year-old man with an isolated undisplaced fracture of the ulna. **c, d** After immobilization in a functional forearm brace for 16 weeks, the anteroposterior and lateral radiographs show massive callus formation and bony union

arguing the biological merits of delayed surgery, we feel that the present methods of internal fixation are so good that the possible added help of delayed surgery is not required. It would be difficult to improve on the present excellent results, namely 97%–98% union, by delaying surgery. The technical difficulties of reduction and the

Also, evacuation of the hematoma, stable fixation of the fracture, and wound drainage allow the patient to move the hand and forearm early, thus eliminating the period of immobilization necessary if surgery is delayed, and aiding early functional recovery.

Surgery may be delayed by general factors, such as the poor state of the polytraumatized patient, in whom other musculoskeletal or visceral injuries have greater priority. Delay may also be necessary if the patient arrives late and the state of the soft tissues would compromise the surgery – for example, if fracture blisters are already present. Under these circumstances, the surgery should be performed at the earliest appropriate time.

We dispute the contention by Smith and Sage (1957) and others that delayed surgery will ensure union more often than immediate surgery, as measured by the formation of increased callus at the fracture site. Without

Fig. 9.3 a–h. Isolated fracture of the ulna – operative management. **a, b** The anteroposterior and lateral radiographs illustrate an isolated fracture in the distal third of the ulna in a 27-year-old urology resident. **c, d** After discussing the options with the patient, it was elected to perform an open reduction and internal fixation using an interfragmental compression screw and a neutralization plate, as shown in the immediate postoperative radiographs. **e, f** At 16 weeks, primary bone union is seen. The patient required no postoperative immobilization and returned to his internship within 2 weeks. **g, h** The implants were removed 24 months after injury. The patient's functional result is excellent

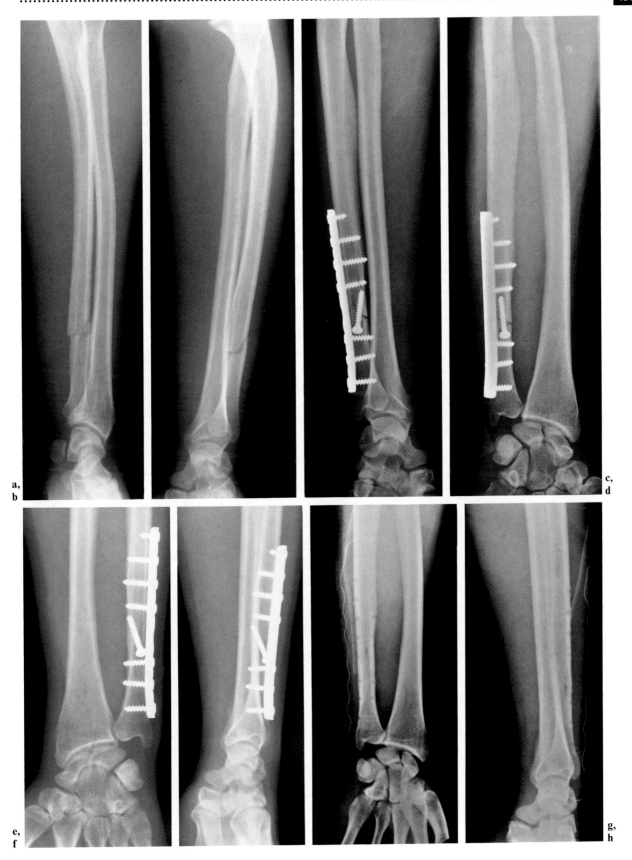

a,
b

c,
d

e,
f

g,
h

delay of functional recovery far outweigh any theoretical benefits in fracture healing.

•••

9.3.4 Surgical Technique

9.3.4.1 Preliminary Considerations

a) Positioning the Patient

In polytrauma, the supine position is most commonly used, especially if other injuries are being fixed simultaneously. For isolated fractures, the prone or lateral position may be used. The arm is placed on an arm board with the shoulder at 90°, allowing the ulna to be approached by pronation and the radius by supination. The same can be achieved by placing the patient in the lateral position with the arm on an arm board. This position is more suitable than the prone position for regional block anesthesia and for obese patients. In isolated fractures of the radius, the supine position is preferable, for isolated ulnar fractures the lateral position or the supine position with the elbow locked.

b) Tourniquet

We prefer a tourniquet in closed fractures to ensure a bloodless field, which reduces the operating time. In open fractures, however, the tourniquet should be in place but not used unless necessary to stop the oozing, which prevents proper identification of the soft tissue structures such as nerves and vessels, increasing the difficulty of anatomical reduction of the fracture.

9.3.4.2 Surgical Approaches

a) Ulna

The approach to the ulna is relatively simple (Fig. 9.4). The ulna is a subcutaneous bone and is easily exposed throughout its length. However, as with other subcutaneous bones, the basic principle of making the skin incision over muscle rather than over bone must be followed. Therefore, we recommend an incision just off the subcutaneous border of the ulna, either on its anterior or posterior aspect, depending on which approach is used for the radius. The correct incision should allow the widest possible bridge between the ulnar and radial incision.

The direct approach to the bone is between the flexor carpi ulnaris and the extensor carpi ulnaris muscles. Periosteal stripping should be kept to a minimum, and all bone fragments with attached soft tissue should be

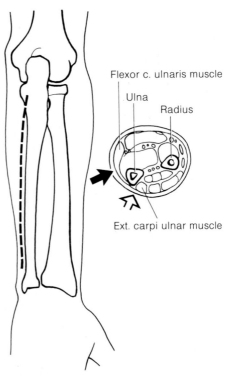

Fig. 9.4. Skin incision for a fracture of the ulna should never be made over the bone itself, but always over soft tissue. This is true for all subcutaneous bones. The cross-sectional illustration indicates the approach between the flexor and extensor carpi ulnaris muscles

handled carefully, to preserve the soft tissue and maintain bone viability.

b) Radius

Anterior Approach (Henry). There are several standard approaches to the radius. We prefer the anterior, as described by Henry (1927) (Fig. 9.5), especially in the proximal and distal thirds, for the following reasons:

1. The approach is extensile, allowing the surgeon to expose the radius from the elbow to the wrist. It is the only approach that allows a major reconstruction of the radius throughout its length.
2. In the upper third, the radial nerve is well protected by the supinator muscle belly during the primary operation. Of even greater importance is the relative safety of the radial nerve in secondary operations such as plate removal.
3. For plate application, this approach is ideally suited to the flat anterior surface of the lower third of the radius. Consideration of tensile versus compressive forces in plate application is not as important in the upper

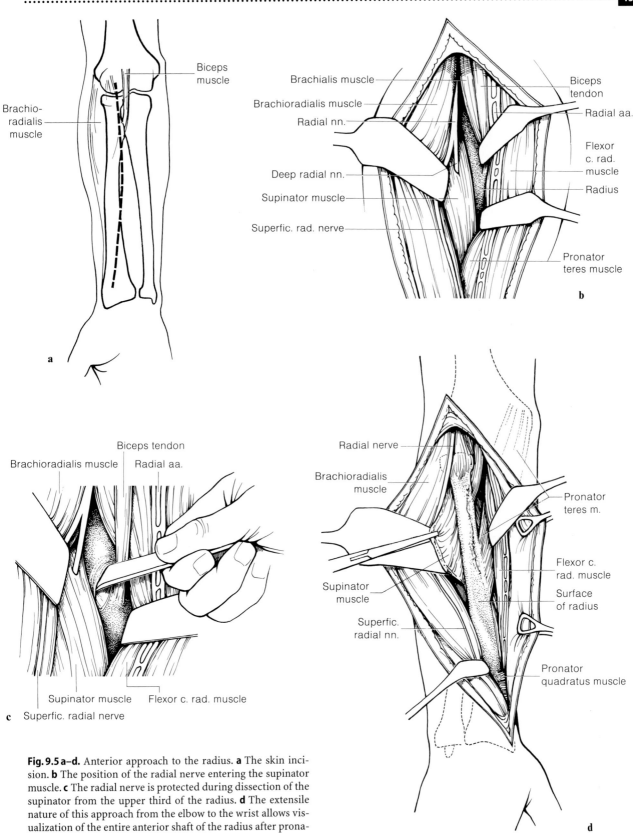

Fig. 9.5 a–d. Anterior approach to the radius. **a** The skin incision. **b** The position of the radial nerve entering the supinator muscle. **c** The radial nerve is protected during dissection of the supinator from the upper third of the radius. **d** The extensile nature of this approach from the elbow to the wrist allows visualization of the entire anterior shaft of the radius after pronation of the forearm

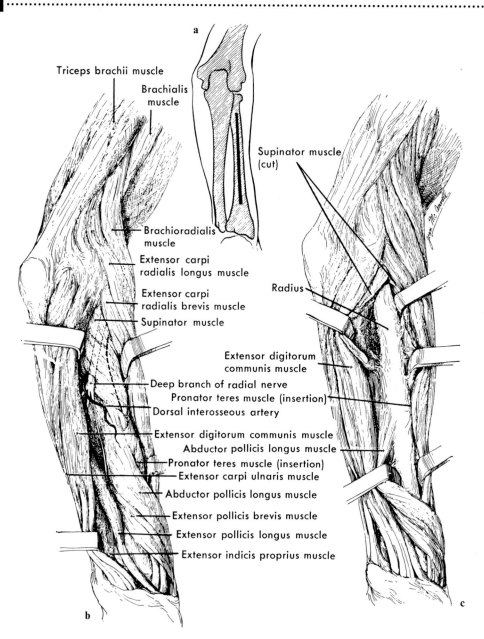

Triceps brachii muscle

Brachialis muscle

Supinator muscle (cut)

Brachioradialis muscle

Extensor carpi radialis longus muscle

Extensor carpi radialis brevis muscle

Supinator muscle

Radius

Extensor digitorum communis muscle

Deep branch of radial nerve

Pronator teres muscle (insertion)

Dorsal interosseous artery

Extensor digitorum communis muscle

Abductor pollicis longus muscle

Pronator teres muscle (insertion)

Extensor carpi ulnaris muscle

Abductor pollicis longus muscle

Extensor pollicis brevis muscle

Extensor pollicis longus muscle

Extensor indicis proprius muscle

Fig. 9.6 a–c. The posterior (Thompson) approach to the proximal middle third of the posterior surface of the radius. **a** Skin incision. **b** Relationship of supinator muscle of the deep branch of the radial nerve at the proximal third of radius. **c** Completed approach. (From Crenshaw 1980)

extremity as in the lower extremity; therefore, even on the curved upper and middle thirds of the radius, application on the anterior or anterolateral surface will not compromise the final results.

4. The technique is relatively easy if precise attention to detail is followed. Remember, an upper-third radial fracture in close proximity to the elbow joint requires a generous incision, extending proximal to the anterior elbow crease. Otherwise, the surgeon will be working in a small "hole" and may damage the important neural structures in the area.

Posterior Approaches. The posterior approach of Thompson (Thompson 1918; Fig. 9.6) is especially suitable for the middle third of the radius, and we occasionally use this. However, it is not suitable for distal-third radial fractures because the posterolateral application of the plate may interfere with the outcropping tendons to the thumb, disturbing their function. Fractures of the upper third of the radius and ulna may also be

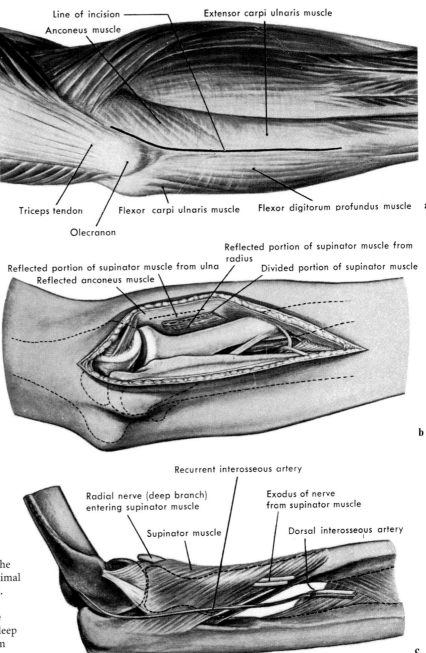

Line of incision
Anconeus muscle
Extensor carpi ulnaris muscle

Triceps tendon
Flexor carpi ulnaris muscle
Flexor digitorum profundus muscle   **a**
Olecranon

Reflected portion of supinator muscle from radius
Reflected portion of supinator muscle from ulna
Divided portion of supinator muscle
Reflected anconeus muscle

b

Recurrent interosseous artery

Radial nerve (deep branch) entering supinator muscle
Exodus of nerve from supinator muscle

Supinator muscle
Dorsal interosseous artery

c

Fig. 9.7 a–c. The Boyd approach to the proximal third of the ulna and proximal fourth of the radius. **a** Skin incision. **b** Approach has been completed. **c** Relation of the deep branch of the radial nerve to the superficial and deep parts of the supinator muscle. (From Crenshaw 1980)

approached by the Boyd technique (Boyd 1940; Fig. 9.7). Care must be taken in this approach to avoid injury to the radial nerve; therefore, it cannot be recommended for routine use.

9.3.4.3 Reduction Techniques

Once the bone has been exposed, great care must be taken to preserve all possible soft tissue attachments during reduction of the fracture. Normally, there is some periosteum stripped by the injury itself, and the surgeon should not add to this stripping. The ideal is achieving the necessary anatomical reduction with minimal soft tissue stripping. Early surgery and the use of indirect reduction techniques will usually allow retention of soft tissue (Fig. 9.8). Especially important is maintaining the periosteal attachment to butterfly fragments (Mast et al. 1989).

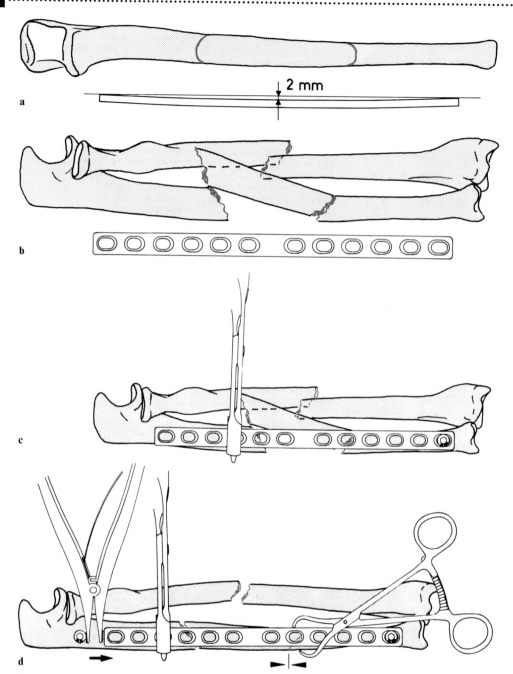

Fig. 9.8. a, b The ulna is more or less straight along its dorsal surface, which is the surface most amenable to plate fixation. From the olecranon distally it presents a slight concavity, then it is straight or gently bowed dorsally until the disalmost portion just proximal to the styloid process. Here again a slight concavity is present. A straight 3.5-cm mini-DCP is compatible with most ulnas. Occasionally, in a large man, the standard DCP should be used. In cases in which indirect reduction is carried out, the ulnar plate is first contoured to provide a very slight amount of concavity to the bone surface of the plate, sufficient to arch the plate away from the straight surface by about 2–3 mm at the apex (**b**). This technique is most useful where a segmental fracture or a large amount of comminution is present. The plate to be used is usually long: 12–16 holes or longer for the 3.5-mm DCP, 8–12 holes for the standard DCP. A

very small amount of convexity in its distalmost portion should be imparted to the bone surface of the plate if it extends to the level of the base of the ulnar styloid. **c** The plate is applied as shown and fixed with a distal screw. A Verbrugge clamp holds the proximal fragments. Care is taken to preserve all blood supply, especially to the segmental fragments. **d** A "push-pull" screw is placed off the proximal end of the plate at a distance of 1 cm from the end of the plate. A medium bone spreader is placed between the push-pull screw head and the end of the plate. Distraction of the plate is carried out. Because of the intact soft tissues, the segmental fracture tends to reduce into the gap between the proximal and distal main fragments. The reduction is fine tuned with the dental pick and held in place with the small pointed reduction forceps (From Mast et al. 1989)

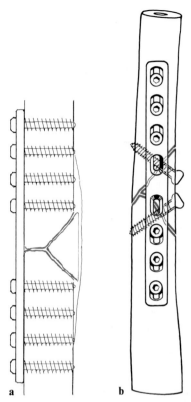

Fig. 9.9. a If the cortex to cortex anatomic reduction can be obtained, the comminuted fragments may be left to ensure rapid bone union. **b** However, if anatomic reduction cannot be obtained, the more traditional technique of fixation of the comminuted fragments is desirable

If cortex to cortex reduction can be achieved, anatomical reduction is assured and the butterfly fragment may be left with its soft tissues (Fig. 9.9 a). Union will usually be rapid. If the comminution involves the entire cortex, then the older techniques of anatomical reduction must be followed (see Fig. 9.9 b).

Indirect reduction is achieved by traction. Direct traction on the fracture without disturbing the soft tissue is achieved by the use of a distractor or traction through a plate (see Fig 9.8 a–d). Forearm clamps should be relatively small and with minimal bulk, such as pointed reduction clamps on the fracture, or a Verbrugge forearm plate for holding the implant (Fig. 9.8 c,d).

9.3.4.4 Technique of Fracture Fixation

a) Principles of Stable Fixation

As previously indicated, to obtain maximum function the surgeon must achieve anatomical reduction and stable internal fixation. Stable internal fixation may be achieved by internal splinting with intramedullary devices or by compression. In the lower extremity, especially the femur, intramedullary fixation is a mainstay of treatment. However, in the forearm, intramedullary devices do not control rotational stability and should therefore rarely be used (Fig. 9.10). Therefore, *compression,* with interfragmental screws or plates under tension, is the method of choice.

b) Methods by Fracture Type

Transverse or Short Oblique Fractures. If the fracture of the radius or ulna is either transverse or short and oblique, a plate under tension may be used to compress the fracture; i.e., the plate is under tension, the fracture under compression. In the forearm, where exposure is often limited, *low contact dynamic compression (LCDC) plates* should be used wherever possible, making the tension device unnecessary.

The application of a plate under tension in a transverse fracture, if carried out correctly, will afford compression to the fracture, thereby stabilizing it and allowing early motion (Fig. 9.11). The same is true of the short oblique fracture. However, in all cases where the obliquity of the fracture allows, a lag screw should be inserted through the plate across the fracture to increase rotational stability (Fig. 9.12).

Spiral Fractures. For spiral fractures, the obliquity is such that one or two lag screws can be used to obtain anatomical reduction, followed by a neutralization plate. An alternative method is to use two carefully placed cerclage wires with minimal soft tissue dissection, followed by a neutralization plate (Fig. 9.13 a–c).

Comminuted Fractures. To achieve anatomical reduction and preserve the soft tissue attachment to bone in comminuted fractures is more difficult. Indirect reduction techniques, as described, should be used (see Figs. 9.8, 9.13). Once the length of the bone has been restored, and the final reduction is achieved, the fracture should be plated without disturbing the soft tissue. If comminution involves the entire shaft, then interfragmental compression with lag screws remains the keystone of treatment, remembering at all times to preserve the soft tissue attachment to the fragments, if possible.

Once interfragmental compression has been achieved, a neutralization plate must be applied to protect the stability of the fracture. Wherever possible, lag screws should be used through the plate and across any of the fracture lines, either in the spiral fracture or in the comminuted fracture, to increase the stability of the system (see Fig. 9.12).

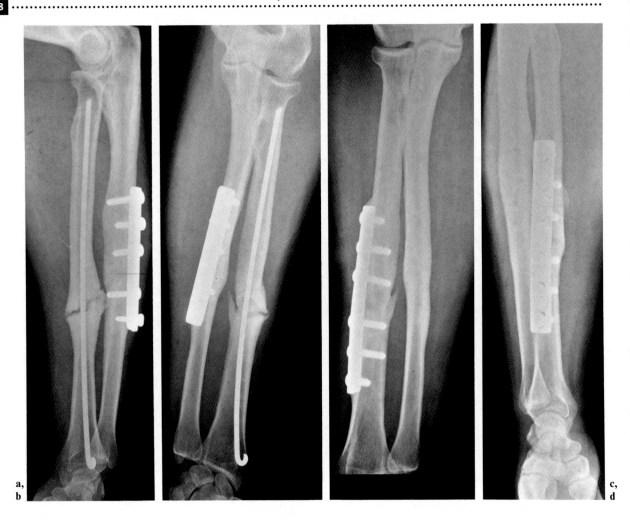

a,
b

c,
d

Fig. 9.10 a–d. Intermedullary splinting of the radius. **a** Lateral and **b** anteroposterior radiographs at 9 months following open reduction and internal fixation of a fracture of both bones of the forearm. The ulna has been plated and has healed, although the distal screw in the plate is loose. The radius was treated with a Rush intermedullary rod and has not united. At this time, the patient had pain on movement and tenderness at the site. The rod was removed and a six-hole dynamic compression (DC) plate applied to this hypertrophic nonunion; the ulnar plate was removed at the same time. **c, d** Complete bony union 1 year after the second operative procedure

c) Implant Selection

For most patients, the 3.5-mm DC or LCDC plates, with 3.5-mm cortical screws in cortex and 4-mm cancellous screws in the metaphysis are the implants of choice. Occasionally in large patients, the narrow 4.5-mm plates may be used.

The length of the plate will depend on the degree of inherent stability in the fracture, as well as the size of the implant and screws. Therefore, comminuted fractures require longer implants to achieve adequate stability and prevent early mechanical overload and failure. In general, at least six to eight cortices into intact diaphysis are necessary for adequate stability, which in comminuted fractures may require an eight- to 12-hole plate. To achieve maximum stability with the long plates, the screws must be inserted at the ends of the plate and as close to the fracture as possible without interfering with the blood supply (Fig. 9.14).

The 3.5-mm DC plates are not only smaller in width and thickness, but also shorter than their counterparts in the larger DC series; for example, an eight-hole large DC plate is 135 mm long, whereas an eight-hole small DC plate is only 97 mm long, as shown in Fig. 9.15 a. Also, the 3.5-mm DC screw has less holding power; therefore, more screws are required to achieve stable fixation (Fig. 9.15 b). A new 3.5-mm cortical screw has recently been introduced and is recommended for use with the 3.5-mm DC plate in the forearm. The holding power of the screw is increased by a larger shank

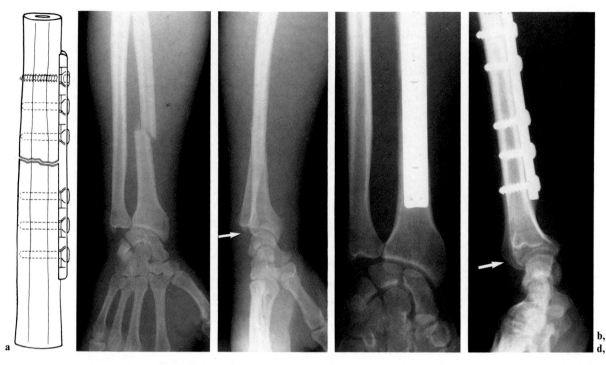

Fig. 9.11 a–e. Fixation of a transverse fracture with a dynamic compression (DC) plate. **a** Application of a six-hole DC plate to a fracture of the radius or ulna. **b** Anteroposterior and **c** lateral radiographs of a 21-year-old man with a displaced fracture of the radius and a subluxation of the distal radioulnar joint *(arrow)*. **d, e** Osteosynthesis of this transverse fracture at 1 year. Primary bone union is complete, the functional result excellent

(2.7 mm) and more threads per length. The instrumentation is characterized by a new 2.5-mm drill. All of the instrumentation has a bronze coloration.

In those instances where small DC plates are chosen, one must be certain that the plate has sufficient length to neutralize the bending forces present and allow firm and rigid immobilization of the fracture. In tall individuals for whom the small 3.5-mm DC plate is chosen, an eight- to 12-hole plate is essential, allowing for the fixation of a minimum of seven cortices on each side of the fracture (see Fig. 9.14). This will provide adequate holding of the plate for a sufficient length of time to allow both early motion of the extremity and sound union of the fracture. Use of the wrong implant may prejudice an otherwise excellent open reduction, as shown in Fig. 9.16, and lead to early failure of the osteosynthesis.

The LCDC plate has many experimental advantages, especially in open fractures. Since the plate surface is indirect and contact between the plate and the bone is kept to a minimum, loss of blood supply to the cortex is minimized (see Fig. 9.17). Most of the cortex remains viable, a marked advantage in open fractures.

Fig. 9.12. Application of a lag screw through the plate and across an oblique fracture, wherever possible, to increase the strength of the fixation

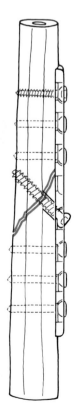

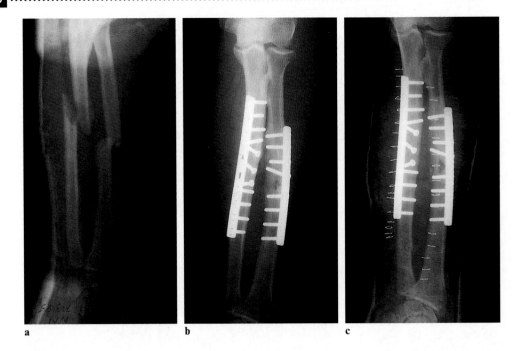

a   b   c

Fig. 9.13. a Radiograph of a forearm fracture. Spiral type ulna and transverse comminuted radius. **b** The ulna was fixed with lag screws and a neutralization plate, the radius with a neutralization plate spanning the comminuted area to preserve its blood supply. **c** The end result at 18 months is excellent

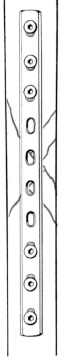

Fig. 9.14. For maximum stability with a long plate on a comminuted fracture, the screw holes at the end of the plate as well as those closest to the fracture must be filled

d) Site of Plate Application

The ulnar plate is applied to the medial border (Fig. 9.18). Occasionally, removal of bony irregularities from this surface will aid in the placement of the plate.

The radial plate application will depend on the surgeon's choice of incision. Since we favor the anterior approach, the radial plate is applied ideally to the flat surface of the lower third of that bone. Through this same anterior approach the plate may be fixed to the anterior or lateral surface of the middle third and the anterior surface of the upper third. Occasionally, difficulty may be encountered in applying the plate laterally through the anterior incision. If posterior approaches are preferred, especially in the middle third of the radius, the plates are fixed to the lateral or dorsolateral surfaces.

e) Bone Grafts

Bone grafts are rarely required in the forearm, if concepts of biological fixation are followed. However, if marked comminution is present with some loss of soft tissues or actual bone loss, as in an open fracture, then a cancellous bone graft is indicated.

The bone graft must not be placed along lacerations in the interosseous membrane, as this may favor a cross-union; it should be placed at sites distant from that membrane, to fill all gaps in the bone and to bridge the fracture (Fig. 9.19 a). Cancellous grafting is especially indicated if there has been significant bone loss in open fractures. In

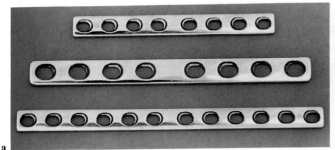
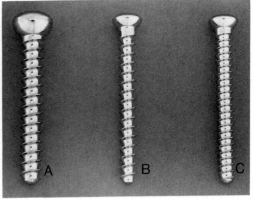

Fig. 9.15. a An eight-hole 3.5-mm dynamic compression (DC) plate, an eight-hole 4.5-mm DC plate, and a 12-hole 3.5-mm DC plate. Note that the length of the 12-hole 3.5-mm plate is approximately equal to that of the eight-hole 4.5-mm DC plate, whereas the eight-hole 3.5-mm DC plate is much shorter. **b** A 4.5-mm cortical screw *(A)*, a 3.5-mm cancellous screw *(B)*, and the new 3.5-mm cortical screw *(C)*

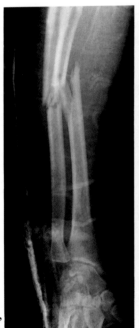
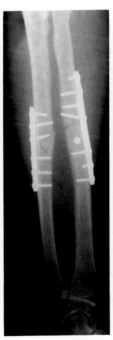
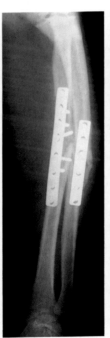
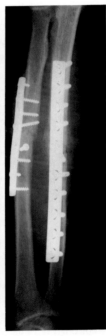
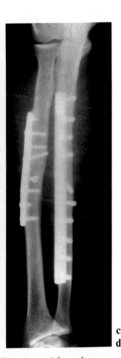

Fig. 9.16 a–e. A short 3.5-mm DC plate on the ulna, resulting in failure. **a** Anteroposterior radiograph of a forearm fracture in a tall 21-year-old man **(b).** The radius was fixed with an eight-hole 3.5-mm DC plate and an interfragmental compression screw. The ulna was fixed with a six-hole 3.5-mm DC plate, with no fixation in the butterfly fragment. Note the short plate compared with the relatively long ulna, allowing a long lever-arm effect. **c** Displacement of the fracture at 10 weeks. **c** Marked limitation of pronation–supination ensued in spite of plaster immobilization. **d** At that time, further surgery on the ulna allowed anatomical reduction and application of a 12-hole 3.5-mm DC plate. No immobilization was necessary; good forearm rotation returned. **e** The final result at 18 months

these instances we prefer internal fixation with a plate to bridge the gap and the use of a cancellous bone graft, usually applied on the fifth to seventh day into a granulating wound, to ensure union (Fig. 9.19 b–e).

On rare occasions, however, an external frame may be used. This method may be applied to the forearm, but it is not recommended, except for comminuted fractures of the distal end of the radius and contaminated open fractures with or without sepsis. If external fixation is used as the definitive treatment in diaphyseal fractures, bone grafting should be used to minimize the risk of nonunion.

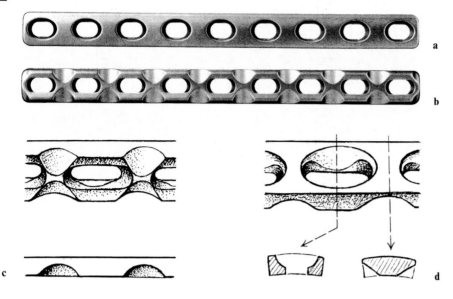

Fig. 9.17 a–d. The LCDC plate. **a** The surface of the plate. **b** The undersurface of the plate. **c** Note the oblique undercuts at both ends of each screw hole. This permits a tilting of the screw of 40° maximum in each direction in the long axis of the bone. **d** Note the trapezoid cross section of the plate and the undercuts between the screw holes. The different undercuts greatly reduce the contact area between the plate and the bone

f) Wound Closure

Skin closure must be carried out using a meticulous atraumatic technique and with no tension. Suction drainage will reduce hematoma formation and is always used postoperatively, where possible. Not infrequently, in fractures of both bones of the forearm, swelling of the forearm muscles makes closure of one incision without tension difficult. Under these circumstances, we do not hesitate to leave a portion of one wound open, even if it leaves a part of the implant exposed. This has been frequent in our practice; therefore, patients should be informed that they may require a secondary closure of one wound. The ulnar wound, located so close to the subcutaneous border, should always be closed. The radial wound, over soft tissues, may be safely left open throughout a portion of its length, since careful placement of the metal implant will bury it under a muscle cover. With early functional rehabilitation, the swelling rapidly disappears from the arm, and it is usually a simple matter to close the wound on the fifth to the seventh postoperative day with sterile tapes or fine sutures. Open treatment of the tense wound prevents necrosis secondary to pressure, prevents sepsis, and has little deleterious cosmetic effect.

Postoperative Care. If, at the end of the procedure, the surgeon feels that anatomical reduction with stable fixation has been accomplished, then early functional rehabilitation should be started. A bulky bandage is applied to the forearm with no plaster cast, and the patient is allowed to move elbow, wrist, and fingers in the immediate postoperative period. In the first 48 h, the arm is elevated on a pillow or a stockinette support and suspended from an intravenous drip pole. The support is

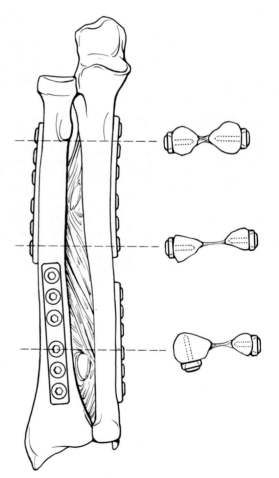

Fig. 9.18. Site of plate application

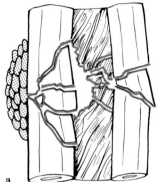

Fig. 9.19a–e. Bone grafts to forearm. **a** The graft should be placed on the surface of the bone opposite the interosseous membrane, which is usually torn, to prevent cross-union. **b** Anteroposterior and **c** lateral radiographs of a 39-year-old police officer who was struck by a bullet and sustained a fracture of his radius. Initial treatment was débridment, open wound treatment, and fixation with pins and plate. Upon referral at 12 weeks, the pins were removed, and after wound healing, a plate was applied to the anterior surface of the radius. **d, e** A massive cancellous bone graft allowed sound union of this fracture and a good functional result

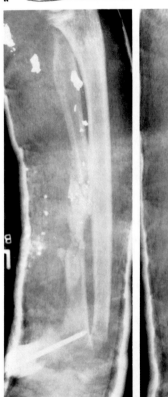
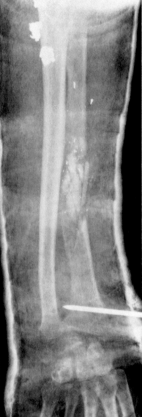
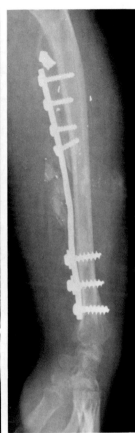
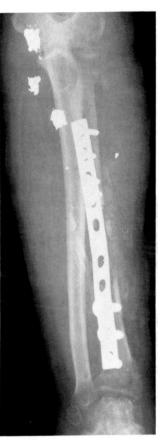

b,
c

d,
e

removed for elbow and wrist exercises. With stable fixation only soft tissue pain is present, and this quickly disappears from the wound area, making early restoration of function the rule. Even in those instances where one wound cannot be closed this program should be instituted, since exercise will reduce swelling and allow early secondary closure.

If the surgeon is concerned about the stability of one or both bones because of comminution or poor bone quality, then the bulky postoperative dressing may be removed on the seventh day and replaced with a small functional forearm splint, as described by Sarmiento et al. (1975). This will allow early motion and still afford protection to the internal fixation.

If the fixation is deemed to be stable, the patient should be encouraged to use the arm for all reasonable activities, but should not, prior to evidence of bony union, take part in sporting activities or do any heavy lifting. The patient should be seen at regular intervals, usually monthly, and follow-up radiographs should be taken. With stable internal fixation, the precise time of bone union is difficult to determine. If no untoward radiographic signs of failure are present, such as irritation callus, bone resorption at the fracture site, or loosening of the screws, and if no clinical signs of failure such as inflammation and pain appear, one may assume that healing is proceeding normally. Radiographic evidence of the fracture line disappearing with no evidence of irritation callus is a positive indication of union. The average time for union to occur will be 8–12 weeks, with delays often arising in markedly comminuted fractures requiring bone grafts. Once union has occurred, the patient is encouraged to resume his or her normal life style.

9.4 Special Considerations

9.4.1 Fractures of Both Bones of the Forearm

Definitive fixation of either fracture should not be carried out prior to the provisional stabilization of both. If either the radius or the ulna is firmly and rigidly fixed before careful reduction of the other fracture, reduction may prove impossible (Fig. 9.20 a). Therefore, we usually provisionally expose and fix the fracture that appears

simpler, either by location (e.g., the ulna rather than the radius) or by its nature (e.g., the transverse or oblique as opposed to the comminuted). Once the first fracture has been carefully exposed using small Hohmann retractors and provisionally fixed with a plate held in place by small reduction or Verbrugge clamps, the other bone is exposed and provisionally fixed in a similar manner (Fig. 9.20 b). At this time the surgeon may proceed with definitive fixation of the fracture.

9.4.2 Fractures of One Bone

9.4.2.1 Fractures of the Radius with Distal Radioulnar Subluxation (Galeazzi)

Displaced fractures of the radius associated with some disruption of the distal radioulnar joint (Fig. 9.21) should be treated by open anatomical reduction and stable fixation (see Fig. 9.11 b–e). This will restore the length of the radius, which in turn ensures the accurate reduction of the distal radioulnar joint, provided prop-

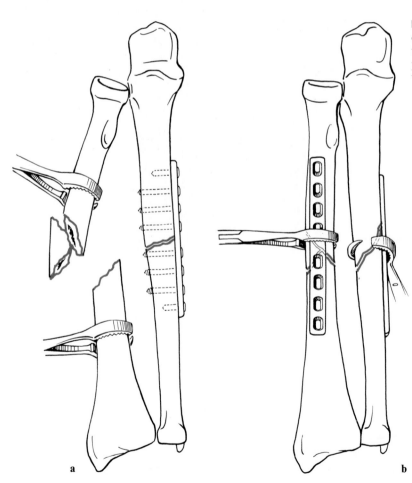

Fig. 9.20. a Fixation of one bone, in this case the ulna, will prevent reduction of the other. **b** Reduction of both bones prior to firm fixation is essential to prevent this intraoperative complication

a   b

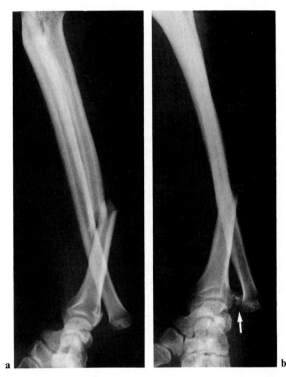

a   b

Fig. 9.21 a, b. Anteroposterior and lateral radiographs of a fracture of the radius with a distal radioulnar subluxation. Note the small intra-articular fracture from the distal ulna *(arrow)*. Open reduction and internal fixation of this fracture are essential

er rotation has been restored. In most cases, no specific treatment is required for this distal injury. If a fracture has occurred through the distal ulna, either through its styloid or distal portion, open reduction and screw fixation in that area will serve to stabilize the distal injury. In most cases, however, the injury occurs through soft tissue, and if the anatomy of the radius is restored by proper open reduction and stable internal fixation, the soft tissues of the distal radioulnar joint will usually heal without major functional impairment. It is essential that the distal ulna is in anatomical position at the end of the fixation procedure for the radius as it can remain dislocated. If it is irreducible and the surgeon is certain that the radius is anatomical, then the distal radial–ulna joint must be operated upon, as the likely cause is soft tissue interposition (tendon or capsule) (Fig. 9.22). The approach, techniques, and implants are as previously described for radial fractures.

Primary wound closure for a solitary radial fracture is usually easy to accomplish and open wound care is rarely required, except for an open fracture.

If stability has been achieved in the radius, the postoperative program consists of a large bulky dressing on the forearm with elevation for the first 48 h and immediate encouragement of elbow, wrist, and hand motion. Patients may be moderately uncomfortable with a wrist injury, but we have not found the use of postoperative splinting to be necessary in most cases.

However, if the distal radioulnar joint is unstable following fixation of the radial fracture, the forearm should be immobilized in supination for 6 weeks.

9.4.2.2 Fractures of the Ulna

a) With Associated Radioulnar Dislocation (Monteggia)

Fractures of the ulna with associated radial head dislocations must be fixed by open anatomical reduction and stable internal fixation to achieve satisfactory results (Fig. 9.23). If the ulna is not anatomically reduced, the radial head will remain in a subluxed position (Fig. 9.24).

In most cases, following anatomical reduction and stable fixation of the ulna, the radial head will anatomically reduce and remain stable (Table 9.1). Therefore, following fixation of the ulna by techniques and implants already described, the surgeon should immediately examine elbow function. Using the image intensifier while the patient is under general anesthetic, he or she should determine the position of stability for the radial head. If the radial head is stable in all positions, then the postoperative program consists of early active motion of the extremity with no external splints.

If the radial head is unstable in various degrees of rotation or extension but stable at 90° of flexion, this

Table 9.1. Treatment of a Monteggia fracture

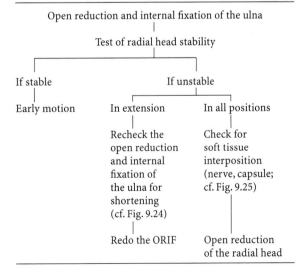

Open reduction and internal fixation of the ulna

Test of radial head stability

If stable	If unstable	
Early motion	In extension	In all positions
	Recheck the open reduction and internal fixation of the ulna for shortening (cf. Fig. 9.24)	Check for soft tissue interposition (nerve, capsule; cf. Fig. 9.25)
	Redo the ORIF	Open reduction of the radial head

146 ·

Chapter 9   **Fractures of the Radius and Ulna**

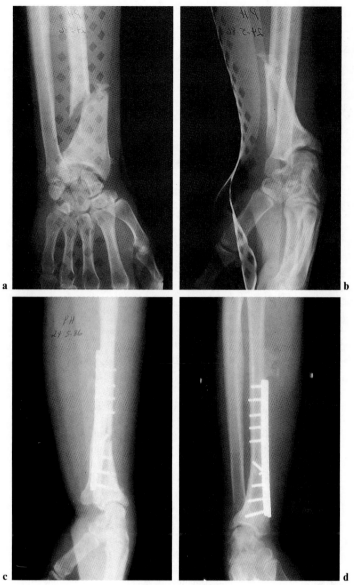

Fig. 9.22 a–d. Irreducible distal radio-ulna joint after ORIF of Galeazzi fracture. **a** Anteroposterior and **b** lateral radiographs of typical fracture of the radius with posterior dislocation of the ulna at the wrist. **c** Intraoperative radiograph showing excellent reduction of the radius, but a persistent dislocation of the distal radioulnar joint. An incision over the distal ulna revealed that the ulnar head had button-holed through the capsule. **d** After reduction, the end result was excellent

usually indicates a malreduced ulna (Fig. 9.24). Either the ulnar length has not been restored or the rotation is not anatomical. The only logical method of dealing with this problem is the "bite the bullet" syndrome, i.e., to take apart the ulnar fixation, start again, and ensure an anatomical reduction. The radioulnar subluxation should reduce fully and be stable in all positions. Occasionally, if concern continues, a cast brace to limit extension in the postoperative period may be used.

If, however, the radial head cannot be reduced or is grossly unstable in all positions except extreme flexion, then a direct operative approach should be made to the radial head to remove any soft tissue interposition – usually a torn annular ligament, but occasionally the radial nerve (Fig. 9.25). The radial head may be approached directly through a separate approach or by extending the ulnar incision proximally toward the lateral epicondyle of the humerus. This posterior approach, reflecting the anconeus and extensor muscle origins anterolaterally, is safe, as it protects the radial nerve. After adequate exposure, the soft tissue interposition must be removed and the radial head reduced. After repair of the annular ligament, the stability of the radial head may be checked under direct vision, and if it is stable, early motion may be instituted, with or without a cast brace.

Gross instability of the radial head occurs in less than 10 % of Monteggia fractures, so those instances requiring an open approach to the elbow are relatively few.

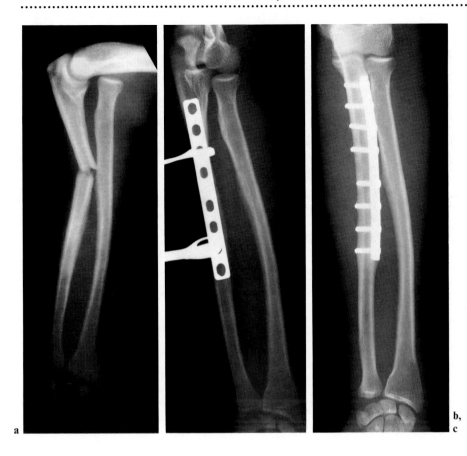

a   b, c

Fig. 9.23 a–c. Fracture of the ulna with dislocation of the proximal radioulnar joint (Monteggia fracture). **a** Radiograph showing a displaced fracture of the ulna with a dislocated radial head. **b** Intraoperative radiograph showing anatomical reduction of the ulna with perfect position of the radial head. **c** At 1 year, sound primary bone union is seen following application of an eight-hole 3.5-mm dynamic compression (DC) plate. Note the perfect position of the radial head. Function in this 22-year-old engineering student was excellent. An injury to the radial nerve at the time of injury recovered in 3 months with no operative intervention to the nerve

However, Monteggia fractures have shown a greater tendency to result in permanent elbow stiffness than any other forearm fracture, as may be expected. Proper reduction of the ulna to restore proximal radioulnar stability and perhaps, in the future, the use of continuous passive motion in the immediate postoperative period may improve these functional results.

b) With Fracture of the Radial Head

In rare instances, a fracture of the shaft of the ulna may be associated with a fracture-dislocation of the radial head. Under these circumstances, the fragments of the radial head may act as a block to pronation and supination and may also prevent stabilization of the proximal radioulnar joint. Therefore, it is almost mandatory to open the elbow joint in this situation and inspect the fracture. If a single fragment is involved, it should be replaced with a lag screw to restore stability of the radial head. If the fracture is grossly comminuted, the only alternative method of treatment available is excision of the radial head and, if necessary, replacement with a silastic or metal radial-head spacer to maintain the stability of the radius until soft tissue healing has occurred (Fig. 9.26).

In summary, the Monteggia fracture is a most challenging forearm injury for the surgeon. Stable anatomical fixation will restore ulnar length. A careful appraisal of the proximal radioulnar joint will aid the surgeon in choosing the most appropriate technique for dealing with the injury and will allow a program of early functional rehabilitation.

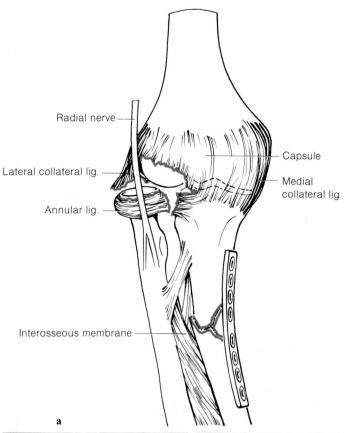

Radial nerve

Lateral collateral lig.

Annular lig.

Capsule

Medial collateral lig.

Interosseous membrane

a

Fig. 9.24a–e. Malreduction of the ulna, causing continuing subluxation of the radial head.
a A fracture of the ulna plated in a valgus position. The radial head remains subluxated.
b Radiograph of a comminuted fracture of the ulna with a displaced radial head. **c** An open reduction and internal fixation of the ulnar fracture resulted in a valgus position, in spite of interfragmental screws and a neutralization plate *(arrowhead)*. Note the subluxation of the head of the radius *(arrow)*. **d** The fracture was allowed to heal with persistent subluxation of the radial head *(arrow)*. **e** Lateral view of the ulnar fracture and its flexed position. The patient had continuing pain in his elbow joint

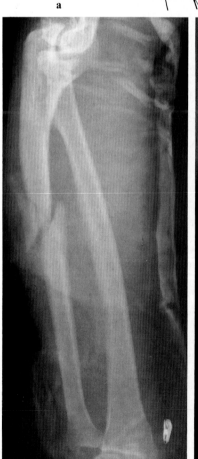

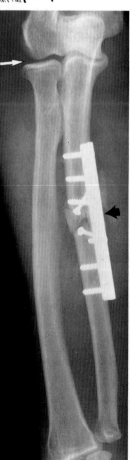

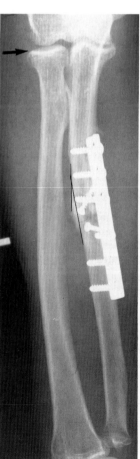

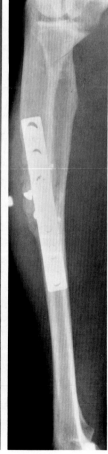

b,
c

d,
e

The postoperative program for these individuals will, of course, vary with the ability of the surgeon to achieve stability of the distal radial fracture. Motion of the elbow and the fingers should always be encouraged. It is only the wrist function that may be compromised in this situation.

9.4.3 Fractures of the Forearm in Adolescents

Most forearm fractures in children should be managed by closed means, whereas almost all such fractures in adults require open treatment. Remodeling of a bone following a fracture in a child is dependent on several factors, including the proximity of the fracture to the joint, the direction of deformity, and the age of the patient. The greatest correction is possible in fractures close to the joint with deformities in the line of joint motion, for example, dorsal angulation in the radius; also, the younger the child, the greater the potential for remodeling.

A diaphyseal forearm fracture is distant from the joint, and the greatest deformity is often rotatory; therefore, there is little chance of complete remodeling in children approaching adolescence. The presence of an open epiphysis will not guarantee a good result by closed means. The surgeon must assess the growth potential of the patient, as in scoliosis management. If growth is unlikely to result in adequate remodeling in the time remaining, then open reduction and internal fixation should be performed.

Most girls over the age of 10 and most boys over the age of 12 are better treated by internal fixation to ensure a perfect functional result, allowances being made, of course, for individual differences.

9.4.4 Open Fractures of the Forearm

The indications for open reduction in the forearm are so strong that we do not vary our technique for an open fracture. The general principles in the management of all open fractures apply. Careful cleansing and débridement are mandatory. Once these have been achieved, we proceed immediately to open anatomical reduction and internal fixation. We feel that the advantages of early stable fixation in the open forearm fracture greatly outweigh the theoretical disadvantages. If exemplary soft tissue management is carried out, there is no increased risk of sepsis. However, the importance of the soft tissue management cannot be overemphasized. If the wound is small, careful assessment of the soft tissues is required in order to choose the appropriate approach. After stabilization of the fracture, the surgical incisions should be closed but the small puncture wound left open.

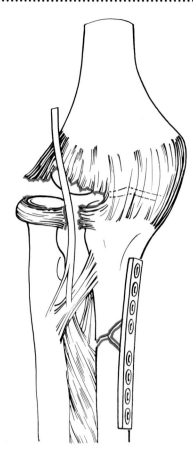

Fig. 9.25. Entrapment of the radial nerve preventing complete reduction of the radial head

c) With Distal Periarticular Radius Fracture

Fractures of the shaft of the ulna associated with distal radial epiphyseal fractures are relatively uncommon, but difficult to manage when they occur. The ulnar shaft fracture does not usually pose a major problem and should be treated as previously indicated. However, the distal radial metaphyseal fracture is often comminuted, unstable, and difficult to fix. If stable fixation of the radius is not achieved, early motion cannot be started, and problems of wrist stiffness and shortening of the radius are common (Fig. 9.27).

Therefore, the distal fracture of the radius requires careful evaluation. If the fracture is not grossly comminuted and the surgeon feels that internal fixation is possible, then this is the ideal treatment. The preferred appliance is the small buttress plate (Fig. 9.28).

In many circumstances, however, the fracture of the distal end of the radius is too grossly comminuted to support a buttress plate. In such cases we favor the use of an external fixation device to maintain continuous traction of the fracture while healing progresses, usually for a period of 6–8 weeks (Fig. 9.29).

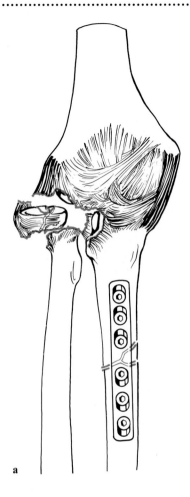

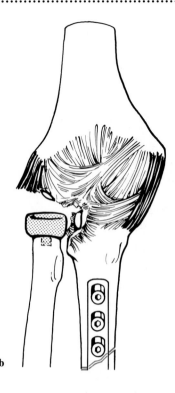

a

b

Fig. 9.26 a, b. Fracture of the proximal ulna with fracture of the radial head and neck. **a** A proximal ulnar fracture with a fracture of the radial neck with intra-articular extension. If the fracture of the radial head is comminuted, the ulnar fracture should be fixed internally and the radial head excised, and if unstable, it should be replaced with a radial head prosthesis (**b**)

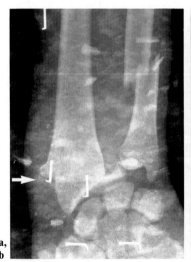

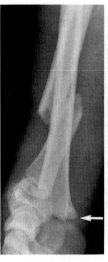

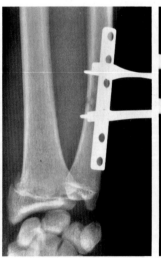

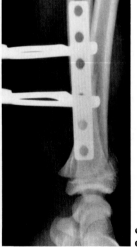

a, b

c, d

Fig. 9.27 a–d. Fracture of the ulna with distal periarticular radial fracture. **a** Anteroposterior and **b** lateral radiographs of a fracture of the distal ulna and an epiphyseal separation of the distal radius in a 16-year-old boy. **c, d** Intraoperative radiographs indicating the dorsal displacement of the radial epiphysis, even with anatomical reduction of the ulna

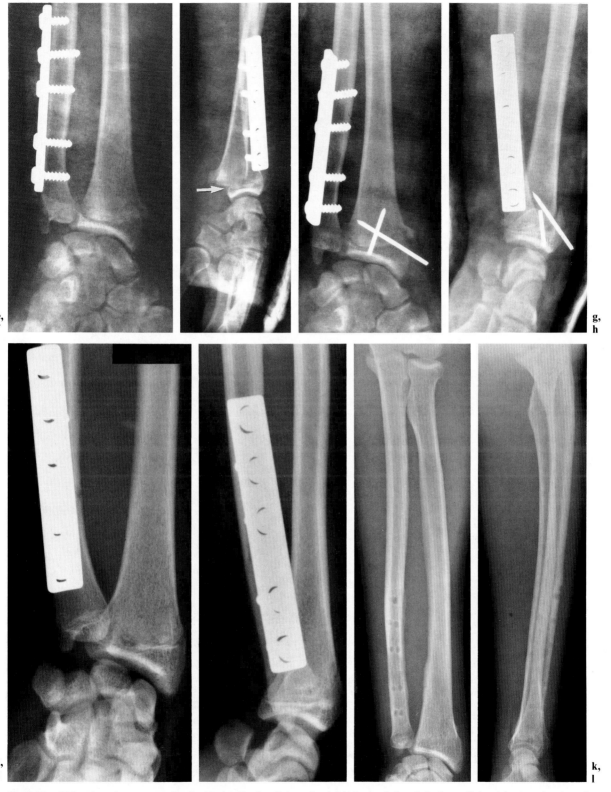

Fig. 9.27. e, f The ulnar fracture was fixed with the distal radial epiphysis displaced 30°. **g, h** Because this patient was almost at the end of his growth, the position was deemed inadequate and an open reduction and internal fixation using Kirschner wires was performed. Reduction was difficult because the ulna was fixed. **i, j** The healed and closing radial epiphysis and union of the ulnar fracture. **k, l** At 2 years the ulnar plate was removed. Note the anatomical reduction of the radius and ulna. At this time, function was excellent

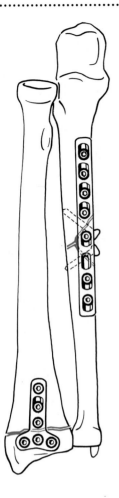

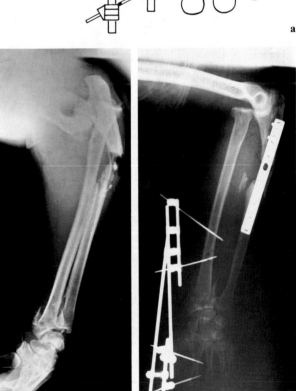

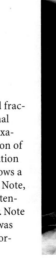

Fig. 9.28. Use of a buttress plate on the distal radius

Fig. 9.29 a–c. Fracture of the ulna with a comminuted fracture of the distal radius. **a** Open reduction and internal fixation of the ulnar fracture, with external skeletal fixation of the distal radial fracture. **b** Severe comminution of the distal radius, with bone loss and severe comminution of the proximal ulnar fracture. **c** The distal radius shows a satisfactory reduction with external skeletal fixation. Note, however, that the malreduction of the ulna with shortening has allowed the radial head to displace anteriorly. Note also the fracture in the radial head. Further surgery was required to lengthen the ulna, correct the flexion deformity, and allow stabilization of the radial head

b,
c

If the wound is large, with varying degrees of skin and soft tissue loss, we again proceed with the necessary fracture stabilization as soon as possible (Fig. 9.30). Careful preoperative planning is essential so that, wherever possible, the metal implant is buried under viable muscle. The skin is left open and covered with a gauze dressing to prevent drying. The patient is returned to the operating room on the third to the fifth postoperative day and the wound inspected.

If there has been no skin loss, and the wound is clean and granulating at that time, wound closure using fine sutures or sterile strips is effected over suction drainage. If the wound is not suitable for resuturing, it is left to granulate by secondary intention or covered by a split-thickness skin graft when it is ready.

If skin was lost at the time of injury, closure may be carried out by split-thickness grafting or other techniques, depending on the depth and extent of the wound. A healthy layer of granulating tissue must, of course, have covered the wound before a skin grafting procedure can be attempted.

In cases with bone loss we prefer to delay the bone-grafting procedure until the first or second dressing change, between the fifth and tenth day after trauma. At that time, only cancellous bone graft may be inserted through the open wound, if it is clean and granulating. No cortical bone must be used, as it does not resist infection well. Again, as previously discussed, if there is no skin loss the wound is closed over suction drainage, but if there is skin loss and a layer of granulating tissue has appeared, the appropriate cover can be used, as outlined above. Occasionally, with complex bone and deep soft tissue muscle loss, a free myocutaneous–osseous flap may be indicated. With or without skin closure, early functional rehabilitation is started. If the fracture fixation is firm, finger and wrist motion is started within 48 h. If a gap exists at the fracture site, or the degree of comminution prejudices the stability of the system, then a simple functional forearm splint will be sufficient to allow early motion.

We have used these techniques even in the face of grossly contaminated wounds with few ill effects, as noted in the large combined series from our center, Sunnybrook in Toronto, and Harborview in Seattle, reported by Moed et al. (1986; Duncan et al. 1992).

In summary, we feel that the management of open fractures of the forearm should consist of the following principles:

- Careful cleansing of the soft tissues and bone
- Antitetanus and antibiotic treatment, instituted immediately
- Careful cleansing and débridement of the soft tissues in the operating room
- Anatomical open reduction and stable fixation of the fractures
- Open management of the soft tissues, with the metal implants buried under muscle where possible
- Secondary skin closure or skin grafting where indicated and secondary bone grafting where necessary
- With major muscle loss, complex myocutaneous or composite myocutaneous–osseous free flaps
- Early functional rehabilitation of the extremity

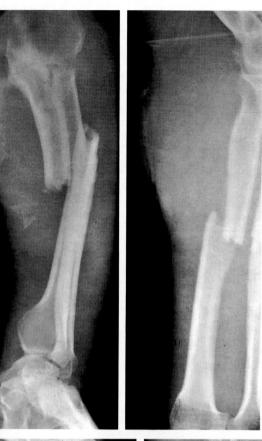

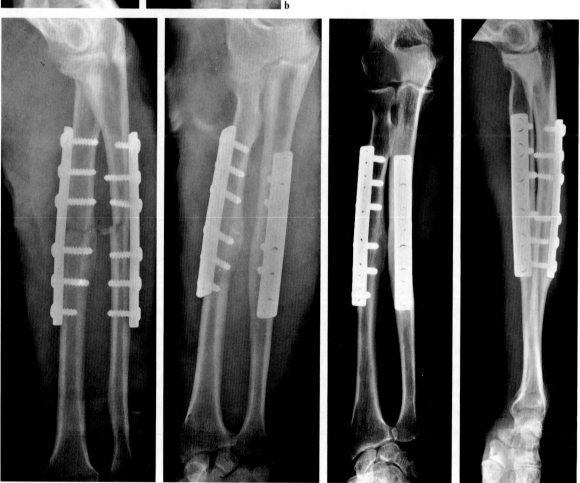

Fig. 9.30 a–h. Open fracture of the forearm. **a** Anteroposterior and **b** lateral radiographs of a 51-year-old man who caught his hand in a garbage incinerator, causing a major soft tissue avulsion and fractures of both bones of the forearm. **c,d** Following thorough cleansing and débridement, both fractures were plated primarily. **e,f** The fractures united in 16 weeks with no evidence of sepsis. The soft tissue lesion was managed with split-thickness skin grafting on the tenth day and primary closure where possible.

g,h The appearance of the forearm is noted with the arm in full ▶ pronation (**g**) and in full supination (**h**)

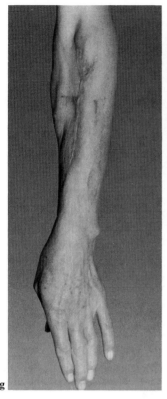

g

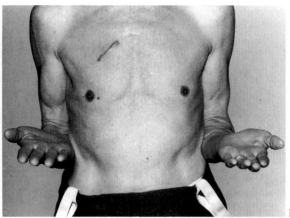

h

9.5 Complications

9.5.1 Radioulnar Synostosis

Radioulnar synostosis is an unfortunate complication that may occur with 1%–8% of fractures of the forearm and may greatly distress both the patient and the surgeon. Among our first 60 reported cases we had two examples (Tile and Petrie 1969). Anderson et al. (1975) reported an incidence of 1.2%, and Teipner and Mast (1980), 4.8%. Botting (1970) reported ten cases from the Birmingham Accident Hospital but gave no incidence. This complication may occur with any method of treatment, but it is more common in severely comminuted or open fractures and more common with open reduction (Vince and Miller 1987). We believe that delayed open treatment of a forearm fracture increases the risk of synostosis considerably. In seven of Botting's ten cases there was delay of internal fixation, and this was also true in the Teipner and Mast series. In one of our two cases there was delayed open reduction (Fig. 9.31); in the other, an unusual case of "wrenched" elbow, synostosis was perhaps unavoidable, considering the magnitude of the injury (Fig. 9.32). To avoid this complication, we recommend immediate primary surgery for the fractures, with great care being taken to refrain from placing bone-graft

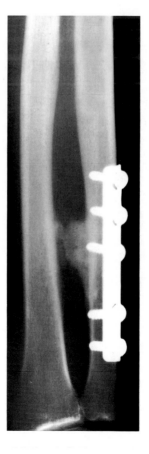

Fig. 9.31. Cross-union. Anteroposterior radiograph of a 39-year-old man with an isolated fracture of the ulna treated with a five-hole plate. No bone graft was used. Note the massive cross-union developing 24 weeks following injury

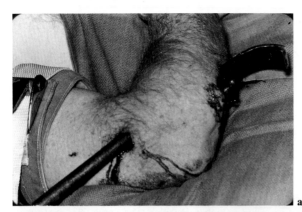

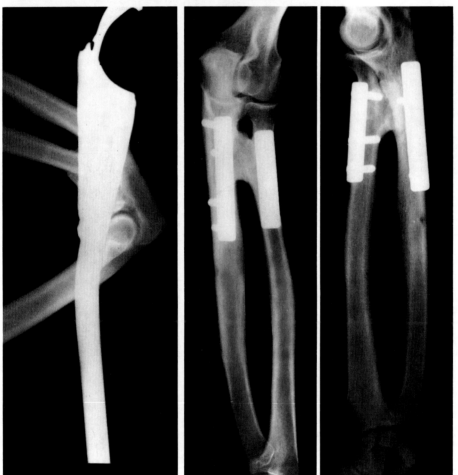

Fig. 9.32. a Cross-union due to open injury. A workman's arm was impaled by a flying wrench, shown in the clinical photograph (**a**) and the radiograph (**b**). After removal of the wrench, both bones were plated (**c**). A solid cross-union developed. (Courtesy of Dr. G.A. McDonald)

material around the disrupted interosseous membrane. Any bone graft should be placed as far from that membrane as possible.

9.5.2 Stress Fracture

Stress fractures may occur at the ends of either plate. The use of a single screw through the proximal and distal hole may reduce this incidence by allowing a more gradual stress distribution.

9.5.3 Refracture and Plate Removal

We cannot be dogmatic about the question of plate removal in the forearm following bone union. In general, we do not routinely remove plates from upper extremities. We suggest removal in young individuals or in patients who have some pain, especially due to the subcutaneous ulnar plate or to the lower screw of the radial plate, which often interferes with the function of the extensor pollicis longus muscle. The plates should never be removed until the cortex has returned to a normal radiographic appearance – in general, a minimum of 2 years following injury. Early removal of the plate has resulted in many refractures, which are most embarrassing to the surgeon and most difficult for the patient (Rumball and Finnegan 1990). If a plate is to be removed, the patient should be immobilized in a functional forearm splint for a 6-week period. This will help to reduce the number of refractures, but will not completely prevent them.

References

Anderson LD, Sish TD, Tooms RE, Park WI (1975) Compression plate fixation in acute diaphyseal fractures of the radius and ulna. J Bone Joint Surg 57-A:287–297

Böhler J (1936) Treatment of fractures. Wright, Bristol, p 421

Botting TD (1970) Post-traumatic radioulna cross-union. J Trauma 1:16–24

Boyd HB (1940) Surgical exposure of the ulna and proximal third of the radius through one incision. Surg Gynecol Obstet 71:86

Chapman MW, Gordon JE, Zissimos A (1989) J Bone Joint Surg 71A/2:159–169

Charnley J (1961) Closed treatment of common fractures, 3rd edn. Livingstone, Edinburgh

Crenshaw AH (1980) Surgical approaches. In Edmonson AS, Crenshaw AH (eds) Campbell's operative orthopaedics, 6th edn. Mosby, St. Louis

Danis R (1947) Théorie et pratique de l'ostéosynthèse. Masson, Paris

DePedro JS, Garci-Navarete F, DeLucas FG (1992) Internal fixation of ulnar fractures by locking nail. Clin Orth Rel Res 283:81–85

Duncan R, Geissler W. Freeland AE et al. (1992) Immediate internal fixation of open fractures of the diaphysis of the forearm. J Orth Trauma 6/1:25–31

Gebuhr P, Holmich P, Orsnes T et al. (1992) Isolated ulnar shaft fractures. J Bone Joint Surg 47B/5:757–759

Goel SC, Raj KB, Srivastava TP (1991) Isolated fractures of the ulnar shaft. Butterworth–Heinemann, London, p 212

Henry AK (1927) Exposure of the long bones and other surgical methods. Wright, Bristol

Hughston JD (1957) Fractures of the distal radial shaft, mistakes in management. J Bone Joint Surg 39-A:249–264

Knight RA, Purvis GD (1949) Fractures of both bones of the forearm in adults. J Bone Joint Surg 31-A:755–764

Mast J, Jakob R, Ganz R (1989) Planning and reduction technique in fracture surgery. Springer, Berlin Heidelberg New York

Moed BR, Kellam JF, Foster RJ, Tile M, Hansen ST Jr (1986) Immediate internal fixation of open fractures of the diaphysis of the forearm. J Bone Joint Surg [Am] 68(4):1008–1017

Rumball K, Finnegan M (1990) Refractures after forearm plate removal. J Ortho Traum 4/2:124–129

Sarmiento A, Cooper JS, Sinclair WF (1975) Forearm fractures. J Bone Joint Surg 57-A:297–304

Schemitsch EH, Richards RR (1992) The effect of manunion on functional outcome after plate fixation of fractures of both bones of the forearm in adults. J Bone Joint Surg 74A/7:1068–1078

Smith H, Sage FP (1957) Medullary fixation of forearm fractures. J Bone Joint Surg 39-A:91–98

Teipner WA, Mast JW (1980) Internal fixation of forearm diaphyseal fractures: double plating versus single compression (tension-band) plating – a comparative study. Orthop Clin North Am 3:381–391

Thompson JE (1918) Anatomical methods of approach in operations on the long bones of the extremities. Ann J Surg 68:309

Tile M, Petrie D (1969) Fractures of the radius and ulna. J Bone Joint Surg 51-B:193

Vince KG, Miller JE (1987) Cross-union complicating fracture of the forearm J Bone Joint Surg 69A/5:640-653

10 Fractures of the Distal Radius

T.S. Axelrod

10.1 Distal Radius Fractures

It remains a mystery as to why the management of this complex group of fractures is still so often directed by a statement made by Abraham Colles over 180 years ago (1814): "One consolation only remains, that the limb will, at some remote period, enjoy perfect freedom in all its motions, and be completely exempt from pain. The deformity, however will remain undiminished through life."

Advances in the understanding of fracture patterns, options in management, and the results that can be expected are nevertheless beginning to exert an impact on the status quo. Patients' expectations continue to escalate, and with this comes the obligation to improve our understanding of these fractures and to offer treatment accordingly. The young and elderly have "forgiving" anatomy and can accommodate themselves to the changes caused by these fractures. The victims of high-energy injuries, on the other hand, especially those with intra-articular extension require special attention.

Several prospective studies have highlighted the relationship of anatomy to function (Howard et al. 1989; van der Linden and Ericson 1991; Cooney et al. 1980; Porter and Stockley 1987). The results relate more to the quality of and the maintenance of the reduction than to the method of immobilization or fixation used to achieve this end result. If closed means can achieve and maintain an adequate reduction, then these are satisfactory.

Function becomes impaired when the deformity exceeds 20° of dorsal angulation, less than 10° of radial inclination, or a radial shift of over 2 mm. Shortening is a major problem. Although the exact distances are difficult to quantify, it appears that radial shortening of 6 mm or more results in an ulna plus deformity sufficient to cause significant ulnar-sided wrist pain secondary to ulnocarpal impingement. This degree of shortening is sufficient to disrupt the distal radial ulnar joint and restrict forearm rotation (Short et al. 1987) (Fig. 10.1). The change in loads across the triangular fibrocartilage disc with radial shortening have been quantified by Palmer (1987).

The intra-articular deformity is yet another issue in the management of these injuries. Impaction fractures of the lunate facet have been termed "die-punch" injuries by Scheck (1962). These intra-articular disruptions occur predominantly in young patients, as the result of high-energy trauma. Any residual intra-articular malalignment of greater than 2 mm is associated with the inevitable development of post-traumatic osteoarthritis (Knirk and Jupiter 1986).

10.1.1 Classification

Historical classifications and eponymic descriptions of these fractures still abound in current publications. As noted by Müller et al. (1987), for any classification system to be useful it must consider the type and severity of the fracture and must serve as a basis for treatment and the evaluation of the outcome of treatment. In 1967 Frykman established a classification system based on radiocarpal/radioulnar joint involvement with or without ulnar styloid fracturing. This system, however, is of limited value in establishing treatment or determining the prognosis of the injury. Many authors, including Cooney et al. (1979), Weber (1987), and Melone (1984), have contributed classification systems for these fractures. Isani and Melone (1988) and McMurtry and Jupiter (1992) developed specific systems that detail the intra-articular fracture of the distal radius.

The AO classification is ideally suited to these fractures (Müller et al 1987). Three major types exist: type A is extra-articular, type B intra-articular partial, and type C intra-articular complete. These types are divided into groups and subgroups reflecting increasing severity and complexity of the injury (Fig. 10.2). This classification system becomes quite complex. Studies of inter- and intraobserver variability indicate that classification beyond the basic type level is reliable and valid only for those with extensive expertise in dealing with these fractures (Kreder et al. 1995).

Fernandez (1987) has proposed a mechanistic classification of these fractures which has been widely adopted in recent years:
- Bending fractures occur with tensile forces resulting in metaphyseal failure (Colles; Smith).

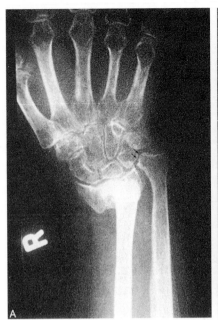

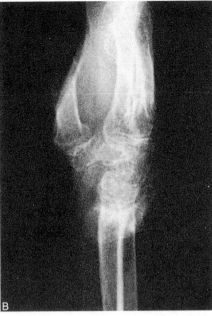

Fig. 10.1. X-ray of a neglected distal radius fracture with severe shortening; radial deviation. Results were very poor

– Compression fractures occur with failure of the joint surface and impaction of the subchondral and metaphyseal bone (die-punch).
– Shearing fractures involve large fragments of the joint surface with simple fracture lines (Barton's, radial styloid).
– Avulsion fractures involve either the radial styloid or the ulnar styloid.
– Combination fractures arise as a combination of the above types, usually from high-energy trauma.

10.1.2 Imaging

Radiographs must include posteroanterior (PA), true lateral, and pronated oblique views. Clearer appreciation of intra-articular step deformities and fragmentation can be obtained with trispiral tomography. Computed tomography (CT) is not needed for most fractures, however, it does provide the best assessment of the distal radioulnar joint (DRUJ).

10.1.3 Closed Treatment

Simple closed treatment involves the provision of adequate analgesia. This can be achieved by the instillation of a xylocaine hematoma block or the use of regional anesthesia. On rare occasions general anesthesia may be preferred. Axial traction and disimpaction of the fracture fragments followed by slight flexion, ulnar deviation, and pronation often achieves a good reduction. Initial immo-

bilization in a dorsal-radial plaster splint provides sufficient support. Postreduction X-rays are mandatory.

It is suggested that close follow-up be instituted with weekly X-ray checks for the first 3 weeks and, if the results are acceptable, immediately prior to final cast removal after 6 weeks. We prefer to leave the initial plaster slab in place for at least 2 weeks before conversion to a cylindrical plaster. The splint can be tightened or rein-

→

Fig. 10.2. The AO/ASIF classification system for distal radius fractures. **A** Extra-articular fractures. *A1,* fracture of the ulna, radius intact (A1.1, styloid process; A1.2, metaphyseal simple; A1.3, metaphyseal multifragmentary). *A2,* fracture of the radius, simple and impacted (A2.1, without any tilt; A2.2, with dorsal tilt, Pouteau-Colles; A2.3, with volar tilt, Goyrand-Smith). *A3,* fracture of the radius, multifragmentary (A3.1, impacted with axial shortening; A3.2, with a wedge; A3.3, complex). **B** Partial articular fractures. *B1,* fracture of the radius, sagittal (B1.1, lateral simple. B1.2, lateral multifragmentary; B1.3, medial). *B2,* fracture of the radius, dorsal rim, Barton (B2.1, simple; B2.2, with lateral sagittal fracture; B2.3, with dorsal dislocation of the carpus). *B3,* fracture of the radius, volar rim, reverse Barton, Goyrand-Smith II (B3.1, simple, with a small fragment; B3.2, simple, with a large fragment; B3.3, multifragmentary). **C** Complete articular fractures. *C1,* fracture of the radius, articular simple, metaphyseal simple (C1.1, posteromedial articular fragment; C1.2, sagittal articular fracture line; C1.3, frontal articular fracture line). *C2,* fracture of the radius, articular simple, metaphyseal multifragmentary (C2.1, sagittal articular fracture line; C2.2, frontal articular fracture line; C2.3, extending into the diaphysis). *C3,* fracture of the radius, multifragmentary (C3.1, metaphyseal simple; C3.2, metaphyseal multifragmentary; C3.3, extending into the diaphysis)

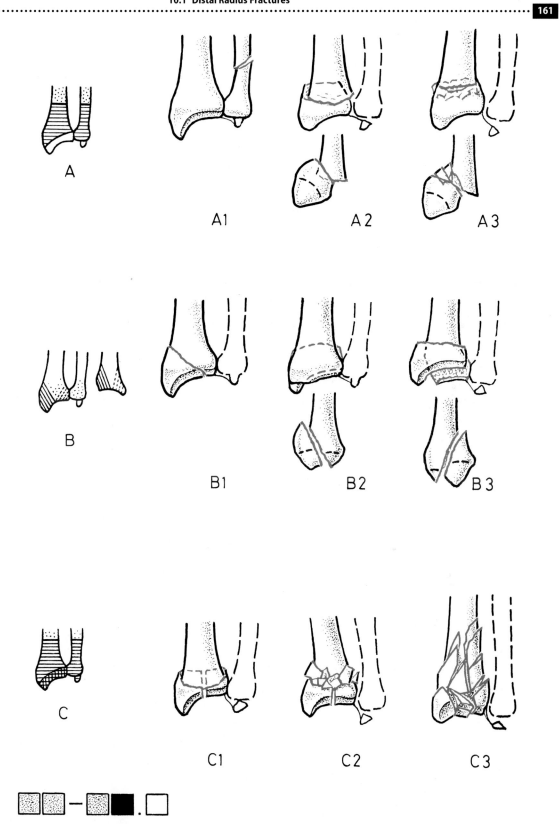

forced as needed. The aim is to avoid losing the initial reduction if the splint is changed before the fracture has a chance to begin to heal. It is important to check the weekly X-rays against those immediately following the initial reduction. Since some loss in reduction is inevitable, and is gradual, the radiographs should not only be compared to those from the previous week.

Surgical intervention can be instituted at any time once a loss in reduction is recognized, but after 3–4 weeks this becomes increasingly difficult.

10.1.4 Management and Decision Making

Determining the ideal management for these injuries one must consider the patient, the limb, and the fracture pattern. Treatment must thus be tailored to the needs of the individual patient. A deformity that is acceptable in a low-demand, elderly individual may not be ideal in a younger, physically active patient with a demanding occupation. Limb considerations include open wounds,

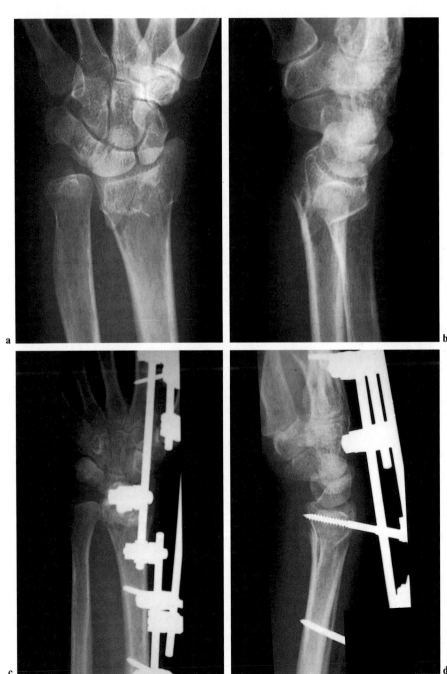

Fig. 10.3 a–d. Radiographs illustrating the use of an extra 3.0-mm Schantz pin to correct the remaining fracture angulation not reduced by ligamentotaxis alone.
a,b Extra-articular distal radius fracture with significant volar angulation through the fracture site. This did not reduce via ligamentotaxis alone.
c,d Use of an additinal Schantz pin to manipulate the distal fragment and linkage onto the standard external fixator frame

soft tissue (tendon, ligament) injuries, and nerve compression syndromes. All of these influence the decision making.

Discussion of the approach to these fractures must first detail the management options and the roles that these play. An algorithm can be used to approach these fractures in a useful surgical format.

10.1.4.1 Percutaneous Pinning

Described as early as 1952 by De Palma, this technique has value in the extra-articular or incomplete articular dorsal or radial shear fracture. Kapandji (1991) has recently described a technique of intrafocal pinning in which the pins serve as buttresses preventing redisplacement of the fracture. For complex, complete articular fractures and for fractures with extensive metaphyseal fragmentation these pinning techniques are not useful in isolation. They may be combined with external fixation in some situations.

10.1.4.2 Pins and Plaster

Treatment by means of pins and plaster is largely of historical value, with complication rates as high as 53 % (Weber and Szabo 1986; Raskin 1994). These have been replaced by metallic external fixation devices.

10.1.4.3 External Skeletal Fixation

By providing firm fixation in the skeleton (2nd or 3rd metacarpal, distal one-third radius) the pins of the external fixator allow precise, firm distraction of the wrist joint and associated fracture fragments. Soft tissue elements pull on small bone fragments (ligamentotaxis), aligning them. On occasion even impacted articular fragments are pulled by the capsular and ligament attachments and align satisfactorily. New pin designs, low-profile frames, and better surgical technique have reduced the complications from these techniques. The use of external fixation has become widespread. This

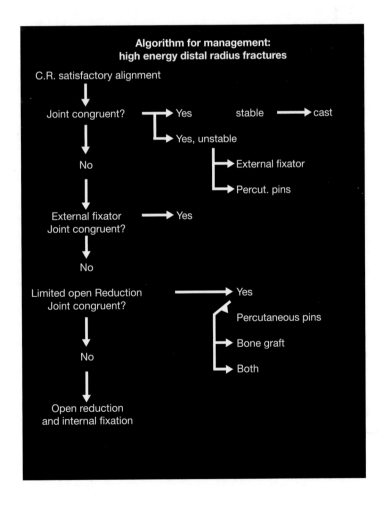

Fig. 10.4. Algorithm for the management of distal radius fractures

technique is excellent for restoring length and radial inclination. The palmar tilt is less well reduced but can be aided by the use of additional K wires or a Shantz pin (Fig. 10.3). External fixation is ideal for compression type fractures. Dynamic mobile fixators have not been shown to be of benefit for these fractures (Raskin 1994; Clyburn 1987).

10.1.4.4 Limited Open Reduction

This technique involves the disimpaction and fine manipulation of depressed articular fracture fragments through a small dorsal incision under fluoroscopic control (Axelrod et al. 1988). This is as an adjunct to external fixation or percutaneous pinning in dealing with compression-type fractures in which the articular segments fail to reduce through indirect means (ligamentotaxis).

10.1.4.5 Open Reduction and Internal Fixation

Formal open reduction and internal fixation is ideal for shear-type articular fractures. Large articular fragments can be reduced and stabilized through interfragmentatary compressive lag screws and/or buttress plates. With severely fragmented compression or combination fractures the use of open reduction, bone grafting, buttress plate, and fine K wire fixation can serve as an adjunct in satisfactorily reducing and maintaining the joint surface. This is a demanding technique in this particular subgroup of fractures and carries a high complication rate (Axelrod and McMurtry 1990; Jupiter and Lipton 1993; Porter and Stockley 1987).

10.1.4.6 Algorithm for Treatment

As seen in the algorithm (Fig. 10.4), a step-wise approach to the surgical management of distal radius fractures is advised. The approach begins with a careful assessment of the fracture configuration. Shearing-type fractures are best treated with immediate open reduction and internal fixation; in all other distal radius fractures it is suggested to begin with a closed reduction. If the reduction is satisfactory and seems relatively stable, cast treatment may suffice. This is rare in high-energy, widely displaced, or multifragmented fracture patterns; more likely the fracture reduces but remains unstable. If the joint is congruent and the extra-articular parameters acceptable, application of an external fixation device is advised. Alternatively, if there is no joint involvement and metaphyseal fragmentation is not excessive, one of the percutaneous pinning techniques may suffice.

The joint reduction must be reassessed again following closed reduction with or without application of an external fixator. If it is satisfactory, no further intervention is needed. If the joint surface remains incongruent, as is often the case with compression fractures, it is advised to perform a limited open reduction (percutaneous elevation) of the depressed joint segment under fluoroscopic control. The reduction is maintained with percutaneous subchondral Kirschner (K) wires. If a major metaphyseal defect exists after reduction, cancellous bone grafting is advised. Bone substitutes may play a role in providing this support in the next few years.

If the limited open technique fails to reduce the fragments, which usually occurs only in high-energy combination injuries, the surgeon is advised to move to a formal open reduction and internal fixation. The surgical approach is dictated by the fracture pattern, but the volar exposure usually allows excellent visualization of the pathology and can be combined with an often needed median nerve decompression. The external fixator is usually left in place as a neutralization device, preventing axial overload of the small joint fragments.

10.1.5 Surgical Technique

Generally, the sooner (in days) that these fractures are operated upon, the better is the result. It is much easier to reduce the fragments through ligamentotaxis early before the hematoma organizes. Soft tissue considerations such as median nerve compression, compartment syndrome, and an open fracture may suggest immediate intervention or advise a short delay in the case of severe swelling.

Surgery can be performed under regional anesthesia except in cases requiring an iliac crest bone graft. A radiolucent hand table or arm boards can be used to support the hand and wrist. A tourniquet is advised, either arm or proximal forearm. Fluoroscopic control is essential. The new low-radiation mini-image intensifers are ideal for these fractures.

In the case of an extra-articular fracture with minimal metaphyseal comminution, the fracture can be held well with two crossed 1.6-mm K wires inserted percutaneously. One is placed through the radial-volar aspect of the radial styloid and the other through the dorsal ulnar region of the metaphysis. The crossed-wire technique provides the best biomechanical support of the various structural pinning methods (Collicutt et al. 1994). The technique of Kapandji (1991) involves inserting three K wires directly into the fracture sight perpendicular to the radius (Fig. 10.5). Once into the fracture the pins are tilted distally, reducing the distal fragment vis-à-vis length and dorsal tilt. The K wires are then power-advanced into the volar proximal cortex where

Fig. 10.5. a,b Extra-articular unstable displaced distal radius fracture (AO type A3). Unsatisfactory following closed reduction. **c,d** Kapandji intrafocal pinning maintained the reduction well. **e,f** Follow-up after pin removal. The fracture has healed anatomically without loss of reduction after pin removal at 6 weeks

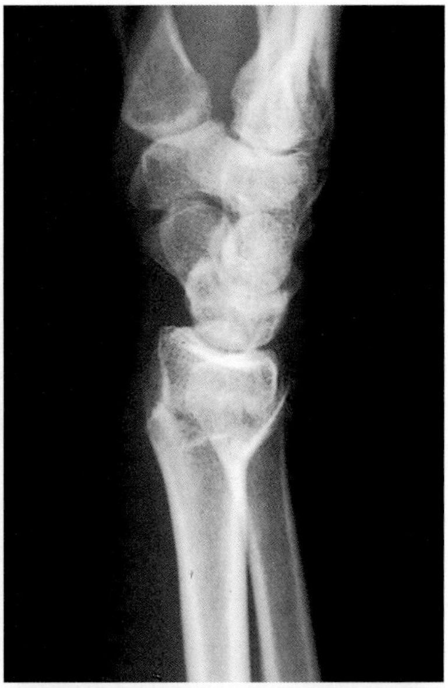

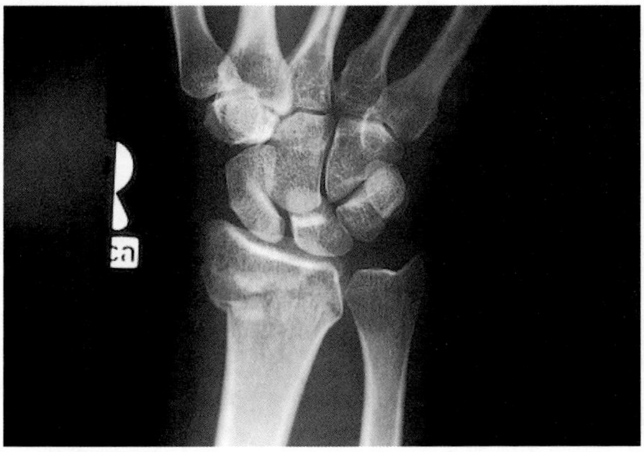

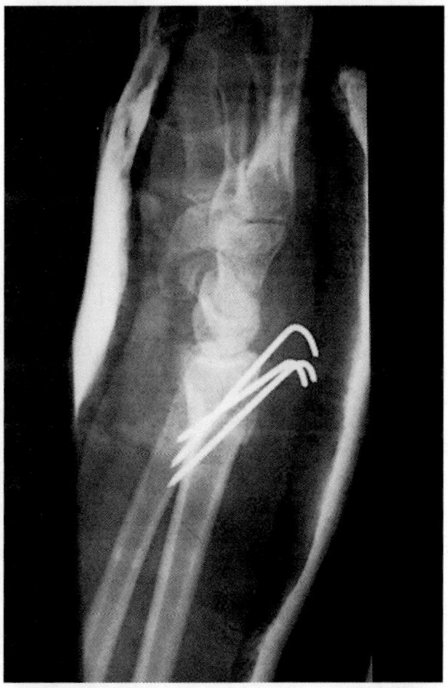

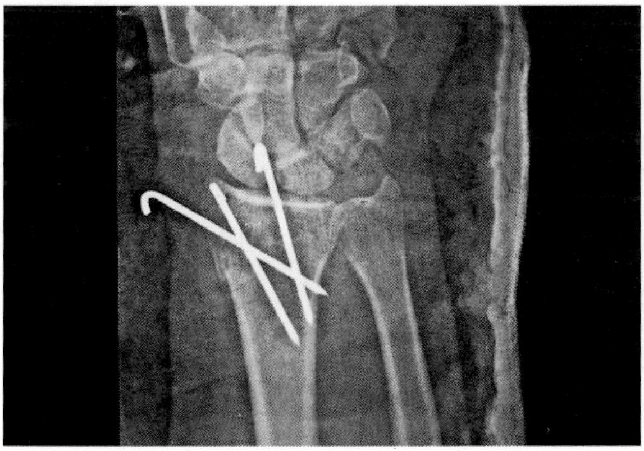

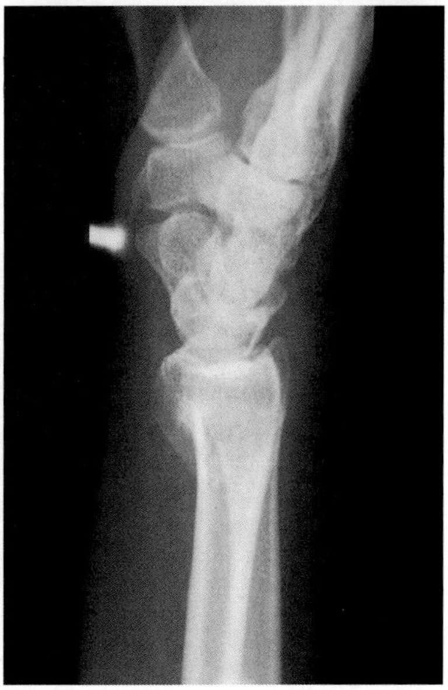

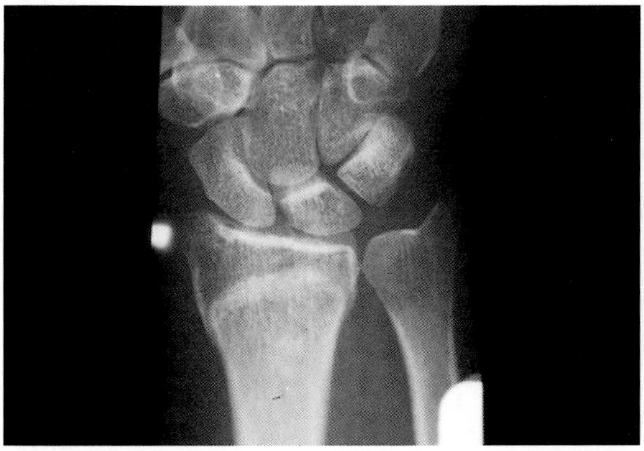

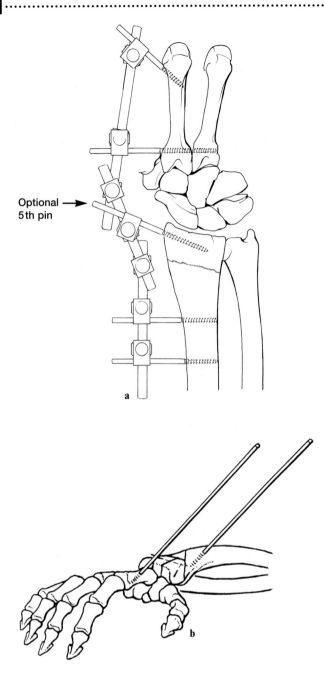

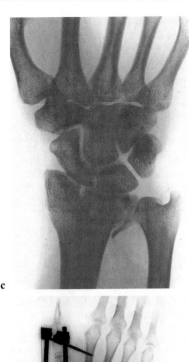

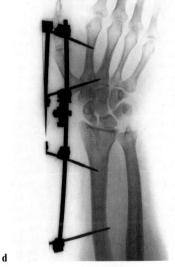

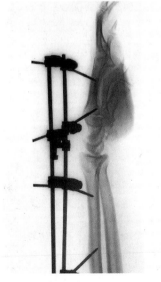

Fig. 10.6. a,b One technique for construction of the small AO external fixator for distal radius fractures. The 2.5-mm Schantz pins are used distally, 3.0-mm proximally. The frame can be constructed in a variety of ways; this frame allows for maximal variability of wrist positioning. **c** A young Swiss man with an AO type C2 intra-articular distal radius fracture. **d,e** The joint displacement was perfectly reduced by ligamentotaxis after application of a simple external fixation frame

they are anchored. A cast is generally applied for several weeks; however, the originial description suggests that casting may not be needed.

10.1.5.1 External Fixation Application

A limited open pin placement technique is advised to reduce the incidence of radial sensory branch injury. Shantz pins of 2.5 mm are placed into the second metacarpal with predrilling (2.0 mm). In individuals with a large skeleton the 3.0-mm pins have a role. With osteopenic individuals it is advised to place the proximal metacarpal pin horizontally and transversely to engage the base of the third metacarpal as well. The universal nature of the AO small fixator allows for this. The pins are placed so as to be slightly divergent and enter the bare area on the dorsal-radial aspect of the metacarpal. Full metacarpal joint flexion is maintained during pin insertion to reduce extensor tendon adherence to the pins.

The proximal two Shantz pins are usually 3.0 mm in diameter. These are placed approximately 6–8 cm proximal to the fracture site under direct visualization. A small cutaneous 1.0-cm incision is made. Subcutaneous and fascial tissues are opened by spreading of a small blunt-tipped instrument. Small right-angle retractors are placed into the wound to allow direct visualization of the dorsal radial surface of the radius. Predrilling is advised, and the pins are inserted by hand.

The frame is assembled as demonstrated in Fig. 10.6, and fracture manipulation is performed. Fine adjustments are made to the fracture. A second connecting bar is advised to control rotation through the frame.

If the fracture reduces well but remains unstable, with the frame in place, supplemental percutaneous crossed K wires can help. Finally, if the volar tilt of the distal fragment is not restored to neutral, a fifth Shantz pin can be inserted directly into the distal fragment by hand and then flexed forward, reducing the fracture, and thereafter linked to the main frame assembly (Fig. 10.7).

It is of prime importance not to overdistract the wrist joint. This is thought to be associated with capsular contracture and extrinsic tendon tightness resulting in postoperative stiffness. If a substantial distraction is needed to hold the wrist reduced, consider supplemental K wire fixation to support the fracture directly. This should allow the overdistraction to be released and still maintain the fracture reduction.

The pin sites are loosely closed with nylon sutures and dressed with proviodine-soaked gauze strips. Supplemental plaster support is usually not used.

Postoperatively, early finger motion is encouraged, as are forearm rotation exercises. Referral to physiotherapy or hand therapy is often needed to effect this early on.

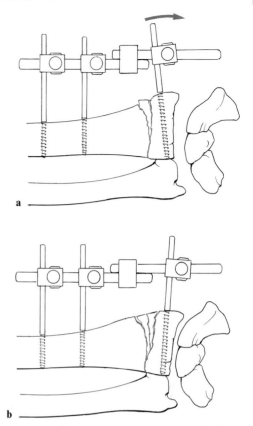

Fig. 10.7 a,b. Direct manipulation of the distal articular fragment into better position using an additional 3.0- or 4.0-mm Schantz pin

Radiographic assessments to confirm alignment are made biweekly until the frame is ready to be removed. The external fixator is usually removed in the clinic at 6 weeks after X-ray control confirms sufficient healing. It is rarely, if ever, left on for more than 8 weeks.

10.1.5.2 Limited Open Reduction

A simple direct manipulation can be performed if the articular surface fails to reduce anatomically after the external fixator has been applied. This usually applies to the compression or die-punch fracture pattern.

A small 1 cm incision is made 1 cm proximal to the metaphyseal fracture line dorsally, directly in line with the depressed joint segment. Blunt spreading takes the surgeon to the dorsal surface of the distal radius. A blunt elevator (Howarth) is introduced and gently manipulated directly into the metaphyseal fracture line. Under fluoroscopic guidance the elevator is used to tease the depressed segment back into anatomical alignment (Fig. 10.8). Percutaneous K wires (1.6 mm) are inserted from radial to ulnar, directly below the subchondral

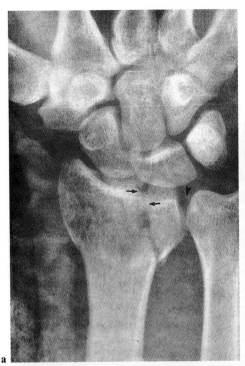

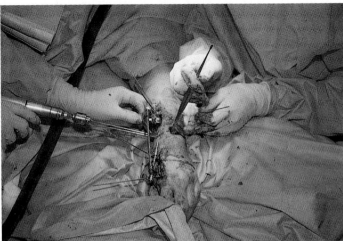

Fig. 10.8. a "Die-punch" fragment was unreduced by indirect means after external fixator was applied. **b** A small dorsal incision is made, inserting an elevator. **c** Using fluoroscopic control, a small elevator is used to directly manipulate the fragment into place. **d** Once reduced, the fragment is pinned into place and supported with bone graft

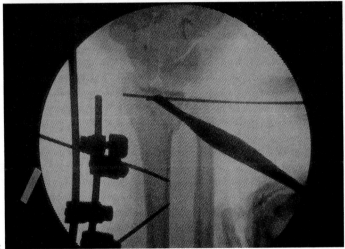

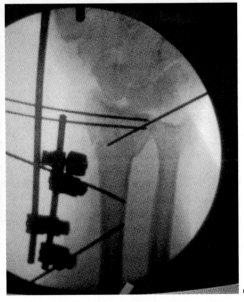

bone surface to support the reduction. A large metaphyseal defect should be filled with cancellous bone graft (iliac crest) to buttress the joint surface. Two percutaneous pins are generally used to support the surface.

The external fixator serves to neutralize the compressive loads across the wrist. The small pins are thus sufficient in most cases to prevent redisplacement of the depressed segments.

A recent review of our experience indicates that this supplemental technique has been used in approximately 20 % of our distal radius fractures treated with external fixators. All have maintained the reduction and have healed without settling of the joint.

The percutaneous pins are left protruding from the skin and bent over, facilitating removal in the clinic setting 4–6 weeks following insertion.

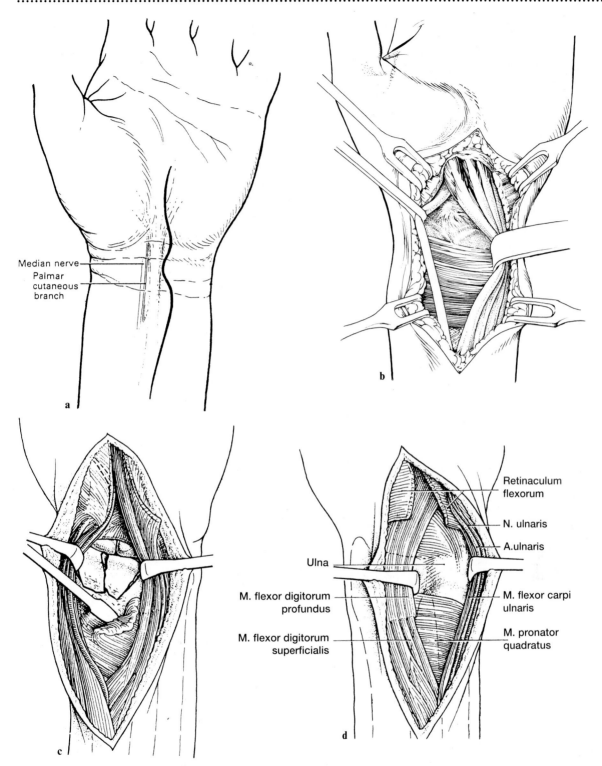

Fig. 10.9 a–d. Extended carpal tunnel exposure to the volar aspect of the distal radius. **a** The skin incision crosses the wrist and creases in a zig-zag fashion. **b** The flexor tendons can be mobilized with the median nerve, developing the interval between the flexors and the nerve. **c** The pronator quadratus muscle is incised on the radial border and retracted to the ulnar side. **d** Alternatively, the interval between the ulnar neuromuscular bundle and the tendons can be developed. The pronator is reflected off the radius, exposing the volar surface proximal to the joint. This provides excellent exposure of the ulnar side of the distal radius volar surface

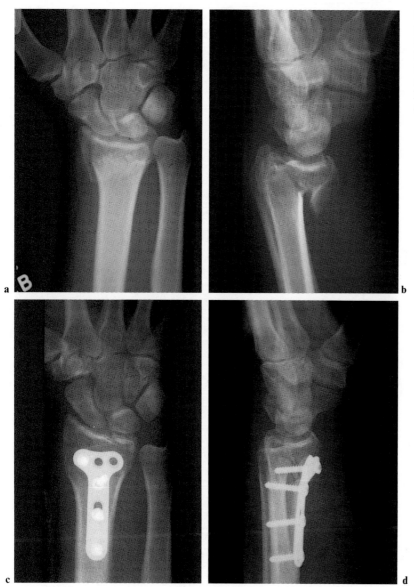

Fig. 10.10. a,b AO type B3, volar; Barton's intra-articular distal radius fracture. Carpus is unstable and subluxes volarward with the volar articular fragment. **c,d** Simple buttressing with a small-fragment T plate will reduce and hold the joint. Distal lag screws are optional

10.1.5.3 Open Reduction and Internal Fixation

Shear Fractures (Volar Barton's, Radial Styloid)

If displaced, as is usually the case, these fractures are best treated with immediate open reduction and internal fixation. The external fixator does not sufficiently control the carpal subluxation inherent in these fractures. Open reduction and plating facilitates early wrist motion and can be the more conservative approach.

One of two volar exposures are used for the AO type B3 (volar Barton's) fracture. We favor a proximal extension of the Russe approach if the injury is a low-energy one, if it occurred a few days previously, and if there is minimal to moderate swelling without clinical evidence of median nerve compression. This is a development of the interval between flexor carpi radialis longus and the radial artery. The pronator quadratus is elevated from radial to ulnar off the radius, and the fracture is exposed.

If there is evidence of median nerve compression, or if the injury is a high-energy one with moderate to severe edema, it is advised to decompress the median nerve through the carpal tunnel. A proximally extended carpal tunnel release can afford excellent access to the distal radius (Fig. 10.9). The median nerve is mobilized and retracted to the radial side and the flexor tendons to the ulnar side. Care is needed not to retract too aggressively on the median nerve. As an alternative the flexor tendons and the median nerve can be taken to the radial side, creating a window of access between the ulnar neurovascular bundle and the flexor tendons. This provides excellent visualization of the ulnar side of the distal radius but limits visualization of the styloid. One should feel free to mobilize the flexor tendons as needed and work through windows radial or ulnar to the tendons for the optimal exposure.

The wrist capsule is not routinely opened. This is to avoid devascularization of the fracture fragments and destabilization of the critical volar wrist ligaments.

The fracture fragments are usually large and have a simple metaphyseal shear-type extension. They can be reduced by extending the wrist over a rolled-up towel and then teased gently into position. There is seldom intra-articular complexity, and with extra-articular reduction the joint therefore reduces perfectly. Provisional fixation with K wires is helpful, followed by the application of a buttress plate. The small T distal radius plate is ideal. This requires some undercontouring to assure compression of the joint surface. The plate is placed quite distally, within 2 mm of the volar rim of the distal radius joint surface. Strictly speaking, only proximal fixation is required for maximal buttress effect. If the bone quality is satifactory, placing one or two lag screws distally through the plate can supplement the fixation and help to control rotation and shift of the

Fig. 10.11 a–c. Shear type of distal radius fracture (AO type B1) in a 23-year-old athelete. Open reduction and internal fixation affords an anatomic reduction of the joint. Lag screw fixation alone will suffice for this shearing type of fracture

joint fragments. Image intensifiers aid in the fracture reduction and plate positioning (Fig. 10.10).

Postoperative casting is needed actually only for 2–4 weeks, followed by early active wrist exercises. The rehabilitation after this treatment is usually simple and uncomplicated. It seems to entail less trouble than that after an external fixator.

The radial styloid shear fracture is approached through a dorsal exposure between the first and second dorsal wrist compartments. Care must be taken to avoid injury to the superficial radial nerve branches in this region. In contrast to the volar fractures, here it is helpful to perform a limited arthrotomy at the edges of the fracture margin to visualize the joint reduction. Two 3.5-mm cortical lag screws, cannulated or otherwise, serve to maintain the reduction well (Fig. 10.11).

Shear Plus Compression

Volar shear fractures occasionally involve disruption of the dorsal metaphyseal cortex, indicating a combined shear plus compression type injury. The buttress plate no longer has an intact dorsal cortex to compress against, loosing its biomechanical advantage. With undercontouring the plate can push the fracture into a dorsally displaced, volar angulation position. To counteract this it is suggested to reestablish the effect of a dorsal cortex by using an external fixator as a tension band, working against the buttress afforded by the volar plate (Fig. 10.12). In addition the plate should not be undercontoured, but rather should follow the shape of the volar metaphysis of the distal radius.

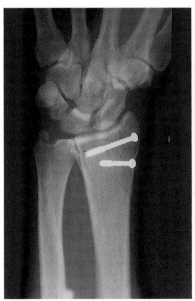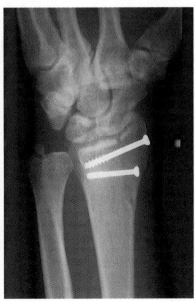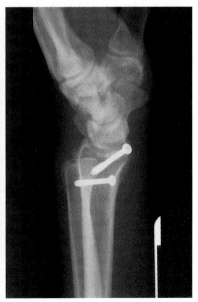

a–c

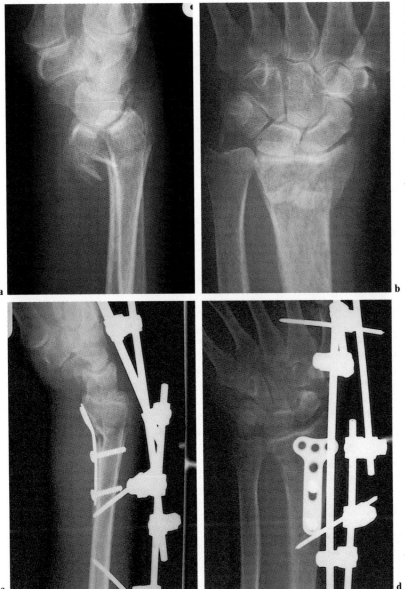

Fig. 10.12. a,b An elderly woman with an unstable volar AO B3 multifragmentary distal radius fracture. Note the dorsal fragmentation. **c,d** With application of the volar buttress plate, the fracture displaced dorsally producing a Colles type deformity. This occurred because the fracture did not have an intact dorsal cortex for the plate to buttress the volar fragments up against. This is corrected by applying the external fixator dorsally, working as a tension band flexing the fragments over the volar plate

Multifragmentary Combined Fractures

These are the most difficult fractures to manage. The small size of the fracture fragments, combined with the extensive soft tissue injuries, make reconstruction a demanding and frustrating task. These can often be dealt with by the techniques described above. If the more limited approaches fail to reduce the joint surface adequately, the next step is open reduction and internal fixation. The external fixator is left in place and serves as a neutralization device.

In most cases the extensile volar exposure as described above is used (Fig. 10.9), combining an extended carpal tunnel release well into the forearm with exposure of the distal radius. The aim is to work within the fracture site, minimizing any additional soft tissue stripping of the small fragments. A small capsulotomy is usually, but not always, needed as it is possible to reflect the metaphyseal fragments distally based on their capsular attachments much, as with a lateral tibial plateau fracture. Working within the fracture, the depressed joint fragments are elevated, supported with iliac crest bone graft, and pinned into position. Small-diameter K wires (1.1–1.25 mm) are useful. The larger volar fragments are then reduced, closing over the central joint fragments, and held in place with a distal radius buttress plate. Where possible, interfragmentary compression is obtained with lag screws. The external fixator is adjusted to unload the joint from compressive loads. A slightly flexed position is ideal. An additional shear fracture of the radial styloid is well held with a percutaneous cannulated 4.0-mm screw inserted just proximal to the anatomical snuff box. Care of the soft tissue structures is essential in placing this screw.

10.2 The Distal Radioulnar Joint

The distal radioulnar joint (DRUJ) is an area of growing interest. Work by Palmer (1987), Bower (1988), and others has provided us with a better understanding of the biomechanics of this complex region.

Many distal radius fractures involve the DRUJ. Displacement of the distal radial metaphysis without an associated ulnar shaft fracture must result in a partial or complete disruption of the distal radial ulnar articulation.

Fortunately, with reduction of the radius, the sigmoid notch usually realigns well with the ulna, and the problem is resolved. This, however, cannot be taken for granted as one of the most common problems in long-term follow-up of distal radius fractures relates to dysfunction of the the DRUJ.

The distal radius is dealt with first, as described with any of the techniques above. The distal radial-ulnar articulation is then checked manually by assessing the anterior-posterior stability of the DRUJ in the operating room in full pronation, full supination, and midposition. If the joint glides well, and the distal ulna feels stable, no more intervention is needed. This is the case in the vast majority of cases. The presence or absence of an ulnar styloid fracture is of no consequence in this situation.

If the ulnar head reduces in one position and feels stable (usually supination) yet is unstable or subluxated in another position, it is advised to immobilize the arm and forearm with an above elbow splint in the stable position. This is achieved using an above elbow plaster splint, which is converted within days to a hinged cast-brace to facilitate elbow rehabilitation. It must be worn full time for 4–6 weeks to allow healing of the soft tissues of the DRUJ. An alternative is cross-pinning of the radius to the ulna in the reduced position. A large K wire of 2.0 mm is used and is passed just proximal to the ulnar head, avoiding the articular cartilage of the sigmoid notch. Our preference remains using the cast brace – provided the DRUJ is stable in supination.

Lastly, the soft tissue and boney damage may be such that the ulnar head is not stable in any position. This usually occurs with the combined multifragmentary fractures. In this situation two paths can be followed. If there is a small or no ulnar styloid fracture, the ulna is held reduced in the most stable position (supination, midpronation, etc.) and cross-pinned to the radius. Direct repair of the triangular fibrocartilage complex (TFCC) back to the ulnar styloid is possible, but sutures cannot afford enough strength to hold the repair without the tremendous torque of the forearm being neutralized by the ulnar-radial cross-pinning. The surgical approach for this repair is the same as that described below for reattaching the ulnar styloid. The TFCC is reattached to the base of the ulnar styloid with heavy nonabsorbable sutures that pass through the fibrocartilage disk and anchor through drill holes in the ulna metaphysis.

In the presence of a moderate to large ulnar styloid fracture the option to cross-pin is satisfactory. However, it has become our preference to perform a tension band wire repair of the ulnar styloid. This is performed through a separate incision, releasing the distal portion of the extensor carpi ulnaris (ECU) tendon and approaching the ulnar styloid directly through the floor of the extensor carpi ulnaris sheath. Care is needed to identify and preserve the dorsal sensory branch of the ulnar nerve in making the skin incision (Fig. 10.13). The fragment and with it the TFCC is reduced and held with a single 1.25-mm K wire. A small loop of gauge 22 stainless steel wire is passed through the ulnar carpal ligament portion of the TFCC, deep to the K wire, and then secured through a small drill hole in the distal ulnar metaphysis. The wire is tightened by twisting it; double twists are not needed. The ulnar head shows remarkable stability after this simple repair. The forearm is immobilized postoperatively in the most stable position to protect this repair for 4–6 weeks. In a recent series 11 of 12 patients treated with this technique showed a stable DRUJ with excellent restoration of pronation and supination; no nonunions of the ulnar styloid occurred (Axelrod and Cheng 1995).

10.3 Postoperative Care

The major concerns of postoperative care involve the surgical incision site and pin site care and avoiding the problems of finger stiffness and occasional frank reflex sympathetic dystrophy. Pin site care is performed daily with betadine or hibitane soaked gauze. Physiotherapy is usually instituted prior to patient discharge (even in the outpatient surgery department if the procedure is carried out as a day case). The aim is to begin aggressive early finger mobilization and to begin work on pronation-supination. If this is begun early, a reduction in stiffness may be seen.

174 ·

Chapter 10   **Fractures of the Distal Radius**

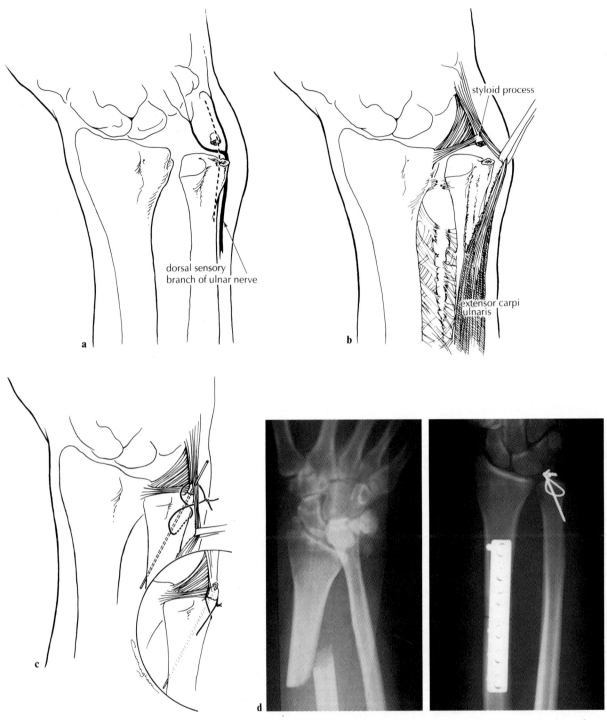

Fig. 10.13. a–c Surgical technique for open reduction and internal fixation of the ulnar styloid process. **a** The incision is made along the ulnar side of the wrist, and care is taken to preserve the dorsal ulnar sensory nerve. **b** The extensor carpi ulnaris sheath is opened and the floor incised. The ulnar styloid fragment is found and left attached distally to the ulnar carpal ligament of the triangular fibrocartilage complex (TFCC). **c** The styloid is reduced and held with a 1.25-mm K wire. A fine gauge wire is passed through the ulnar carpal ligament and around the K wire. It is looped into a drill hole in the ulna and tightened down. **d** Radiographs of a 44-year-old woman with a severe Galeazzi injury illustrating complete dislocation of the distal radioulnar joint. Following internal fixation of the radius, the DRUJ remained unstable in all planes. **e** Open reduction and tension band fixation of the ulnar styloid provided excellent DRUJ stabilization. Uneventful union of all fractures occurred in 8 weeks

10.4 Complications

Complications around distal radius fracture surgery are common; however, most are relatively straightforward to manage.

10.4.1 Pin Site Infection

Pin site infection occurs in about 20 % of all pins (Shantz and K wires) and depends on the length of time that the pins are in place. If pins are left more than 8–10 weeks, probably all become infected. General wound care usually deals with this problem through a local release of the adherent skin and soft tissues. Daily pin care is continued, and oral antibiotics may be needed. One should watch for lymphangitis and cellulitis, the occurrence of which requires the intravenous administration of antibiotics and possibly removal of the offending pin. If the pins are almost ready to come out, simply removing them 1–2 weeks early usually solves the problem.

10.4.2 Median Nerve Compression

Postoperative median nerve compression poses a significant problem and must be dealt with readily. If the nerve function is worse than that preoperatively, and the nerve was not decompressed, dressings are split and the hand elevated and observed for a short time. If there is no improvement within 1–2 h, it is urgent that the nerve be decompressed. The ulnar nerve is less frequently involved. If the wrist is dramatically swollen, and median nerve decompression is indicated, it is simple to decompress the ulnar nerve through Guyon's canal at the same time through the same incision.

10.4.3 Reflex Sympathetic Dystrophy

This condition occurs acutely after management of a distal radius fracture and is often associated with median nerve compression (Jupiter 1992). A median nerve decompression should be considered. The mainstay for dealing with a severely stiff, painful hand after surgery consists of physiotherapy and the use of brachial plexus anesthesic blocks. Coordination between the pain service and the physiotherapy department is essential. This continues to be a major problem; the full solution still eludes us.

10.5 Conclusions

Fractures of the distal radius are very common, and the majority are amenable to simple cast treatment. A subgroup of patients with difficult fractures require special attention to prevent a poor outcome. Using a variety of surgical techniques and devices, these fractures can be reduced and held in relatively anatomical position until healing. Poor results still occur with the severe combined (AO type C3.3) injuries involving articular cartilage damage and the inability to achieve satifactory reduction. In other cases, for reasons not yet clear, the soft tissues may react poorly to the injury, resulting in problems of finger and wrist stiffness even in the presence of an excellent fracture reduction.

References

Axelrod TS, Cheng SL-T (1995) Complex dislocations of the distal radioulnar joint. J Hand Surg [Am]

Axelrod TS, McMurtry (1990) Open reduction and internal fixation of comminuted intraarticular fractures of the distal radius. J Hand Surg [Am] 15:1–11

Axelrod TS, Paley D, Green J, McMurtry RY (1988) Limited open reduction of the lunate facet in comminuted intraarticular fractures of the distal radius. J Hand Surg [Am] 13:372–377

Bower WH (1988) The distal radioulnar joint. In: Green DP (ed) Operative hand surgery, 2nd edn. Lippincott, Philadelphia, pp 939–989

Clyburn TA (1987) Dynamic external fixation for comminuted intra-articular fractures of the distal end of the radius. J Bone Joint Surg Am 69:248–254

Colles A (1814) On the fracture of the carpal extremity of the radius. Edinburgh Med Surg J 10:182–186

Collicutt J, McGillivary G, Gross M, Johnson J (1994) A biomechanical analysis of percutaneous pinning for unstable extra-articular fractures of the distal radius. J Bone Joint Surg Br 76 [Suppl 1]:23

Cooney WP III, Linscheid RL, Dobyns JH (1979) External pin fixation for unstable Colles' fractures. J Bone Joint Surg Am 61:840–845

Cooney WP III, Dobyns JH, Linscheid RL (1980) Complications of Colles' fracture. J Bone Joint Surg Am 62:613–619

De Palma A (1952) Comminuted fractures of the distal end of the radius treated by ulnar pinning. J Bone Joint Surg Am 34:651–662

Fernandez DL (1987) Avant-bras segmental distal. In: Mueller ME, Nazarian S, Koch P (eds) Classification AO des Fractures. I. Les os longs. Springer, Berlin Heidelberg New York, pp 106–115

Heim U, Pfeiffer KM (1988) Internal fixation of small fractures. Technique recommended by the AO-ASIF group, 3rd edn. Springer, Berlin Heidelberg New York

Howard PW, Stewart HD, Hind RE et al (1989) External fixation or plaster for severely displaced comminuted Colles' fractures? A prospective study of anatomical functional results. J Bone Joint Surg Br 71:68–73

Isani A, Melone CP Jr (1988) Classification and management of intra-articular fractures of the distal radius. Hand Clin 4:349–360

Jupiter JB (1992) Fractures of the distal radius. In: Eilert RE (ed) Instructional course lectures, vol XLI. American Academy of Orthopaedic Surgeons, Baltimore

Jupiter JB, Lipton H (1993) Operative treatment of intraarticular fractures of the distal radius. Clin Orthop 292:48–61

Kapankji AI (1991) "Reduction-effect" ARUM type intra-focal pins in the osteosynthesis of fractures of the lower end of the radius. Ann Chir Main Memb Super 10(2):138–145

Knirk JL, Jupiter JB (1986) Intra-articular fractures of the distal end of the radius in young adults. J Bone Joint Surg Am 68:647–659

Kreder HJ, Hanel D, McKee M, McGillivary G, Jupiter JB, Swiontkowski M (1995) Consistency of the AO classification for distal radius fractures. Presented at the Annual Meeting of the Canadian Orthopaedic Association, Halifax

McMurtry RY, Jupiter JB (1992) Fractures of the distal radius. In: Browner B, Jupiter J, Levine A, Trafton P (eds) Skeletal trauma. Saunders, Philadelphia

Melone CP Jr (1984) Articular fractures of the distal radius. Orthop Clin North Am 15:217–236

Müller ME, Nazarian S, Koch P (1987) Classification AO des fractures. I Les os longs. Springer, Berlin Heidelberg New York

Palmer AK (1987) The distal radioulnar joint: anatomy, biomechanics and triangular fibrocartilage complex abnormalities. Hand Clin 3:31–40

Porter M, Stockley I (1987) Fractures of the distal radius: intermediate and end results in relation to radiologic parameters. Clin Orthop 220:241–252

Raskin KB (1994) Advances in external fixation. Presented at the AO/ASIF Advanced Hand Symposium, Telluride, Colorado, August

Scheck M (1962) Long-term follow-up of treatment of comminuted fractures of the distal end of the radius by transfixation with Kirschner wires and cast. J Bone Joint Surg Am 44:337–351

Short WH, Palmer AK, Werner FW et al (1987) A biomechanical study of distal radius fractures. J Hand Surg [Am] 12:529–534

Smith RJ, Peimer CA (1977) Injuries to the metacarpal bone and joints. Adv Surg 2:341–374

van der Linden W, Ericson R (1981) Colles' fracture: how should its displacement be measured and how should it be immobilized? J Bone Joint Surg Am 63:1285–1288

Weber ER (1987) A rational approach for the recognition and treatment of Colles' fractures. Hand Clin 3:13–21

Weber SC, Szabo RM (1986) Severely comminuted distal radial fracture as an unsolved problem: complications associated with external fixation and pins and plaster techniques. J Hand Surg [Am] 11:157–165

Part III   Fractures of the Spine, Pelvis, and Acetabulum

11 Fractures of the Spine

R. Hu

11.1 Introduction

Injury to the spinal column and its associated neurological structures occurs commonly and can have devastating effects on the function of individual. The rate of new spinal injury within a population has been estimated at approximately 64 in 100 000 per year (Hu, in press). This rate varies with the age and sex of the individual, with men sustaining a disproportionate occurrence of spinal injury in the younger age groups. With aging, women begin to experience greater rates of spinal column injury as a result of osteopenic fractures. Injuries in younger patients are more likely caused by significant trauma and to have other areas of injury in the body (Hu, in press; Saboe et al. 1991). Injury to the spinal column has the worst functional outcome and the highest rate of long term disability of injuries to all organ systems in the human body (MacKenzie et al. 1988).

The care and treatment of the patient with spinal injury must be guided by an accurate and logical clinical and radiological assessment. The majority of patients with spinal column injury do not require operative treatment (Gertzbein 1992). When encountering a patient with a spinal column injury, two major concerns should be kept in mind: (1) assessment and protection of the neurological status of the patientand (2) assessment and maintenance of mechanical integrity. What effects will operative or nonoperative intervention have on the neurological and mechanical structures of the spine? Although separate issues, these two concerns are indivisible and must be assessed and treated in a parallel fashion. Action to address one aspect of the spinal injury will always affect the other.

11.2 History

Treatment of patients with spinal column and neurological injury was surrounded by pessimism until the middle of the twentieth century. The inevitable course of patients with neurological injury was death from early respiratory failure (Van Buren and Wagner 1994) or subsequent urinary sepsis and renal failure. Skin breakdown and contractures from prolonged recumbent care caused significant morbidity and mortality in those patients able to survive the renal and respiratory complications.

11.2.1 Internal Fixation and Fusion

In the latter part of the eighteenth century, there were reports of treatment of spine fractures with spinous process wiring. In the early twentieth century, the use of spinal fusion for infection of the spine was reported Hibbs (1911) and by Albee (1911). During and following the Second World War, Sir Ludwig Guttman established the first multidisciplinary spine units, and his model of treatment of the spinal cord injury patient has been the basis of most modern treatment centers (Guttman 1949).The goals of spinal cord injury care changed as life expectancy improved. The operative treatment of spine fractures was still rare, while postural treatment in specialized spinal cord injury units lowered the mortality associated with these devastating injuries. Prevention of deformity and maximization of function became as important as survival following the initial injury.

Holdsworth (1970) reviewed his patients and was able to differentiate injury patterns that were stable with nonoperative treatment from those that would have progressive deformity or worsening neurological function. In those patients with unstable injury, surgical stabilization was advocated.

Once the concept of stable and unstable spinal injuries became widely acknowledged, internal fixation and fusion was a natural progression. In parallel with concepts being developed in other areas of the treatment of musculoskeletal injury, stable internal fixation with solid fusion gradually became the goal of surgical spine treatment. In the post World War II decade, internal fixation of the spine was limited to spinous process plating or wiring and did not provide stable fixation allowing early mobilization of the patient. Treatment of neurological injuries often included laminectomy, which contributed to the instability at the site of the fracture.

11.2.2 Distraction Rod Fixation

The modern era of internal fixation of the spine began in the late 1950s with the Harrington distraction rod. This rod, with distraction hooks at either end, allowed the in situ correction of deformities and was a quantum leap in the care of the spinal patient. Harrington rods provided the surgeon with a relatively stable internal fixation device that had a significant mechanical ability to correct and apply forces to the spinal column. Although many surgeons were initially quite skeptical of this new method of spinal fixation, the superiority of this system when combined with spinal fusion produced widespread use in scoliosis and further expansion into the spinal fracture arena (Dickson et al. 1978; Reibel et al. 1993). Unfortunately, the greater instability of spinal injury compared to the scoliotic spine was not initially appreciated, and assessment of the injury mechanism and its effect on stability was not clearly defined. The use of the distraction rods in very unstable injuries led to hook dislodgement and rod failure or to unwanted over-distraction of the spinal injury (Gertzbein et al. 1982; McAfee and Bohlman 1985). Despite these problems, the Harrington rod became the mainstay of internal fixation of the unstable spine until the early 1980s.

11.2.3 Segmental Sublaminar Wires

In the early 1980s, sublaminar wiring as reported by Luque provided a method of fixation that did not depend upon hooks at the extremes of the stabilization rod. Segmental sublaminar wiring provided multiple points of fixation throughout the construct, allowing distribution of reduction forces and solid fixation (Luque et al. 1982). Luque rods were widely used in scoliosis; however, with the more widespread use in unstable spine injury, kyphosis and collapse on the rod continued to be a problem (Huckell et al. 1994). A combination of the distraction effects of the Harrington rods with supplemental sublaminar wires provided an excellent compromise to the deficiencies of both systems. Further refinements of the Harrington system occurred with the production of square-ended hooks that allowed contouring of the rods to accommodate the sagittal alignment of the spine (Munson et al. 1984). Edwards and Levine (1986) developed a set of plastic sleeves that increased the reductive force at the fracture site and decreased the length of fusion necessary for instrumentation of the fracture.

11.2.4 Short-Segment Fixation

The necessity to decrease the extent of fusion was becoming clear as more patients experienced accelerated degeneration of segments adjacent to the fusion. With fewer segments fused, more residual motion segments are available to accommodate the normal range of motion encountered in the spine. In an endeavor to minimize motion segments fused, screw fixation of the spine was developed. Facet joint fixation with screws was described by King (1948) and Boucher (1959). These methods had a high rate of pseudoarthrosis and better methods were developed. From 1963 onward, Raymond Roy-Camille described the use of vertebral pedicle screws attached to posterior plates (Roy-Camille et al. 1986). This method of fixation was advocated as a stable method of internal fixation that minimized the length of spinal fusion. Dick (1987) and Magerl (1984) further developed systems and methods of fixation of the spine using pedicular screws connected to rods. Pedicle screw fixation has been further refined and has become a mainstay of internal fixation in patients with thoracolumbar fractures. While pedicle screw fixation was enjoying an explosion in interest, further refinements of the hook rod constructs were being made, fuelled by the concepts popularized by Cotrel et al. (1988) in patients with scoliosis. With multiple hooks connected to rods, the spine could be manipulated and reduced with a high degree of accuracy and controllability. Stability of these constructs was excellent, and these instruments (and their many permutations) were soon being used in the care of spinal fracture patients (Fabris et al. 1994).

Similarly in the cervical spine, short-segment fusion has become common with the advent of posterior facet plating, as advocated by Roy-Camille (Roy-Camille et al. 1992) and Magerl (An et al. 1991a; Heller et al. 1991). Rigid fixation with short segment fusion and less limitation of motion was a percieved advantage. Anterior plate fixation as advocated by Caspar et al. (1989) has become increasingly popular, and as bicortical screw fixation in the cervical spine has been superseded by unicortical locking screws this has become a routine method of stabilization of the fractured cervical spine. Anterior internal fixation has become the sole method of fixation of spinal fractures in the hands of some surgeons (Aebi et al. 1986, 1991).

11.3 Initial Assessment and Management

The first priority in treating patients with suspected spinal injuries is to identify life-threatening conditions that must be treated immediately. During medical stabilization, the patient is immobilized so that assessment and treatment can be safely performed. The patient is placed on a firm "back board" and sandbags are placed beside the head and neck to immobilize the cervical spine. A hard cervical collar may also be applied. Complaints of pain should raise the suspicion of spinal injury. Even with low-energy trauma, fracture can occur in patients with poor-quality bone. Care must be taken to rule out injury, particularly in patients with an altered level of consciousness or intoxication. In these individuals, symptoms may be masked by the mental state and catastrophic events may occur if the injury is not identified. Facial lacerations and fractures are often associated with cervical spine injuries (Bohlman 1979). Rib cage injuries, multiple rib fractures, or sternal injury may be associated with thoracic spine injury. Thoracolumbar junction and lumbar injuries can be associated with intra-abdominal injuries. (Anderson et al. 1991; Saboe et al. 1991).

11.3.1 Physical Examination

Physical examination should be thorough once the primary survey of the patient has been completed and the

patient is hemodynamically stable. Examination of the spinal column with careful inspection of the back for abrasions, contusions, or deformity should be performed. Bruising of the back or flank region or of the anterior abdomen as a result of a seatbelt should raise the suspicion of spinal column injury (Fig. 11.1 a,b). Palpation of the spinous process to outline the contour and integrity of the posterior elements must be performed (Fig. 11.2). Palpable steps or gaps indicate injury to the posterior elements and are important in the subsequent decision making for surgical treatment.

11.3.1.1 Neurological Examination

A complete neurological examination must be performed. This may be difficult to complete in patients who have multiple extremity injuries or are uncooperative, unconscious, or in pain. Nevertheless, it is important to perform the examination in as complete a fashion as possible. Sensation, motor function, and reflex function must be assessed in the upper and lower extremities. This should be done in a systematic fashion, working from proximal muscle groups and moving distally ensuring that all myotomal levels are examined. (Table 11.1).

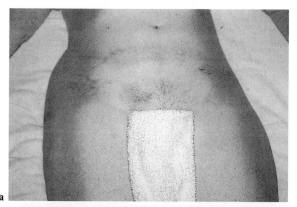

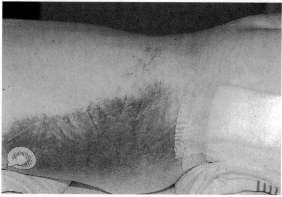

Fig. 11.1. a Anterior abdomen of patient with traumatic lumbosacral dislocation demonstrating bruising from seat belt along the anterior abdominal wall. **b** Demonstrates lateral flank bruising as the result of tracking of blood from the posterior injury

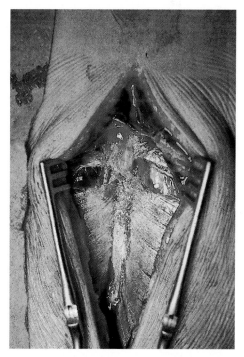

Fig. 11.2. Intraoperative photograph of disruption of the lumbodorsal facet and intraspinous ligaments secondary to a flexion injury and palpation of this prior to surgery would demonstrate tenderness as well as a palpable gap and possibly a deformity as a result of this injury

182

Chapter 11   Fractures of the Spine

Table 11.1. Sensory, motor and reflex findings by anatomical level

Anatomical level	Sensory	Motor	Reflex
C4	Lateral shoulder	Deltoid	N/A
C5	Lateral arm	Brachialis / Biceps	Bicipital
C6	Radial forearm and first webspace	Biceps, pronator teres, brachioradialis	Bicipital
C7	Middle finger	Extensor carpi radialis, triceps	Triceps reflex
C8	Ulnar border of hand	Flexor carpi ulnaris, deep finger flexors	
T1	Ulnar border of forearm	Intrinsics, abduction/ adduction fingers	
T4	Nipple level		
T10	Umbilicus		
L1	Inguinal crease		
L2	Anterior thigh	Hip flexors	
L3	Anterior distal thigh	Hip Adductors/ flexors	
L4	Anterior knee, medial calf	Quadriceps, foot dorsiflexions	Quadriceps reflex
L5	Dorsum of foot	Extensor hallucis longus, hip abductor	
S1	Lateral heel	Plantar flexors of feet	Achille's reflex
S2-S3-S4	Perianal sensation	Rectal tone	Bulbo- cavernosus

Sensation testing must also be performed in a continuous systematic manner from cranial to caudal. The torso and abdominal regions are often overlooked in this assessment, and it should be remembered that the cervical dermatomes extend to the proximal torso just distal to the clavicles. Thoracic neurological injury can only be accurately located by a thorough sensory examination. Reflex examination must be performed in the upper and lower extremities assessing for presence or absence. Asymmetry of response will indicate the side of maximal injury. If deep tendon reflexes are brisk and plantar responses are upgoing, injury to the spinal cord may have occurred. More commonly, these findings of hyperreflexia represent a more chronic process causing an upper motor neuron lesion secondary to compression of the spinal cord. In acute spinal cord injury, flaccid paralysis with absent reflexes is most common.

11.3.1.2 Sacral Reflexes

Sparing of spinal cord function may only be demonstrated by preservation of sacral sensation. Sacral reflexes, such as the anal wink or bulbocavernosus reflex, will provide the earliest evidence of resolution of spinal shock. When this occurs, an accurate prognosis for spinal cord recovery can be rendered. If no return of neurological function has occurred following the resolution of spinal shock, the potential for functional recovery following spinal cord injury is negligible.

11.3.1.3 Corticosteroids

If spinal cord injury has occurred, maintenance of spinal cord perfusion is important to prevent further damage to the cord. High-dose corticosteroid administration should be performed; in a multicenter randomized, controlled clinical trial it has been demonstrated to be effective in improving neurological recovery following spinal cord injury. Megadose steroid administration must be administered within 8 h of injury. An initial bolus of 30 mg/kg body weight followed by an infusion of 5.4 mg/kg for 23 h following injury is recommended. Some controversy remains concerning the extent of neurological recovery as well as the potential side effects of high-dose corticosteroid therapy (Bracken et al. 1990; Ducker and Zeidman 1994).

11.3.2 Initial Radiological Assessment

Radiological assessment should be done after stabilization of life-threatening injuries. X-rays should include orthogonal views of the entire spinal column in the head-injured or intoxicated patient. In the conscious and alert patient, the cervical spine should be X-rayed as well as any other area that is painful or tender. Once a suspicious area has been identified, a determination of stability should be made. If insufficient information exists on the plain radiographs to make this decision, then further imaging should be done.

11.3.2.1 Plain Films and Tomography

Plain radiographs remain the mainstay of assessment of patients with spinal injury. Tomography is still a helpful method to delineate lesions that are not clear on plain films. Although computed tomography (CT) examination is the preferred next step in the imaging of bony injury, tomography can provide a view of the spine in the sagittal dimension that provides more useful information than axial CT or reformatted sagittal views.

Table 11.2. Clinical instability in the middle and lower cervical spine

Element	Point value[a]
Anterior elements destroyed or unable to function	2
Posterior elements destroyed or unable to function	2
Positive stretch test	2
Radiographic: (resting films) Sagittal plane displacement > 3.5 mm Sagittal plane angulation > 11°	4
Abnormal disc narrowing	1
Developmentally narrow spinal canal Sagittal diameter < 13 mm Pavlov ratio < 0.8	1
Spinal cord damage	2
Nerve root damage	1
Dangerous loading anticipated	1

From White and Panjabi (1990).
[a] A total of 5 points or more is regarded as unstable.

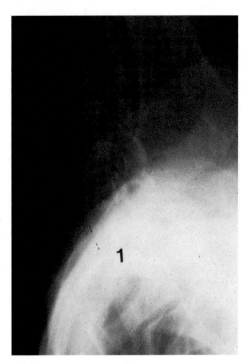

Fig. 11.4. Lateral swimmer's view with markers on the vertebral body of C7 and T1 *(1)* demonstrating satisfactory alignment

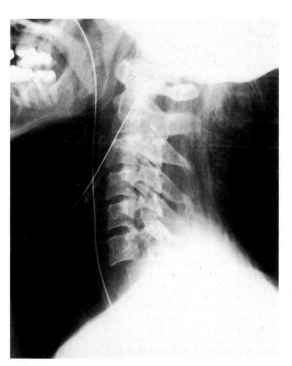

Fig. 11.3. Lateral cervical spine X-ray with translation of C6 on C7

Tomography is also useful in identifying odontoid fractures or facet injuries in the lower cervical spine. Fractures and changes in alignment in the lower cervical and upper thoracic spine may also be seen more readily on lateral tomography.

The plain radiographs should be assessed in a systematic way. The anterior and posterior vertebral body alignment should proceed in a gentle arc with no sharp transitions in sagittal alignment. The individual vertebral bodies are then inspected for injury. Anterior translation of the cephalad body in relation to the caudad body should be assessed and compared to acceptable limits (Table 11.2). Soft tissue swelling in the area anterior to the cervical spine may represent hematoma or soft tissue injury. The acceptable width of soft tissue is up to 7 mm anterior to C3 and up to 20 mm anterior to C5, C6, and C7 (Penning 1981). Variation in the outline of the vertebral body on anteroposterior view may represent fracture or deformity.

In the cervical spine lateral (Fig. 11.3), anteroposterior and open mouth odontoid views are necessary. If the cervicothoracic junction is not visible on the lateral, a transthoracic swimmers view is mandatory (Fig. 11.4). If the radiographs are negative, yet the patient has significant pain or tenderness to palpation of the cervical spine, flexion extension views should be performed. These must be done under the supervision of a physician and the patient must be entirely cooperative. Until the patient is conscious and cooperative the spine cannot be completely "cleared."

The upper thoracic spine is particularly difficult to visualize in heavyset individuals. The lateral view will often be obscured by the bulk of the shoulder and other

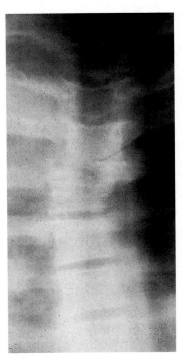

Fig. 11.5. Anterior posterior tomography of the upper thoracic spine demonstrating a lateral translation and a fracture through the vertebral body of T4

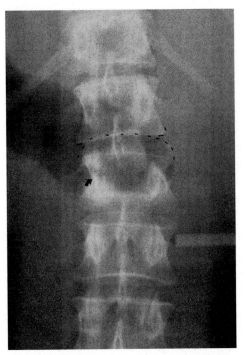

Fig. 11.7. Change in alignment that can be assessed from an anterior posterior view. Note the body of L2 has an oval appearance as demonstrated by the *cross-hatch marks.* The body of L1, however, remains rectangular in appearance. This indicates a kyphotic deformity with malaligmnent of L1 and L2. Note the fracture through the pedicle of L2 as demonstrated by the *arrow*

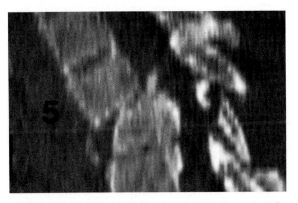

Fig. 11.6. Sagittal reconstruction of computed tomography examination demonstrating anterior translation of T5 *(5)* on T6. Note also the posterior element fracture with comminution of the facet joint

methods of imaging such as tomography or CT scan with sagittal reconstructions should be done (Figs. 11.5, 11.6). Injuries in the axial plain may not be adequately visualized by CT axial cuts only, and reconstructions are necessary. The anteroposterior views of the thoracic spine may provide a great deal of information. A sudden change of vertebral body outline from rectangular to oval indicates that there is a marked change in sagittal alignment, possibly indicating a kyphotic deformity. This radiographic appearance results from the relative orientation of the vertebrae from anteroposterior (rectangular) to oblique (viewing the anterior body in more profile and thus seeing an oval outline) (Fig. 11.7). Mediastinal widening can indicate thoracic injury as a result of paraspinal hematoma (Bolesta and Bohlman 1991; Fig. 11.8). Rotation or malalignment of the spinous processes or offset of the pedicles indicates that there has been significant rotatory injury to the thoracic spine.

At the thoracolumbar junction, widening of the pedicles on the anteroposterior view is pathognomonic of the burst fracture (Martijn and Weldhuis 1991). In these injuries the lateral view can demonstrate a cortical rim of retropulsed bone within the spinal canal (McGrory et al. 1993; Fig. 11.9). Kyphosis and percentage crush of the vertebral body is readily obtained on the lateral view. The normal sagittal alignment of the thoracolumbar junction is neutral with no kyphosis or lordosis.

The lumbosacral spine is well visualized with plain radiography. Anteroposterior and lateral views are sufficient in this region, and oblique views are seldom necessary. Rotation of vertebral bodies as demonstrated by offset of the spinous processes is an important indicator

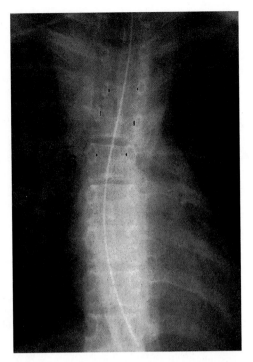

Fig. 11.8. Fracture dislocation of T5 on T6. Of particular note is the malalignment of the pedicles from T4 to T6 and one can see a widening of the T5 pedicle as well as a translation of this vertebral body

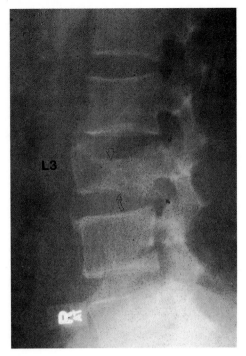

Fig. 11.9. This burst fracture of *L3* demonstrates retropulsion of bone into the spinal canal as illustrated by the *solid arrows*. Also, injury to the superior and inferior endplates indicates loss of integrity of the vertebral body as demonstrated by the *open arrows*

of injury, as is widening of the interspinous distance (Fig. 11.10). The sacral spine is often overlooked as an area of injury, and the symmetry of the sacral foramen should be reviewed. The arches of the foramen are continuous and symmetrical bilaterally. These injuries are often associated with pelvic injuries, and the sacral foramen should be outlined to ensure that no injury has occurred.

11.3.2.2 Computed Tomography Scan

CT examination is often done following plain film identification of a suspicious area in the spine. CT images are computer-generated averages of X-ray data obtained in the axial plane (McAfee et al. 1983). As a result there are limitations to the information that the CT scan can provide. Injuries that are predominantly in the axial plane can be overlooked (Fig. 11.11). The amount of canal occlusion is best demonstrated by CT scan of the injured level (Keene et al. 1989). Three-dimensional and sagittal reconstructions are often performed to assist in visualizing complex fractures and these images may prove helpful (Figs. 11.12, 11.13). The CT examination is of particular importance when planning surgical approach and instrumentation technique (McAfee et al. 1983).

11.3.2.3 Myelography

The majority of spinal injuries are adequately visualized with plain film and CT examination and do not require myelography. Myelography should be performed when neurological deficit is incompatible with the plain film injury or when the neurological deficit is progressing. Myelography should always be accompanied by CT examination. One other clear indication for imaging the neurological elements is in those patients with potential disc extrusion following bilateral facet subluxation or dislocation in the cervical spine . Imaging can be done with myelography or magnetic resonance imaging (MRI), whichever is most readily available. In the thoracolumbar spine, flexion distraction injuries may similarly cause injury to the disc, allowing extrusion into the canal (Fig. 11.14). Care should be taken to identify this possibility and decompress the canal prior to reduction of the deformity.

11.3.2.4 Magnetic Resonance Imaging

MRI investigation is now becoming common in the assessment of patients with acute spinal injury. The

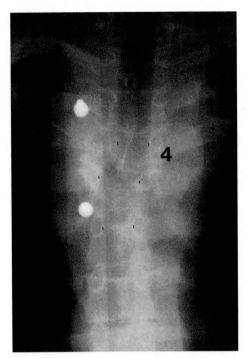

Fig. 11.10. This anterior posterior view of the upper thoracic spine again demonstrates a rotation of the vertebral bodies and lateral translation indicating a complete fracture dislocation

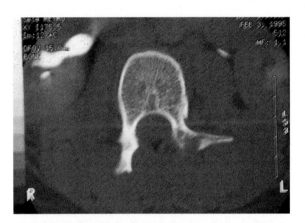

Fig. 11.11. Axial view of a flexion distraction injury. Despite the severity of the injury there is relatively little damage to the body of the vertebra. One should, however, note the evidence of an empty facet and this would indicate that there has been some degree of kyphosis or dislocation and no remaining posterior element integrity

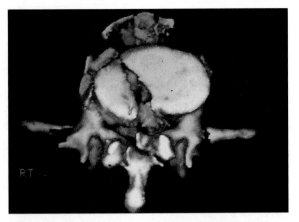

Fig. 11.12. Three-dimensional reconstruction of the fractured vertebral body demonstrates a complete occlusion of the spinal canal as well as evidence of posterior facet and laminar injury. This assists in assessment of the integrity of the vertebral body

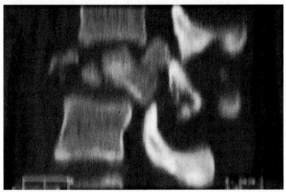

Fig. 11.13. Sagittal reconstruction of the previously noted fracture, again demonstrating complete canal encroachment as well as vertebral body comminution

appearance of the spinal cord on MRI has prognostic value in terms of completeness and recoverability of cord injury. The presence of hematoma within the cord is a poor prognostic indicator for functional recovery (Bondurant et al. 1990). Identification of ligamentous injury is also of great value when spinal injury has

occurred. Often the bony injury is not exceptional, yet ligamentous injury is extensive on MRI and the decision to stabilize is clarified (Brightman et al. 1992; Emery et al. 1989). Bony injury will not be satisfactorily demonstrated with MRI only, and CT is still the method of choice in this situation. Use of MRI in those patients with multiple injuries and needing ventilator support is still technically complex and requires appropriate ventilators and life-support apparatus.

Once the injury has been identified and the patient stabilized, the decision about operative intervention must be made. This will be based on evidence gathered from the clinical and radiological investigations.

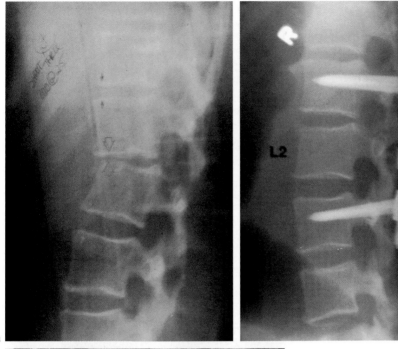

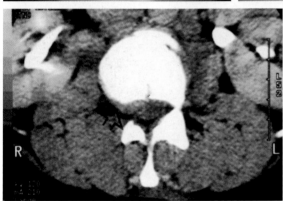

Fig. 11.14. a Lateral lumbar spine X-ray with a narrowing of the intervertebral disk space at the level of the injury as demonstrated by the large open arrows. This is compared to the disc space above and below. This narrowing of disc space is suspicious of a disk injury and in flexion distraction injury through soft tissue one should be aware of this. **b** Computed tomography scan of this injury with evidence of disk extrusion at the night posterior lateral corner. Decompression should be performed prior to fixation

11.4 Classification

A classification system is useful only if it can facilitate communication, help in decision making, and truly differentiate those fractures that are prone to further neurological and mechanical deterioration from those injuries that are trivial. Sir Frank Holdsworth used a mechanistic method to classify fractures (Holdsworth 1970). He described an anterior column comprised of the vertebral body and associated ligaments and disc structures and a posterior column including the facet joints, lamina, spinous processes, and associated ligaments. Fractures could be differentiated depending upon the columns injured. Denis (1984) extended this classification by describing a third column that included the posterior half of the vertebral body and its associat-

ed annulus and disc. This third column was implicated as the distinguishing figure of the burst fracture and became more evident with the advent and popularization of the CT scanner. The anterior column and the posterior column can be biomechanically demonstrated; however, the middle column is not a separate mechanical entity. Ferguson and Allen used a mechanistic classification to describe fractures of the cervical and thoracolumbar spine (Allen et al. 1982; Ferguson and Allen 1984). Their classification system is useful to understand the injuring forces and has some utility in planning treatment. Louis (1983) has used a classification schema that uses three pillars as the basis of description. The vertebral bodies are stacked one upon another as a multisegmented pillar; similarly the facet joints are paired, multisegmented pillars contributing to the overall stability of the spine. The AO group has recently devised

Table 11.3. Checklist for clinical instability in the thoracic and thoracolumbar spine

Element	Point value[a]
Anterior elements destroyed	2
Posterior elements destroyed	2
Disruption of costovertebral articulations	1
Radiographic: (resting films) Sagittal plane translation > 2.5 mm (2 points) Sagittal plane angulation > 5° (2 points)	4
Spinal cord or cauda equina damage	2
Dangerous loading anticipated	1
Total of 5 or more=unstable	

From White and Panjabi (1990).
[a] A total of 5 points or more is regarded as unstable.

Table 11.4. Checklist for clinical instability in the lumbar spine

Element	Point value[a]
Anterior elements destroyed	2
Posterior elements destroyed	2
Radiographic: (resting films) Sagital plane translation > 4.5 mm or 15% Sagital plane angulation > 22°	4
Cauda equina damage	3
Dangerous loading anticipated	1

From White and Panjabi (1990).
[a] A total of 5 points or more is regarded as unstable.

Table 11.5. Cervical spine injury and treatment

Cervical level	Neurological deficit	Anterior approach	Posterior approach	Nonoperative
Occiput C1 injury	Usually fatal if present		Occipital cervical fusion with internal fixation	
C1-C2 transverse ligament injury	Partial injuries result of impingement of C1 arch on spinal cord		Stabilization C1-C2 fusion; wire/bone graft or transfacetal screws	
Odontoid fracture type II i) Undisplaced <4 mm ii) Anterior displacement iii) Posterior displacement	25%-40% fatal at accident scene	iii) Odontoid compression screw	ii) Wire/bone graft fusion or transfacetal screws	i) Halo
Acute C2 spondylolisthesis i) Undisplaced ii) Displaced iii) Angulated/displaced iv) Disc/facet disruption		iii) Anterior plating C2-3 iv) Anterior plating C2-3	iii) Posterior C1-3 fusion	i) Hard collar ii) Halo iii) Halo then if displaces operatively
C3-C7 i) Anterior element disruption ii) Facet dislocation/ fracture (i.e., posterior disruption)	+ Anterior compression – Neurological deficit – Anterior compression + Root compression from facet fracture	i) Anterior decompression and plating fusion	ii) Closed reduction, then posterior fixation; wiring or facet plating	Halo immobilization

a classification system based upon a mechanistic description of the radiological appearance (Magerl et al. 1994). Three major injuring forces are included: type A (compression forces), type B (distraction forces), and type C (torsion forces). Injuries are not exclusively one type or another, and combinations of injury mechanism can occur. Further subclassification divides these injuries into increasingly severe levels of damage. Type A1 injuries affect the vertebral body only and are the result of axial compression or flexion; they are described in other classifications as compression fractures. A2 injuries have a vertebral body split in the coronal or sagittal plane and the posterior elements are generally not involved. The A3 injuries consist of burst fractures with retropulsion of bone into the canal. Type B1 injuries have predominantly posterior element distraction and have been described in other schemata as flexion distraction injuries through the disc or ligament. B2 inju-

Table 11.6. Thoracic and lumbar injury

Level	Neurological deficit	Anterior approach	Posterior approach
T1-T3	Negative		Hook rod fixation lower cervical to midthoracic spine
T1-T3	Positive	Anterolateral approach to cervical with sternal osteotomy with or without plate	With or without posterior hook rod fixation
T3-T5	Negative or positive complete cord injury		Hook rod fixation three levels proximal and three levels distal
T3-T5	Positive partial cord injury	Anterior thoracotomy, parascapular approach decompression plus+ plating	
T5-T11 i) Type A ii) Type B posterior iii) Type C	Negative or complete cord injury		Types A and C: Posterior hook rod three above three below Type B: compression hook rod
T11-L2 i) Type A ii) Type B posterior iii) Type C	Negative		Types A and C: posterior pedicle screw reduction and fusion Type B: compression hook rod
T11-L2 i) Type A ii) Type B posterior iii) Type C	Positive	Type A: Anterior thoracoabdominal decompression and stabilization and bone graft strut	Type B: compression or pedicle screw Type C: posterior stabilization
L3-L5	Positive		Posterior pedicle screw fixation and posterolateral decompression
L3-L5	Negative		Posterior pedicle screw fixaton

ries occur through bone, and B3 lesions are anterior distraction injuries through the disc as a result of hyperextension forces. Type C injuries are injuries of the anterior and posterior elements with rotation in combination with a type A or B injury and are commonly described as fracture-dislocations. These are the most unstable and require stabilization.

White and Panjabi (1990) have developed an objective quantifiable check list of criteria for clinical instability. Throughout the spinal column specific amounts of anterolisthesis and kyphosis have been shown to correlate with instability in a laboratory setting. These guidelines imply an inability to bear a physiological load (Tables 11.3–11.6).

The upper cervical spine is an anatomically distinct region. Fractures and injuries in this area have specific classifications that relate to injury mechanism and subsequent treatment. Thoracic and lumbar injuries are descriptively classified as follows:

- Compression injuries, which involve the vertebral body with little effect upon the spinal canal and low likelihood of posterior ligamentous injury. These are the result of flexion forces on the spine.
- Burst fractures, which involve the spinal canal with retropulsion of the posterior vertebral cortex and and result from a combination of axial loading and flexion.
- Flexion distraction or Chance-type injuries, which involve posterior element distraction secondary to flexion about a center of rotation anterior to the abdomen.
- Fracture-dislocations, which involve large-magnitude forces in flexion, rotation, or shear that disrupt all spinal elements causing displacement.

The underlying questions that all of these classifications attempt to address are the integrity of the anterior compressive column, the integrity of the posterior elements, and the effects upon the neurological elements (Pope and Panjabi 1985). Although we routinely use Denis' classification system to describe fractures of the thoracolumbar spine, the decision to operatively stabilize is not based solely upon the radiographic classification. Both clinical and radiological diagnosis must be examined rationally to treat the spinal injury.

11.5 Operative Decision-Making with Neurological and Biomechanical Goals

The objective of care of the spinal-injured patient is to have a stable, pain-free spine, to prevent increased neurological deficit, and to provide conditions for the improvement of neurological deficit. The neurological and biomechanical goals are separate but interrelated and must be thought of in parallel rather than sequential fashion. Rehabilitation of the patient will be optimal if these objectives can be met. One should strive to prevent unnecessary surgery, while simultaneously preventing catastrophes.

11.5.1 Indications

There are clear indications for surgical treatment of spinal injury. Progressive neurological deficit is an emergency situation and identification of the cause of deterioration by imaging of the spinal canal with CT, myelography, or MRI should be done expeditiously. If compression of neurological structures is demonstrated, decompression is done on an emergency basis. Stabilization is done in conjunction with decompression since the stability of the spine is often compromised by the same injuring event.

Injuries with complete neurological deficit will usually require stabilization. The potential for recovery of a complete spinal cord injury is low. However, the spine is generally unstable as a result of the magnitude of force required to cause complete injury of the neurological elements. These injuries require operative stabilization for early rehabilitation.

Controversy exists in patients who have no neurological deficit or a stable partial deficit. In an attempt to approach these injuries logically, the following questions should be considered.

11.5.1.1 Does the Patient Have a Neurological Deficit? If so, to What Degree?

Greater amounts of force are required to produce complete neurological deficits and greater amounts of instability result. Complete lesions routinely require stabilization. A nerve root injury implies that less displacement of the spine has occurred following injury and the magnitude of injuring force is less than in a complete cord injury. Although still a serious injury, the spinal column may retain more stability than in the patient with complete cord injury. Incomplete neurological deficit, either cord or root, will likely have some improvement with nonsurgical treatment; however, there is strong opinion that optimal recovery can best be achieved through decompression of these neurological elements in those patients with demonstrated compression. In the cervical spine, sparing of even one nerve root level will have significant effect upon the function of a quadriplegic patient, and surgery to achieve this goal through decompression of the nerve root and cord can be justified. (Anderson and Bohlman 1992; Bohlman and Anderson 1992; Clohisy et al. 1992) (McAfee et al. 1985).

11.5.1.2 Are the Anterior Elements Intact?

In cancellous bone with straightforward compression injuries, the strength of the remaining bone is 60% stronger than the original cancellous bone (White and Panjabi 1990). Therefore, potential further collapse is minimal. This is likely true in those patients with only superior endplate involvement; however, one should be cautious in those patients who have a bursting type that affects both superior and inferior endplates of the vertebral body. In such cases extrusion of the anterior portion of the vertebral body is often seen, indicating loss of cortical integrity. The vertebral body will not withstand normal physiological loads and internal fixation must be performed (McCormack et al. 1994). Vertebral body compression with superior and inferior endplate involvement is often associated with a loss of vertebral height of greater than 50%, and operative fixation should be considered. In addition, if kyphosis of the injured segment exceeds 30° in the thoracolumbar spine, then sagittal alignment is compromised and compensatory changes in alignment elsewhere in the spine must occur. Patients with greater than 30° of kyphosis have poorer functional results following treatment than patients with less deformity (Gertzbein 1992). Rotational malalignment on the anteroposterior film indicates an injuring force that was significant and stabilization should be considered.

Assessment of the anterior vertebral body must be followed by assessment of the posterior elements of the spine.

11.5.1.3 Are the Posterior Elements Intact?

Posterior element injury indicates that the spine is more unstable; however, undisplaced or minimally displaced laminar fractures such as in burst injuries are not indicators of disruption of the posterior ligamentous structures. Major injury to the posterior elements usually occurs through distraction or rotation forces.

Physical examination may reveal a palpable defect, malalignment of the spinous processes, bruising, or severe tenderness on palpation of the spine. Review of the anteroposterior or lateral plain radiographs may demonstrate widening of the interspinous distance, fracture of the lamina or pars interarticularis, or rotational malalignment of the spinous processes. CT examination can demonstrate asymmetry or gaping of the facet joints, indicating injury to the posterior ligamentous or bony structures. The stabilizing function of the posterior elements are lost and the residual stability of the anterior elements are relied upon to maintain spinal column integrity. Posterior element injury rarely occurs in isolation and usually have an associated anterior column injury. Injury through ligament or disc has a poorer prognosis with nonsurgical treatment. Lesions through bone may heal adequately when treated with bracing.

11.5.1.4 What Information to Assess with Imaging?

Good-quality imaging is essential for good-quality decision making. Adequate, well-centred, technically good plain films will be the first imaging method to contribute to the decision. This is most often followed by CT examination. CT can clearly define injury of the posterior bony elements. It provides information concerning the size of bony fragments, size of vertebral pedicles (for insertion of pedicle fixation), and the extent of vertebral destruction. The CT scan, however, cannot clearly demonstrate soft tissue injury. Patients with injuries where the plane of tissue disruption is parallel to the axial CT images may have their injuries underestimated or overlooked. The amount of bony retropulsion into the spinal canal does not form a definite indication for operative decompression of the neurological elements. Patients with almost complete occlusion of the spinal canal may have no deficit, and patients with minimal occlusion may have complete deficits. The CT scan is only a "snapshot" in time and there may have been more spinal canal compression that has subsequently recoiled since the time of injury (Keene et al. 1989; McAfee et al. 1983). If neurological deficit secondary to bony compression is identified, then decompression should be performed. If no neurological deficit is present, then operative treatment should not be based solely on the CT scan that demonstrates "significant" canal occlusion.

11.5.1.5 Will the Patient Tolerate Operative or Nonoperative Treatment?

Surgical treatment of spinal injury is not a minor procedure. Surgery may be prolonged, blood loss may be significant, and increasing damage to the neurological elements can occur from the preoperative or intraoperative care of these individuals. Conversely, the prolonged recumbent treatment of patients with unstable injuries is unsatisfactory as a result of the potential effects of pulmonary decompensation, thromboembolic disease, and general debility that will occur.

11.6 Preparation for Surgery

Once the decision for operative treatment has been made further preparation is necessary to ensure an optimal outcome. Decisions must be made concerning:

1. Timing of surgery
2. Preoperative planning and preparation
3. Surgical approaches
   – For decompression
   – For stabilization
4. Stabilization methods

11.6.1 Timing of Surgery

Timing of surgery remains a controversial topic. With all patients with neurological deterioration, surgery should be performed on an emergency basis. The primary goal in this case is rapid decompression of the neurological elements and stabilization of the spinal column. In patients with neurological deficits that are stable, the patient may benefit from decompression and stabilization in the first 24 h. Although neurological recovery has not be definitively related to the rapidity of decompressive procedures, complications such as respiratory dysfunction and pressure sores are decreased with early fixation and mobilization. In the multiply injured patient, early decompression and stabilization is desirable, although the logistics of a complex, occasionally lengthy operation may overwhelm the resources available. We prefer to operate at the earliest possible time when somatosensory evoked potential monitoring (SSEP), experienced nursing staff, and surgical assistants are available. With the increasing complexity of spinal instrumentation systems, this is becoming more important for the efficient intraoperative care of the spinal-injured patient. Fatigue, inexperience with internal fixation systems, and unprepared assistants lead to frustration on the part of the surgeon, and care can be suboptimal as a result of these factors. Anesthesia must also be prepared for the treatment of these patients, and particularly in cervical spine injuries the availability of an experienced anesthesiologist capable of fiberoptic intubation is a necessity. The patient is usually taken to the operating room between 24 h and 3–4 days following injury.

We use SSEP monitoring in those patients with an incomplete neurological lesion who are undergoing decompression of the spinal canal. SSEP monitoring is also used in neurologically normal patients who have significant deformity and who will require reduction of this deformity. Evoked potential monitoring is an accurate method of evaluating the function of the spinal cord and in experienced hands will allow the operating surgeon the ability to correct any reversible lesions that may occur as a result of positioning or reduction of the spinal injury. Decreases in peak-to-peak amplitude of greater than 50% sustained for more than 15 min indicates that a significant event has occured (Nash and Brown 1989). Anesthetic agents should be reviewed for changes in dosage that can be related to the SSEP monitoring. Electrodes must be examined to ensure that these have not been dislodged, and if there is no other reason for the amplitude changes, the reduction maneuver must be relaxed. If caught early, lesions are reversible if they result from sudden changes in position or distraction and the inciting event is altered.

11.6.2 Patient Positioning

Patient positioning is critical in the execution of any operative procedure. The surgical approach used, whether or not decompression is performed, and stabilization will all have a bearing on patient positioning. General aspects of the prone position to keep in mind are that with cervical posterior approaches the head must be securely stabilized in a neutral position in relation to the torso. This can be done with the use of a Mayfield tongs or with a halo ring attached to the anterior portion of the vest. Care must be taken to pull the shoulders distally with tape to allow satisfactory X-ray of the lower cervical spine. The arms must be tucked along the sides and well padded at the elbow and wrist. The body should be supported with bolsters that minimize pressure on the abdomen. The bed can be placed in a slightly reverse Trendelenburg to assist in the view of the field.

Anterior approaches to the cervical spine necessitate the use of a small bolster beneath the shoulders to allow slight physiological extension of the neck. The head should have traction applied preferably through Gardner-Wells tongs. The head can be turned slightly away from the side of approach. Shoulders should also be taped to allow visualization of the lower cervical spine on X-ray. Arms are tucked by the side and a slight reverse Trendelenburg position can be used.

Posterior approaches to the thoracic and lumbar spine should be performed with the patient positioned on firm bolsters across the chest and pelvis. These will allow the abdomen to hang free to decrease pressure in the intra-abdominal veins and bleeding from the epidural veins. We do not use a Relton-Hall or Wilson frame

because of the inability to image through these frames. The operating table we use is radiolucent and allows anteroposterior and lateral image intensification without obscuring of the spine.

With anterior approaches to the thoracic and lumbar spine, the patient is positioned in the lateral decubitus position. Care must be taken to ensure that the coronal plane of the spine is perpendicular to the floor. This will serve as an indirect guide to the instrumentation that may be implanted. It must be ensured that vertebral screws be implanted away from the spinal canal. This can only be ensured if the orientation of the spinal canal is known. Flexion of the table is helpful to open the lateral flank or thoracic incision. This position must be borne in mind when definitive fixation is performed, since scoliosis can occur from the flexion. Straightening the operating table prior to the closure will make closure easier.

11.6.3 Intraoperative Blood Loss

Intraoperative blood loss can be minimized and limited by a number of different methods. Appropriate operative positioning must be done to prevent excess intra-abdominal pressure. If bolsters are used, they should be large enough to allow the abdomen to hang free. Judicious use of monopolar and bipolar cautery is essential. In cases that require extensive exposure and dissection, such as hook rod fixation of the thoracic spine or combined anteroposterior fixation cases, where blood loss is expected to exceed 500 ml, the cell saver should be used to salvage and reinfuse blood from the surgical field.

11.7 Anatomy as Related to Surgical Approaches

11.7.1 Posterior Approach

Surgical approaches to the spine are thought to be straightforward and simple. Almost all procedures in the past were performed through a midline posterior incision. The exposure from the upper cervical spine to the lumbosacral junction is similar, with subperiosteal dissection of the paraspinal musculature to the transverse process regions simple to perform. There are some regions that provide more challenge and require some preoperative planning to minimize intraoperative difficulties. Particularly in transition areas such as the occipitocervical, cervicothoracic, and lumbosacral regions, proper wide draping and generous exposure are necessary to facilitate fixation of these regions.

The posterior approach can be used for decompression of neural elements in specific indications where compression of neural elements from posterior structures occurs.

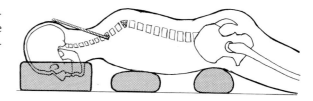

11.7.1.1 Cervical Spine Posterior Approach

To allow safe instrumentation of the occipitocervical region, care must be exercised during the positioning of the patient. With the head extended, the space between the occiput and lamina of C1 is almost nonexistent. Without placing the head in a neutral or slightly flexed position, the laminar space will be impossible to instrument. The upper cervical region requires increased care when dissection over the arch of C1 is being performed. At this level the vertebral arteries are at risk and are approximately 1.5 cm from the midline of the lamina as they enter the posterolateral foramen magnum.

11.7.1.2 Cervical Spine Decompression

Patients with nerve root lesions in the cervical spine secondary to facet joint fracture should have posterior decompression of the nerve root followed by stabilization of the spine. When anterior compression of the spinal cord is present, anterior decompression should be performed. The cord responds poorly to retraction, and a complete decompression of anterior structures from the posterior approach can produce catastrophic results from retraction of the neural elements.

11.7.1.3 Thoracic Spine Posterior Approach

Similarly, when instrumenting upper thoracic fractures, the instrumentation must often extend into the lower cervical region. Because of the transition from kyphosis to lordosis, the lamina are difficult to approach and placing laminar hooks over the lamina in this region is frustrating. Long-handled instruments will tend to abut against the cervical spine, making insertion increasingly difficult (Fig. 11.15). In this situation, preoperative preparation of the entire mid- and lower cervical spine will allow extension of the skin incision and facilitation of placement of fixation devices.

11.7.1.4 Lumbosacral Junction Posterior Approach

In the lumbosacral junction region there is a similar transition from the lordotic region to kyphotic region. Placement of fixation devices in this region may prove challenging. Overhang of the posterior iliac crest may

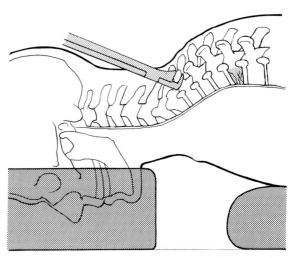

Fig. 11.15. Line drawing illustrating the difficulty of placing internal fixation as well as instrumentation in the upper thoracic spine following an upper thoracic injury. Abutment against the base of the skull may occur because of the deformity as well as the change in sagittal alignment from kyphosis to lordosis in this region. Care should be taken to adequately expose this area to allow safe placement of internal fixation

make placement of pedicle screws into the sacral pedicle difficult, and sacral ala fixation may be necessary. In addition, some instrumentation devices may not be suited for the lordosis of this level, and placement of the fixation may be impossible without appropriate connectors. Notwithstanding the need to gain adequate exposure to facilitate instrumentation, as little dissection of the paraspinal musculature as possible should be performed to allow maximal functional recovery. The patient's functional results are felt to correlate with amount of paraspinal dissection and denervation. To minimize dissection, prevent the wrong level from being instrumented, and decrease denervation of muscle, a lateral plain radiograph should always be performed with a radiological marker on a readily identifiable bony structure.

11.7.2 Thoracolumbar and Lumbar Spine Decompression

At the thoracolumbar junction and caudad to this level, the spinal cord is smaller or has ended and retraction of the thecal sac has less predilection for neural damage. Decompression through a posterolateral approach or a transpedicular approach can be done relatively safely. However, it must be kept in mind that a decompression done in this manner will add to the instability of the fracture and fixation becomes even more necessary to prevent further complications.

If the decision to decompress posteriorly has been made, the preoperative CT scan is used to plan the proce-

dure. Care should be exercised when dissecting muscle from the lamina. Often a fracture of the lamina and disruption of the posterior ligaments has occurred. Inadvertent entry into the spinal canal can occur with subsequent damage of the neural elements. Exposure of the transverse processes to identify landmarks and prepare for fusion is done prior to the decompression. This will provide some protection to the neural elements. The spinal canal should be entered at the interlaminar level between the cephalad vertebrae and the injured vertebrae (Garfin et al. 1985; Hardaker et al. 1992). This is contrary to the degenerative case where entry into the spinal canal occurs at the named level of the disc (i.e., L4–5 discs enter at L4–5 interlaminar space). This difference in entry point is appropriate, since the majority of burst

Fig. 11.16. a Entrance into the canal proximal to the named interlaminary space. **b** If a burst fracture of L1 occurs then entrance into the canal is obtained from the T12-L1 interlaminary space. This is as a result of the relationship of the retropulse bone to the pedicle bone of the injured vertebrae. **c** Initial decompression through the pedicle and removal of cancellous bone from this region. **d** Care should be taken to leave the posterior cortical margin. **e** Further reduction of this cortical rim can be performed after the cancellous bone has been removed and gentle impaction of the cortical fragment can then be accomplished

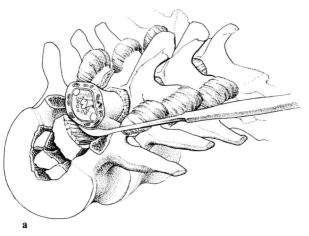

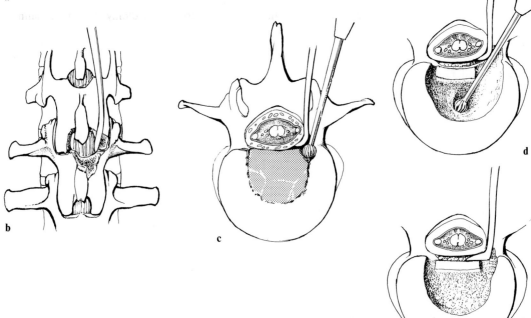

fractures have retropulsed bone originating from between the pedicles of the vertebrae. The pedicles are cephalad to the lamina of the injured level. Once the canal has been entered, the pedicle is identified. In patients with neurological deficits and a laminar fracture on CT scan, dural tears may be present and must be repaired (Cammisa et al. 1989). As a result of tenting of neural elements over retropulsed bone, the pedicle may have to be removed using a high-speed dissecting burr. This allows room to decompress the retropulsed vertebral fragment without undue tension on the thecal sac and its contents. The burr is used to undercut the vertebral body, and the remaining cortical shell of bone is then gently impacted into the space created. Special angled bone punches may be used for this purpose. Once sufficient decompression of one side of the spinal canal has been performed, the contralateral side can be done. It may not be necessary to remove the pedicle on the contralateral side, since tension on the neural elements will be less after a partial decompression of the sac. Careful palpation of the floor of the canal should then be done with an angled instrument to ensure complete decompression (Fig. 11.16).

There is great controversy concerning the approach for decompression of the spinal canal in patients with a thoracolumbar bursting-type fracture. Advocates of anterior and posterior approaches provide reasoned arguments for both approaches, and this will be touched upon further in this chapter.

11.7.3 Anterior Approach

As surgical and anesthetic techniques have become more refined, the anterior approaches to the spine have become more popular. The surgeon must be familiar with the relevant anatomy of the anterior cervical spine, the thoracic cavity, and the retroperitoneal structures in the abdomen. Although all vertebrae in the spinal column can be reached from an anterior approach, some are more difficult to reach and have greater potential complications than others.

11.7.3.1 Cervical Spine

Cervical vertebrae from C3 to C7 can be reached through a standard anterolateral approach to the cervical spine. This utilizes the interval medial to the carotid sheath and anterior to the sternocleidomastoid. The pretracheal and prevertebral fascia medial to the dissection is identified and bluntly divided to expose the anterior cervical vertebral bodies. In the upper cervical spine at the level of the hyoid bone, the hypoglossal nerve may be visible as it runs along the lower border of the digastric muscle. The superior laryngeal nerve can be identi-

fied at the superior horn of the hyoid bone and is just distal to the lingual artery. At this point it is in contact with the prevertebral muscles. The phrenic nerve is located lateral to the vascular bundle and can occasionally be seen if retraction is aggressive. Vascular structures that may be at risk or that may require ligation include the inferior thyroidal vein in the lower neck, and in the upper neck a common venous trunk may require sectioning. The inferior thyroid artery may also be encountered in the lower part of the exposure at the level of the tubercle of C6. This vessel may not require ligation because of its length. In the upper dissection the superior thyroidal courses across the dissection, as does the lingual. These vessels rarely require sectioning.

11.7.3.2 Cervicothoracic Junction

Exposure of the cervicothoracic junction and upper thoracic spine becomes more problematic. In the thin individual it may be possible to reach these vertebrae through the traditional anterolateral approach to the cervical spine. However, in those individuals with thick short necks or barrel chests, exposure of the C7–T1 junction becomes almost impossible. In this situation, osteotomy of the manubrium may be performed to allow further exposure (Kurz et al. 1991).

11.7.3.3 Thoracic Spine

The majority of the thoracic spine may be approached anteriorly with ease. Thoracotomy should be planned through the bed of the rib two spaces above the injured vertebrae. This is necessary because of the downward slope of the ribs. Levels from T6 to T10 can be reached in this way. Preoperative anteroposterior chest or thoracic X-rays (Fig. 11.17) can be used to assess the downward slope of the ribs and the possible exposure obtained by going through different rib beds. Choice of rib bed may be altered if the ribs are particularly horizontal or vertical.

When injury has occurred in the upper thoracic spine above T4, the approach is more technically demanding. With upper thoracic injury, a periscapular dissection of the rib cage with resection of one or more ribs may be necessary to expose the vertebral bodies at this level (Fessler et al. 1991). Even when exposed, this area is somewhat difficult to work within because of the transition between kyphosis and lordosis of the cervical spine. When instrumentation must extend to the first or second thoracic body, the surgeon should consider using an extended anterolateral approach with osteotomy of the manubrium (Kurz et al. 1991).

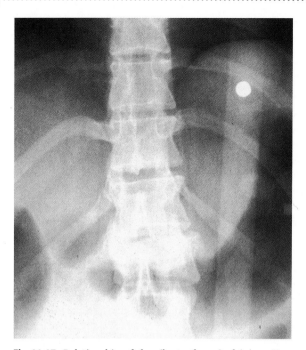

Fig. 11.17. Relationship of the ribs to the spinal injury. Preoperative assessment of the obliquity of the ribs will assist in deciding the appropriate approach to the anterolateral body. More oblique ribs will make fixation difficult in the proximal normal vertebral body and a higher rib level should be chosen. In this case a twelfth rib approach would allow access to the normal proximal vertebrae

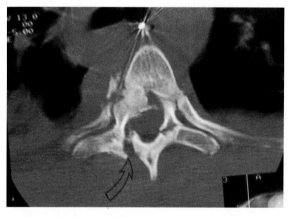

Fig. 11.18. Computed tomography scan demonstrates the great vessels anterior to the vertebral body. The majority of the vertebral body is obscured bv the aorta on the left. Surgical approach and internal fixation from the right would be appropriate in this individual

Costotransversectomy has been used for approach to the thoracic spine. This approach, however, is quite limited and adequate exposure for internal fixation is difficult to obtain. Decompression of the contralateral neural elements may also be less than optimal because of the limited exposure. Internal fixation and stabilization of the spine is necessary following these procedures.

The choice of side of approach is determined by the side with greatest neurological injury. The position of the great vessels in relation to the lateral vertebral body must also be assessed. In the midthoracic spine, the left-sided approach to the lateral vertebral body is often obscured by the aorta(Fig. 11.18). In addition, prominent hardware may erode the great vessels if they are adjacent to prominent internal fixation devices.

11.7.3.4 Thoracolumbar Junction

Optimal exposure of the thoracolumbar junction anteriorly is obtained through a thoracoabdominal approach (Bohlman and Eismont 1981; Bohlman 1985; McAfee et al. 1985). This is performed through the bed of the tenth rib. The retroperitoneal space is entered following blunt dissection of the layers of the abdominal muscles just distal to the costal chondral cartilage. The diaphragm is isolated from both the thoracic and retroperitoneal cavities. Detachment of the diaphragm is performed 1 cm medial to the rib cage. Care should be taken to leave sufficient lateral diaphragm to allow reattachment during closure. Stay sutures positioned at 5–10 cm intervals are highly recommended to allow accurate repair of the diaphragm.Once the crus of the diaphragm has been identified at its insertion into the spine, these fibers can be bluntly dissected from the spine using a Cobb periosteal elevator. The psoas muscle at the thoracolumbar junction is relatively small and can be swept posteriorly using the cobb elevator.

Exposure using this approach is adequate for levels from T11 to L4. If instrumentation must exceed these levels, then another approach must be used.

11.7.3.5 Lumbar Spine

The lumbar spine from L2 to the L4–5 disc space can be approached through a 12th rib subdiaphragmatic approach. This is analogous to the retroperitoneal portion of the thoracoabdominal approach, and the interval is identified as in that approach with blunt dissection of the abdominal musculature to enter the retroperitoneal space. The exposure at these mid- and lower lumbar levels is often obscured by the psoas muscle. This muscle bulk is dissected posteriorly from the anterolateral body of the vertebrae, and relaxation of the muscle can be assisted by flexion of the lower extremity. The L4–5 intervertebral disc level is the practical distal extent of exposure, since at this level bifurcation of the iliac vein obscures the region, as occasionally do ascending iliolumbar veins.

11.7.3.6 Lumbosacral Junction

The lumbosacral junction must be reached through a transperitoneal approach through the midline. Dissection between the common iliac bifurcation will allow good visualization of this area. The need for a laparotomy makes use of this approach impractical in most acute clinical situations. There may be rare instances where this is appropriate (Finkelstein, in press).

11.7.4 Decompression Anterior Approach

There are certain common issues that arise when performing anterior decompression of the thoracolumbar spine. Preoperative imaging provides a guide for the extent of decompression necessary as well as the side with the most neurological compression.

Once the lateral aspect of the vertebral body has been exposed, the segmental vessels must be identified, ligated, and divided. These vessels are easily identified in the "valleys" of the vertebrae between the avascular regions of the discs, "the hills" of the spinal column. Once these vessels are controlled, the periosteum is stripped posteriorly to the level of the pedicle to provide a landmark for the spinal canal. In the thoracic spine, the base of the rib occasionally has to be removed to allow dissection to the level of the pedicle. The neural foramen can be palpated caudad to the pedicle, and the spinal canal will be deep to this region (Fig. 11.19).

Once the pedicle has been identified, the vertebral resection can be performed (Bohlman and Eismont 1981). Resection of the body is done first, and decompression of the canal is then performed. The posterior cortex of the vertebral body and the retropulsed fragment remains as corticocancellous bone. By using a high-speed burr, the cancellous bone can be gently removed, leaving a cortical shell that can easily be removed by pulling into the space of the resected verte-

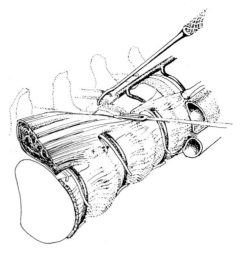

Fig. 11.19. The location of the segmental vessels and the dorsal extent of dissection. The dissector is palpating the edge of the neural foramen which is the posterior margin of decompression of the vertebral body

bral body. Care should be exercised to not allow rebound of the fragments back into the thecal sac during this portion of the procedure. In addition, the surgeon should attempt to decompress the contralateral side first so that the bulging decompressed thecal sac does not obscure the subsequent decompression (Fig. 11.20).

Fig. 11.20. Decompression of the vertebral body from an anterior approach. Illustration to the *left* demonstrates initial decortication and removal of bone from the lateral cortex. The *middle view* demonstrates a cancellectomy on the vertebral body, leaving a cortical rim that this retropulsed. Illustration on the *right* demonstrates removal of bone beginning on the contralateral cortical surface to prevent obstruction of the view by a bulging thecal sac

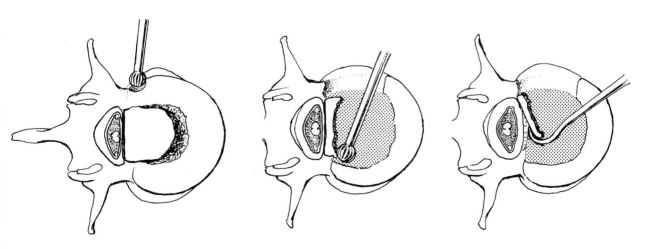

11.8 Fractures and Specific Management

11.8.1 Upper Cervical

Occipitocervical injuries are rarely survivable and these patients are not seen in the emergency department. Seventy-two percent of patients with fatal craniospinal injuries have neck lesions, with a significant number of ligament injuries occurring in the upper cervical region (Bohlman 1979). Radiological identification of these patients is often delayed if they survive the initial scene of the accident. In the normal individual, the tip of the odontoid will point to the clivus at the base of the skull on lateral radiograph of the cervical spine. If this alignment is disrupted, cranial cervical injury should be suspected. Care should be taken to avoid overzealous traction of the cervical spine because of the potential complication of distraction through the zone of injury. Treatment of these patients consists of a fusion of the occiput to cervical spine (McAfee et al. 1991; Wertheim and Bohlman 1987). This can be performed with a closed Luque rectangle and subcortical and sublaminar wires. Unicranial cortical screw and plate fixation of the occiput to cervical spine has also been described. Five of 32 patients described by Sasso et al. (1994) were treated successfully with this technique.

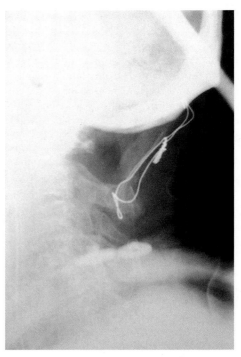

Fig. 11.21. This patient had evidence of occipital cervical instability and subsequently had a posterior occipital cervical fusion using cortical cancellous bone grafting and wirng technique

11.8.1.1 Atlas Injury

Injury to the atlas occurs following an axial load to the ring of the atlas. The resultant injury is described as a Jefferson or burst fracture of the atlas. On the open mouth odontoid view, if combined displacement of the lateral masses of the atlas exceeds 7.0 mm, then this is presumptive evidence of instability (disruption of the transverse ligament) (Fielding et al. 1974). CT examination will show whether injury to the insertion of the transverse ligament has occurred, demonstrated by flakes of avulsed bone. Treatment of patients with stable atlantal injuries with displacement of less than 7 mm on open mouth odontoid view is done with hard collar immobilization. If greater displacement has occurred and CT or MRI confirms injury to the ligament or flexion extension lateral cervical spine X-rays demonstrate greater than 4 mm of motion, stabilization with a posterior occiput to C2 fusion is necessary (Fig. 11.21). An alternative method would be to treat for 8 weeks in halo immobilization until bone healing. Flexion extension lateral cervical spine films can then be performed as well as CT examination to assess the amount of healing of the ring. If flexion extension films demonstrate instability and CT demonstrates bony healing of the ring, an atlan-

toaxial fusion can be performed (Effendi et al. 1981). This minimizes the resultant loss of motion from fusion of the upper cervical spine.

11.8.1.2 Atlas and Odontoid Injury

Occasionally, odontoid fractures occur in conjunction with atlas injuries. Treatment with halo immobilization until C1 arch healing has occurred, followed by fusion with wiring of C1– C2 posterior elements, is one method of dealing with this combination of injury. If stabilization of the odontoid is critical to the care of the patient and halo immobilization is not practical, then anterior odontoid screw fixation is an appropriate method of fixation (Geisler et al. 1989). Alternatively, posterior transfacetal fixation of the C1–C2 facets, as described by Magerl, can be performed (Grob et al. 1991; Marcotte et al. 1993; Figs. 22 a–d, 23). Loss of motion using odontoid screw fixation will be minimal, since no motion segments are fused. Transfacet screws will cause loss of rotation secondary to atlantoaxial immobilization.

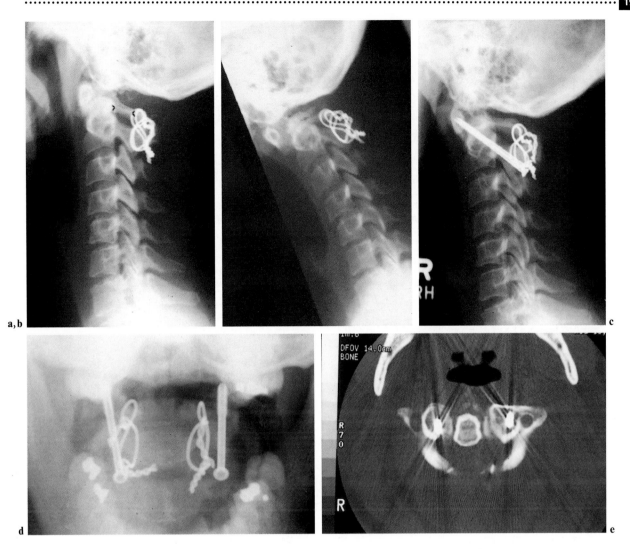

a,b

c

d

e

Fig. 11.22. a,b Flexion and extension of a failed posterior fusion of C1-C2. Note evidence of atlantoaxial instability with narrowing of the spinal canal as demonstrated by the *arrows*. **c** Anterior posterior open mouth view illustrating a transarticular facet screw fixation of Cl-C2. **d** Lateral X-ray demonstrating position of transarticular screws. **e** Postoperative computed tomography examination demonstrating placement of screws within the lateral masses of Cl

11.8.1.3 Odontoid Injury

Odontoid fractures are divided by Anderson and D'Alonso (1974) into those above the transverse ligament (type I), which are inconsequential and should be treated symptomatically, those at the base of the odontoid (type II), which are most commonly associated with nonunion and malunion, and those fractures occurring through the body of the axis (type III). These latter injuries heal readily with halo immobilization. Of the type II injuries, age greater than 40 years, angulation of the fracture, and displacement of the fracture, particularly posteriorly, are prognostic indicators for nonunion of the odontoid. Approximately 30 % of type II injuries go on to nonunion (Clark and White 1985). Traditional treatment for these injuries in patients with displacement has been posterior Gallie C1–C2 wire and bonegraft fusion. This technique tends to displace fractures posteriorly. When posterior displacement is of concern, fusion can be performed with sublaminar wires beneath the arch of C1 and C2 with an interposition bone graft between the lamina, as described by Brooks and Jenkins (1978).

Anterior odontoid screw fixation has become more popular as a method to treat patients with posteriorly displaced odontoid fractures, as well as patients with

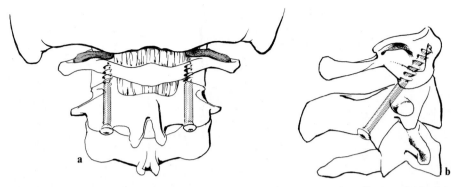

Fig. 11.23 a,b. Orientation and placement of transarticular screw fixation of C1 and C2. Care should be taken to place these screws in a direct sagittal orientation to prevent injury to the spinal cord medially and injury to the vertebral arteries laterally

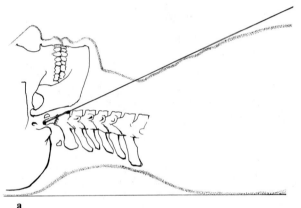

Fig. 11.24. a Lateral line drawing demonstrating the ideal position of an odontoid screw and the line projected from this position along the rib cage and anterior chest. A long radiopaque marker should be placed beside the neck along this track with the aid of lateral image intensification. If the radiopaque marker is below the level of the anterior chest wall then placement in this ideal position will be difficult interoperatively. **b** Anterior posterior and lateral image intensification. These two views should be obtained simultaneously and therefore two image intensifiers are necessary for ideal placement of screws

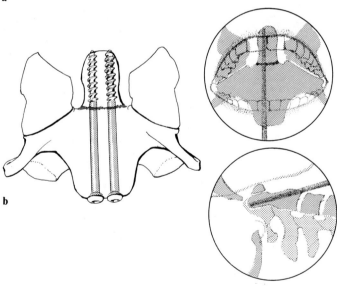

associated C1 arch injuries. If this method is proposed, a careful preoperative assessment of the patient must be performed. The fracture must be able to be reduced without flexing the head and neck to a great degree. Reported results indicate that this method has a low incidence of neurological injury and a high incidence of union of the odontoid (Bohler 1982; Esses and Bednar 1991; Geisler et al. 1989; Fig. 24). However, the technical challenges of this method should not be forgotten. The patient cannot have a very large chest or have a very lordotic cervical spinal alignment. These factors will make placement of the odontoid screw in an ideal position impossible (Fig. 11.25). A rapid way of assessing these factors is to preoperatively place a straight radiopaque marker aimed at the tip of the odontoid and along the proposed track of instrumentation and use lateral image intensification to confirm the position. If this straight marker cannot be placed into the proposed position of the odontoid screw because of the anatomical limitations mentioned above, then the surgeon should use a posterior method for stabilization of the odontoid. Magerl transfacet screws may also be used posteriorly for odontoid fractures.

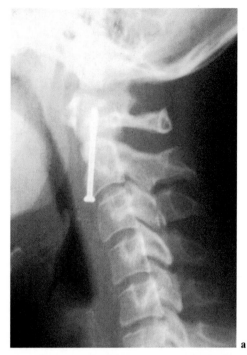

a

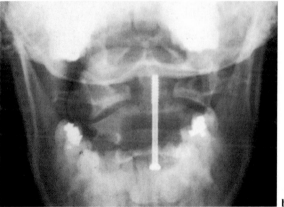

b

Fig. 11.25 a,b. Lateral and posterior views of anterior odontold screw fixation of a type II odontoid fracture

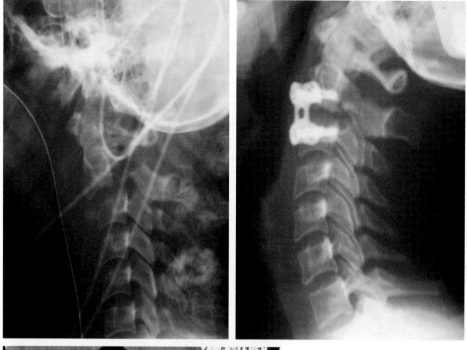

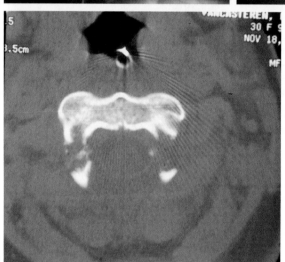

Fig. 11.26 a–c. This patient had a traumatic spondylothesis of C2 on 3 with angulation and displacement. **b** A computed tomography scan demonstrates a fracture of the posterior elements of C2. **c** Lateral view of anterior plating of C2 on C3

11.8.1.4 C2 Injury

Traumatic spondylolisthesis of the C2 may occur as a result of sudden flexion or sudden extension of the neck. Undisplaced fractures can be treated with external orthosis such as a hard collar. Nonangulated fractures with up to 3 mm of displacement (type I) are satisfactorily treated with a halo. Type II fractures are those with angulation or displacement. Those with angulation only can be treated with traction reduction and halo vest application. In those patients with disruption of the facet joint and disc space (type III), stabilization should

be performed with anterior plate stabilization and fusion (Fig. 11.26).

11.8.2 Lower Cervical Spine

Injuries in the lower cervical spine are commonly of flexion distraction or flexion axial compression injury. The majority of these injuries may be treated quite adequately with halo vest immobilization. Those patients with facet dislocations or other ligamentous injury will not do well with nonoperative halo vest treatment, with

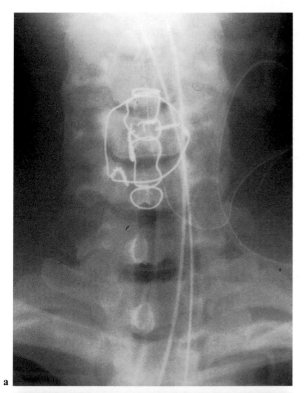

a

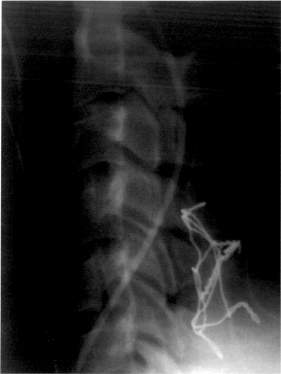

b

Fig. 11.27 a,b. Anterior posterior and lateral views of a C5 on 6 dislocation treated with posterior triple wire technique and bone graft fusion

only 21.4% of patients having satisfactory results (Sears and Fazl 1990). If radiological assessment confirms anterior compression of neurological structures (which often happens with bursting type), then an anterior decompression and iliac crest bone graft strut with plate fixation is the optimal method to address both neurological and mechanical aspects of the injury (Aebi et al. 1986, 1991; Caspar et al. 1989; Garvey et al. 1992). If the injury is predominantly ligamentous without bony compression of the neurological elements, then a posterior stabilization can be performed. Simple wire fixation and bone grafting is an efficient, strong, and low-risk method of spine stabilization (Fig. 11.27). Posterior plate fixation has been increasing in popularity; however, it is a technically more demanding method of fixation, with the possible risks of damaging underlying cervical nerve roots deep to the facet joints (An et al. 1991a; Heller et al. 1991; Roy-Camille et al. 1992). In those patients with injured spinous processes or laminar injuries, plating would provide superior fixation compared to wiring methods (Figs. 11.28, 11.29).

As mentioned previously, the approaches to the cervicothoracic junction anteriorly present particular difficulties when instrumentation must be performed. If the goal is instrumentation of these levels, then the surgeon should be prepared to perform an osteotomy of the manubrium and expose the upper thoracic spine. Anterior plating systems can be used for stabilization.

11.8.3 Thoracic Spine

Decisions concerning treatment of thoracic spine fractures are based primarily upon the neurological deficit of the patient. Complete cord injury is usually associated with a biomechanically unstable injury such as a fracture dislocation. These injuries may be purely a result of flexion injury or may have a rotatory component. Since recovery of neurological function in these individuals is unlikely, the primary goal is realignment and stabilization of the spinal column to allow early rehabilitation. These goals can be met quite readily with a posterior instrumentation of the thoracic spine. Upper thoracic spinal injuries requiring posterior fixation are best dealt with using a hook rod construct. There may be instances where injury has occurred to the posterior elements such that extension of stabilization must be done into the lower cervical spine. This transition zone is difficult to instrument, as previously mentioned. In the midthoracic spine instrumentation methods can include hook rod constructs in the neurologically intact patient (Fig. 11.30). Distraction rods with sublaminar wires are used in complete spinal cord injuries. The added risk of worsening neurological deficits from sublaminar wires in the complete spinal cord injury patient is minimal.

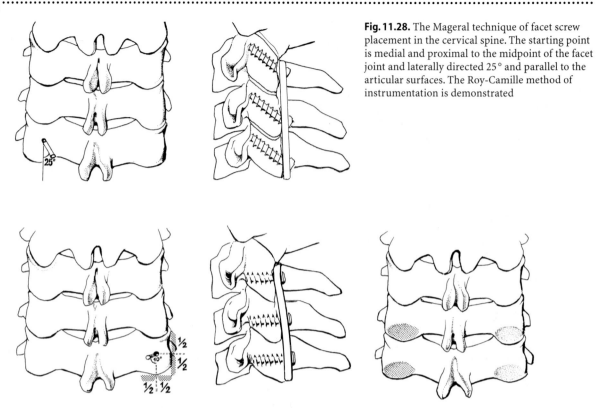

Fig. 11.28. The Mageral technique of facet screw placement in the cervical spine. The starting point is medial and proximal to the midpoint of the facet joint and laterally directed 25° and parallel to the articular surfaces. The Roy-Camille method of instrumentation is demonstrated

Fig. 11.29. More horizontal placement of the screw perpendicular to the posterior cortex and at the midpoint of the articular surfaces medially and laterally. The screws are inclined laterally at 10°

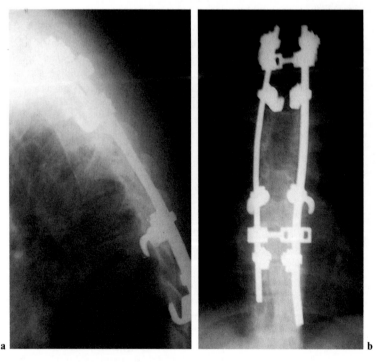

Fig. 11.30 a,b. Postoperative views of hook rod fixation of mid-thoracic fracture in a neurologically intact patient

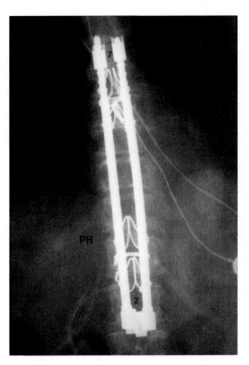

Fig. 11.31. Anterior posterior view of a midthoracic fracture is treated with Harrington distraction rods with sublaminar wires

This method of fixation is simple and provides immediate stability of the spine. The techniques are also widely known, and fixation devices are inexpensive and commonly available. We prefer to perform this method of fixation in such patients (Fig. 11.31 a–c).

When neurological deficit is incomplete, as can occur from a burst fracture of the thoracic spine, identification of bony compression of the neurological elements may dictate the need for anterior decompression and stabilization. If this is the case, a transthoracic approach to the spine is used. Anterior instrumentation in the mid- and upper thoracic spine is limited by the size of the vertebrae. In smaller individuals, the mid- and upper thoracic spine is often 2–3 cm in diameter and most fixation devices designed for the thoracolumbar spine are too bulky (Fig. 11.32). In this region application of a 4.5- or 3.5-mm dynamic compression plate (DCP) can be done and a posterior fixation may be necessary to allow early mobilization of the patient. Bone graft strut fusion should be done in conjunction with the decompression and fixation (Fig. 11.33 a–c). Fortunately, the majority of forces that the bone graft encounters in the thoracic spine are flexion, and this serves to compress the grafts. During the anterior procedure, reduction of kyphosis is often difficult to assess. To ensure adequate reduction, care must be taken to distract the decompression site enough to make the endplates of the vertebrae above

and below the decompression site parallel. Provided the anterior longitudinal ligament has been left intact, distraction will provide good reduction and return of alignment. The anterior ligament will also act as a gauge for overall sagittal alignment.

11.8.4 Thoracolumbar Junction

The thoracolumbar junction, from T10 to L2, presents a number of distinct issues for treatment of spinal injury. The majority of injuries at this level are of an axial loading nature resulting in a burst fracture. As a result, neurological deficits are a result of retropulsion of bone from the posterior vertebral body between the pedicles. This bone is often firmly attached to the annulus fibrosis of the superior disc and endplate. If neurological injury has occurred, then an anterior decompression with strut grafting and stabilization is chosen. This is done through a thoracoabdominal approach based upon the tenth rib. This approach will allow excellent visualization of T11, T12, and L1. If injury has occurred at T10 or T11 and instrumentation must be performed to T9, then the diaphragm may be spared and the dissection can occasionally be carried out using a thoracotomy only. Similarly, in those individuals who have injury of L2, a 12th rib approach may be all that is required to expose the L1–L3 vertebrae. If a 12th rib approach has been done but exposure is not adequate, the alternatives include subperiosteal dissection of the crus of the diaphragm or a limited detachment of the diaphragm from the lateral chest wall. This, however, does limit the actual ability to place instrumentation properly in the spine because of the overhanging rib cage blocking a perpendicular placement of instrumentation (Fig. 11.34 a–f).

Distractive injuries of the posterior elements may occur in the lower thoracic and lumbar spine. These variants of Chance fractures will respond to conservative management if the majority of injury has occured through bone. However, when significant injury to the soft tissues has occured, posterior fixation and fusion should be performed. This can be in the form of compression rods or of pedicle fixation in a compression mode (Fig. 11.35).

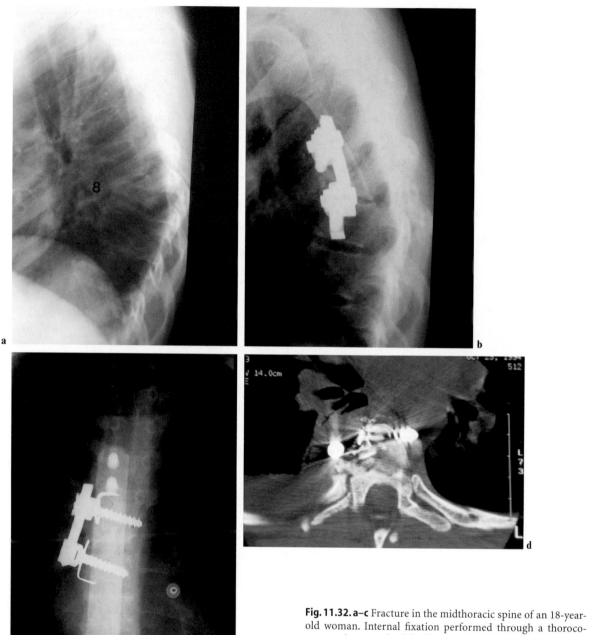

Fig. 11.32. a–c Fracture in the midthoracic spine of an 18-year-old woman. Internal fixation performed through a thoroco-tomy using vertebral bodies screws and rods demonstrate the difficulties of instrumentation in smaller individuals. **d** Demonstrates protrusion of the screw through the contra-lateral vertebral body immediately adjacent to the aorta. This instrumentation was subsequently removed

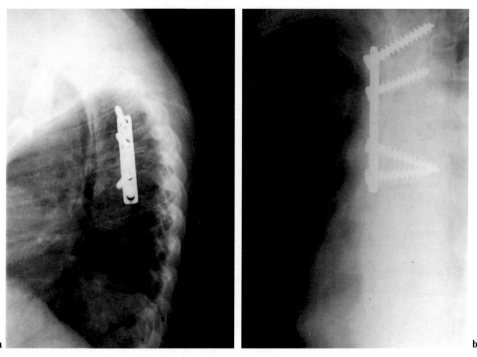

Fig. 11.33. a Lateral and **b** anterior posterior view of a pathological fracture of T6 treated with a 4.5-DC plate for stabilization of this fracture

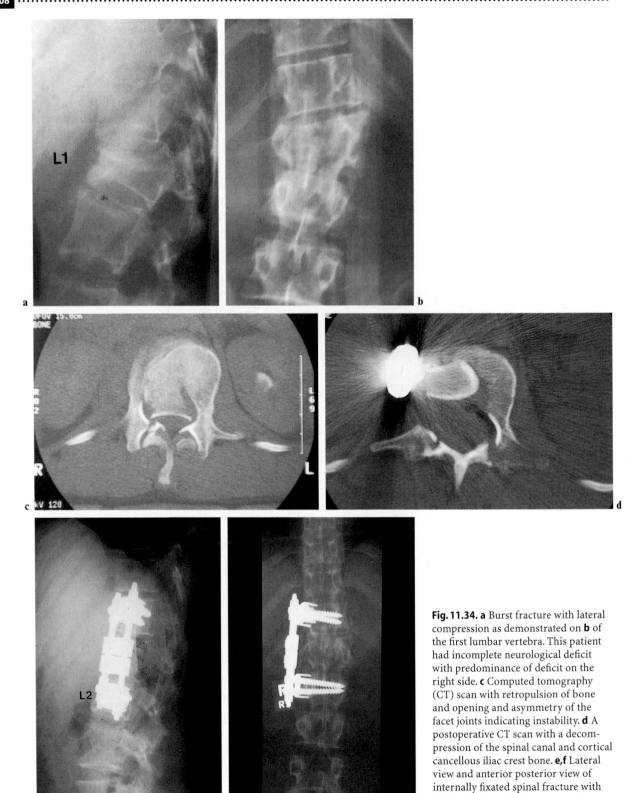

Fig. 11.34. a Burst fracture with lateral compression as demonstrated on **b** of the first lumbar vertebra. This patient had incomplete neurological deficit with predominance of deficit on the right side. **c** Computed tomography (CT) scan with retropulsion of bone and opening and asymmetry of the facet joints indicating instability. **d** A postoperative CT scan with a decompression of the spinal canal and cortical cancellous iliac crest bone. **e,f** Lateral view and anterior posterior view of internally fixated spinal fracture with cortical cancellous strut

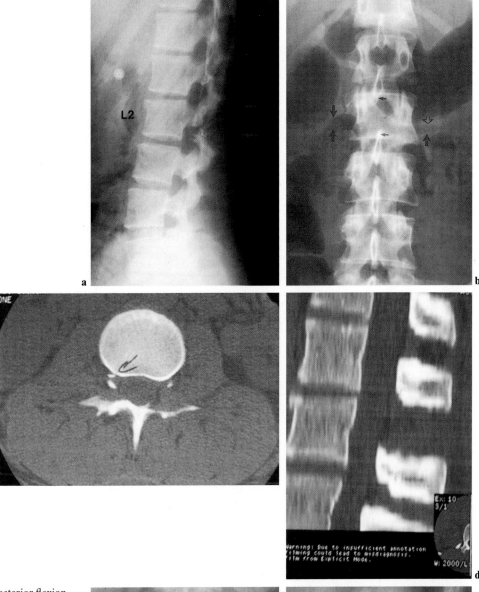

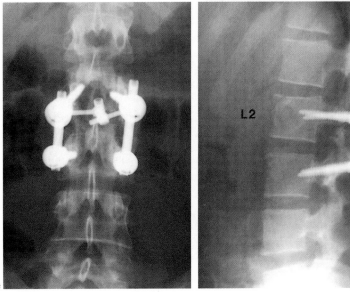

Fig. 11.35. a Anterior posterior flexion view of flexion distraction injury. Note the increased distance of the interspinous distance *(small closed arrow)*. There is also evidence of fracture of the transverse process as demonstrated by *larger arrows* and *open arrow*. **b** The lateral view demonstrates fracture to the pars interarticularus at L2. **c** Computed tomography examination with what appears to be very minimal damage of the vertebral body. This is somewhat deceptive and more clearly demonstrated amount of distraction of the spinous process can be seen on the sagittal reconstruction views in **d. e,f** Postoperative views with posterior pedicle screw fixation in a compression mode demonstrated by the anterior posterior (**e**) and lateral (**f**) views

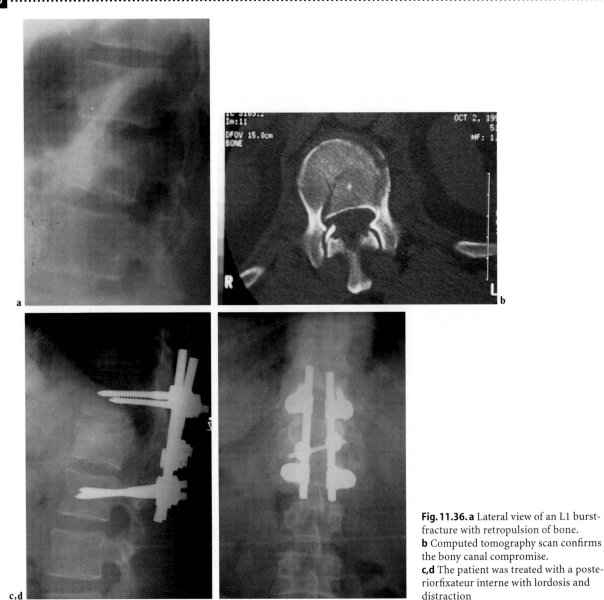

Fig. 11.36. a Lateral view of an L1 burst-fracture with retropulsion of bone.
b Computed tomography scan confirms the bony canal compromise.
c,d The patient was treated with a posteriorfixateur interne with lordosis and distraction

11.8.4.1 Internal Fixation

Internal fixation at the thoracolumbar junction must be strong and versatile (Zdeblick et al. 1993). Plates affixed to the spine without a stable screw plate connection have a propensity to loosen, and disassembly of the plate from the screws can occur. Fixation with solid connection between screws and longitudinal members can be in the form of plates or screw rod constructs. Our preference has been to use the Kaneda fixator (Kaneda et al. 1984). This provides excellent immediate fixation; however, it should be kept in mind that this, or any, fixator is unable to stabilize injuries with complete disruption of the anterior and posterior elements as occurs in fracture-

dislocation. In these cases, combined anterior and posterior fixation is necessary.

In neurologically intact patients with biomechanically unstable burst fractures of the thoracolumbar junction, posterior fixation in the form of pedicle screw fixation one level above and one level below the lesion is done (Magerl 1984; Dick 1987; Carl et al. 1992). The pedicle fixation must provide the ability to axially distract the spine as well as realign the spine in lordosis. We have used the internal fixator for this purpose, because of the long lever arms that the Shanz pins provide. These pins allow significant lordotic force to be applied through the pedicles. In combination with this lordotic force, distraction can be done along the internal fixator rods

Fig. 11.37. a,b Anteroposterior and lateral view of an L3 burst fracture with incomplete neurological deficit.
c Computed tomography scan demonstrates canal encroachment.
d Posteroperative views of solid fusion and spontaneous anterior fusion

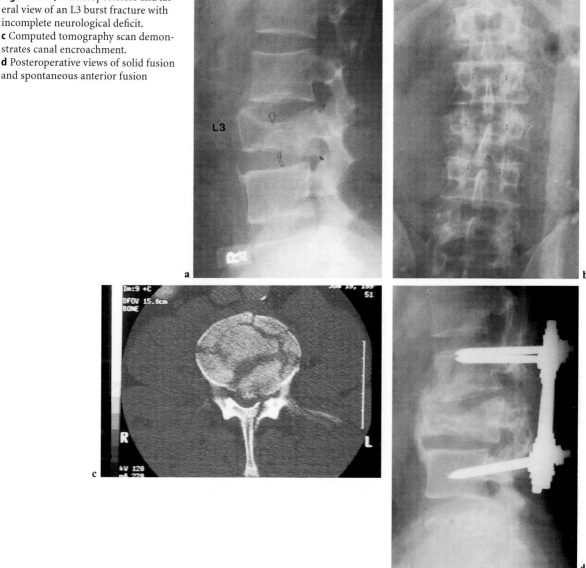

(Fig. 11.36 a–c). Reduction of retropulsed fragments can occur, although the total percentage of reduction and the probability of reduction remain controversial. Preoperative CT scans are necessary to provide an estimate of the size of the pedicle in the lower thoracic and upper lumbar spine. The L1 vertebrate routinely has the smallest pedicle diameter in the thoracolumbar junction, and these pedicles may be so small in small individuals as to make pedicle screw insertion hazardous (Hou et al. 1993). If this is the case, then use of a posterior hook rod construct is preferred. It should be remembered that the goal in these neurologically intact patients is to realign the spine to 0° of kyphosis at the thoracolumbar junction (Fig. 11.37). Postsurgery collapse may occur following posterior fixation. This may occur in the face of a solid fusion and may represent the continued absence of the anterior weight-bearing column with plastic deformation of the posterolateral fusion (Fig. 11.38). Alternatively, fusion may not be solid and collapse may represent pseudoarthrosis and failure of the instrumentation at the bone screw interface.

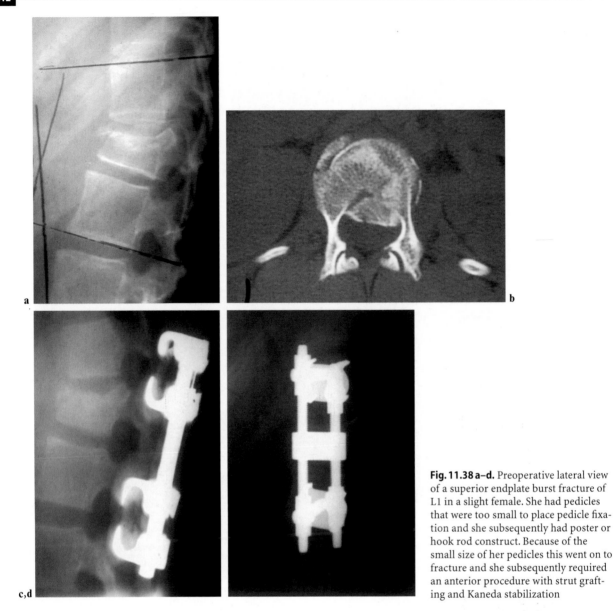

Fig. 11.38 a–d. Preoperative lateral view of a superior endplate burst fracture of L1 in a slight female. She had pedicles that were too small to place pedicle fixation and she subsequently had poster or hook rod construct. Because of the small size of her pedicles this went on to fracture and she subsequently required an anterior procedure with strut grafting and Kaneda stabilization

11.8.5 Lumbar Spine

With the advent of pedicle screw fixation, the treatment of lumbar fractures was greatly simplified. If neurological injury has occurred and decompression is necessary, then this can be performed through a posterior approach. Decompression can be done by removing the pedicle at the level of compression and removing the offending bony or soft tissue compressive material using appropriate hand and power instruments. Since the spinal cord ends at the L1–L2 intervertebral space, decompression of the lumbar spine beneath L2 is much less hazardous to the neurological elements. Complete and adequate decompression can be performed through the posterior approach. The anterior approach in the mid-lumbar spine is more difficult because of the abdominal contents, the psoas muscle overlying the lateral aspects of the vertebral body, and the depth within the pelvis of the vertebral bodies. As the intervertebral disc of L4–L5 is approached, the bifurcation of the inferior vena cava overlies the area of dissection. In addition, large ascending branches of the iliolumbar vein cross this area and make exposure difficult if fixation must be applied. Even for decompression of the vertebral body, the exposure is limited and occasionally not sufficient to meet the goals of adequate decompression and fixation of the spine (Fig. 11.39).

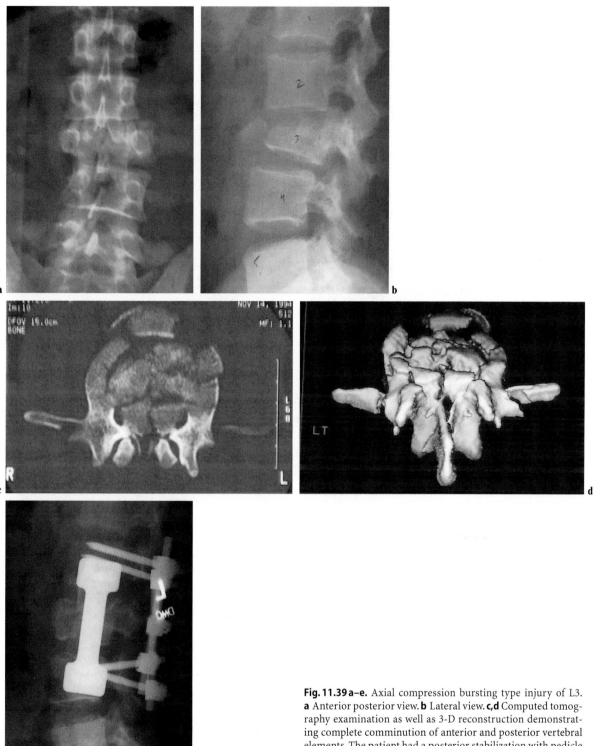

Fig. 11.39 a–e. Axial compression bursting type injury of L3. **a** Anterior posterior view. **b** Lateral view. **c,d** Computed tomography examination as well as 3-D reconstruction demonstrating complete comminution of anterior and posterior vertebral elements. The patient had a posterior stabilization with pedicle screw fixation and an anterior bone graft strutting with plate fixation. This was necessary to stabilize this three-column injury

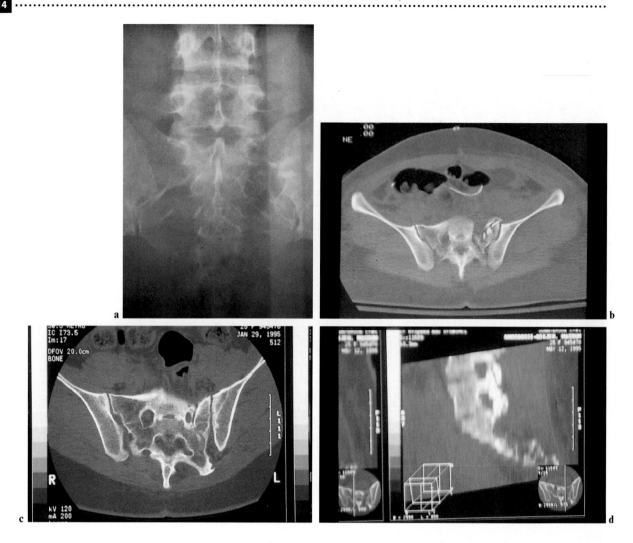

Fig. 11.40 a–d. Anterior and posterior views of a sacrum following a pelvic fracture. Note the disruption of the sacral foraminal arches on the left side. **b** Immediate computed tomography (CT) scan demonstrates a fracture through sacral foramina. **c** There is a narrowing of the sacral foraminum with an Sl radiculopothy. The patient had a posterior decompression and sacral foraminotomy as demonstrated in the reconstruction of the CT scan in **d**

11.8.6 Sacral Fractures

Fractures of the sacrum are often overlooked because of the other associated injuries such as pelvic fracture. The sacrum has a complex three-dimensional anatomy, and plain films are often not sufficient to define these injuries. Denis et al. (1988) have divided these injuries into those lateral to the sacral ala, those at the sacral foramen, and those through the body. The fractures through the foramen are most commonly associated with neurological deficit. These neurological deficits are usually sacral root deficits and confusion can occur as to the cause of these deficits, particularly if the sacral fracture is not suspected on clinical and radiological examination (Denis et al. 1988). If the neurological deficit is identified as a result of bony compression within the foramen, decompression can be performed. This is done through a posterior approach (Fig. 11.40) Stability of the sacrum

The lumbosacral junction is similarly best approached for decompression and stabilization through a posterior approach. Pedicle screw fixation allows short segment stable fixation with satisfactory ability to perform decompression. In rare cases anterior fixation or decompression is necessary. This is done through a transperitoneal approach and allows limited access to the lumbosacral disc.

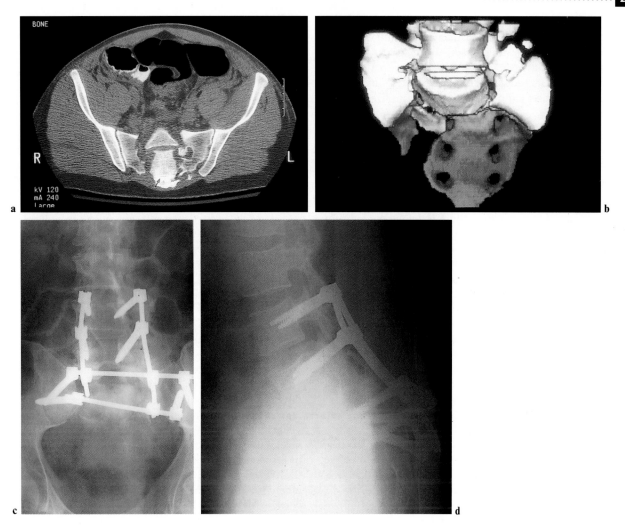

Fig. 11.41 a–d. This 25-year-old man had an injury secondary to a fall from a height and a computed tomography (CT) scan demonstrates bilateral sacral fractures and the 3-D reconstruction illustrates the rotational effect of this injury. **c,d** Because of the instability of pelvis to spine it was necessary to perform iliac fixation in conjunction with a lower lumbar fixation to provide satisfactory stabilization

is intimately related to stability of the pelvis, and a complete assessment of this should be performed. Complete dissociation of the sacrum from the pelvis can occur, and these are complex problems best dealt with through the combined expertise of the spine and pelvic surgeon (Fig. 11.41).

11.9 Postoperative Care

In patients with cervical injury, an assessment of the intraoperative stabilization will dictate the postoperative care. Halo fixation may still be required in those patients who have had fixation with a wiring construct or who have poor bone quality. If fixation is solid, such as can be obtained with posterior facet plating, then a firm collar is all that is necessary.

11.9.1 Brace Wear

In thoracolumbar spinal injuries, the patients are routinely placed in an external orthosis. These range from total contact thoracolumbosacral orthosis, to hyperextension braces, to chairback braces. The primary function of most of these braces in the face of stable internal fixation is to remind the patient and to limit his or her motion rather to provide added stability to the spinal column. It has been our practice to place patients with lower thoracic and thoracolumbar injuries in hyperextension braces and those with lumbar injuries in chair-back braces.

11.9.2 Mobilization

The patients are mobilized as soon as possible following surgical stabilization. The patient is allowed in a chair in the first 24 h and following this, if the patient is neurologically normal, ambulation is begun. Brace wear is encouraged whenever the patient is out of bed and is continued for an average of 3 months after surgery.

11.9.3 Complications and Their Prevention

Prevention of complications in patients with spinal column and cord injury requires careful attention to details in all phases of the treatment of these patients. Preoperative care and assessment, intraoperative management, and postoperative care are integral in the minimization of adverse outcomes in spine fracture care (Albert et al. 1991; Baker et al. 1993; Esses et al. 1993).

Assessment of the stability of the fracture has been previously discussed. Very unstable injuries such as fracture dislocation have different requirements than injuries that have moderate instability such as flexion distraction injuries. Combined anterior and posterior fixation is most appropriate in the former, whereas posterior fixation is satisfactory in the latter. These decisions can be made preoperatively and resources should be marshaled accordingly.

11.9.4 Pedicle Screw Insertion

Pedicle screw fixation is able to provide stable fixation while also minimizing length of fusion. However, pedicle screw insertion is associated with some increased risk to the neurological elements. It is estimated that up to 5.2 % of pedicle screws are associated with neurological injury (Esses et al. 1993). To minimize complications, knowledge of the anatomy of the vertebrae and pedicles at different levels of the spine is essential. The angle of pedicle inclination and the position of the pedicle in relation to the transverse processes varies at different levels of the spine. Inclination to the midline of the pedicles is 0° in the lower thoracic and L1 and L2 vertebrae. In the mid-lumbar vertebrae, inclination is close to 15°, and in L5 and the sacrum inclination can be 20° and 30°, respec-

tively. In the sacral region, overhang of the posterior superior iliac spine and iliac crest may make insertion of a screw into the midpoint of the pedicle and sacral body impossible. The size of pedicles varies significantly throughout the lower thoracic and lumbar spine. The largest pedicles are at L5 and may measure 15 mm in diameter at their narrowest point. In the upper lumbar spine, the pedicle may measure only 4–5 mm in small individuals. Choice of pedicle screw and instrumentation method must be made with this in mind.

Starting points for insertion of pedicle screws are not constant throughout the spine, and it is our practice to use image intensification to aid in identification of the pedicles. This is particularly true if spinal decompression is not performed and the pedicles are not readily palpable. This is done in both the anteroposterior and lateral planes to view the pedicles. Prior to beginning the surgery, the surgeon must ensure that the patient is on an appropriate radiolucent table and the image intensifier can be positioned appropriately. The intensifier must be able to provide an anteroposterior view as well be able to swing in the sagittal plane such that the image beam will be parallel to the vertebral pedicle and endplates in areas of lordosis and kyphosis. Anteroposterior views are varied to allow rotation about the spine to obtain a direct "end-on" view of the pedicle, much as is done during distal locking of an intramedullary nail. The amount of inclination of the image machine is related to the inclination of the pedicle at the level of interest. It should be kept in mind that if a screw is placed in the pedicle of the sacrum in a sagittal plane, it will likely traverse the junction of the sacral body and alae where the bone is particularly narrow. Care should be exercised not to place an overly long screw in this region.

11.9.5 Thromboembolic Disease

Thromboembolic disease occurs in 68 % of patients with spinal cord injury (Geerts et al. 1994). Postoperative thromboembolism prophylaxis with low-dose heparin is carried out in all these patients. In neurologically intact patients, deep-vein thrombosis (DVT) occurs in relation to other musculoskeletal injuries, and all patients admitted with multiple trauma are begun on thromboembolism prophylaxis with low-dose heparin. With more body systems injured the potential for DVT is greater. Seventy-three percent of patients with extremity injuries with spinal injuries have DVT. In neurologically normal patients who will be out of bed within 2–3 days, antiembolism stockings are used routinely. Patients with spine fracture who will not become mobile early should have DVT prophylaxis. Major spinal surgery predisposes patients to DVT and prophylaxis should be considered (Smith et al. 1994).

11.9.6 Urinary Care

Urinary care in the form of intermittent catheterization is instituted early in the care of these patients. In complete spinal cord injury, this is begun soon after surgical stabilization. In neurologically normal patients, indwelling Foley catheters are removed after the first 48 h. This is done to allow more accurate assessment of urinary control as well as to decrease the potential for urinary sepsis.

11.10 Outcomes of Treatment of Spinal Injury

Functional recovery following injury to the spinal column and cord is directly related to the severity of injury. Return to work and the percentage of patients convalescing after minor spinal injury has been demonstrated to be 75% and less than 5% at 1 year, respectively. Return to work of patients with neurological injuries was only 11%. Only 43% of one group of patients with spinal injury had no limitations at 1 year following injury. This overall rate of patients with functional limitations is the highest rate when compared to other body system injuries following trauma (MacKenzie et al. 1988).

Nonoperative care of patients with spinal trauma occurs in those patients who have less severe injury. Generally these patients are neurologically normal with no biomechanical instability. In the cervical spine, many patients are treated nonoperatively although they have evidence of neurological and mechanical instability. The functional results of these patients are most dependent upon the neurological status and less so on the method of definitive treatment. If stability has been obtained, either through operative or nonoperative means, results in terms of pain are satisfactory. However, functional limitation and return to work are affected by more than the anatomical pathology and are measures that may reflect psychosocial factors that are not readily addressed by the surgical management.

In the thoracic and thoracolumbar spine, nonoperative treatment of compression fractures of the spine that are not unstable may still lead to persistent back pain. Between 40% and 75% of patients with compression fractures following spine fracture continued to have back pain (Young 1973). Presence and severity of pain appears to be related to deformity, with patients with greater than 30° of kyphosis having significantly more pain than those patients with less than 30° kyphosis, regardless of whether they were treated operatively or nonoperatively. These symptoms are independent of the severity of the fracture. Nonoperative treatment of burst fractures of the thoracolumbar junction has been shown to be efficacious and have satisfactory outcomes,

although direct comparison of individual fractures is difficult (Reid et al. 1988; Mumford et al. 1993; Cantor et al. 1993). Lumbar spine burst fractures without neurological deficit can also be treated nonoperatively with 90% good or excellent results (An et al. 1991b). Neurological status does not deteriorate in those patients chosen for nonoperative treatment. In general, those patients with more severe fractures and with neurological deficit are treated operatively.

In surgically treated patients, severe pain is less common than in nonoperatively treated patients. Neurological recovery appears to better following anterior decompression compared to posterior decompression in patients with partial deficit. Pain postoperatively is as likely as in those patients with nonsurgical treatment, although severe pain may be less common. It appears that pain after treatment is most likely in patients with deformity greater than 30° (Gertzbein 1992). Increase of deformity occurs less frequently following surgery because of the surgical reduction that is performed at operation, although increases following the first 3 months of treatment are not different when operative and nonoperative methods are compared.

11.11 Conclusion

The operative treatment of spinal injury is technically challenging. However, the most difficult part of care of spinal-injured patients is the decision making that is necessary to provided optimal management of the mechanical and neurological components of the injury. Patients most likely to benefit from operative treatment are those that have neurological deficit as a result of injury. Partial neurological injuries will likely improve if bony decompression is peformed when impingement of the neurological structures is identified. Complete lesions will require operative stabilization, since the majority of these patients will be unstable secondary to their trauma. Neurologically intact patients with facet dislocations or ligamentous injury in the cervical spine will benefit from operative stabilization. In the thoracic and lumbar spine, patients with greater than 30° of kyphosis and 50% vertebral body crush will benefit from operative stabilization. When disruption of vertebral elements has occurred through soft tissue and ligaments, the potential for stable healing is diminished and operative stabilization should be considered.

Even with optimal management, significant long-term sequelae in the form of loss of function and persistent pain will be present in many patients following injury.

References

Aebi M, Mohler J, Zach GA, Morscher E (1986) Indication surgical technique and results of 100 surgically-treated fractures and fracture-dislocations of the cervical spine. Clin Orthop Related Res 203:244–257

Aebi M, Zuber K, Marchesi D (1991) Treatment of cervical spine injuries with anterior plating. Spine 16(3S):S38-S45

Albee FH (1911) Transplantationof a portion of the tibia into the spine for Pott's disease. J Am Med Assoc 57:885

Albert TJ, Levine MJ, Balderston RA, Cotler JM (1991) Gastrointestinal complications in spinal cord injury. Spine 16(10S):S522-S525

Allen JBL, Ferguson RL, Lehmann TR, O'Brien RP (1982) A mechanistic classification of closed indirect fractures and dislocations of the lower cervical spine. Spine 7(1):1–27

An H, Gordin R, Renner K (1991 a) Anatomic considerations for plate-screw fixation of the cervical spine. Spine 16(10S): S548-S551

An HS, Vaccaro A, Cotler JM, Lin S (1991 b) Low lumbar burst fractures. Comparison among body cast harrington rod luque rod and Steffee plate. Spine 16(8 s):S440-S444

Anderson LD, D'Alonzo RT (1974) Fractures of the odontoid process of the axis. J Bone Joint Surg 56-A:1663–1674

Anderson P, Bohlman HH (1992) Anterior decompression and arthrodesis of the cervical spine: long-term motor improvement. II. Improvement in complete traumatic quadriplegia. J Bone Joint Surgery 74-A(5):683–692

Anderson PA, Rivara FP, Maier RV, Drake C (1991) The epidemiology of seatbelt-associated injuries. J Trauma 31(1):60–67

Baker J, Reardon PR, Reardon MJ, Heggeness MH (1993) Vascular injury in anterior lumbar surgery. Spine 18(15): 2227–2230

Bohler J (1982) Anterior stabilization for acute fractures and nonunions of the dens. J Bone Joint Surg 64-A(1):18–27

Bohlman HH (1979) Acute fractures and dislocations of the cervical spine. An analysis of three hundred hospitalized patients and review of the literature. J Bone Joint Surg 61-A(8):1119–1142

Bohlman HH (1985) Current concepts review: treatment of fractures and dislocations of the thoracic and lumbar spine. J Bone Joint Surg 67-A(1):165–169

Bohlman HH, Anderson PA (1992) Anterior decompression and arthrodesis of the cervical spine: long-term motor improvement. I. Improvement in incomplete traumatic quadriparesis. J Bone Joint Surg 74-A(5):671–681

Bohlman HH, Eismont FJ (1981) Surgical techniques of anterior decompression and fusion for spinal cord injuries. Clin Orthop Related Res 154:57–67

Bolesta MJ, Bohlman HH (1991) Mediastinal widening associated with fractures of the upper thoracic spine. J Bone Joint Surg 73-A(3):447–450

Bondurant FJ, Cotler HB, Kulkarni MV, McArdle CB, Harris JH (1990) Acute spinal cord injury. A study using physical examination and magnetic resonance imaging. Spine 15(3):161–168

Boucher H (1959) A method of spinal fusion. J Bone Joint Surg 41-B:248–259

Bracken MB, Shepard MJ, Collins WF et al (1990) A randomized controlled trial of methylprednisolone or naloxone in the acute treatment of acute spinal cord injury: results of the second National Acute Spinal Cord Injury Study. N Engl J Med 322:1405–1411

Brightman RP, Miller CA, Rea GL, Chakeres DW, Hunt WE (1992) Magnetic resonance imaging of trauma to the thoracic and lumbar spine. The importance of the posterior longitudinal ligament. Spine 17(5):541–549

Brooks AL, Jenkins EB (1978) Atlanto-axial arthrodesis by the wedge compression method. J Bone Joint Surg 60A:279–284

Cammisa FP Jr, Eismont FJ, Green BA (1989) Dural laceration occurring with burst fractures and associated laminar fractures. J Bone Joint Surg 71-A(7):1044–1052

Cantor JB, Lebwohl NH, Garvey T, Eismont FJ (1993) Nonoperative management of stable thoracolumbar burst fractures with early ambulation and bracing. Spine 18(8): 971–976

Carl AL, Tromanhauser SG, Roger DJ (1992) Pedicle screw instrumentation for thoracolumbar burst fractures and fracture-dislocations. Spine 17(8S):S317-S323

Caspar W, Barbier D, Klara P (1989) Anterior cervical fusion and Caspar plate stabilization for cervical trauma. Neurosurgery 25(4):491–502

Clark CR, White AA (1985) Fractures of the dens A multicenter study. J Bone Joint Surg 67-A(9):1340–1348

Clohisy JC, Akbarnia BA, Bucholz RD, Burkus JK, Backer RJ (1992) Neurologic recovery associated with anterior decompression of spine fractures at the thoracolumbar junction (T12-L1). Spine 17(8S):S325-S330

Cotrel Y, Duboussett J, Guillaumatte M (1988) New universal instrumentation spinal surgery.Clin Orthop 227:10–23

Denis F (1984) Spinal instability as defined by the three-column spine concept in acute spinal trauma. Clin Orthop Related Res 189:65–76

Denis F, Davis S, Comfort T (1988) Sacral fractures: an important problem. Retrospective analysis of 236 cases. Clin Orthop Related Res 227:67–81

Dick W (1987) The fixateur interne as a versatile implant for spine surgery. Spine 12:882–900

Dickson J, Harrington PR, ErwinWD (1978) Results of reduction and stabilization of the severely fractured thoracic and lumbar spine. J Bone Joint Surg 60-A:799–805

Ducker T, Zeidman SM (1994) Spinal cord injury. Role of steroid therapy. Spine 19(20):2281–2287

Edwards CC, LevineAM (1986) Early rod sleeve stabilization of the injured thoracic and lumbar spine. Orthop Clin North Am 17(1):121–146

Effendi B, Roy D, Cornish B, Doussalt RG, Laurin CA (1981) Fractures of the ring of the axis. A classification based on the analysis of 131 cases. J Bone Joint Surg 63-B(3):319–327

Emery SE, Pathria MN, Wilber RG, Masaryk T, Bohlman HH (1989) Magnetic resonance imaging of posttraumatic spinal ligament injury. J Spinal Disorders 2(4):229–233

Esses SI, Bednar DA (1991) Screw fixation of odontoid fractures and nonunions. Spine 16(10S):S483-S485

Esses S, Sachs BL, Dreyzin V (1993) Complications associated with the technique of pedicle screw fixation. A selected survey of ABS members. Spine 18(15):2231–2239

Fabris D, Costantini U, Gentilucci G, Ricciardi A (1994) Cotrel-Dubosset instrumentation in thoracolumbar seat belt-type and flexion-distraction injuries. J Spinal Disorders 7(2): 146–152

Ferguson RL, Allen BL (1984) A mechanistic classification of thoracolumbar spine fractures. Clin Orthop Related Res (189):77–88

Fessler RG, Dietze DD, MacMillan M, Peace D (1991) Lateral parascapular extrapleural approach to the upper thoracic spine. J Neurosurg 75:349–355

Fielding JW, Cochran GVB, Lawsings III JF, Hohl M (1974) Tears of the transverse ligament of the atlas. A clinical and biomechanical study. J Bone Joint Surg 56-A:1683–1691

Finkelstein J, Hu R, Al-Harby T (in press) Open posterior dislocation of the lumbosacral junction. Spine

Garfin SR, Mowery CA, Guerra J, Marshall LF (1985) Confirmation of the posterolateral technique to decompress and fuse thoracolumbar spine burst fractures. Spine 10(3):218–223

Garvey TA, Eismont FJ, Roberti LJ (1992) Anterior decompression structural bone grafting and Caspar plate stabilization for unstable spine fractues and/or dislocations. Spine 17(10S):S431–S435

Geerts WH, Code KI, Jay RM, Chen E, Szalai JP (1994) A prospective study of venous thromboembolism after major trauma. N Engl J Med 331:1601–1606

Geisler FH, Cheng C, Poka A, Brumback RJ (1989) Anterior screw fixation of posteriorly displaced type II odontoid fractures. Neurosurgery 25(1):30–38

Gertzbein SD (1992) Scoliosis Research Society multicenter spine fracture study. Spine 17(5):528–540

Gertzbein S, MacMichael D, Tile M (1982) Harrington fixation as a method of fixation in fractures of the spine. A critical assessment of deficiencies. J Bone Joint Surg 64-B(5):526–529

Grob D, Jeanneret B, Aebi M, Markwalder T-M (1991) Atlantoaxial fusion with transarticular screw fixation. J Bone Joint Surg 73-B(6):972–976

Guttman L (1949) Surgical aspects of the treatment of traumatic paraplegia. J Bone Joint Surg 31-B(5):399–403

Hardaker WT, Cook WA, Friedman AH, Fitch RD (1992) Bilateral transpedicular decompression and harrington rod stabilization in the management of severe thoracolumbar burst fractures. Spine 17(2):162–171

Heller JG, Carlson GD, Abitbol J-J, Garfin SR (1991) Anatomic comparison of the Roy-Camille and Magerl Technique for screw placement in the lower cervical spine. Spine 16(10S):S552–S557

Hibbs RA (1911) An operation for progressive spinal deformit. NY Med J 93:1013

Holdsworth F (1970) Fractures dislocations and fracture-dislocations of the spine. Review article. J Bone Joint Surg 52-A(8):1534–1551

Hou S, Hu R, Shi Y (1993) Pedicle morphology of the lower thoracic and lumbar spine in a chinese population. Spine 18:1850–1855

Hu R, Mustard C, Burns C (in press) Incident spine fractures in a complete population. Spine

Huckell C, Powell JN, Eggli S, Hu R (1994) A comparative analysis of distraction rods versus luque rods in high thoracic spine fractures. Eur Spine J 3:270–275

Kaneda K, Abumi K, Fujiya M (1984) Burst fractures with neurological deficits of the thoracolumbar-lumbar spine. Results of anterior decompression and stabilization with instrumentation. Spine 9(8):788–795

Keene JS, Fischer SP, Vanderby R, Drummond DS, Turski PA (1989) Significance of acute posttraumatic bony encroachment of the neural canal. Spine 14(8):799–802

King D (1948) Internal fixation for lumbosacral fusion. J Bone Joint Surg 30-A:560–565

Kurz LT, Pursel SE, Herkowitz HN (1991) Modified anterior approach to the cervicothoracic junction. Spine 16(10S):S542–S547

Louis R (1983) Surgery of the spine. Springer, Berlin Heidelberg New York

Luque E, Cassis N, Ramirez-Wiella G (1982) Segmental spinal instrumentation in the treatment of fractures of the thoracolumbar spine. Spine 7:312–317

MacKenzie EJ, Siegel JH, Shapiro S, Moody M, Smith RT (1988) Functional recovery and medical costs of trauma: an analysis by type and severity of injury. J Trauma 28(3):281–297

Magerl F (1984) Stabilization of the lower thoracic and lumbar spine with external skeletal fixation. Clin Orthop 189:125–142

Magerl F, Aebi M, Gertzbein SD, Harms J, Nazarian S (1994) A comprehensive classification of thoracic and lumbar injuries. Eur Spine J 3:184–201

Marcotte P, Dickman CA, Sonntag VKH, Karahalios DG, Drabier J (1993) Posterior atlantoaxial facet screw fixation. J Neurosurg 79:234–237

Martijn A, Veldhuis EFM (1991) The diagnostic value of interpediculate distance assessment on plain films in thoracic and lumbar spine injuries. J Trauma 31(10):1393–1395

McAfee PC, Bohlman HH (1985) Complications following Harrington rod instrumentation for fractures of the thoracolumbar spine. J Bone Joint Surg 67-A(5):672–686

McAfee PC, Yuan HA, Fredrickson BE, Lubicky JP (1983) The value of computed tomography in thoracolumbar fractures. An analysis of one hundred consecutive cases and a new classification. J Bone Joint Surg 65-A(4):461–473

McAfee PC, Bohlman HH, Yuan HA (1985) Anterior decompression of traumatic thoracolumbar fractures with incomplete neurological deficit using a retroperitoneal approach. J Bone Joint Surg 67-A(5):672–686

McAfee PC, Cassidy JR, Davis RF, North RB, Ducker TB (1991) Fusion of the occiput to the upper cervical spine. A review of 37 cases. Spine 16(10S):S490–S494

McCormack T, Karaikovic E, Gaines RW (1994) The load sharing classification of spine fractures. Spine 19(15):1741–1744

McGrory B, Van der Wilde RS, Currier BL, Eismont FJ (1993) Diagnosis of subtle thoracolumbar burst fractures. A new radiographic sign. Spine 18(15):2282–2285

Mumford JWJN, Spratt KF, Goel VK (1993) Thoracolumbar burst fractures. The clinical efficacy and outcome of nonoperative management. Spine 18(8):955–970

Munson G, Satterlee C, Hammond S, Betten R, Gaines RW (1984) Experimental evaluation of Harrington rod fixation supplemented with sublaminar wires in stabilizing thoracolumbar fracture-dislocations. Clin Orthop Related Res 189:97–102

Nash CL, Brown RH (1989) Current concepts review: spinal cord monitoring. J Bone Joint Surg 71A:627–630

Penning L (1981) Prevertebral haematoma in cervical spine injury: incidence and etiologic significance. Am J Roentgenol 136(3):533–561

Pope MH, Panjabi M (1985) Biomechanical defintions of spinal instability. Spine 10(3):255–256

Reibel G, Yoo JU, Frederickson BE, Yuan HA (1993) Review of Harrington rod treatment of spinal trauma. Spine 18(4):479–491

Reid D, Hu R, Davis LA, Saboe L (1988) The non-operative treatment of burst fractures of the thoracolumbar junction. J Trauma 28(8):1188–1194

Roy-Camille R, Saillant G, Mazel C (1986) Internal fixation of the lumbar spine with pedicle screw plating. Clin Orthop Related Res 203:7–17

Roy-Camille R, Saillant G, Laville C, Benazet JP (1992) Treatment of lower cervical spinal injuries C3-C7. Spine 17(10S):S442-S446

Saboe LA, Reid DC, Davis LA, Warren SA, Grace MG (1991) Spine trauma and associated injuries. J Trauma 31(1):43–48

Sasso R, Jeanneret B, Fischer K, Magerl F (1994) Occipito-cervical fusion with posterior plate and screw instrumentation. A long-term follow-up study. Spine 15:2364–2368

Sears WA, Fazl M (1990) Prediction of stability of cervical spine fracture managed in the halo vest and indications for surgical intervention. J Neurosurg 72:426–432

Smith MD, Bressler EL, Lonstein JE, Winter R, Pinto MR, Denis F (1994) Deep venous thrombosis and pulmonary embolism after major reconstructive operations of the spine. A prospective analysis of three hundred and seventeen patients. J Bone Joint Surg 76-A(7):980–985

Van Buren RL, Wagner Jr FC (1994) Respiratory complications after cervical spinal cord injury. Spine 19(20):2315–2320

Wertheim SB, Bohlman HH (1987) Occipitocervical fusion. Indications techniques and long-term results in thirteen patients. J Bone Joint Surg 69-A(6):833–836

White III AA, Panjabi MM (1990) Clinical biomechanics of the spine, 2 nd edn. Lippincott, Philadelphia

Young MH (1973) Long-term consequences of stable fractures of the thoracic and lumbar vertebral bodies. J Bone Joint Surg 55-B(2):295–300

Zdeblick T,Warden KE, Zou D, McAfee PC, Abitbol JJ (1993) Anterior spinal fixators. A biomechanical in vitro study. Spine 18(4):513–517

12 Fractures of the Pelvis

M. Tile

12.1 Introduction

In the past two decades, traumatic disruption of the pelvic ring has become a major focus of orthopedic interest, as has the care of polytraumatized patients. This injury forms part of the spectrum of polytrauma and must be considered a potentially lethal injury with mortality rates of 10%–20%. The stabilization of the unstable pelvic ring in the acute resuscitation of multiply injured patients is now conventional wisdom.

With respect to the long-term results of pelvic trauma, conventional orthopedic wisdom held that surviving patients with disruptions of the pelvic ring recovered well clinically from their musculoskeletal injury. However, the literature on pelvic trauma was mostly concerned with life-threatening problems and paid scant attention to the late musculoskeletal problems reported in a handful of articles published prior to 1980. In spite of the clinical impressions that most patients do well, some authors have suggested otherwise.

Holdsworth (1948) reported on 50 pelvic fractures and indicated that of the 27 patients with a sacroiliac dislocation, 15 had significant pain and were unable to work, whereas those with a sacral or iliac fracture had more satisfactory results. Pennal and Sutherland (1959), in a large, unpublished study of 359 cases, further suggested that patients with unstable vertical shear injuries had many late complications. Slätis and Huittinen (1972) and Monahan and Taylor (1975) both confirmed the significant percentage of late musculoskeletal problems.

In reading the literature, the case mix for each series must be determined; otherwise the conclusions may be erroneous. Pelvic fractures must be classified according to their degree of instability or severity. If a series contains a large number of stable, inconsequential fractures, the overall results with simple treatment will be excellent, whereas if it contains a high percentage of displaced, unstable pelvic disruptions, the results with simple treatment will be quite different (Fig. 12.1). Therefore, in reading the literature, we must be certain that we are not comparing apples with oranges or chalk with cheese. An understanding of this injury is the key to logical decision making.

12.2 Understanding the Injury

In order to better understand our proposed classification and rationale of management, some knowledge of pelvic biomechanics is essential.

The pelvis is a ring structure made up of two innominate bones and the sacrum. These bones have no inherent stability, and the stability of the pelvic ring is thus due mainly to its surrounding soft tissues.

The stabilizing structures of the pelvic ring are the symphysis pubis, the posterior sacroiliac complex, and the pelvic floor. Although the anterior structures are important, contributing 40% of the stiffness to the ring (Hearn et al. 1991), the integrity of the posterior sacroiliac complex is most important in maintaining pelvic ring stability (see Fig. 12.6).

12.2.1 Ring Structure of the Pelvis

The pelvis is a true ring structure. It is self-evident that if the ring is broken in one area and displaced, then there must be a fracture or dislocation in another portion of the ring. Thus the vast literature describing anterior or posterior pelvic fractures suggesting that they appear in isolation is misleading. Gertzbein and Chenoweth (1977), in a series of patients with *undisplaced* anterior pelvic fractures noted that a technetium polyphosphate bone scan of the posterior sacroiliac complex gave a positive reading in every case, indicating the definite presence of a posterior lesion (Fig. 12.2). This was further confirmed in the publication by Bucholz (1981), in which posterior lesions at autopsy were found in all patients with pelvic trauma even when the radiograph had revealed only an anterior lesion.

12.2.2 Anatomical Lesions

The anterior pelvic lesion may be a symphysis pubis disruption or overlap, or pubic rami fractures unilaterally or bilaterally. A symphysis disruption may also occur in combination with pubic rami fractures.

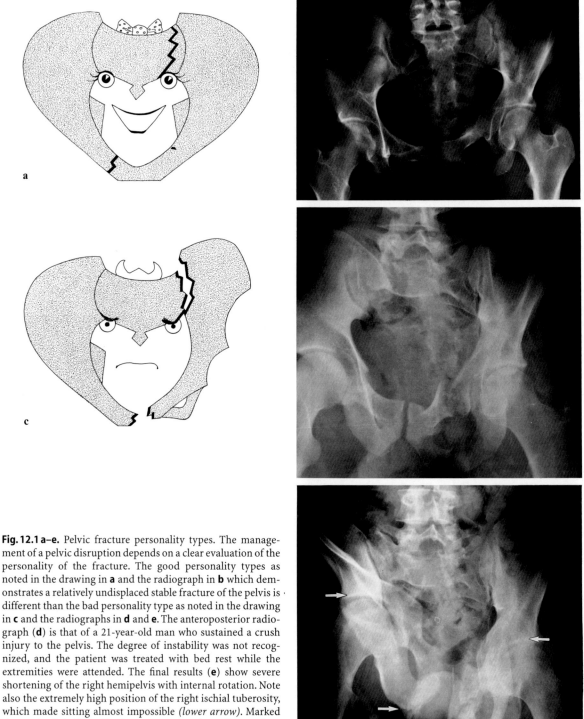

Fig. 12.1 a–e. Pelvic fracture personality types. The management of a pelvic disruption depends on a clear evaluation of the personality of the fracture. The good personality types as noted in the drawing in **a** and the radiograph in **b** which demonstrates a relatively undisplaced stable fracture of the pelvis is different than the bad personality type as noted in the drawing in **c** and the radiographs in **d** and **e**. The anteroposterior radiograph (**d**) is that of a 21-year-old man who sustained a crush injury to the pelvis. The degree of instability was not recognized, and the patient was treated with bed rest while the extremities were attended. The final results (**e**) show severe shortening of the right hemipelvis with internal rotation. Note also the extremely high position of the right ischial tuberosity, which made sitting almost impossible *(lower arrow)*. Marked shortening is indicated by the *upper arrows* above. Comparison of these two cases is like comparing apples to oranges or chalk to cheese

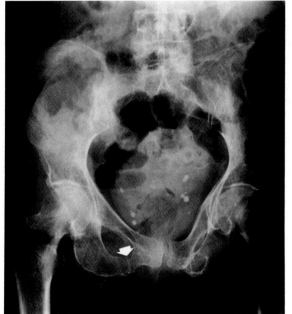

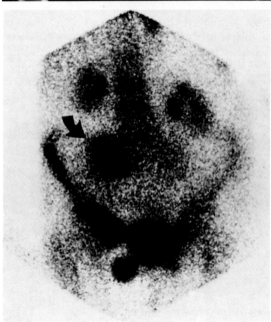

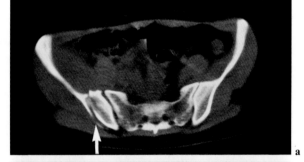

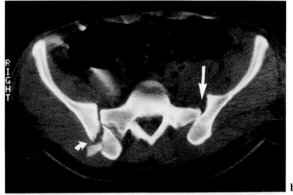

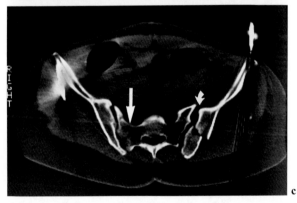

Fig. 12.3 a–c. Injuries to the posterior pelvic complex. The posterior injury may be a fracture through the ilium (**a**), a pure dislocation of the sacroiliac joint (**b**, *straight arrow*), or a fracture through the sacrum (**c**, *straight arrow*). A common pattern is a fracture dislocation through the sacroiliac joint, as shown by the *small curved arrows* in **b** and **c**

Fig. 12.2. a Radiograph of a patient with an apparently undisplaced fracture of the inferior and superior pubic ramus on the right side *(white arrow)*. No lesion is seen posteriorly. The deformity of the left hemipelvis represents a malunion of an old left acetabular fracture. **b** Technetium polyphosphate bone scan of the same patient clearly showing the increased uptake of the superior and inferior pubic ramus fracture anteriorly, but also a massively increased uptake at the right sacroiliac joint, indicating a posterior lesion *(black arrow)*. (From Tile 1984; courtesy of Dr. S.D. Gertzbein)

The posterior lesion may be a fracture of the ilium, often in the coronal plane, a dislocation or fracture-dislocation of the sacroiliac joint, or a fracture through the sacrum (Fig. 12.3). The commonest lesion is a sacral fracture followed by a combined injury, i.e., a fracture-dislocation of the sacroiliac joint, usually with a portion of the ilium remaining attached to the main sacral fragment.

Sacral fractures, in turn, may be classified as lateral, medial, or through the foramena or as complex types (H types).

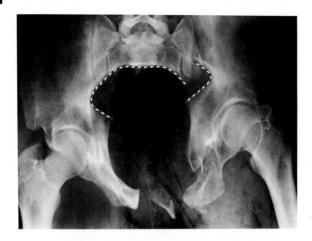

Fig. 12.4. The *dotted line* on the *right* represents the sacroglu-teal line on the inlet view of the pelvis. Any break in the conti-nuity of this line, as shown on the *left*, represents displacement of the posterior complex, an ominous prognostic indicator. (From Tile 1984)

Of greater importance than the site of the posterior lesion is the degree of displacement of the posterior sac-roiliac complex. This can best be seen on the inlet radio-graph showing posterior displacement of the so-called sacrogluteal line (Fig. 12.4) and is best confirmed by computed tomography (CT) scan. Therefore, the poste-rior lesion, although present, may be undisplaced and have intact posterior ligaments, often associated with a sacral crush, or may be displaced with a major ligamen-tous disruption of the posterior pelvic complex (Fig. 12.5).

12.2.3 Stability of the Pelvis

The anatomical lesions are important for surgical management, but the stability factor is more important for overall decision making in the management of patients.

Stability may be defined as the ability of the pelvis to withstand physiological forces without significant displacement. It is obvious that pelvic stability is dependent not only on the bony structures, but also on the strong ligamentous structures binding together the three bones of the pelvis, i.e., the two innominate bones and the sacrum. If these ligamentous structures are removed, the pelvis falls into its three component parts. Moreover, stability is a spectrum: at one end of the spectrum is the intact pelvic ring, at the other end a completely unstable pelvis, an *internal hemipelvectomy*. In our pelvic classification based on stability, the fractures at the stable end are type A, at the unstable

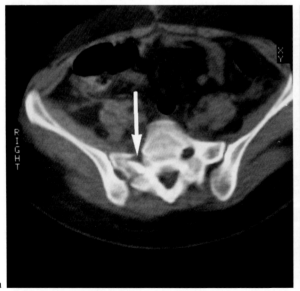
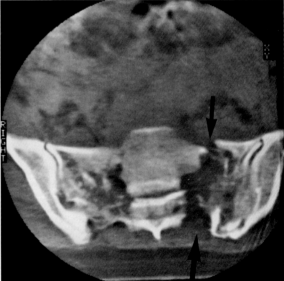

Fig. 12.5 a,b. The posterior lesion may be stable or unstable. **a** The impacted right sacrum is clearly seen *(white arrow)*. There is at least 1 cm of overlap between the two fragments. This posterior lesion is stable and cannot be moved. **b** The left

sacral lesion is grossly unstable *(black arrows)*. As well as the displacement at the fracture, all soft tissues are disrupted. (From Tile 1984)

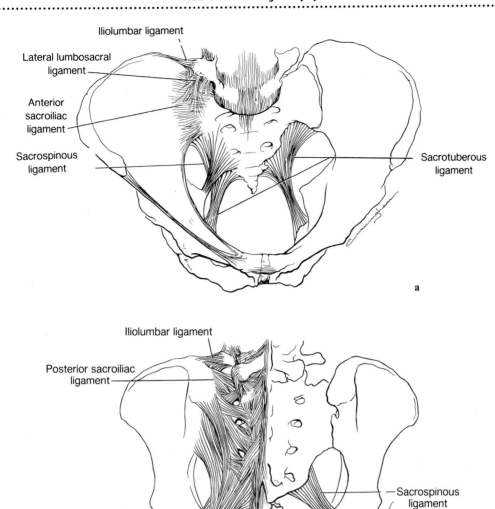

Iliolumbar ligament

Lateral lumbosacral ligament

Anterior sacroiliac ligament

Sacrospinous ligament

Sacrotuberous ligament

a

Iliolumbar ligament

Posterior sacroiliac ligament

Sacrospinous ligament

Sacrotuberous ligament

b

Fig. 12.6 a, b. The major posterior stabilizing structures of the pelvic ring, as seen from the anteroposterior (**a**) and posterior view (**b**). The anteroposterior view (**a**) indicates the sacrospinous ligament as a strong triangular ligament lying anterior to the sacrotuberous ligament, a strong band extending from the lateral portion of the dorsum of the sacrum to the ischial tuberosity. These two ligaments form part of the pelvic floor, which is also supported by the pelvic floor muscles and fascia. The anterior sacroiliac ligament is flat and not as strong as the posterior sacroiliac ligamentous structures noted in the drawing (**b**). The posterior sacroiliac ligament, the sacrotuberous ligaments, and the sacrospinous ligaments are the major posterior stabilizing structures of the pelvic ring, that is, the posterior tension band of the pelvis. The ipsilateral sacroiliac complex often shows a compression through the sacrum. The pelvic floor integrity is usually maintained by the implosion force, thereby buckling the ligaments on the pelvic floor as noted. (From Tile 1984)

end type C, and those with partial stability in the middletype B.

The stability of the pelvic ring depends upon the integrity of the posterior weight-bearing sacroiliac complex (Fig. 12.6) and the pelvic floor. The major ligaments are the sacroiliac, the sacrotuberous, and the sacrospinous.

12.2.3.1 Sacroiliac Complex

The intricate posterior sacroiliac complex is a masterly biomechanical structure able to withstand the transference of the weight-bearing forces from the spine to the

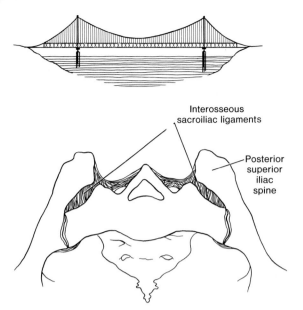

Fig. 12.7. The suspension bridge-like appearance of the ligaments binding the posterior sacroiliac complex. Note the vertical direction of the interosseous posterior sacroiliac ligaments, noted by Grant to be the strongest in the body, as well as the transverse component acting as the suspension, joining the pillars, represented by the posterior superior or iliac spines, to the sacrum. (From Tile 1984)

lower extremities. The ligaments have a major role as posterior stabilizers, because the sacrum, contrary to what is expected, does not form the shape of a keystone in a Roman arch, but is quite the reverse. Therefore, the strong posterior sacroiliac interosseous ligaments have

been described as the strongest in the body, maintaining the sacrum in its normal position in the pelvic ring. Also, the iliolumbar ligaments join the transverse processes of L5 to the iliac crest, and the intervening transverse fibers of the interosseous sacroiliac ligaments further enhance the suspensory mechanism. The entire complex looks and functions like a suspension bridge (Fig. 12.7).

The anterior sacroiliac ligaments are flat and strong and resist external rotation and shearing forces, although they do not have the strength of the posterior ligaments.

12.2.3.2 Pelvic Floor

The pelvic floor, with its muscular layer covered by investing fascia, also acts as a stabilizer of the pelvic ring. Two major ligaments also form part of the pelvic floor, namely the sacrospinous and sacrotuberous.

The strong sacrospinous ligament, with fibers running transversely from the lateral edge of the sacrum to the ischial spine, resists external rotation of the pelvic ring (Fig. 12.8). The complex sacrotuberous ligament arises from most of the sacroiliac complex posterior to the sacrospinous ligament and extends to the ischial tuberosity. This strong ligament, positioned in the vertical plane, resists vertical shearing forces applied to the hemipelvis (Fig. 12.9). Therefore, these two supplementary ligaments, the sacrospinous and sacrotuberous, placed at 90° to each other, are well adapted to resist the two major forces acting upon the pelvis, i.e., external rotation and vertical shear. In this way, they supplement the posterior sacroiliac ligaments.

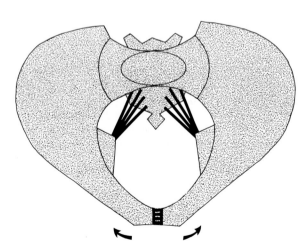

Fig. 12.8. The sacrospinous ligaments, joining the sacrum to the ischial spines, resist external rotatory forces *(arrows)*. (From Tile 1984)

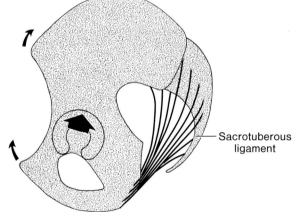

Fig. 12.9. The sacrotuberous ligament, joining the sacrum to the ischial tuberosity, resists a shearing rotatory force *(arrows)*. (From Tile 1984)

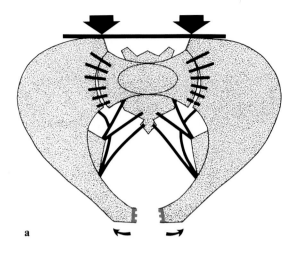

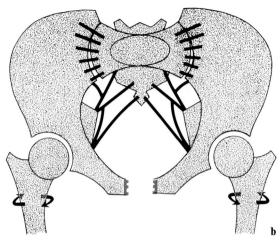

Fig. 12.10. a A direct blow to the posterior superior iliac spines will cause the symphysis pubis to spring open. **b** External rotation of the femora or direct compression against the anterior

superior spines will also cause springing of the symphysis. (From Tile 1984)

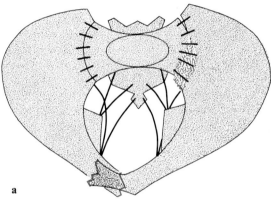

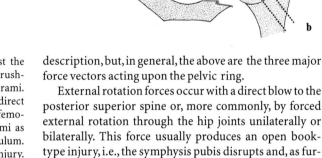

Fig. 12.11. a A lateral compressive force directed against the iliac crest will cause the hemipelvis to rotate internally, crushing the anterior sacrum and displacing the anterior pubic rami. **b** Lateral compression injury may also be caused by a direct force against the greater trochanter. In that situation, the femoral head acts as a battering ram, dividing the pubic rami as shown, often through the anterior colum of the acetabulum. The ipsilateral sacroiliac complex is also crushed in this injury. Note that the sacrospinous and sacrotuberous ligaments generally remain intact along with the pelvic floor in this lateral compression-type injury. (From Tile 1995)

12.2.4 Types of Injurious Forces Acting on the Pelvis

Most forces acting on the pelvis are either (a) external rotation, also called anteroposterior compression, (b) internal rotation (lateral compression), or (c) shearing or translational forces in the vertical plane. In the complex high-energy trauma seen in our society, some forces defy

description, but, in general, the above are the three major force vectors acting upon the pelvic ring.

External rotation forces occur with a direct blow to the posterior superior spine or, more commonly, by forced external rotation through the hip joints unilaterally or bilaterally. This force usually produces an open booktype injury, i.e., the symphysis pubis disrupts and, as further force is applied, the sacrospinous ligament and the anterior ligaments of the sacroiliac joint may also open (Fig. 12.10). Eventually, impingement of the posterior ilium on the sacrum occurs. At this point, the posterior sacroiliac ligaments still confer stability to the ring and translation vertically or posteriorly is not possible.

The force of internal rotation or lateral compression may be transmitted by a direct blow to the iliac crest, often causing an upward rotation of the hemipelvis or the so-called bucket-handle fracture, or through the femoral head, often causing an ipsilateral injury (Fig. 12.11). In this pattern, the anterior structures, usu-

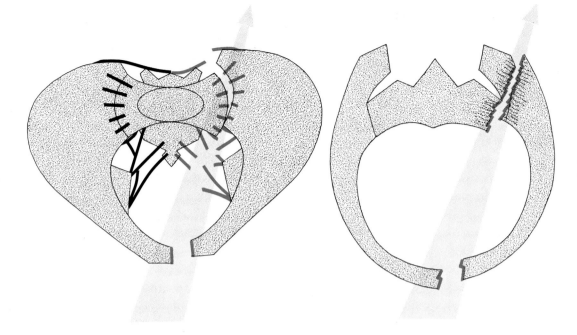

Fig. 12.12. A shearing force *(arrows)* crosses perpendicular to the main trabecular pattern of the posterior pelvic complex in the vertical plane. These forces cause marked displacement of bone and gross disruption of the soft tissues, resulting in major pelvic instability. (From Tile 1995)

ally the rami, break and the hemipelvis rotates internally. If the posterior ligaments remain intact, the anterior sacrum will compress. If the posterior ligaments tear, stability is still maintained by the pelvic floor.

Shearing forces in the vertical plane cross the main trabecular pattern of the posterior sacroiliac complex, whereas a lateral compressive force causes impaction of the cancellous bone and usually allows retention of the ligament integrity. However, external rotation and lateral compression forces may be so great that they overcome the restraining effect of the ligament. Therefore, a completely unstable pelvic ring may be caused by complex forces acting on the pelvis. The term "shear" is synomonous with these complex forces. Shearing forces cause marked displacement of bone and gross disruption of the soft tissue structures (Fig. 12.12), including the pelvic floor. Continuation of these forces beyond the yield strength of the soft tissues produces an unstable pelvic ring with major anterior and posterior displacement. No finite point is reached with these shearing forces; therefore, the entire hemipelvis may be avulsed from the body, occasionally resulting in a traumatic hindquarter amputation.

12.2.5 Effect of Forces on Soft Tissue

External rotation and shear forces tend to tear soft tissue; therefore, the injuries caused by these forces are usually major: tearing viscera and arteries and causing traction injuries to nerves. Lateral compression forces (internal rotatioin) tend to puncture viscera and compress nerves (Dalal et al. 1989).

12.3 Classification (Table 12.1)

By combining the concepts of stability, force direction, and pathoanatomy, a meaningful classification may be developed to aid in patient management. No classification can answer all the question regarding a specific injury. Since the first edition of this book, and since our publication in *The Journal of Bone and Joint Surgery* in January 1988 (Tile 1988), refinements have been made to our original classification to allow acceptance as the comprehensive classification of pelvic fractures.

All classifications should serve as guides to treatment and should allow centers to compare like cases. The management of individual patients requires careful specific assessment, and the surgeon must be able to draw the fracture lines on a dry skeleton as well as determine the degree of soft tissue injury.

The classification also follows the A,B,C nomenclature of the comprehensive classification (Müller et al. 1990), with increasing severity of injury from A to C. It must also be remembered that the types A, B, and C based on stability form a spectrum rather than a rigid

Table 12.1. Classification of pelvic ring disruption

Type A: Stable pelvic ring injury
  A1: Avulsion of the innominate bone
  A2: Stable iliac wing fracture or stable minimally
      displaced ring fractures
  A3: Transverse fractures of the sacrum and coccyx

Type B: Partially stable
  B1: Open book injury
  B2: The lateral compression injury
      B2.1: Ipsilateral type
      B2.2: Contralateral type (bucket-handle)
  B3: Bilateral B injuries

Type C: Unstable (vertical shear)
  C1: Unilateral
      C1.1: Ilium
      C1.2: Sacroiliac dislocation or fracture dislocation
      C1.3: Sacrum
  C2: Bilateral, one side B, one side C
  C3: Bilateral C lesions

The Qualifications of the anterior arch lesions C1) to C9) are identical for all subgroups of the Types B and C:

C1) unilateral pubis / rami fx, ipsilateral
C2) unilateral pubis / rami fx, contralateral
C3) bilateral pubis / rami fx
C4) symphysis pubis disruption, $\leq$ 2.5 cm
C5) symphysis pubis disruption, > 2.5 cm
C6) symphysis pubis disruption, locked
C7) symphysis + ipsilateral pubis / rami fx (tilt) (yes)
C8) symphysis + contralateral pubis / rami fx
C9) symphysis + bilateral pubis / rami fx
C10) no anterior lesion

black and white concept. For the purpose of this classification, the posterior pelvis is located posterior to the acetabulum, and the anterior arch anterior to it. The fracture type is based on the posterior lesion, which is more important for stability, and the anterior lesions are denoted by modifiers.

Stability is defined as the *ability* to withstand physiological forces without deformation. Therefore, at one end of the stability scale, the type A pelvic lesions do not displace the ring, only involving the avulsions of the iliac wing or transverse sacral fractures, really spinal injuries. In all these cases the pelvis remains intact. At the other end of the spectrum, the type C fractures are unstable, with complete disruption of the posterior arch, the pelvic floor, and usually the anterior arch. The type B fractures retain some posterior stability and are therefore partially stable; they cannot, by definition, translate vertically or posteriorly.

A and B types generally comprise about 70% of the total fractures, even in trauma centers; the remainder are unstable type C; (Pohlemann et al. 1995).

The partially stable (type B) injuries are of two varieties: the open book or anteroposterior compression injury, caused by external rotation, and the lateral compression injury, caused by internal rotation. It should be remembered that the open book injury caused by an external rotatory force is unstable in external rotation, whereas the lateral compression injury may be unstable in internal rotation or may be rigidly impacted, but neither is unstable in the vertical plane unless a force which disrupts the posterior ligamentous structures is present. Also, it is self-evident that unstable pelvic injuries may be produced by any force vector which overcomes the yield strength of the soft tissues.

12.3.1 Type A Stable Fractures (Table 12.1)

In the type A injury, the pelvic ring is stable and cannot, by definition, displace by physiological force. These injuries include type A1 avulsion fractures, which usually occur in adolescents and do not involve the pelvic ring. The type A2 fractures involve the iliac wing or the anterior arch without a posterior injury, a rare occurrence. The type A3 fractures are transverse fractures of the sacrum and coccyx and should more correctly be considered as spinal injuries.

12.3.2 Type B – Partially Stable Fractures (Table 12.1)

12.3.2.1 Open Book (Anteroposterior Compression) Fractures (B1, B3.1)

External rotatory forces applied to the pelvis usually cause a disruption of the symphysis pubis; however, they may also cause an avulsion fracture of the pubis adjacent to the symphysis or a fracture through the pubic rami, the symphysis avulsion or disruption being more common. Since the force is a continuum and may stop at any point, several possibilities exist.

First, an opening of the symphysis pubis less than 2.5 cm permits stability to be retained in the pelvic ring, a situation not dissimilar to that observed during delivery of a baby. In the rare traumatic injury, the sacrospinous and anterior sacroiliac ligaments remain intact (Fig. 12.13). Therefore, a CT scan will show no opening of the sacroiliac joints.

Second, continuation of the external rotatory force will reach a finite end point when the "book" opens to the extent that the posterior iliac spines abut upon the sacrum. In this particular circumstance, the sacrospinous ligaments and the anterior sacroiliac ligaments are torn, but the strong posterior sacroiliac ligaments remain intact (Fig. 12.14). Occasionally, the posterior injury may be a fracture of the ilium or sacrum.

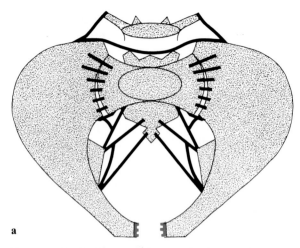
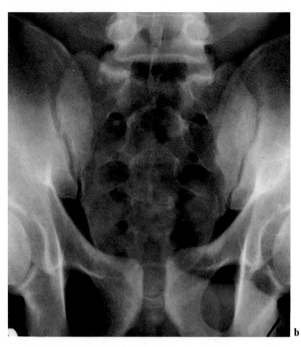

Fig. 12.13 a,b. The first stage of an open book injury (type B1) is a disruption of the symphysis pubis only with no involvement of the sacroiliac joints (**a**). The patient in **b**, a hockey player who sustained a direct blow to the posterior sacroiliac area bilaterally, noted immediate pain anteriorly at the symphysis pubis. His radiograph indicates a symphysis pubis separation of 1.5 cm with no opening of the sacroiliac joints posteriorly. (From Tile 1995)

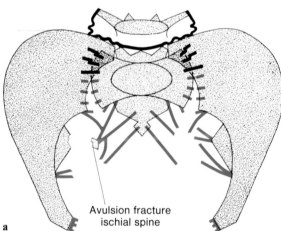
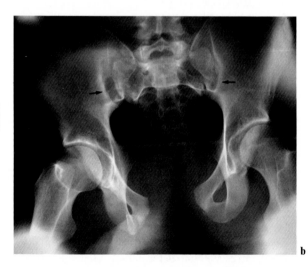

Avulsion fracture
ischial spine

Fig. 12.14 a,b. The second stage of an open book injury. **a** In this diagram note that the symphysis pubis has disrupted more than 2.5 cm. If that occurs, the sacrospinous ligaments tear or an equivalent avulsion of the adjacent sacrum or ischial spine occurs, as well as an avulsion of the anterior sacroiliac joints, causing a wide anterior opening of the sacroiliac joints. However, pelvic stability is maintained by the intact posterior ligamentous structures, indicated by the *black lines*. The endpoint is reached when the posterior iliac spines abut the sacrum. **b** A typical radiograph showing the disruption of the symphysis pubis and the markedly widened sacroiliac joints anteriorly *(arrows)*. (From Tile 1984)

Therefore, this injury is unstable in external rotation, but as long as the force does not continue beyond the yield strength of the posterior ligaments, stability can be returned to the pelvic ring by internal rotation.

It is extremely important to realize that the external rotatory force may in fact continue beyond the yield strength of the posterior ligament, causing a complete avulsion of the hemipelvis. This is no longer an open book configuration but is now an unstable fracture of the worst variety (Fig. 12.15). In fact, as previously indicated, a complete traumatic hemipelvectomy may ensue. Therefore, the presence of a symphysis disruption does

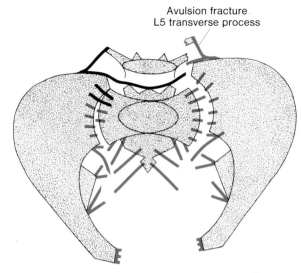

Avulsion fracture
L5 transverse process

Fig. 12.15. The presence of a symphysis disruption does not imply a stable configuration; in fact, most symphysis disruptions are associated with unstable posterior lesions, as shown. Note the telltale avulsion fracture of the L5 tranverse process, indicating instability and posterior displacement of this fracture. (From Tile 1984)

not always imply an open book fracture. Careful assessment is required to be certain that vertical instability is not also present.

Ultimately, with this type of force, a symphysis disruption as well as involvement of the pelvic soft tissues such as the vagina, the urethra, the bladder, or the rectum may occur.

In the classification, the anterior lesion is designated by modifiers (Table 12.1). In the open book injury typical varieties of open book fracture may occur with fractures anteriorly through the pubic rami unilaterally or bilaterally.

12.3.2 Partially Stable Fractures (Type B2)

12.3.2.1 Lateral Compression Fractures

There are several types of lateral compression injury depending upon the site of the anterior and posterior lesion (Table 12.1). The anterior and posterior lesions may be on the same side or ipsilateral (type B2.1), or they may be on opposite sides, producing the so-called bucket-handle type of injury (type B2.2).

Fig. 12.16 a–c. Lateral compression fracture, type B2.1: ipsilateral. The diagram (**a**) shows a typical ipsilateral type of lateral compression injury. Note the anterior crush to the sacrum and the overlap of the pubic rami. In this particular case there is posterior disruption, but stability is afforded by the crush in the sacrum and the intact pelvic floor. The force necessary to produce this seemingly minimally displaced fracture is often underestimated because of the elastic recoil of the pelvis. This fracture, barely perceptible on the inlet radiograph (**b**, *arrow*), was obviously grossly displaced at the moment of injury, since the bladder was pulled back into it, as shown in the cystogram (**c**, *arrow*). (From Tile 1984)

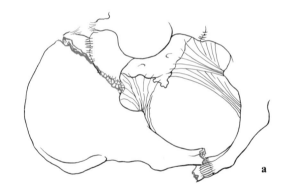

a

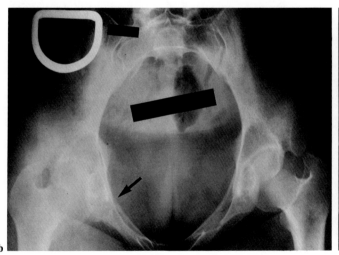

b

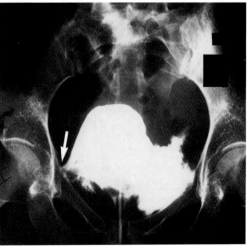

c

a) Type B2.1 – Ipsilateral Fractures

An internal rotation force applied to the ilium or, more commonly, a direct blow to the greater trochanter may cause a typical lateral compression or internal rotation fracture of the hemipelvis. The superior and inferior rami break, and a crush may then occur anteriorly at the sacroiliac joint or through the sacrum, but, commonly, the posterior ligamentous structures do not disrupt (Fig. 12.16 a). The entire hemipelvis may be forced across to the opposite side, thereby rupturing the bladder or blood vessels within the pelvis. The elastic recoil of the tissues may deceive the examiner and the fracture appear undisplaced in the radiograph. However, the radiographs in Fig. 10.16 b, c show the bladder being drawn back into the fracture site by the recoiling pelvis.

If the bone is stronger than the ligaments, the posterior ligaments may disrupt, but stability may be retained by an intact pelvic floor, not disrupted by the *implosion* force.

The anterior injury designated by the modifiers may be as follows (see Table 12.1):

- *Fractures of both rami.* This is the most common injury, with a spike of bone possibly penetrating the pelvic viscera.
- *Locked symphysis.* This rare injury is a form of ipsilateral lateral compression type. As the hemipelvis internally rotates, the symphysis disrupts and locks, making reduction extremely difficult (Fig. 12.17).
- *Tilt fracture.* The tilt fracture consists of a symphysis disruption and a fracture of the superior ramus, with possible impingement of the bone into the vagina of young females (Fig. 12.18).

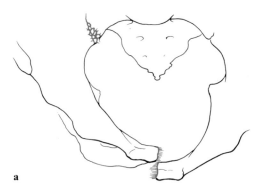

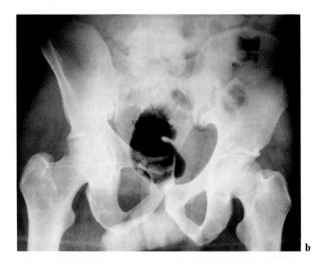

Fig. 12.17 a, b. Locked symphysis. **a** Diagram and **b** anteroposterior radiograph showing an unusual type of lateral compression injury where the symphysis becomes firmly locked anteriorly. (From Tile 1984)

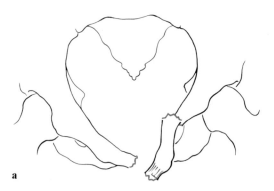

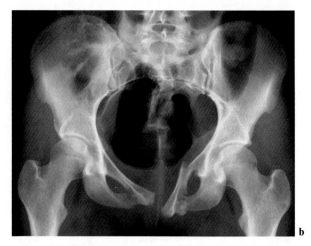

Fig. 12.18. a A variant of the type I injury often seen in young women. The lateral compressive force fractures the superior ramus, often through the anterior column of the acetabulum. Continuing lateral compression rotates the distal fragment through the symphysis pubis, thereby disrupting it. This distal fragment assumes a vertical position and may impinge on the perineum, as demonstrated in the anteroposterior radiograph (**b**). (From Tile 1984)

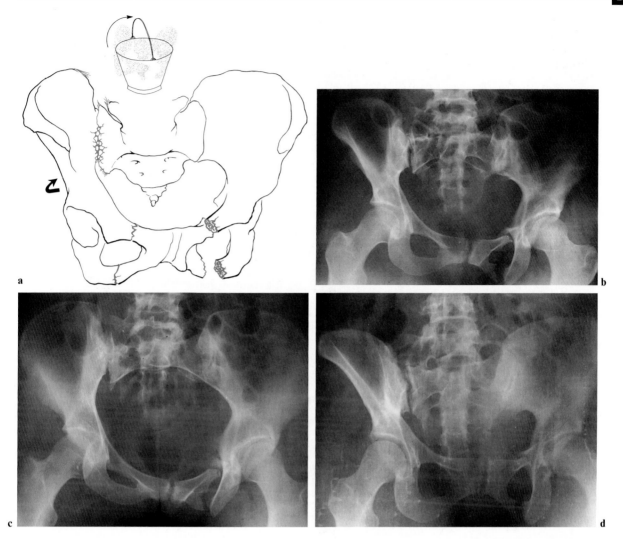

Fig. 12.19 a–d. Type B2.2 lateral compression injury. The diagram (**a**) demonstrates a typical type B2.2 lateral compression injury, characterized by compression of the posterior sacroiliac complex associated with a straddle or butterfly fracture of the four pubic rami anteriorly. The anteroposterior (**b**), inlet (**c**), and outlet (**d**) views of this 19-year-old woman show this classic lesion with upward rotation and impaction of the right hemipelvis. Even under general anesthesia, this hemiplevis could not be moved on the third day following injury, indicating severe posterior impaction

b) Type B2.2 – Contralateral: Bucket-Handle Injuries

The bucket-handle type of injury is usually caused by a direct blow to the ilium. The anterior fracture may be on the opposite side to the posterior lesion (contralateral type) or all four rami may fracture anteriorly but the anterior displacement is on the side opposite the posterior lesion. Another combination might be a symphysis disruption with two rami fractures.

This injury has particular characteristics that may seem confusing. The affected hemipelvis rotates anteriorly and superiorly like the handle of a bucket (Fig. 12.19). Therefore, even if the posterior structures are relatively intact, the patient may have a major leg length discrepancy. Very often, the posterior structures are firmly impacted, the deformity being clearly noted on physical examination. Reducing these fractures and thereby the leg length discrepancy requires derotation of the hemipelvis rather than pure traction in the vertical plane.

With continued internal rotation, the posterior structures may yield, producing some instability. However, the anterior sacroiliac crush is usually so stable that reduction is difficult and some stability is maintained by the intact pelvic floor and the sacrospinous and sacrotuberous ligaments.

This is akin to the situation with a vertebral fracture, where the vertebral body may be crushed by flexion forces but the posterior spinous ligament has ruptured.

234 •••

Chapter 12   **Fractures of the Pelvis**

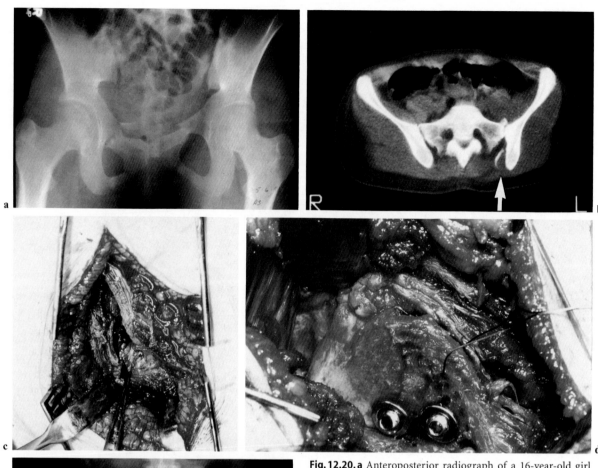

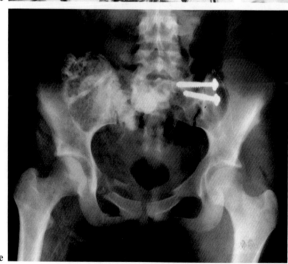

Fig. 12.20. a Anteroposterior radiograph of a 16-year-old girl with a type B2.2 bucket-handle fracture. The fracture involves all four pubic rami and the left sacroiliac joint. **b** Computed tomography (CT) clearly outlines the essential features of this fracture. Note the anterior crush of the sacrum, the internal rotation of the left hemipelvis, and, in this case, the avulsion of the iliac apophysis which had not yet fused to the ilium *(arrow)*. **c** Clinical appearance at surgery of this apophysis avulsion (outlined by the probe, *arrow*). **d** Appearance after reduction and fixation with two lag screws crossing the sacroiliac joint. **e** Postoperative radiographic appearance

Posteriorly, the arrow points to the avulsion of the posterior iliac apophysis (Fig. 12.20 b, c). At surgery, the apophysis was clearly avulsed but the posterior sacroiliac ligaments were completely intact. After posterior reduction of the fracture and fixation by two screws, the pelvis is anatomically reduced (Fig. 12.20 d, e).

c) Type B3 – Bilateral Partially Stable Injuries

The B3 bilateral injuries may be the classical open book type (B3.1), or one side B1 and one side B2 (B3.2), or bilateral B2 (B3.3).

An excellent example of this is shown in Fig. 12.20 a. The original radiograph of this 16-year-old girl shows the internal rotation of the left hemipelvis and the posterior impaction. All four rami are broken anteriorly and the leg length discrepancy is seen. The CT scan (Fig. 12.20 b) again shows the left hemipelvis to be internally rotated and the anterior portion of the sacroiliac joint crushed.

12.3.3 Type C – Unstable Fractures – Complete Disruption of the Posterior Arch (see Table 12.1)

An unstable pelvic disruption implies disruption of the posterior sacroiliac arch as well as a rupture of the pelvic floor, including the posterior structures as well as the sacrospinous and sacrotuberous ligaments (Fig. 12.21). The unstable injury may be unilateral (type C1), affecting one posterior iliac complex, or may be bilateral (type C2 or C3), affecting both.

The unilateral lesions may be fractures of the ilium (type C1.1) through the sacroiliac joint, or either a pure dislocation or a fracture-dislocation with involved ilium or sacrum (type C1.2), or a fracture of the sacrum (type C.1.3).

The bilateral types C2 include one side unstable (C) and one side partially stable (B), while the C3 lesions include bilaterally unstable types.

Telltale radiographic signs of instability include avulsion of the transverse process of the L5 vertebra or of either attachment of the sacrospinous ligament (Fig. 12.22). Greater than 1 cm of posterior or vertical translation is noted. The CT scan shows the radiographic appearance of the unstable posterior complex better than the plain radiograph and should be obtained in all cases.

A comparison of the CT scans (Fig. 12.23) shows clearly the difference between the impacted stable posterior complex and the grossly unstable complex of the vertical shear injury.

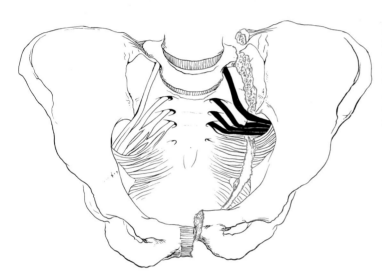

Fig. 12.21. Unilateral unstable vertical shear fracture. Shearing forces cause massive disruption of the pelvic ring, including the pelvic floor. Note the avulsion of the ischial spine and the tip of the transverse process of L5, both signs of pelvic instability. Note also the stretch of the lumbosacral plexus, commonly injured in this pattern of injury. (From Tile 1984)

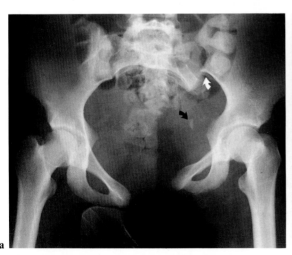

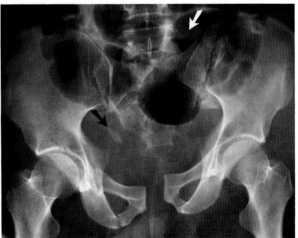

a   b

Fig. 12.22 a,b. Telltale signs of instability. **a** Avulsion of the ischial spine *(black arrow)* and posterior displacement of the ilium *(white arrow)*. **b** Avulsion of the sacral end of the sacro- spinous ligament *(black arrow)* and the tip of the transverse process of L5 on the opposite side *(white arrow)* in this bilateral injury. (From Tile 1984)

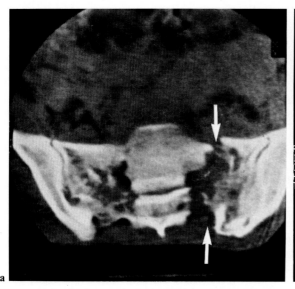
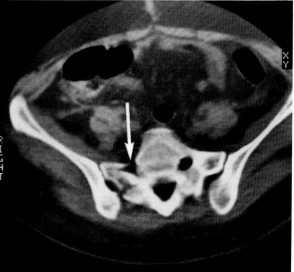

a   b

Fig. 12.23. a Computed tomography (CT) scan showing marked disruption and instability of the left sacrum as a result of a shearing force. **b** CT scan showing impaction of the right sacrum from a lateral compression injury. This young woman sustained an acetabular fracture as well, confirming the mechanism of injury. Note the marked overriding of the sacral fragments on the fractured side as compared to the normal left side. Impaction was so rigid that no abnormal movement of the hemipelvis was detected on physical examination with image intensification. (From Tile 1984)

12.3.4 Unusual Types of Fracture

a) Complex Fractures

Many severe types of fracture dislocation of the pelvis defy precise classification because of the complex forces causing the injury. In these cases, the pelvic ring may be disrupted in a very bizarre fashion. Because of the high-energy forces involved, the pelvic ring is usually unstable; since most are bilateral, most will fall into the C3 classification.

b) Bilateral Sacroiliac Dislocation with an Intact Anterior Arch

This unusual injury is usually caused by hyperflexion of the legs (for example, two of our cases were in young women who were crushed in the hyperflexed position under a horse which reared and fell backwards). In this particular situation, the anterior complex remains intact but both sacroiliac joints dislocate posteriorly (C3).

c) Pelvic Disruptions Associated with Acetabular Fractures

If a pelvic ring disruption is associated with an acetabular fracture, the prognosis will clearly change and will be more dependent upon the acetabular component than upon the pelvic ring disruption. These complex injuries are relatively common. CT scanning of acetabular fractures has indicated a significant number of sacroiliac injuries and pelvic ring disruptions associated with acetabular fractures. In the comprehensive classification, the pelvic ring component is classified separately from the acetabulum (see Chap. 13).

12.4 Natural History

In an attempt to further elucidate the incidence and severity of the early and late musculoskeletal complications of this injury, we undertook a clinical study in association with R. Lifeso, D. Dickinson, and R. McBroom (Dickinson et al. 1982). The purpose of this study was to place the management of this injury in perspective by determining which pelvic fractures had the poorest prognosis. With the current trend to internal fixation of the pelvis, a study of the natural history of this injury is even more important, in order to place that trend in perspective, for without a knowledge of the natural history, logical decision making becomes impossible. The results of our review of 248 cases are shown in Tables 12.2–12.6.

In this study, every patient was recalled, personally interviewed, examined, and radiographed using the inlet, outlet, and anteroposterior views. The conclusions may be summarized as follows:

Table 12.2. Comparison of series A and series B patients[a] (from Tile 1984)

	Series A (n=148)	Series B (n=100)
1. Age (range)	34.2 years (15-81)	30.9 years (14-85)
2. Sex		
Male	91	55
Female	57	45
3. Injury types		
Motor vehicle accidents	89 (60%)	81
Fall	17 (11.5%)	11
Crush	34 (23%)	4
Miscellaneous	8 (5.5%)	4
4. Workmen's Compensation Board	43 (29%)	5
5. Associated injuries		
CNS	31 (21%)	38
Chest	19 (13%)	15
Gastrointestinal	10 (6.6%)	20
Bladder	17 (11%)	8
Urethra	6 (4%)	4
Nerve	12 (8%)	3
Musculoskeletal	63 (43%)	10
6. Follow-up average	60 mo	2 years

[a] In Tables 12.2–12.6, series A is a group of 148 cases of pelvic fracture managed in Toronto teaching hospitals and in non-teaching hospitals in Ontario, retrospectively reviewed; series B consists of the first 100 cases of pelvic fracture treated at the Sunnybrook Medical Center, Toronto, prospectively reviewed.

Table 12.3. Factors resulting in unsatisfactory results (from Tile 1984)

	Series A: 37/148	Series B: 35/100
Pain	37	32
Leg length discrepancy > 2 cm	7	2
Nonunion	5	3
Permanent nerve damage	9	3
Urethral symptoms	5	1
Deaths		17

1. *Stable* injuries gave few major long-term problems. Pain, if present, was usually mild or moderate.
2. By contrast, patients with *unstable* pelvic disruptions had many problems at review. Approximately 30% of this group had continuing pain, including 3% with nonunion of the posterior complex and 5% with malunion, defined as having a greater than 2.5-cm leg length discrepancy. In addition, 5% had permanent nerve damage, and 3% continuing urethral problems following urethral rupture.

The pain, when present, usually arose from the posterior sacroiliac joint area or from the lower lumbar spine. CT has shown lumbar spine involvement in significant numbers of patients with pelvic disruption. The pain in these cases was more severe, and usually associated with an unreduced sacroiliac dislocation or a nonunion.

In summary, the natural history of pelvic trauma depends on the degree of violence, the type of injury, the method of treatment, and the presence or absence of complications such as a urethral tear, permanent nerve damage, malunion, malreduction of the sacroiliac joint, or nonunion. The unstable vertical shear injury results

Table 12.4. Pain (moderate and severe) (from Tile 1984)

	Series A (n=148)				Series B (n=100)			
	No.	Nil	Moderate	Severe	No.	Nil	Moderate	Severe
Incidence	53 (36%)	–	–	–	35	–	–	–
Location								
Posterior	47 (32%)	–	–	–	32	–	–	–
Anterior	6 (4%)				3			
Severity								
Anteroposterior compression	23	14	8	1	6	3	3	
Lateral compression	86	47	35	4	69	53	16	
Unstable (shear)	9	4	2	3	25	9	13	3
Total	118a	65	45	8	100	65	32	3

[a] Thirty cases with major acetabular involvement were not considered in this total.

238 ·

Chapter 12   **Fractures of the Pelvis**

Table 12.5. Leg length discrepancy (malunion) (from Tile 1984)

Amount (cm)	Series A (%)	Series B (%)
0	64	68
0–1	19.5	19
1–2	11.5	11
>2	5	2

Table 12.6. Results by fracture type (from Tile 1984)

	Series A (*n*=148)					Series B (*n*=100)				
	Total No.	Satisfactory		Unsatisfactory		Total No.	Satisfactory		Unsatisfactory	
		(n)	*(%)*	*(n)*	%		*(n)*	%	*(n)*	%
Anteroposterior compression	23	18	78	5	22	6	3	50	3	50
Lateral compression	114	79	69	35	31	69	53	77	16	23
Unstable (shear)	9	5	56	4	44	25	9	36	16	64

in a significant number of permanent problems resulting in posterior pain.

Therefore, it is obvious that most of our energies should be directed to the management of the unstable vertical shear injury, especially if the sacroiliac joint is dislocated or subluxated, since more stable injuries achieve good to excellent results when managed by simple means, as will be described.

· ·

12.5 Management of the Pelvic Disruption

Management of a pelvic disruption depends on the "personality" of the injury as well as that of the associated injuries (see Fig. 12.1) and may be considered under the following four headings: assessment, resuscitation, provisional stabilization, and definitive stabilization, which, although considered separately, form a continuum of care.

· ·

12.5.1 Assessment

12.5.1.1 General Assessment

It is beyond the scope of this chapter to detail the general assessment of the polytraumatized patient. Suffice it to say that a polytraumatized patient with a pelvic fracture represents a therapeutic challenge to the treating surgeon because the mortality rate remains approxi-

mately 10%. The necessity of a planned treatment protocol for the polytraumatized patient cannot be overemphasized. The patient must have immediate appropriate treatment from the time of injury until stabilization in an appropriate intensive care unit. The central theme of system management during resuscitation is *simultaneous* rather than *sequential* care. We recommend the treatment protocol of the American College of Surgeons in the Advanced Trauma Life Support (ATLS) Program (Aprahamian et al. 1981).

In the primary survey, problems involving the airway, bleeding (shock), and the central nervous system have the highest priority. Immediate life-saving resuscitation, therefore, must be directed to both the airway and the presence of shock. In pelvic trauma, shock may be profound due to retroperitoneal arterial or venous hemorrhage.

The secondary survey following the primary resuscitation includes further examination of the airway, bleeding, the central nervous system, the digestive system, the excretory system, and, finally, the fracture. For further study in the management of polytrauma patients, we refer the reader to the excellent monograph on this subject by the American College of Surgeons mentioned above.

12.5.1.2 Specific Musculoskeletal Assessment

For the management of the musculoskeletal injury, assessment is directed to the determination of the stability of the pelvic ring.

a) Clinical Assessment

As in all areas of clinical medicine, an accurate history is essential; patients who have sustained a high-energy injury from motor vehicle trauma or falls from a height are much more likely to have an unstable pelvic injury than those who have sustained low-energy trauma.

The physical examination is at least as important as the radiographs in determining pelvic stability. The

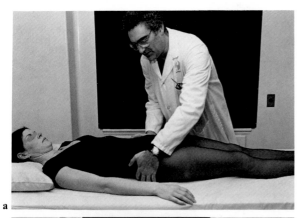

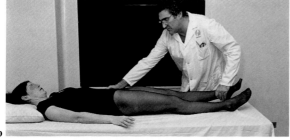

Fig. 12.24. a Direct palpation of the iliac crest will reveal crepitus or abnormal motion, which, if present, is the best indicator of instability of the pelvis. **b** With one arm controlling the injured hemipelvis and the second arm applying traction, the amount of instability present can be determined. (From Tile1984)

essence of the physical examination is to inspect the patient for major bruising or bleeding from the urethral meatus, vagina, or rectum. If these latter two areas are not carefully inspected, occult lacerations may be overlooked, with dire consequences, since these lacerations always mean an *open* fracture of the pelvis.

The pelvic area and the lower extremities should be examined with the patient undressed, so that displacement and limb shortening can be detected. In the absence of a lower extremity fracture, rotatory deformity or limb shortening usually implies an unstable pelvic injury.

Determination of pelvic stability can simply be done by the physician applying his or her hands to the anterior superior spine and moving the affected hemipelvis (Fig. 12.24 a). Open book injuries are maximally externally rotated and can be closed by compression of both anterior iliac spines. Lateral compression injuries are usually in an anatomical recoiled position unless they have been impacted. Further internal rotation by compression of the iliac crests will displace the fracture. Finally, by applying one hand to the pelvic iliac crest and using the other to apply traction to the leg, displacement in the vertical plane can usually easily be diagnosed

(Fig. 12.24 b). This maneuver may require two examiners, one to apply traction and the other to palpate the iliac crests. If possible, these manipulations should be done under image intensification to verify the type of displacement and whether displacement in the vertical plane is present.

b) Radiographic Assessment

Plain Radiographs. As a routine in the acute situation, a single anteroposterior radiograph as commonly used in most trauma centers is usually sufficient to determine the presence or absence of pelvic ring instability. Although this radiograph will suffice in the acute injury during the resuscitative phase, a single anteroposterior radiograph may be misleading. Therefore, for accurate assessment of pelvic ring displacement, an inlet and an outlet view should be added (Fig. 12.25). The inlet view, taken by directing the X-ray beam 60 ° from the head to the midpelvis, is the best radiographic view to demonstrate posterior displacement. The outlet view, taken by directing the X-ray beam from the foot of the patient to the symphysis at an angle of 45 °, demonstrates superior or inferior migration of the hemipelvis.

These views are now also used for radiographic control of iliosacral screw placement; therefore, a knowledge of the skeletal landmarks is important.

CT Scan. The CT scan is the best single investigative tool for determining pelvic instability, since the sacroiliac area is best visualized by this technique. Stable impacted fractures of the sacrum can be clearly differentiated from grossly unstable ones by this method (Figs. 12.3, 12.5). In pelvic ring trauma, three-dimensional CT is helpful in assessing the overall injury pattern, but not nearly as much as in acetabular trauma.

12.5.1.3 Diagnosis of Pelvic Instability

Careful clinical and radiographic assessment will allow the surgeon to determine the personality of the pelvic injury, i.e., whether the musculoskeletal injury is more to the stable or to the unstable end of the stability scale. The completely unstable (type C) can usually be diagnosed clinically by the lack of a firm endpoint in rotation or traction. Radiographically, a displacement or gap on plain X-ray or CT equivalent to 1 cm and the presence of avulsion fractures of the ischial spine or sacrum all suggest instability.

Patients with partially stable (type B) have a firm endpoint on palpation, be it external rotation (B1) or internal rotation (B2). In the latter, the pelvis may be impacted in the internally rotated position (see Fig. 12.19).

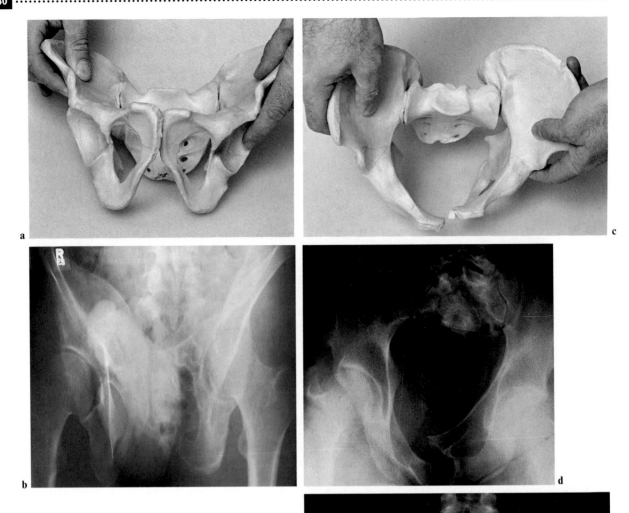

Fig. 12.25 a–e. With the standard anteroposterior radiograph, inlet and outlet views may be very helpful. The outlet view as shown on the skeleton (**a**) and the radiograph (**b**) is the best view for visualizing the sacrum, the sacroiliac joints, and the sacral foramina, caudad and cephalad displacement is seen as well. The inlet view, as noted in the skeleton (**c**) and radiograph (**d**) best delineates posterior displacement of the hemipelvis. **e** Note the different information obtained from the above views compared to the anteroposterior view. (From Tile 1984)

12.5.2 Resuscitation

Hemorrhage in pelvic trauma may be life-threatening. The site of bleeding is determined by peritoneal lavage, portable ultrasound, or CT. In the resuscitative phase, control of hermorrhage must be rapid and may be life-saving.

Patients with an unstable pelvic disruption are at much greater general risk than those with a stable pelvis. In our first prospective study of 100 patients, 12 of the 15 mortalities were in this unstable group (McMurtry et al. 1980). Their blood transfusion requirements were three times greater (15.5 units versus 5.5 units), their injury severity score was 37 (as against 29 in those with a stable

Table 12.7. Pneumatic antishock garment (PSAG; from Tile 1984)

Advantages
Simple
Rapid
Reversible
Splint fractures
Accessible and available
Safe

Disadvantages
Decreased visibility of abdomen and lower extremities
Decreased access to abdomen and lower extremities
Complication of abuse
Exacerbation of congestive heart failure (congestive cardiac failure is an absolute contraindication to the use of PSAG)
Decreased vital capacity
Compartment syndrome

pelvis), and their overall complication rate was three times higher.

Patients suffering this complication require *massive fluid replacement*, as outlined by the American College of Surgeons' ATLS protocol. Early management of shock should include the pneumatic antishock garment (PASG). The advantages and disadvantages of the PASG are listed in Table 12.7. In our opinion, the advantages outweigh the disadvantages, the only notable disadvantage being restriction of access to the abdomen. The garment must not be precipitously released. During gradual release of the garment, the blood pressure must be carefully monitored. Any drop greater than 10 mmHg in the systolic blood pressure is a contraindication to further deflation. Other guidelines of importance include inflation of the legs prior to the abdominal portion and reversing that order during deflation. In transfer situations, great care must be taken to prevent lengthy inflation periods, which may cause compartment syndromes in the lower extremity.

Fracture stabilization belongs in the resuscitative phase of management. There is a growing body of evidence to suggest that the application of a simple anterior external frame will reduce retropelvic venous and bony bleeding to the extent that other intervention is rarely required. Therefore, pelvic stabilization should be performed early. Pelvic clamps which can be applied in the emergency room with direct skeletal fixation are now available and are being assessed (Ganz et al. 1991). It is hoped that this will reduce mortality by allowing the volume of the pelvis to decrease to its normal size, thereby restoring the tamponade effect of the bony pelvis and helping to stop the venous bleeding. The precise method for early fracture stabilization will be discussed in the next section.

We have found *embolization* of the pelvic vessels to be of little overall value in the management of these patients. In our trauma unit, we have narrowed its use to those patients who are bleeding mainly from a small-bore artery such as the obturator or the superior gluteal arteries. It is of little value in hemodynamically unstable patients in extremis with massive bleeding from the major vessels of the internal iliac system, because the emboli cannot control this type of hemorrhage, and the patient may die during the attempt. It is also, of course, of no value in venous or bony bleeding.

Small-bore artery bleeding may be assumed if, although the patient can be well controlled using the above methods of fluid replacement, PASG, and fracture stabilization, he or she goes back into a shocked state each time the fluid is slowed down. In those circumstances, after hemodynamic stability has been achieved, the patient is moved to the vascular suite, an arteriogram performed, and if a smallbore artery is lacerated it is embolized with Gelfoam (Upjohn Pharmaceutic Co.) or other embolic material.

Direct surgical control is rarely indicated and is usually unsuccessful. However, currently, urgent laparotomy and packing the pelvis in patients in extremis is becoming widely used, especially in Europe, and will be evaluated (Pohlemann et al. 1993). Open surgery is also indicated for open fractures.

Very high mortality rates have been reported with open pelvic fractures (Richardson et al. 1982). However, the type of open pelvic injury, be it posterior or peroneal, is of great prognostic significance, and all open pelvic fractures cannot therefore be lumped together. It must be recognized that some pelvic fractures are really traumatic hemipelvectomies, and, rarely, completing the hemipelvectomy may be lifesaving (Lipkowitz et al. 1982).

12.5.3 Provisional Stabilization

Provisional stabilization is required only for those fractures that potentially increase the volume of the pelvis, i.e., the wide open book injury (B1, B3.1) or the unstable pelvic fracture (C). It is rarely required for lateral compression injuries (B2), which make up a large percentage of the total number of pelvic disruptions.

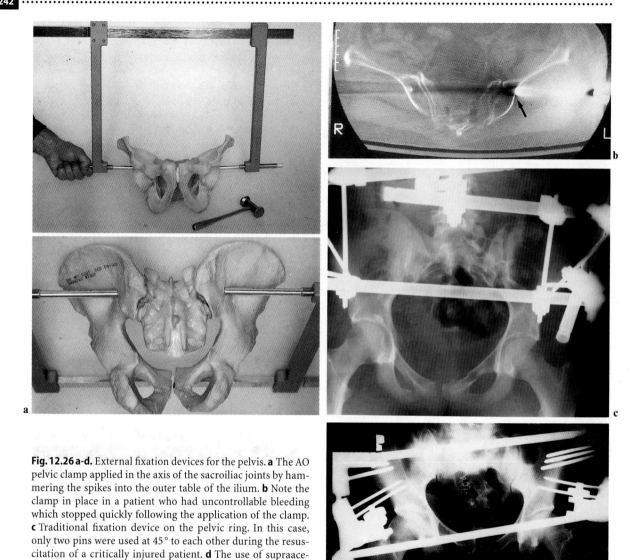

Fig. 12.26 a-d. External fixation devices for the pelvis. **a** The AO pelvic clamp applied in the axis of the sacroiliac joints by hammering the spikes into the outer table of the ilium. **b** Note the clamp in place in a patient who had uncontrollable bleeding which stopped quickly following the application of the clamp. **c** Traditional fixation device on the pelvic ring. In this case, only two pins were used at 45° to each other during the resuscitation of a critically injured patient. **d** The use of supraacetabular pins which must be inserted with image intensification to avoid intering the hip joint

12.5.3.1 External Fixation or Pelvic Clamp

Provisional fixation can be obtained by a pelvic clamp or by an anterior external skeletal fixator. Whichever is used, it should be applied quickly.

The presently available pelvic clamps (Fig. 12.26 a,b; Ganz et al. 1991; B. Browner, personal communication) were designed to be used in the resuscitation room, to be applied quickly, to reduce the pelvic volume, and to impart some stability to the pelvis, thereby reducing bleeding. At the moment, they are being evaluated biomechanically and clinically. Although the concept is good, the results to date are confusing and show no major advantage over more traditional frames.

The anterior frame will reduce the volume of the pelvis, thereby reducing venous and bony bleeding. An added beneficial effect is a major reduction in pain and the ability to induce the upright position in order to better ventilate the patient in the intensive care unit. Since such patients are usually extremely ill, we believe that a simple configuration will suffice – two pins percutaneously place in each ilium at approximately 45° to each other, one in the anterior superior spine and one in the iliac tubercle, joined by an anterior rectangular configuraton (Fig. 12.26).

Recently, especially in older patients, there has been a trend towards the use of one pin in the supra-acetabular area (Fig. 12.26 b). There is good bone in this area, but

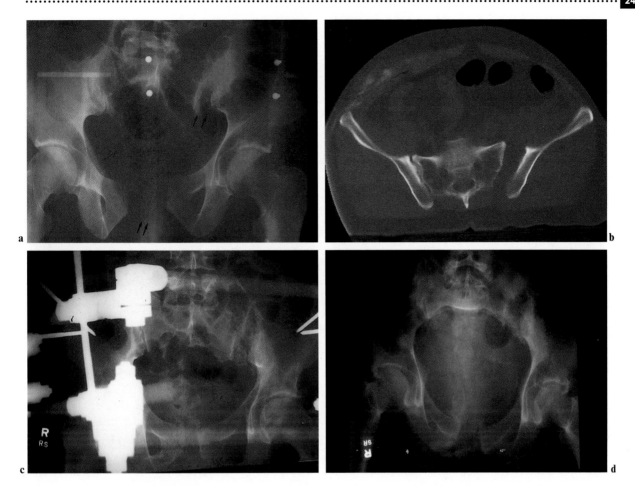

Fig. 12.27 a–d. This 39-year-old patient sustained an unstable pelvic disruption with abdominal and head injuries. An external fixator was applied as a life-saving measure, as was a skeletal traction pin in the left femur. Note the wide posterior gap at the sacroiliac joint in spite of the external fixator and the traction. Attempts were made on three separate occasions to take this patient back for internal fixation of the posterior sacroiliac complex but he was so medically unstable that on two occasions he had cardiac arrests in the intensive care unit prior to surgical intervention. Because of that it was decided to continue his pelvic treatment. At 6 weeks there was massive callus in the left sacroiliac joint. Traction was continued for 8 weeks. The left sacroiliac joint healed with no shortening and a good outcome. **b** Computed tomography showing a wide opening of the sacroiliac joint

care must be taken to avoid penetration of the hip joint. The pin must be confirmed to be extra-articular on image intensification.

Biomechanical studies performed in our laboratory and elsewhere have shown that simple frames can give good stability in the open book fracture (Fig. 12.27). However, in the unstable pelvic disruption, even the most elaborate frames cannot fully stabilize the pelvic ring if the patient is to be ambulated (Fig. 12.28). In our opinion, sophisticated frames requiring dissection to the anterior inferior spine are contraindicated in the acute resuscitation period. They have some biomechanical advantage, but this advantage is so slight that the added risk of the operative procedure is not worth taking. At present, as mentioned, the supra-acetabular pin is usually inserted by closed percutaneous techniques.

12.5.3.2 Skeletal Traction

Since the frames or clamps cannot restore stability to unstable type C fractures, a temporary traction pin in the distal femur may be very helpful until definitive treatment is initiated. With the frame or clamp in place, 15–20 kg of traction will prevent the hemipelvis from shortening. In the event that the patient is extremely ill and internal fixation is undesirable or unsafe, this may become definitive and lead to a good outcome (Fig. 12.27). The question of timing of external frames is an open question at this time. However, in most cases of unstable pelvic fractures, the frames or clamps should be

244 ·

Chapter 12   **Fractures of the Pelvis**

Fig. 12.28 a–c. Stable lateral compression injury (type B2.2). **a** Anteroposterior X-ray of a 16-year-old girl with a stable lateral compression injury. Note the fracture in the left ilium *(arrow)* and all four pubic rami. **b** Cystogram of the same patient showing a ruptured bladder. **c** Final result at 1 year was excellent. Treatment consisted of 8 weeks of complete bed rest followed by ambulation with partial weight bearing for a further 4 weeks. Note that all fractures are healed and the position is good

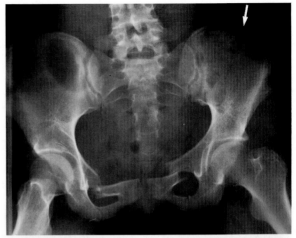

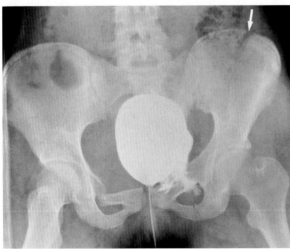

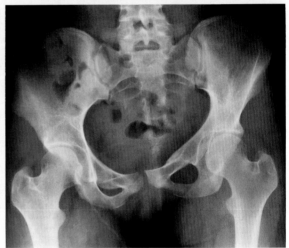

applied rapidly and in such a way that they do not interfere with laparotomy. This is desirable in almost all instances, unless it is certain that the life-threatening hemorrhage is intraperitoneal.

12.5.3.3 Early Internal Fixation

What is the role of internal fixation in the early resuscitative phase of treatment? Present literature reports show increased complications (McGowan et al. 1987; Schied et al. 1991). However, early internal fixation may be indicated as follows:

a) *Anterior stabilization of the symphysis and medial rami.* If the patient is undergoing laparotomy and a symphysis disruption is present, plating will greatly simplify the further treatment. This is also true for medial rami fractures. Lateral rami fractures at this time are better treated by an external frame. If a urologic procedure has been performed, the urologist should use a suction drain

and catheter, not a suprapubic tube, which is a risk factor for sepsis. Two plates at 90° to each other will give excellent stability to the unstable pelvis when combined with an external frame and may be definitive care in some very sick patients.

b) *Posterior stabilization.* At this time, early posterior fixation is risky and should only be done in pelvic centers. However, with future improvement in guidance systems (CT, wands), the technique may become safer.

12.5.4 Definitive Stabilization

Definitive stabilization of the musculoskeletal injury depends upon a precise diagnosis of the fracture configuration. No matter what the configuration, if the pelvic ring is stable and undisplaced or minimally displaced, symptomatic treatment only is necessary. Patients with this injury may be mobilized quickly and the pelvic fracture, i.e., the musculoskeletal injury, largely ignored.

12.5.4.1 Stable Fractures (Type A)

Therefore, virtually all type A fracture can be managed symptomatically with the following exceptions. Avulsion fractures (A1) of the iliac crest, especially in young athletes, can be simply fixed with lag screws if widely displaced. Fractures of the iliac wing with wide displacement (A2) may, with full informed consent, be fixed with standard techniques, especially in young women, as this injury can leave a malalignment of the iliac crest. Transverse sacral fractures (A3) should be considered as spinal injuries; therefore, with wide displacement and a sacral plexus neurological deficit, reduction of the fracture with or without decompression is usually required.

a) Open Book (Anteroposterior Compression) Fractures (Type B1, B3.1)

This lesion may be unilateral or bilateral, but the treatment is more dependent on the extent of the injury overall. The anterior disruption is indicated in the classification by a modifier: $\alpha4$ indicates a symphysis disruption of less than 2.5 cm, and $\alpha5$ of more than 2.5 cm.

In the open book fracture, with the symphysis pubis open less than 2.5 cm ($\alpha4$), no specific treatment is indicated. Patients with this injury usually have no posterior disruption and have intact sacrospinous ligaments (Fig. 12.13). Therefore, the situation is somewhat akin to the stretching of the symphysis pubis that takes place during pregnancy. With simple symptomatic treatment, i.e., bed rest until comfortable, healing is usually adequate and few patients complain of any symptoms.

If the symphysis pubis is open more than 2.5 cm (Fig. 12.14), several options are available to the surgeon.

External Fixation. We prefer stabilization of the pelvis with a simple anterior external frame, as described above (Fig. 12.26). The pins should remain in place for approximately 6–8 weeks; the frame should then be loosened and radiographs taken under stress to see whether healing has occurred and whether there is stability across the symphysis. If healing is adequate, the pins are removed at this stage. If not, the anterior frame is reattached for a further 4-week period. With no vertical displacement possible, the patients may be quickly ambulated. Reduction is best obtained in the lateral position or in the supine position with both legs fully internally rotated.

Internal Fixation. If the patient has a visceral injury necessitating a paramedian midline or Pfannenstiel incision, internal fixation using a 4.5-mm plate will restore stability. In this particular injury with partial stability, a single four-hole plate placed across the superior surface of the symphysis pubis will restore stability. The type of plate will vary with the specific injury: 3.5-mm low-contact dynamic compression (LCDC) plate or curved reconstruction, occasionally 4.5 mm. This should be done immediately after the abdominal procedure prior to closure of the skin. In this instance a double plate, recommended for symphysis fixation of unstable fractures, is unnecessary, since the open book fracture is inherently stable.

Spica or Sling. The patient with an open book fracture may also be treated with either a hip spica with both legs internally rotated or in a pelvic sling. These two methods are better suited to children and adolescents than to adults, and we much prefer external fixation as definitive treatment for this fracture configuration. Nursing care with these options is difficult, and long periods of bed rest are required, with the ensuing complications.

b) Lateral Compression Fractures (Type B2)

Lateral compression fractures are usually partially stable, and therefore surgical stabilization is rarely required; it is called for only if reduction is necessary to correct malalignment or leg length discrepancy. Since these injuries often result in an impacted posterior complex, an intact pelvic floor, and hence a relatively stable pelvis, disimpaction and reduction should only be done if the clinical state of the patient warrants it. This will vary with the age of the patient, the general medical state, the degree of rotation of the hemipelvis, and the amount of leg length discrepancy. In a young individual, a leg length discrepancy of more than 2.5 cm or marked internal rotation which cannot be compensated by external rotation of the hip are indications to reduce the lateral compression injury. This is especially true in bucket-handle injuries. However, we must stress again that the vast majority of lateral compression injuries may be treated with bed rest alone and do not require any external or internal fixation (Fig. 12.28).

If reduction is desirable for the above reasons, it may be effected manually with external rotation (Fig. 12.29 a) or with the aid of external skeletal pins placed in the hemipelvis (Fig. 12.29 b, c). By placing a handle on the cross-rod and applying an external rotation force, the bucket-handle fracture may be reduced by derotation externally and posteriorly, allowing disimpaction of the posterior complex. In some instances, reduction is impossible and the surgeon must decide whether open reduction, the only remaining option, is necessary. Undue force applied to the pins may dislodge them from the bone; therefore, the major reduction force must be on the bone itself, not the pins.

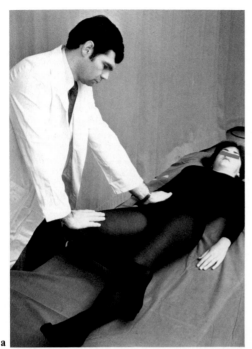

a

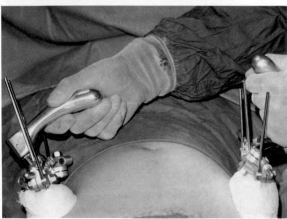

b

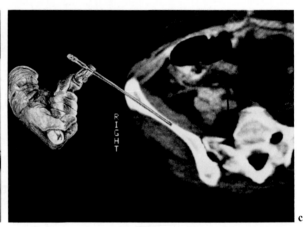

c

Fig. 12.29. a Closed reduction of a lateral compression-type injury is performed by external rotation of the hip with the knee flexed and direct pressure on the hemipelvis, as shown. **b** The type of leverage that can be obtained by placing handles on the crossbars of the external fixation device to allow for both internal and external rotation of the unstable hemipelvis. **c** Diagrammatic representation on a CT scan indicating the type of direct leverage that can be obtained on the affected hemipelvis. (From Tile 1984)

If *external skeletal pins* have been used to help with reduction, a simple rectangular anterior frame should be applied at the end of the maneuver to hold the hemipelvis in the external rotated position.

In polytrauma patients, a simple external skeletal frame is indicated to relieve pain, to allow some movement in bed, and even the upright position, which in turn allows for easier nursing care. In this pattern, good stability is obtained with the anterior frame.

Internal fixation of a lateral compression injury is rarely indicated except in the atypical type with bony protrusion into the perineum, especially in women. In that particular case, a short Pfannenstiel incision will allow derotation of the superior ramus, and fixation with a threaded pin is ample (Fig. 12.30). The pin may be removed at 6 weeks in the stable configuration. Rarely, if

deformity is great and cannot be reduced closed, open reduction and internal fixation is indicated.

Warning: Pelvic slings are contraindicated in lateral compression and unstable vertical shear injuries since they will cause further major displacement (Fig. 12.31).

12.5.4.3 Unstable Fractures (Type C)

In unstable shear fractures, simple anterior frames will not be adequate for definitive management, as an attempt to ambulate the patient will often result in redisplacement (Fig. 12.32). Therefore, the two options open to the surgeon are either the addition of femoral supracondylar skeletal traction or internal fixation.

Fig. 12.30. a The original radiograph demonstrates the rotated superior ramus of the left pubis through a disrupted symphysis pubis. **b** Since the posterior complex is stable, open reduction and internal fixation with a threaded Steinman pin restored stability. **c** Union occurred quickly, and the pin was removed at 6 weeks. (From Tile 1984)

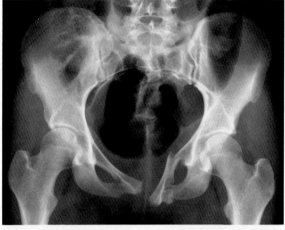

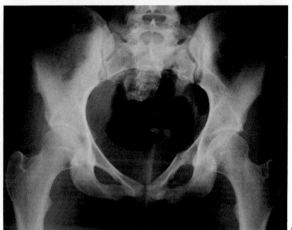

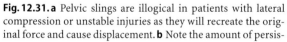

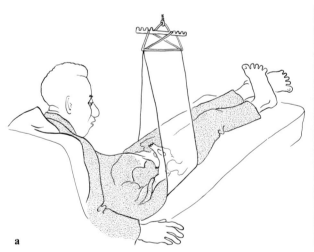

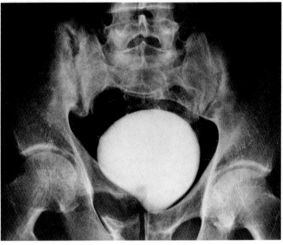

Fig. 12.31. a Pelvic slings are illogical in patients with lateral compression or unstable injuries as they will recreate the original force and cause displacement. **b** Note the amount of persis- tent displacement and impingement on the bladder. Note also that neither the superior ramus nor the fracture through the sacrum is united. (From Tile 1984)

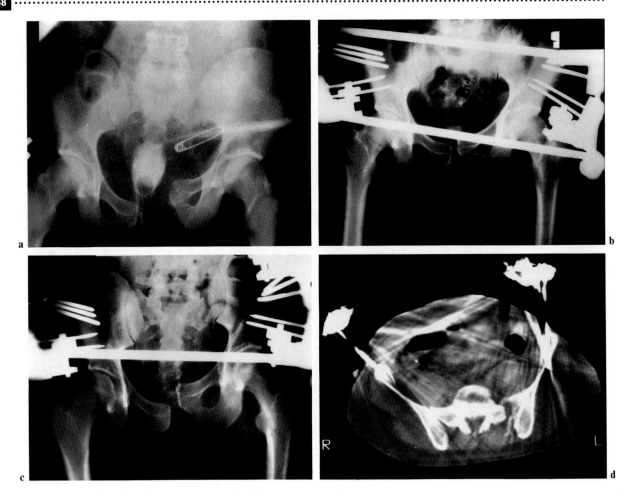

Fig. 12.32. a Anteroposterior cystogram showing an unstable fracture of the pelvic ring including a symphysis disruption and fracture through the left sacrum. Treatment consisted of a double-cluster frame. **b** The postreduction radiograph shows adequate position. **c,d** After ambulation, however, redisplacement occurred, as shown on the radiograph (**c**) and computed tomography (CT) scan (**d**). Anterior frames do not afford sufficient stability to allow early ambulation in unstable pelvic ring disruptions. (Case courtesy of Ronald E. Rosenthal, M.D., Long Island, New York)

a) Skeletal Traction with External Fixation

Isolated, unstable shear injuries may be safely and adequately managed by the addition of a supracondylar femoral traction pin to a pelvis stabilized with an anterior external frame (Fig. 12.33). In our clinical review, patients managed in this fashion, especially those with fractures of the sacrum, fracture-dislocations of the sacroiliac joint, or fractures of the ilium had satisfactory long-term results. Redisplacement, if it occurred, was minimal and rarely clinically significant. Internal fixa-

tion may be a preferred option, but in many instances this may be undesirable because of the poor accessibility to a surgeon or center with expertise in pelvic surgery. In those circumstances, since internal fixation of the posterior pelvic complex is fraught with many complications, it is far safer for the general orthopedist to manage pelvic trauma, especially isolated pelvic trauma, in this manner, than attempt ill-advised open reductions (Fig. 12.34).

The traction must be maintained for 8–12 weeks and the patient monitored with anteroposterior and inlet radiographs as well as CT scans, where indicated. A major problem in the past has been too early ambulation of these patients, who require a longer period of recumbency to allow for sound bony union.

b) Open Reduction and Internal Fixation

Internal fixation of the pelvis, especially the posterior sacroiliac complex, was virtually unreported prior up to 1980, with almost no literature on this subject except for

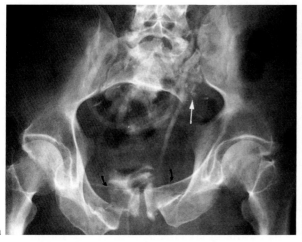

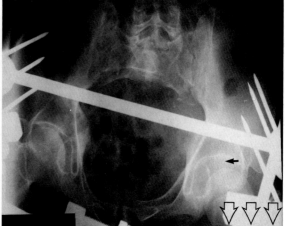

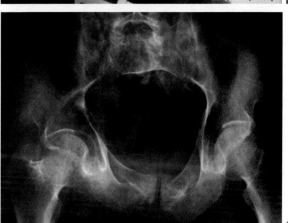

Fig. 12.33 a–c. Unstable pelvic disruption treatment with external frame and traction. **a** Anteroposterior intravenous pyelogram of a 59-year-old man who sustained a grossly unstable pelvic ring disruption in a motor vehicle accident. The *white arrow* indicates the marked disruption of the left sacrum with posterior displacement of 2.5 cm, causing an injury to the lumbosacral nerve plexus. The two *black arrows* show the avulsion of the rectus abdominus muscle anteriorly through the symphysis. **b** Restoration of alignment was possible with an anterior frame and 30 lb (about 13.5 kg) of supracondylar traction on the left leg *(broad arrows)*. Note the distraction of the left hip joint *(black arrow)*. **c** Final result showing healing of all fractures and adequate restoration of the pelvic ring. The clinical result was good except for a permanent nerve damage in the left leg. (From Tile 1984)

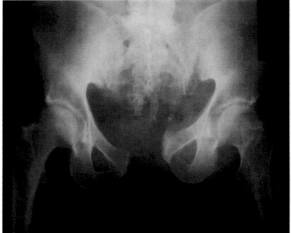

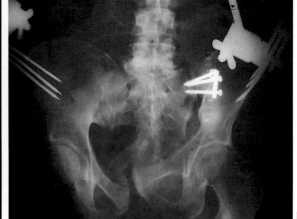

Fig. 12.34. Anterior posterior radiograph indicating an unstable left hemipelvis through a symphysis disruption and left sacroiliac disruption. Initial treatment with an external fixator and traction showed an acceptable reduction. An attempt made at open reduction and internal fixation using screw fixation redisplaced the fracture with the resulting significant rotational malunion and leg length discrepancy

Table 12.8. Indications for open reduction and internal fixation of the pelvis

A. Anterior internal fixation
  Disrupted symphysis pubis
    In unstable (type C) pelvic disruption
    Symphysis open greater than 2.5 cm
    Locked symphysis
  Rami fractures
    Associated with femoral artery or nerve injury
    Tilt fracture with ramus protruding into vagina
    Marked displacement (unstable type C disruption)

B. Posterior internal fixation
Unreduced posterior complex with >1 cm of displacement, especially if through the sacroiliac joint
Open fractures with posterior (not perineal) wound
Unstable posterior complex associated with acetabular fractures

sporadic case reports. There are reports of plating and wiring of the anterior symphysis complex but few of the posterior complex. The past 5 years have brought a marked increase of internal fixation of the pelvis, and we must examine whether this is justified or not. We have seen from our study of the natural history of pelvic fractures that the stable injuries, which comprise approximately 70% of the total number of cases, have few indications for internal fixation. For unstable disruptions, many patients can be safely and adequately managed by external fixation and skeletal traction. Therefore, posterior internal fixation of the pelvis should be done infrequently and only in cases showing significant indications (Table 12.8).

Advantages. The advantages of pelvic internal fixation are as follows:

1. Anatomical reduction and stable fixation would allow easier pain-free nursing of the polytraumatized patient, since excellent stability may be restored to the pelvic ring, as shown in Fig. 12.35 a.
2. Modern techniques of internal fixation (especially compression) would be useful on the large cancellous surfaces of the pelvis to avoid malunion and nonunion.

Disadvantages. The disadvantages include the following:

1. *Loss of tamponade and the possibility of massive hemorrhage.* The superior gluteal artery is commonly injured during pelvic trauma, but the injury may be unrecognized because the artery may clot. With the massive blood transfusions required in these patients, the clotting mechanism may be defective on the fifth–tenth postoperative day when surgical

exploration is performed. Reinjury to the artery during exposure of the fracture may result in massive hemorrhage.
2. *Sepsis.* Posterior incisions in the acute trauma situation have resulted in an unacceptably high rate of skin necrosis (Fig. 12.36). Even without posterior incisions, we have seen skin breakdown in many of our patients with severe unstable vertical shear injuries (Fig. 12.37). At surgery, the gluteus maximus muscle is often torn from its insertion, leaving no underlying fascia to nourish the skin. Skin breakdown has been frequent in spite of meticulous technique, adequate nutrition, and preoperative antibiotics (Fig. 12.37).
3. *Neurological damage.* We have now seen seven cases of neurological damage caused by screws entering the first sacral foramen or the spinal canal. These injuries have occurred in patients previously neurologically normal (Fig. 12.38). The insertion of screws posteriorly across the sacroiliac joint must be precise in order to avoid that complication.

Indications. The indications for open reduction and internal fixation of the pelvis are listed in Table 12.8.

Fig. 12.35. a Results of the biomechanical testing show the superior stability afforded the pelvis by posterior fixation in the unstable vertical shear injury. (Adapted from Tile 1984). **b** *Graph* indicates the main stiffness of the pelvis (in newton meters) achieved with various forms of anterior fixation, noted by the *bars*; namely, one inferior plate on the symphysis pubis, one superior plate on the symphysis pubis, two plates, and external fixation. In each case, the anterior fixation was associated with anterior sacroiliac plates, lag screws, and transiliac (sacral bars). Note that no matter what form of posterior fixation was used, two plates across the symphysis *(dark bars)* yielded the highest values of overall ring stiffness, stressing the importance of stable anterior fixation in this model. (From Hearn et al. 1991). **c** Schematic representation of displacement transducers and target, aligned with three orthogonal sacroiliac axes. **d** Mean displacement, in micrometers per newton applied axial load (±SD), in the medial–lateral axis, corresponding to sacroiliac joint separation. Values are grouped by posterior fixation, showing anterior fixation within each group (*n*=8). **e** Mean anteroposterior displacement (±SD), in micrometers per unit of applied load, corresponding to interfragmentary shear in the direction of an axis aligned normal to the posterior sacral surface. Values are grouped by posterior fixation, showing anterior fixation within each group (*n*=8). **f** Mean vertical displacement (±SD), in micrometers per newton applied axial load, corresponding to shear displacements of the sacroiliac joint in the direction of the longitudinal axis of the sacrum. Values are grouped by posterior fixation, showing anterior fixation within each group (*n*=8). (From Hearn et al. 1991)

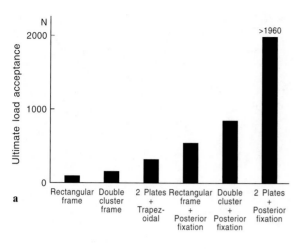

a

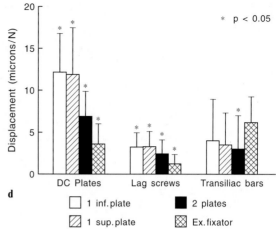

d

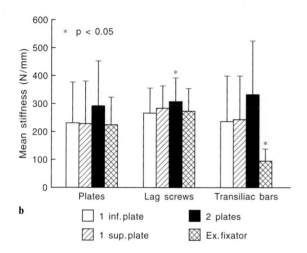

b

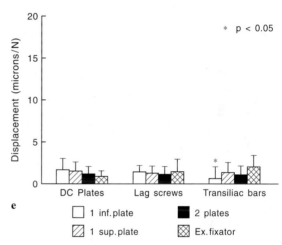

e

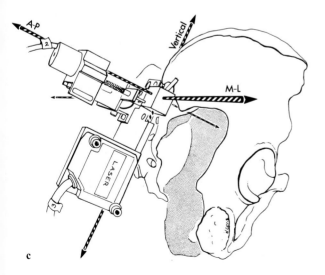

c

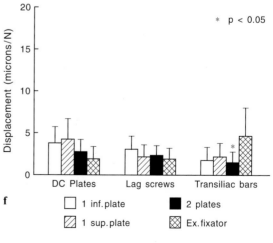

f

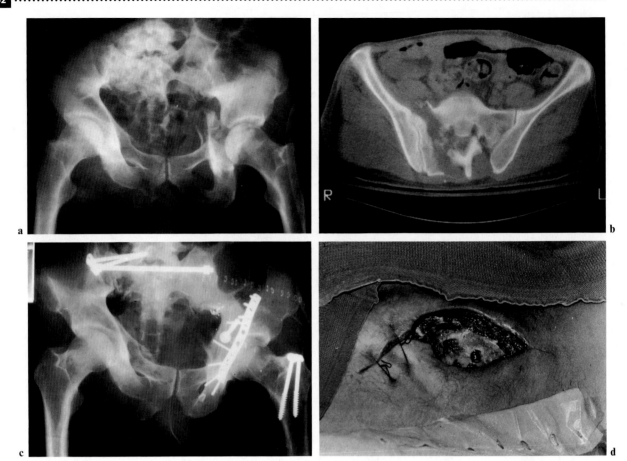

Fig. 12.36. a Anteroposterior radiograph showing a fractured left acetabulum and right sacrum taken 5 weeks following injury. The disruption of the right sacrum is better seen on computed tomography (**b**). **c** The left acetabular fracture was openly reduced and internally fixed, as was the right sacroiliac joint, with two screws and a sacral bar. At the time of surgery, the gluteus maximus muscle was completely avulsed from its insertion on the ilium. The skin was avascular, and the underlying muscle fibrous and atrophied. The wound edges necrosed, but the patient refused further surgery and eventually the entire wound was covered with granulation tissue (**d**)

1. Anterior internal fixation

a) *Symphysis disruption.* If the patient has a disrupted symphysis pubis and the general surgeons, urologists, or trauma surgeons are proceeding with a laparotomy or exploration of the bladder, then plating the symphysis pubis in a reduced position will greatly simplify the management of the case. If the fracture pattern is a stable open book variety, a short two- or four-hole plate can be placed on the superior surface of the symphysis pubis to restore stability. If the symphysis pubis disruption is part of an unstable pelvic ring pattern, then double plating to prevent displacement in the vertical and anteroposterior

planes is preferable (Fig. 12.37). When combined with an external frame, stability will be restored, as shown in Fig. 12.35; therefore, it may be used as definitive treatment in some cases. This is especially true with dual plating, which is biomechanically superior to a single plate (Fig. 12.35). However, plates should not be used in the presence of fecal contamination or the proposed use of a suprapubic tube; in that situation, external fixation is usually the safer and preferred option.

b) *Displaced fracture in the perineum* (see Fig. 12.18). In the atypical type of lateral compression injury, with rotation of the superior pubic ramus through the symphysis into the perineum, i.e., the tilt fracture, a limited Pfannenstiel approach, derotation of the fragment, and fixation with a threaded pin will maintain the fracture until healing has been completed, usually a period of 6 weeks for this stable fracture.

c) *Associated anterior acetabular fracture.* If a fracture of the anterior column of the acetabulum or a transverse fracture is associated with a symphysis disruption, a displaced sacroiliac joint, or a fracture in the ilium, an ilioinguinal approach can be used to fix both components of the fracture, as shown in Fig. 12.39. This case represents an unusual configuration of an open book

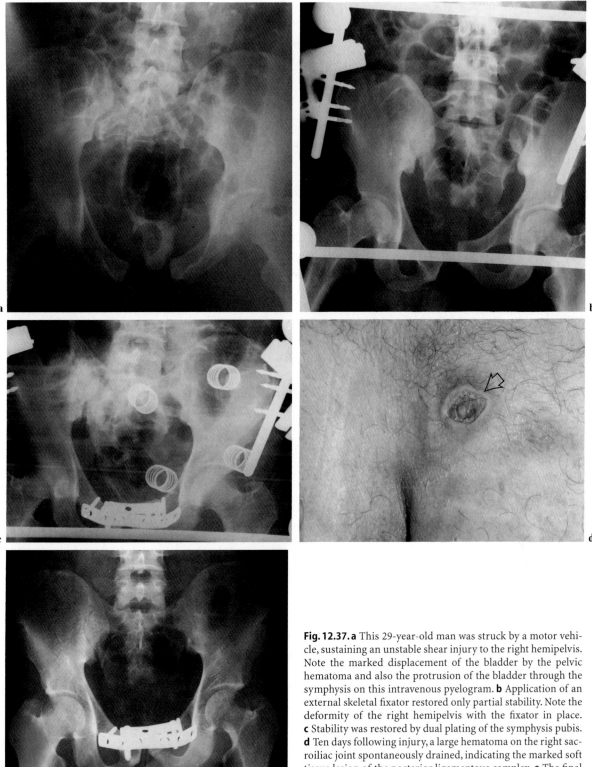

Fig. 12.37. a This 29-year-old man was struck by a motor vehicle, sustaining an unstable shear injury to the right hemipelvis. Note the marked displacement of the bladder by the pelvic hematoma and also the protrusion of the bladder through the symphysis on this intravenous pyelogram. **b** Application of an external skeletal fixator restored only partial stability. Note the deformity of the right hemipelvis with the fixator in place. **c** Stability was restored by dual plating of the symphysis pubis. **d** Ten days following injury, a large hematoma on the right sacroiliac joint spontaneously drained, indicating the marked soft tissue lesion of the posterior ligamentous complex. **e** The final result was good, with sound healing of the right sacroiliac joint and no displacment of the pelvic ring. (From Tile 1984)

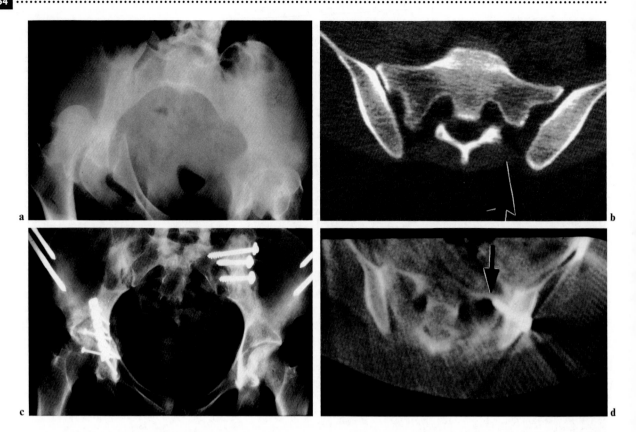

Fig. 12.38. a Anteroposterior radiograph showing a fracture dislocation of the right hip and a dislocation of the left sacroiliac joint. **b** This is better seen on the computed tomography (CT) scan. Treatment consisted of open reduction and internal fixation of the right acetabular fracture, internal fixation of the left sacroiliac joint, and an anterior frame. **c** Note the position of the screws. **d** Postoperative CT showing the tip of the screw in the first sacral foramen *(arrow)*

injury with a massive symphysis disruption, an anterior opening of the right sacroiliac joint, and an external rotation injury to the left ilium extending into the anterior column of the acetabulum with major displacement. This fracture was approached through an ilioinguinal incision and all components fixed as shown.

In acute trauma, an open approach to the laterally placed pubic rami fractures is impractical and usually unnecessary. Recently, percutaneous techniques have been developed to fix these fractures retrograde from the symphysis; however, the technique is still experimental, risks penetration of the hip, and should only be done in expert centers.

2. Posterior internal fixation.

a) *Malreduction of the posterior sacroiliac complex.* This is difficult to define, but greater than 1 cm of dis-

placement of the posterior sacroiliac complex, especially in pure sacroiliac dislocation, may be an indication for posterior internal fixation. If posterior fracture with or without dislocation is noted, some displacement may be acceptable because healing of the fracture may lead to a satisfactory outcome.

However, there may be instances where the fracture itself cannot be reduced, thus requiring open reduction, as shown in Fig. 12.40. In this particular case, the patient was injured in a collision between a motor bike and a motor vehicle. Note the external rotation of the left hemipelvis. This unusual injury caused by an external rotatory force on the left hemipelvis has fractured the ilium and driven the iliac portion of the sacroiliac joint anteriorly until it rested on the front of the sacrum. The lumbosacral plexus was injured but gradually recovered, except for the fifth nerve root, which was permanently damaged. When seen at 6 months following injury, the left hemipelvis was externally rotated 45° and the fracture dislocation was not united. The patient had significant pain on sitting or standing. All four rami were fractured anteriorly, the right ones not being united but the left being united. Utilizing two teams of surgeons with the patient in the right lateral position, the sacroiliac joint was approached from both the inside and the outside of the pelvis. The fracture could not be reduced until

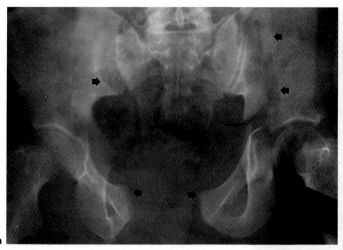
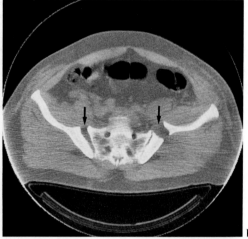

a

b

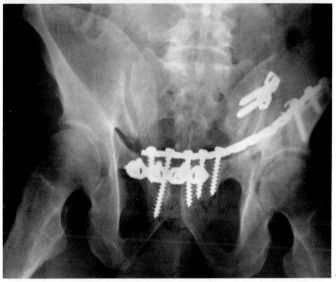

c

Fig. 12.39. a Anteroposterior radiograph demonstrating a left acetabular fracture associated with a pelvic ring disruption. Note the left acetabular fracture *(long arrow)* and the massive symphysis pubis disruption associated with a fracture of the left ilium and an anterior opening of the right sacroiliac joint, a variation of an open book fracture *(short arrows).* **b** The open right sacroiliac joint and left iliac fracture are best seen on the computed tomography (CT) scan. **c** Open reduction and internal fixation were performed through an ilioinguinal approach with fixation as shown. (From Tile 1984)

the left anterior pubic rami fractures, which were healed, were osteotomized. At that point, the left hemipelvis could be reduced and held with three anterior plates placed across the sacroiliac joint. One long anterior plate across the symphysis pubis and the rami fractures fixed the anterior complex.

b) *Polytrauma treatment.* Current surgical wisdom requires polytraumatized patients to be nursed in the upright position to improve chest ventilation. If the pelvic fracture is so unstable that this becomes impossible, then open reduction may aid in the post-trauma care of the patient. Since stabilization with an anterior external frame will usually allow nursing in the upright position for the first few days with or without a traction pin in the femur, when this position is often lifesaving, this indication would be relative rather than absolute.

c) *Open posterior fracture.* In those uncommon instances when the posterior sacroiliac complex is dis-

rupted and the posterior skin has been lacerated from within, the same principles applied to other open fractures can be applied here. With the wound already open, the surgeon should take the opportunity to stabilize the posterior complex in a manner described later in this chapter. In those instances, the wound may be left open and closed secondarily.

However, if the open wound is in the perineum, then all forms of internal fixation are usually contraindicated. Both the rectum and the vagina must be examined carefully for lacerations to rule out occult open fractures of the pelvis. Open fractures into the perineum are dangerous injuries and result in a high mortality rate. Treatment for the open pelvic fracture should include cleansing and careful débridement of the wound followed by open wound care. The fracture should be stabilized in the first instance with an external skeletal frame. Both bowel and bladder diversion with a colostomy and

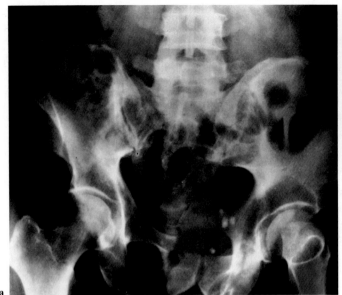

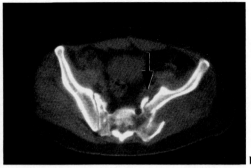

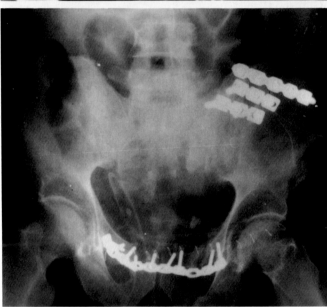

Fig. 12.40. a Anteroposterior radiograph of an unstable pelvic ring disruption. The injury looks relatively innocuous; however, note that the left hemipelvis is externally rotated approximately 45° compared to the right. The left hemiplevis shows an iliac oblique view, the right an anteroposterior view. **b** This is more clearly seen on the computed tomography (CT) scan. Note that the hemipelvis anterior to the iliac fracture has rotated externally and has compressed into the sacrum *(arrow)*. The patient had a lumbosacral nerve plexus injury. **c** The pelvis failed to unite, and 7 months after the original injury, because of severe pain, a combined anterior and posterior approach was employed and resulted in reduction of the pelvis and fixation as shown. Stability was restored and the final result is good

cystostomy are essential. Occasionally, minimal internal fixation, especially across the anterior arch or symphysis, may be very helpful; however, this requires much experience and surgical judgment.

d) *Associated posterior acetabular fractures.* Transverse or posterior fractures of the acetabulum associated with pelvic ring disruption are also an indication in some instances for posterior fixation of the pelvic ring and acetabulum. This requires careful decision making and preoperative planning. The acetabular fracture cannot be reduced anatomically until the pelvic portion is reduced.

12.5.4.4 Surgical Techniques

a) General Aspects

Timing. In general, we prefer to wait with pelvic open reduction until the patient's general state has improved, which is usually between the fifth and the seventh posttrauma day. During this initial period, relative stability is maintained with the external fixator and skeletal traction.

Exceptions to this rule are instances when a laparotomy or bladder exploration has been carried out, so that the symphysis is already exposed; it should then be internally fixed primarily. Secondly, in the rare instance of a vascular injury to the femoral artery necessitating vascular repair, associated with a pelvic factor, the incisions may be carefully planned with the vascular surgeon to allow stabilization of the anterior pubic rami.

As previously mentioned, a posterior open fracture may also be a rare indication for immediate open reduction and internal fixation.

With percutaneous techniques and better guidance systems, earlier surgery may become prevalent in the next decade.

Antibiotics. Prophylactic antibiotics are routinely given for these major operative procedures. A first-generation cephalosporin is given intravenously just prior to surgery and continued for 48 h or longer if necessary.

Antithrombotic Therapy. Recent epidemiological studies (Geerts et al. 1990) have shown that 60 % of patients with pelvic trauma develop deep-vein thrombosis. The specific balance between clots and further pelvic bleeding is delicate; suffice it to say that some form of therapy is indicated when the threat of further hemorrhage is appreciably over.

b) Implants

Plates. Because of the difficulty in contouring the standard plates in the several directions required, we recommend the 3.5-mm and 4.5-mm reconstruction plates for pelvic fixation (see, e.g., Figs. 12.38, 13.41). These plates can be contoured in two planes and are most useful. In general, the 3.5-mm plates are used on most women and smaller men, and the 4.5-mm plates on larger men. Preshaped reconstruction plates are available for the anterior column fractures.

Screws. The 3.5-mm fully threaded cancellous screws and the 6.5-mm fully threaded cancellous screws are essential components of the fixation system, as well as all the standard lag screws in the two sizes (4.0 mm and 6.5 mm). Screws of exceptional length, up to 120 mm, are required in the pelvis.

Instruments. Since reduction of the pelvic fragments is the most difficult part of the operation, special pelvic clamps are essential. These include the pointed fracture reduction clamps and the large pelvic reduction clamps held in place with two screws (see Fig. 13.33). Other specialized pelvic reduction clamps are also available. We also find the flexible drills and taps as well as the universal screwdriver to be essential for pelvic open reduction and internal fixation. This allows the surgeon to work around corners, especially necessary when working on

anterior fixation of the symphysis pubis in obese individuals.

c) Anterior Pelvic Fixation

Symphysis Pubis Fixation

Surgical Approach. If the abdomen is already open through a midline or paramedian incision, then the symphysis can be simply fixed through that approach. If no incision has been made and the symphysis is being approached primarily, the Pfannenstiel incision transversely offers excellent visualization (Fig. 12.41). In the acute case, the rectus abdominis muscle has usually been avulsed and dissection is easy. The surgeon must stay on the skeletal plane to avoid injury to the bladder and urethra.

Reduction. Reduction of the symphysis is usually easy in the acute case. The medial aspect of the obturator foramen should be exposed and the fracture reduction clamp inserted through the foramen (Fig. 12.41 b). Reduction should be anatomical. Care must be taken to avoid catching the bladder or urethra in the symphysis when closing the clamp.

Internal Fixation. In the stable open book configuration, a simple two- or four-hole 3.5-mm or 4.5-mm reconstruction plate applied to the superior surface of the symphysis will afford excellent stability. An external frame is not essential in this particular injury.

In the symphysis disruption associated with an unstable pelvic disruption, we favor a double-plate technique (Fig. 12.41 c). A two-hole plate, usually 4.5 mm, is fixed to the superior surface of the symphysis with two 6.5-mm cancellous screws (Fig. 12.41 d) immediately adjacent to the symphysis pubis. To avoid displacement in the vertical plane, an anterior plate, usually a 3.5-mm reconstruction plate in women or a 4.5-mm one in men, fixed with the appropriate screws and applied anteriorly will often offer increased stability. Restoration of this anterior tension band will allow the previously inserted anterior frame to compress the posterior complex by externally rotating the hemipelvis at the time the clamps are closed. Good stability may be obtained and the patient may assume the upright position. In addition, if later fixation of the posterior injury is attempted, the position of the injury will be relatively reduced.

Pubic Rami Fractures
Although technically possible, we have not favored direct fixation of the pubic rami. If the fractures are laterally placed, the end results of nonoperative care are usually satisfactory; therefore, the indications are limit-

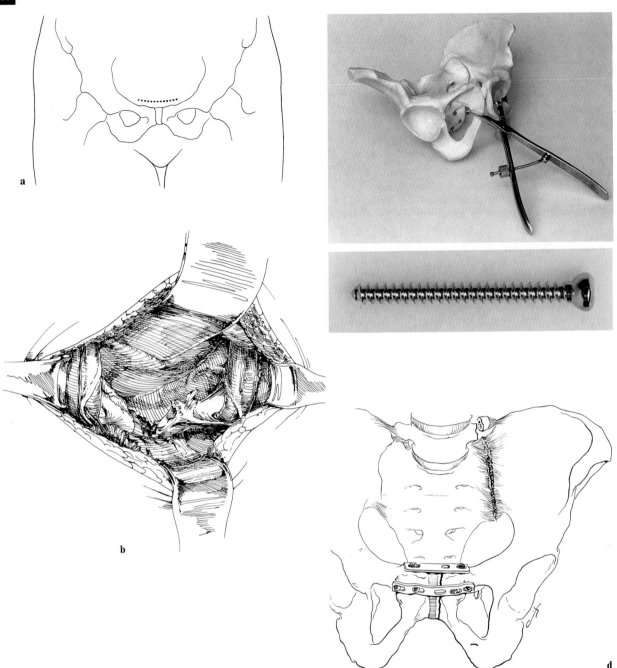

Fig. 12.41. a Open reduction of the symphysis pubis is done through a Pfannenstiel incision. **b** Deep dissection of the symphysis pubis. Usually, in a symphyseal disruption, the dissection is done by the injury; rarely, the rectus needs to be removed from the pubis. The bladder is retracted, as noted, and the inferior epigastric artery and the spermatic cord are protected. **c** A large fracture reduction clamp is inserted around the medial border of both obturator foramina. Closure of the clamp will easily restore the anatomy of the symphysis pubis. **d** Fixation is secured using two 4.5-mm dynamic compression (DC) plates placed at right angles to each other. **e** Fully threaded cancellous screws should be used to anchor the plates to the soft bone of the symphysis. (From Tile 1995)

ed. Open reduction requires major dissection possibly using an ilioinguinal approach. If fractures of the pubic rami are associated with a posterior pelvic disruption, we feel that it would be more prudent to approach the pelvis posteriorly, since restoration of stability in that location is far superior to anterior fixation. Therefore, we see very few indications for fixation of the pubic rami, which can be controlled with an external frame, associated with posterior fixation. Retrograde percutaneous superior ramus screws have now been introduced through the symphysis, but should only be used in expert hands and only for very limited indications. The potential hazard of penetrating the hip joint and/or the femoral artery may be potentially greater than the benefits. Further study is required for this technique.

d) Posterior Pelvic Fixation

The posterior sacroiliac complex may be approached anterior or posterior to the sacroiliac joint. Decision making for either approach is in a state of flux at this time but, in general, the following guidelines may be given. Firstly, the complication rate for posterior incisions in the post-traumatic period is high. In our series, the incidence of wound breakdown from skin necrosis was unacceptable, especially in patients with a crush injury. The posterior skin is often in a precarious state and spontaneously breaks down even without surgery because of the avulsion of the underlying gluteus maximus fascia. Therefore, there is a growing trend toward anterior fixation of the sacroiliac complex. It is of historical interest that our mentor, George Pennal, from whom we learned a great deal about pelvic disruption, originally approached the sacroiliac joint anteriorly, but because of poor fixation methods using staples abandoned the approach. With the use of plates anteriorly, stability can be restored. This more physiological approach is now being advocated with greater frequency.

Therefore, we favor the anterior approach for fixation of sacroiliac dislocations and some fracture dislocations, and the posterior approach for some iliac fractures and sacral crush. Percutaneous techniques are becoming more prevalent and, with better radiographic or wand control, also safer. Skin problems may be avoided, but reduction remains a problem.

e) Anterior Fixation of the Sacroiliac Joint

Surgical Approach. A long incision is made from the posterior portion of the iliac crest to beyond the anterior superior spine. The iliac crest is exposed and the iliacus muscle swept by subperiosteal dissection posteriorly to expose the sacroiliac joint including the ala of the

sacrum (Fig. 12.42 a). If further exposure is required, the incision may be extended distally as for the iliofemoral or Smith-Petersen approach to the hip joint. The greater sciatic notch should be clearly exposed to protect the sciatic nerve.

The L5 nerve root exits from the intervertebral foramen between L5 and S1 and crosses the L5–S1 disc to the ala of the sacrum, where it joins the S1 nerve root as it exits from the S1 foramen (Fig. 12.42 b, c). These nerves are in jeopardy in this approach, and care must be taken not to injure them either by pointed reduction clamps or by plates that are longer than one screw on the sacral portion.

This technique is not suitable for fractures of the sacrum because of the proximity to the nerves; therefore, it can only be used in sacroiliac dislocations or fractures of the ilium. Reduction may be difficult and is aided by longitudinal traction and pointed fracture clamps in the anterior superior spine of the ilium pulling anteriorly. The reduction should be checked anteriorly at the greater sciatic notch.

Two two- or three-hole 4.5-mm plates held by 6.5-mm fully threaded cancellous screws afford excellent fixation (Fig. 12.42 d–e). A rectangular external frame will supplement the posterior fixation if no fixation is present at the symphysis. The wound should be drained and closed.

If the patient is young and good stability has been attained, the upright position may be assumed, but weight bearing should be restricted until healing progresses, a period of approximately 6 weeks.

f) Posterior Fixation of the Sacroiliac Joint

As noted previously, the posterior approach to the sacroiliac joint is safe and straightforward, but the risk of complications such as wound breakdown and nerve damage is significant, and it should therefore be approached with considerable caution. The indications include an unreduced sacral crush, sacroiliac dislocation, and fracture-dislocation. Since no clear indications exist at this time for favoring either the anterior or the posterior approach to the sacroiliac joint, the surgeon's choice of approach can often be guided by personal preference.

Surgical Approach. The incision should be longitudinal just lateral to the posterior superior iliac spine over the belly of the gluteus maximus muscle (Fig. 12.43 a). The subcutaneous border of any bone should always be avoided, especially in this area. The incision is opened to the posterior superior spine and iliac crest area. The gluteus maximus muscle, which is often avulsed, is further dissected by the subperiosteal route to expose the super-

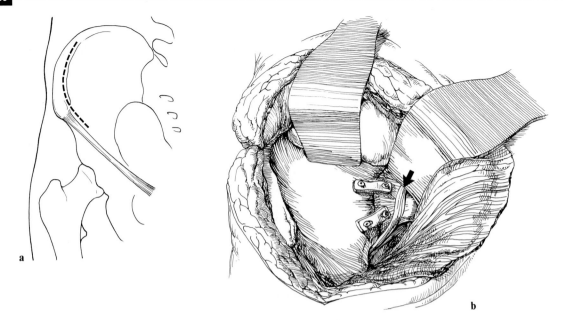

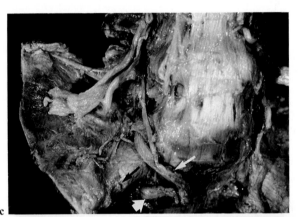

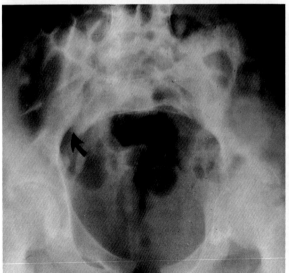

Fig. 12.42 a–e. Anterior fixation of the sacrioiliac joint. **a** Incision just medial to the iliac crest. **b** Subperiosteal dissection of the iliacus muscle will expose the sacroiliac joint. Note the proximity of the L5 nerve root *(arrow)*, which when joined by the S1 nerve exiting through the S1 foramen becomes the sciatic nerve, which leaves the pelvis through the greater sciatic notch, as shown. **c** Anatomical dissection showing the relationship of the L5 nerve root to the sacroiliac joint. The L5 nerve root *(small white arrow)* is seen crossing the ala of the sacrum and joining with the S1 nerve root exiting the first sacral foramen *(broad white arrow)*. The sacroiliac joint is outlined by the *black arrow*. **d** Inlet view showing an unstable right hemipelvis with posterior displacement of the right sacroiliac joint and disruption of the symphysis. **e** Fixation of the right sacroiliac joint with two anterior plates and a single plate on the symphysis pubis

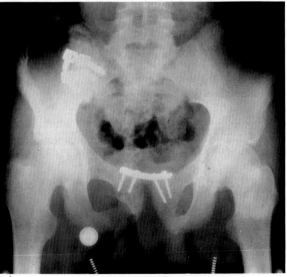

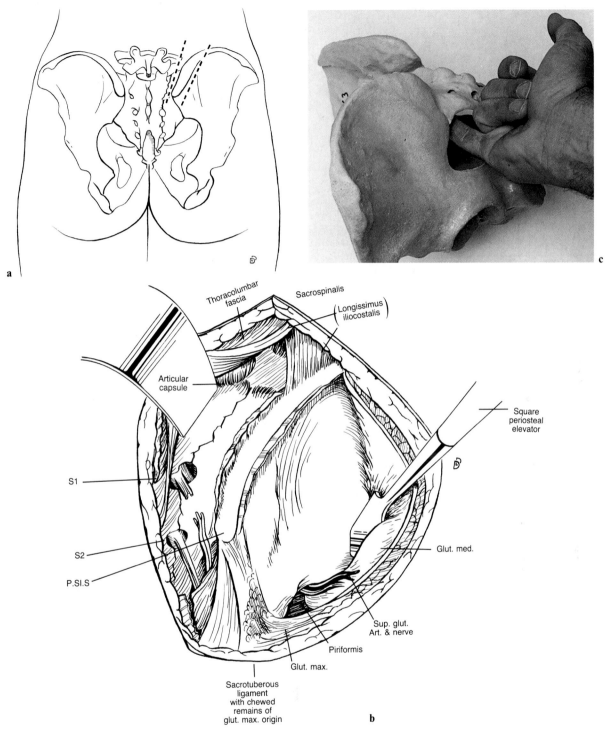

Fig. 12.43 a–c. Posterior pelvic fixation. Note that the surgical incision should be made either 1 cm medial or lateral to the posterior iliac spine and not directly over the subcutaneous border (**a**). Depending on the amount of exposure required posteriorly, the insertion of the gluteus maximus may be dissected from the lateral aspect of the ilium into the greater sciatic notch with an elevator, as noted in the diagram. **b** Note also that the superior gluteal artery and nerve exit from the greater sciatic notch, and great care must be taken when dissecting in that area. If exposure to the posterior aspect of the sacrum is required because of sacral fracture, note the medial dissection and the sacral fracture. Exposure of the posterior foramina may help with reduction. **c** Dissection should allow the palpating finger to explore the anterior aspect of the joint to confirm reduction. (From Tile 1984)

ior gluteal notch. The sciatic nerve must be protected as it exits through the notch. In the unstable fracture for which this incision is indicated, the examining finger can be placed through the notch to explore the anterior aspect of the sacrum (Fig. 12.43 b). Anatomical reduction can be verified only by this maneuver. Image intensification is most desirable, especially if screws are to be used across the sacroiliac joint and the sacral foramina are to be avoided.

g) Open Techniques of Posterior Fixation

Fractures of the Ilium: Screw and Plate Fixation. Posterior fractures of the ilium or fracture dislocations of the sacroiliac joint are best fixed with standard techniques of open reduction of the fracture and primary internal fixation with lag screws across the fracture, followed by the application of a 4.5-mm or 3.5-mm reconstruction plate, as a neutralization plate. Usually two plates are required to prevent displacement (Fig. 12.44).

Sacroiliac Dislocations: Screw Fixation. Screw fixation across the sacroiliac joint affords excellent fixation. The screws can be used alone or through a small plate as a washer, especially in older individuals. The technique of placement of these screws must be precise; otherwise, damage to the cauda equina by penetration of the spinal canal or to the S1 foramen will be unacceptably common. If this technique is to be used, image intensification is essential in two planes as well as a lateral view of the sacrum (Fig. 12.45).

The superior screw should be placed in the ala of the sacrum and across into the area of the S1 body. A 2-mm Kirschner wire should be inserted first and checked on the image intensifier to confirm the position. Across the sacroiliac joint, 6.5-mm cancellous lag screws over washers (Fig. 12.45) or cannulated screws now available must be used.

In a sacroiliac dislocation, a length of 40–45 mm will suffice. However, for a sacral fracture or sacral nonunion, the screw must penetrate the S1 body to cross the fracture line. In those circumstances, longer screws of 60–70 mm must be used, and therefore the position of the screw is critical. The surgeon must have his or her finger over the top of the iliac crest and on the ala of the sacrum as a guide and the drill and guide wire must be inserted under image intensification.

The second screw, again using image intensification, should be inserted distal to the S1 foramen. To avoid the nerve within the foramen, the final screw can be placed distal to the S1 foramen, although in this area it is extremely difficult because of the thinness of the bone. The foramen can be seen on the image intensifier or may be seen directly by posterior disruption and dissection.

Often two screws may be placed proximally and one distally. It is essential that the surgeon embarking on this technique learn it in a manual skills laboratory prior to inserting these screws into a patient.

Sacral Fracture: Transiliac Bar Fixation. In the acute sacral crush requiring open reduction through a posterior approach, the use of sacral bars is safe and adequate. Since the device does not penetrate the sacrum, the neural elements are not at risk unless compression across the fracture is excessive and traps the nerve in the foramen. In all open approaches to sacral fractures, the fracture should be exposed, all fragments removed from the neural foramina, and the reduction as anatomical as possible, lining up the neural foramina. The insertion of two sacral bars will restore excellent stability to the posterior complex, as shown in Fig. 12.46. The addition of the anterior frame will complete the stabilization.

The incision on the side of injury is the same as previously mentioned, just lateral to the posterior superior iliac spine. The posterior spine is exposed, a gliding hole made, and the threaded sacral bar driven through until it hits the opposite posterior iliac spine. The sharp point on the sacral bar is driven through the posterior spine until it emerges on the outer table of the iliac crest. Washers and nuts are inserted and the bars cut off flush at the nut. A second bar is inserted distally. An absolute contraindication is a fracture in the posterior superior spine area. If none exists, good compression may be obtained for the sacral crush without fear of damaging the neural elements. We favor this approach for the acute sacral crush, where necessary. Newer transiliac bars have been developed and are being tested at this time (Gorczyca et al. 1994; Schied et al. 1991).

Iliosacral Screws. In experienced hands, iliosacral screws inserted as previously outlined offer excellent fixation for sacral fractures, if the anterior arch is controlled by either internal or external fixation.

Sacral Plates. Small sacral plates have been developed by the Hannover Group (Pohlemann et al. 1993) and are being tested at this time.

Closed Percutaneous Iliosacral Screws. As previously stated, percutaneous techniques are becoming more common with more experienced pelvic surgeons for the reasons given. Precise placement of the screw is essential to prevent neurological complications (McLaren 1995; Matta and Saucedo 1989), and reduction must be adequate. The patient may be in the supine position, another advantage in polytrauma care, and damage to soft tissues is minimal.

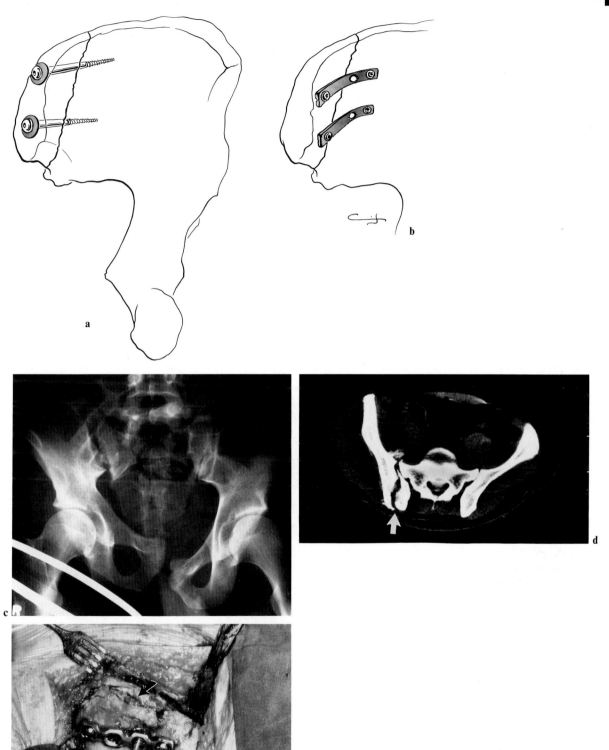

Fig. 12.44. a The use of lag screws to fix a fracture of the ilium. **b** The use of plates to fix the posterior ilium. **c** Anteroposterior radiograph showing a fracture through the ilium. **d** Computed tomography (CT) scan of the same patient. **e** A 4.5-mm reconstruction plate fixing the anatomically reduced fracture in the coronal plane. Note the lag screw fixation being used to compress this fracture. (From Tile 1984)

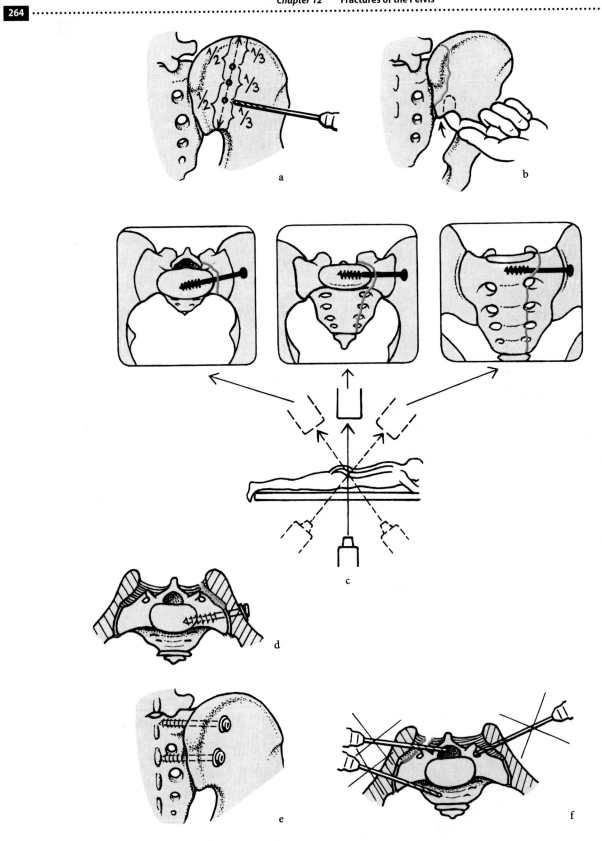

Fig. 12.45 a–f. Fixation of sacroiliac dislocation by 6.5-mm cancellous bone screws (According to Matta). **a** Entry points of cancellous bone screws. **b** Insertion of the index finger through the incisura ischiatica helps in aiming the drill. **c** X-ray controls of screw position. **d, e** Correct position of cancellous bone screws. **f** Drilling directions to be avoided (sacral foramina, spinal canal, great vessels)

Bilateral Sacroiliac Injuries. In bilateral injuries, the sacral bars cannot be used unless supplemented with screw fixation into the sacrum on at least one side to prevent posterior displacement of the entire complex.

12.5.4.5 Postoperative Care

Postoperative care depends entirely on the quality of the bone and the quality of the fixation. If the bone quality is good and fixation is stable anteriorly and posteriorly, ambulation with crutches is possible. However, in most cases, a period of postoperative traction is prudent and may prevent late displacement.

12.5.4.6 Complications

a) Early Complications

Complications of pelvic trauma occur as a result of the injury pattern and /or the operative intervention. The surgeon must ensure that the treatment modality chosen is safe. Prophylactic antibiotics are a necessity to reduce the incidence of sepsis. Wounds must be kept away from areas of skin and soft tissue crush to limit the incidence of wound necrosis. Fixation devices must be carefully placed to avoid penetration of the great vessels or the neurological structures. During surgery, neurological monitoring is desirable.

Pelvic vein thrombosis is common; therefore, antithrombotic prophylaxis is indicated. However, this is extremely difficult in the immediate post-trauma period because of the danger of further bleeding. Therefore, anticoagulants should be used only after the patient's condition has stabilized.

b) Late Complications

Nonunion and Malunion. Since nonunion of the pelvis is not a rare event, occurring in 3 % of cases, the above techniques may prove valuable in the management of these difficult problems. The surgeon must be familiar with all of the above techniques before embarking on the management of a nonunion, especially in the malreduced position. These complex problems require indi-

vidualization and careful preoperative planning. Posterior iliac osteotomies may be required to correct vertical displacement. If major amounts of correction are necessary (more than 2.5 cm), we favor a staged procedure. The first operative procedure should include freeing up of the nonunion and corrective osteotomies posteriorly or anteriorly, as required. The patient should then be placed in supracondylar skeletal traction with a weight of 30–40 lb (14–18 kg) applied to the limb. With the patient awake, correction can be monitored radiographically. Problems with the sciatic nerve may be detected because the patient is awake. At 2–3 weeks following the primary operation, a secondary procedure to stabilize the pelvis may be performed (Fig. 12.47). Occasionally, the large, double cobra plate or a long, contoured DC plate may be helpful for these difficult cases.

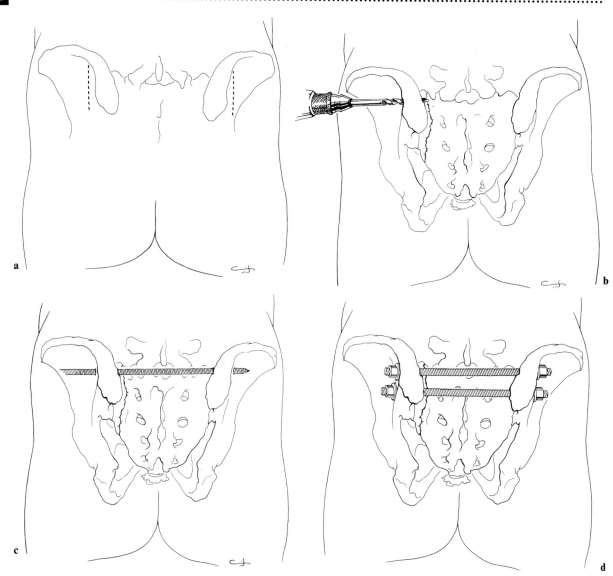

Fig. 12.46 a–g. Transiliac bar posterior fixation. **a** Two slightly curved, vertically placed incisions are made just lateral to the posterior superior spines. **b** After reduction of the fracture dislocation, Kirschner wires are placed across the sacroiliac joint as provisional stabilization. The posterior iliac crest in the region of the posterior spine is predrilled with a 0.25-inch (6.4-mm) drill bit to provide a gliding hole. **c** A second hole is predrilled for the second bar. The sacral bar is then inserted posterior to the sacrum and the sharp trochar point driven into the opposite posterior iliac spine. **d** A standard washer is used to prevent sinking of the sacral rod nut into the bone. Then the nuts are tightened, compressing the sacroiliac joint or the sacral fracture. **e** The two transiliac bars in place on a cadaveric specimen. The tips of the bars should of course be cut short so as not to interfere with the posterior soft tissues. **f** An anteroposterior radiograph of a case of pelvic disruption in a 32-year-old female, showing the two sacral bars stabilizing the posterior lesion and an anterior frame, the anterior lesion. **g** The final result after healing of the fracture and removal of the anterior frame. (From Tile 1995)

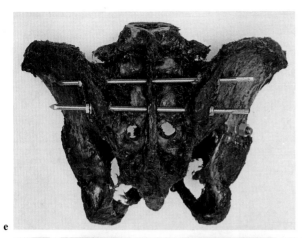

e

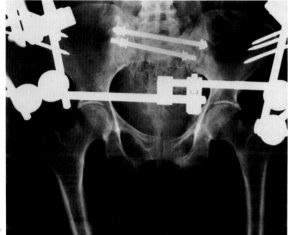

f

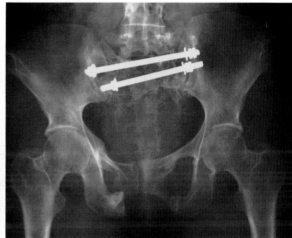

g

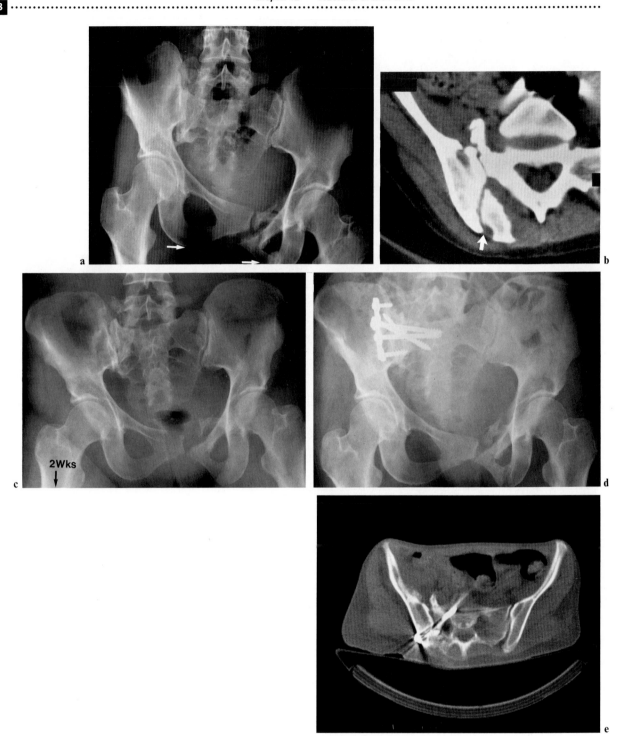

Fig. 12.47. a Anteroposterior radiograph of a 35-year-old woman who sustained an unstable disruption of the pelvic ring 18 months prior to this radiograph. Note the marked internal rotation of the right hemipelvis as well as posterior displacement of greater than 2 cm. Note also the leg length discrepancy, as indicated by the position of the femoral heads. A major problem in these individuals with pelvic nonunion is their difficulty in sitting because of the different planes of the ischial tuberosities *(white arrows)*. Note also the nonunion of the left superior pubic ramus. **b** The nonunion is confirmed on the computed tomography (CT) scan. The fibrous tissue in the posterior nonunion site was divided and the patient placed in traction. **c** After 2 weeks in traction, note on the anteroposterior radiograph that the posterior displacement of the right hemipelvis has been corrected. At this time open reduction and internal fixation through a posterior approach restored stability to the pelvis. **d** Note that three of the long lag screws cross the nonunion site and enter the body of the sacrum. A bone graft was placed around the nonunion, which subsequently healed. **e** The appearance on the CT scan after healing

12.6 Conclusions

Disruption of the pelvic ring is a serious injury with a significant mortality. Early management is directed to the essentials of polytrauma care. Complications of this injury are many, including massive hemorrhage, rupture of a hollow viscus, especially bladder, urethra, and small bowel, and open wounds in the perineum. As the general aspects of the injury are dealt with, the musculoskeletal injury should not be forgotten but should be managed concurrently with the other injuries. The trauma or orthopedic surgeon must carefully plan the early management to include stabilization of the pelvic fracture. A knowledge of the fracture types is essential for logical decision making.

The role of *external* skeletal fixation or a pelvic clamp may be lifesaving in provisional fixation of the unstable pelvic disruption. It should be applied quickly and simply. External skeletal fixation may also be used as definitive treatment in the stable open book (B1) fracture, in the occasional lateral compression injury (B2) which requires reduction by external rotation, or in a patient with polytrauma and in the unstable pelvic disruption (C) in association with supracondylar skeletal traction, or open reduction and internal fixation.

The role of *internal* fixation is becoming clearer, although most cases of pelvic disruption will do well using simpler traction methods. However, internal fixation does afford the advantage of excellent stability to the ring and easier nursing care, as with femoral fractures in polytrauma. Therefore, the indications will widen with improved techniques, percutaneous or open, and improved guidance systems to improve safety. Anterior fixation of symphyseal disruption is desirable. For posterior pelvic fixations we favor the anterior approach to the sacroiliac joint for sacroiliac dislocations and iliac fractures, and the posterior approach for sacral fractures and some fracture dislocations of the sacroiliac joint. For sacral disruptions, we favor the insertion of two transiliac bars posteriorly or iliosacral screws.

Above all, these fractures occur in very ill polytraumatized patients and are often extremely complex. Therefore, management must be individualized and cannot be doctrinaire, since the outcome of this injury, especially the sacral fracture, currently depends more on the injury than on the treatment (Schied et al. 1991). This is especially true if a nerve lesion is present, as it is in 40%–50% of unstable (C) sacral fractures (Schied et al. 1991). The final result in these patients may be disappointing.

Therefore, further study is needed, as well as further refinements of technique, which in the future will, I believe, be with percutaneous techniques. Also needed at this time is careful clinical evaluation to be certain that patients are being helped at minimal risk.

References

Aprahamian C, Carrico CJ, Collicott PE et al (1981) Advanced trauma life support course. Committee on Trauma, American College of Surgeons Park Ridge, IL

Bucholz RW (1981) The pathological anatomy of Malgaigne fracture dislocations of the pelvis. J Bone Joint Surg 63A(l):400–404

Dalal SA, Burgess AR, Siegel JM, Young JW (1989) Pelvic fractures in multiple trauma. Classification by mechanism is key to pattern of organ injuries, resuscitation requirements and outcome. J Trauma 29:981

Dickinson D, Lifeso R, McBroom R, Tile M (1982) Disruptions of the pelvic ring. J Bone Joint Surg 64B(5):635

Ganz R, Krushell R, Jacob R, Kuffer J (1991) The anti-shock pelvic clamp. Clin Orthop 267:71

Geerts WH et al (1990) Venous thrombosis in trauma – a prospective study. Orthop Trans 14: 271

Gertzbein SD, Chenoweth DR (1977) Occult injuries of the pelvic ring. Clin Orthop 128:202–207

Gorczyca J, Varga E, Woodside T, Hearn T, Powell J, Tile M (1994) The strength of iliosacral lag screws and transiliac bars in the fixation of vertically unstable pelvic ring injuries with sacral fractures. Presented at the Orthopaedic Trauma Meeting, Los Angeles

Hearn TC et al (1991) Effects of ligamentous sectioning and internal fixation of bending stiffness of the pelvic ring. In: Proceedings of 13th International Conference on Biomechanics, Perth, W. Australia, 9–13 December, pp 518–520

Holdsworth FW (1948) Dislocation and fracture dislocations of the pelvis. J Bone Joint Surg 3OB:461–466

Lipkowitz G, Phillips T, Coren C, Spero C, Glassberg K, Velcek FT (1982) Hemipelvectomy: a lifesaving operation in severe open pelvic injury in childhood. J Trauma 25 (9):823–827

Matta J, Saucedo T (1989) Internal fixation of pelvic ring fractures Clin Orthop 242: 83–98

McGowan S, Kellam JF, Tile M (1987) Unstable pelvic ring disruptions – results of open reduction and internal fixation. Orthop Trans 11: 478

McLaren AC (1995) In: Tile M (ed) Fractures of the pelvis and acetabulum. Williams and Wilkins, Baltimore, p 150

McMurtry R, Walton D, Dickinson D, Kellam J, Tile M (1980) Pelvic disruption in the polytraumatized patient: a management protocol. Clin Orthop 151:22–30

Monahan PR, Taylor RG (1975) Dislocation and fracture dislocation of the pelvis. Injury 6(4):325–333

Müller ME, Allgower M, Schneider R, Willenegger H (1990) Manual of internal fixation, 3rd edn. Springer, Berlin Heidelberg New York

Pennal GF, Sutherland GO (1959) The use of external fixation. Paper presented at the Canadian Orthopaedic Association Annual Meeting

Pohlemann T, Bosch U, Gansslen A, Tscherne H (1993) The Hannover experience in management of pelvic fractures. Clin Orthop 305:69–80

Richardson JD, Harty J, Amin M et al (1982) Open pelvic fractures. J Trauma 22(7):533–538

Schied DK, Kellam JF, Tile M (1991) Open reduction and internal fixation of pelvic ring fractures. J Orthop Trauma 5:226

Schopfer A, Hearn TC, D'Angelo D, Tile M (1994) Biomechanical comparison of fixation methods of vertically unstable pelvic ring disruption. Int Orthop 18 (2):96–101

Slätis P, Huittinen VM (1972) Double vertical fractures of the pelvis: a report on 163 patients. Acta Chir Scand 138:799–807

Tile M (1984) Fractures of the pelvis and acetabulum, 1st edn. Williams and Wilkins, Baltimore

Tile M (1988) Pelvic fractures: should they be fixed? J Bone Joint Surg. 70B:l

Tile M (1995) Fractures of the pelvis and acetabulum, 2nd edn. Williams and Wilkins, Baltimore

13 Fractures of the Acetabulum

M. TILE

13.1 Introduction

Fractures of the acetabulum are relatively uncommon, but because they involve a major weight-bearing joint in the lower extremity, they assume great clinical importance. The principle of management for this fracture is as for any other displaced lower extremity intra-articular fracture, namely, that anatomical reduction is essential for good long-term function of the hip joint. In some cases, anatomical reduction may be obtained by closed means, but more often, open reduction followed by stable internal fixation allowing early active or passive motion will be required. In the past, the achievement of this ideal, that is, anatomical reduction, has been difficult because of technical problems such as those caused by complicated anatomy, difficulty with surgical exposure, severe comminution in many cases, and major associated injuries. Permanent disability was reported to be high whether open or closed methods were used.

13.1.1 Natural History

A search of the early literature on this subject may seem confusing because it is based on broad generalizations made by lumping all acetabular fractures together. It is important when reading this literature to remember that it is not the overall results that are important, since they may reflect a high proportion of inconsequential fractures. If one is making broad generalizations based on a number of acetabular fractures, a knowledge of the case mix of the series becomes essential. If a large percentage of the cases are of the type shown in Fig. 13.1 a, then one would expect good results from simple closed treatment. On the other hand, if the majority of cases are like the one in Fig. 13.1 b, poor results may be expected from closed treatment. Therefore, it is essential when reading the literature to separate the apples from the oranges, that is, to compare only similar fracture types (Fig. 13.1 c).

For example, in the article by Rowe and Lowell (1961), closed methods using traction were recommended as the treatment of choice for acetabular fractures. However, close scrutiny of this paper describing 93 fractures in 90 patients revealed a large number of inconse-

quential fractures in older individuals with expected good results, and, in examining the high-energy injuries, 26 involved the superior weight-bearing dome of the acetabulum. When anatomical reduction was obtained, 13 of 16 had a good result, but when anatomical reduction of the dome fragment was not obtained, ten out of ten had a poor result. Of the posterior wall fractures, of which there were 17, closed management led to poor results in six out of nine cases, whereas open management led to good results in eight out of eight cases. The undisplaced fractures and the medial wall fractures in elderly individuals without protrusio gave satisfactory results with closed means. Thus, the conclusion from this early series should have been that high-energy displaced fractures involving the posterior wall or the superior weight-bearing dome were best treated by open reduction and internal fixation if the anatomy could not be restored by closed means. Conversely, the study also shows that both-column fractures (in this study called medial wall fractures) as well as some anterior types in elderly patients can be managed nonoperatively with the expectation of a good result.

Judet et al. (1964) recommended open reduction and internal fixation for all displaced acetabular fractures and proposed a classification of these fractures based on the pattern of injury.

Pennal et al. (1980), reporting on 103 fractures of the acetabulum, indicated that of those with a poor reduction, 72 % had clinical and radiographic osteoarthritis at 5-year follow-up, whereas of those with a good reduction, only 30 % had such changes. Although the incidence of osteoarthritis in those with a good reduction in this series may seem high, the severity of the arthritis was much less and the incidence less than half of those with a poor result.

Letournel (1980) reported on 350 fractures of the acetabulum with very good results in 75 %, good results in 8 %, and poor results in 17 %. Of the 74 % of the patients with an anatomically reduced hip joint, 90 % had a good result. Of the 26 % imperfectly reduced, only 55 % had a good result if some incongruity remained, only 11 % if a degree of protrusio remained, and only 9 % if there were major technical failures.

In a review of our own case material (Tile et al. 1984), 227 charts were examined. Ninety-five cases of minor

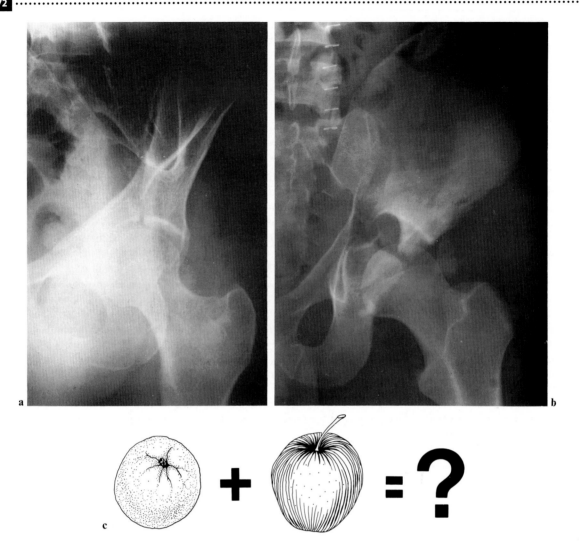

Fig. 13.1 a–c. Comparing the undisplaced acetabular fracture (**a**) to the grossly displaced comminuted acetabular fracture associated with a pelvic ring disruption (**b**) is like comparing an orange to an apple (**c**). (From Tile 1984)

trauma were excluded because displacement was less than 5 mm at the joint. Thus, all inconsequential fractures were removed from this series. Only two of those 95 had any difficulty with their hip at review. There were 13 deaths, eight in the post-trauma period, all in older individuals between 59 and 88 years of age, and five with subsequent trauma, a frequent finding in such a series. Fifteen cases were lost to follow-up, two were treated at 9 and 12 months and thereby excluded from the series, leaving 102 cases. At review, all patients were recalled, personally examined by one of the authors, and standard radiographs taken. Our findings mirrored those in the literature. Excellent results could be attained if anatomical reduction was achieved and complications avoided.

Matta et al. (1986) stressed that anatomical reduction can rarely be achieved by closed means, therefore decision making must be based on the specialized radiographic views of Letournel and Judet (1981). Displacement of greater than 3 mm, especially through the roof of the acetabulum, was considered an indication for open reduction and internal fixation.

Similar conclusions have been reported in the more recent literature (Goulet and Bray 1989, Pantazopoulos and Mousafiris 1989; Powell et al. 1988). Letournel (1993), in the largest series of operatively treated acetabular fractures, followed this same principle. His results, considered the gold standard in 1995, showed variations in the ability to achieve anatomical reduction (Table 13.1), depending on the type and severity of the fracture; even in the most expert hands, anatomical reduction was achieved in only 70 % of fixations.

Thus, the literature is not confusing and, if fractures of a similar type and severity are compared, makes the

Table 13.1. Clinical results of acetabular fractures (from Letournel 1993)

Type of fracture	Clinical results					Total	Percentage of excellent results
	Excellent	Very good	Good	Fair	Poor		
Posterior wall	87	6	3	4	17	117	74
Posterior column	9	–	1	1	–	11	81.82
Anterior wall	6	–	1	1	1	9	66.67
Anterior column	12	1	1	–	2	16	75.00
Transverse	17	1	–	–	1	19	89.47
T-shaped	20	3	–	–	3	26	76.92
Transverse and posterior wall	49	16	10	9	17	101	48.51
Posterior column and posterior wall	5	1	2	1	8	17	29.41
Anterior column and posterior hemitransverse	26	5	4	3	3	41	63.41
Both-column	76	21	14	11	13	135	56.30
Total	307 (62.40%)	54 (10.98%)	36 (7.32%)	30 (6.10%)	65 (13.21%)	492 (100%)	62.40

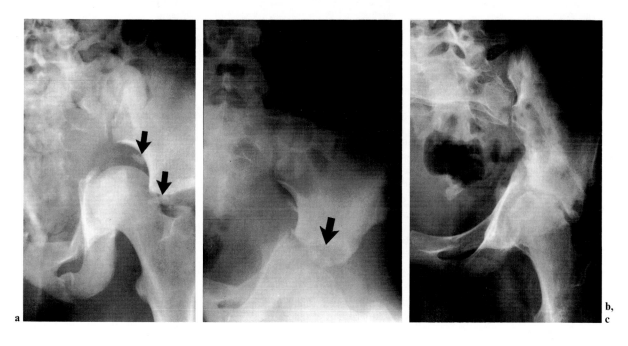

a   b, c

Fig. 13.2 a–c. Anteroposterior radiograph (**a**) of the left hip of a 17-year-old girl demonstrating a transverse fracture of the left acetabulum through the dome with a central dislocation of the hip. The two *arrows* in **a** point to loose bony fragments. Following closed reduction (**b**), the two bony fragments have been retained within the joint *(arrow)*. In spite of traction, reduction is inadequate, with bony fragments in the joint and incongruity between the femoral head and acetabulum. Definitive treatment consisted of traction until the fracture healed. Her result at 18 months is shown in **c**. Note the severe narrowing and erosions on the superior weight-bearing margin of the femoral head. The patient's clinical result was poor. She had a 60° flexion deformity with continuous pain and required an arthrodesis. (From Tile 1984)

following statement with surprising unanimity: joint congruity is essential for good long-term function; however, joint congruity may be difficult to achieve. Joint congruity must be assessed by strict radiographic means, including computed tomography (CT), and must cover all the essential parts of the acetabulum, including the anterior column, the superior weight-bearing portion, and the posterior column. Failure to recognize incongruity caused by displacement of the columns, comminution, or articular impaction will result in early destruction of the hip joint (Fig. 13.2).

If closed reduction fails to achieve congruity, then open reduction is essential, but open reduction and internal fixation will only improve the results if anatom-

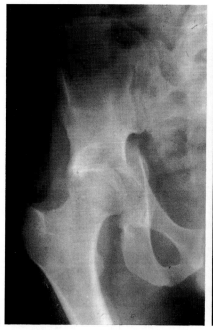
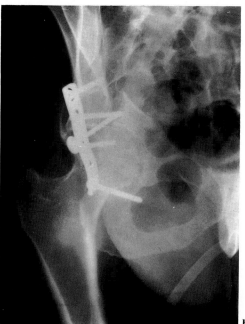

Fig. 13.3. a Radiograph of a 59-year-old man with a transverse fracture of the acetabulum associated with a posterior wall fracture. **b** Postoperative radiograph of the same patient showing a plate placed on the posterior column and one screw in the posterior wall. Note, however, that the fracture is unreduced, the femoral head is subluxated anteriorly, and there is no interfragmental compression between the major fragments of the transverse fracture. This incongruous reduction resulted in a total hip arthroplasty 2 years following the acetabular fracture

ical reduction is achieved and operative complications are avoided. Failure to obtain an anatomical reduction in the patient shown in Fig. 13.3 resulted in an early total hip arthroplasty. Note that the plate is on the posterior column; however, the head is displaced anteriorly and the anterior column remains unreduced as on the preoperative radiograph. The basic tenet of fracture care, that is, interfragmental compression of the major fragments, has been forgotten, with the predictable result.

Surgical treatment of this injury is extremely demanding and requires adequate resources, both human and material. The learning curve may be long, but also remember that it may be very hard on patients with this injury. Because of the considerable technical difficulties, a subspecialty "pelvic-acetabular surgery" has developed. Complex acetabular fractures are uncommon but should only be managed by experienced surgeons working with a knowledgable team. Most large metropolitan areas in the developed world have or should have such a team. The surgical team should have an experienced surgeon as well as a minimum of two qualified assistants and a complete surgical armamentarium including specialized pelvic equipment. Therefore, the natural history of an acetabular fracture may be summarized as follows: if the joint is stable and congruous following reduction, and if complications are avoided, a satisfactory result may be expected; but if the joint is incongruous, joint destruction will ensue.

The major factors affecting the prognosis are as follows:

1. The degree of initial displacement
2. The damage to the superior weight-bearing surface of the acetabulum or the femoral head
3. The degree of hip joint instability caused by a posterior wall fracture
4. The adequacy of reduction, either open or closed
5. The late complications of:
   Avascular necrosis of the femoral head
   Heterotopic ossification
   Chondrolysis
   Sciatic or femoral nerve injury

13.1.2 Surgical Anatomy

The surgeon must be adept at three-dimensional (3D) conceptualization to master the complex anatomy of the acetabulum. From its lateral aspect, the acetabulum is cradled by the arms of an inverted Y (Fig. 13.4 a, b). The posterior column is strong and triangular, with extremely thick bone at the greater sciatic notch. The medial surface forms the posterior aspect of the quadrilateral plate.

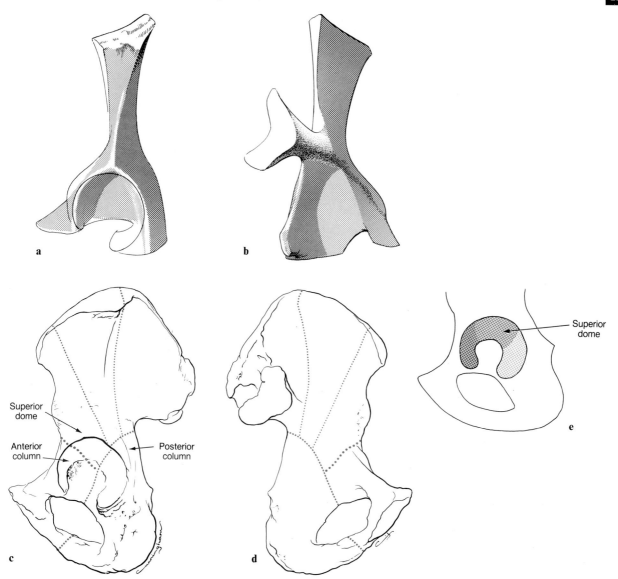

Fig. 13.4. a The acetabulum is cradled by the arms of an inverted Y. **b** The two columns are linked to the sacral bone by the "sciatic buttress" (from Letournel 1993). **c** Lateral aspect of the hemipelvis and acetabulum. The posterior column is characterized by the dense bone at the greater sciatic notch and follows the *dotted line* distally through the center of the acetabulum, the obturator foramen, and the inferior pubic ramus. The anterior column extends from the iliac crest to the symphysis pubis and includes the entire anterior wall of the acetabulum. Fractures involving the anterior column commonly exit below the anterior inferior iliac spine as shown by the *heavy dotted line* or through other areas of weakness in the ilium, between the anterior superior spine and tubercle and behind the tubercle *(dotted lines)*. **d** The hemipelvis from its medial aspect. The area between the posterior column and the heavy dotted line, representing a fracture through the anterior column, is often considered the superior dome fragment, represented by the *middle portion* (**e**). (From Tile 1984)

The anterior column extends from the symphysis pubis to the iliac crest. Fractures of the anterior column may comprise any portion of the column. Most commonly, the anterior column fracture exits below the anterior inferior iliac spine, but the other areas of exit are usually in the weak areas of the iliac crest between the iliac spines, between the anterior superior spine and the tubercle, and a common Y pattern involving the area behind the tubercle. Inspection of the lateral aspect of the acetabulum will indicate the important articular fractures, especially in the weight-bearing dome area (Fig. 13.4 e). This area, although vague anatomically, has great clinical significance, since fractures of this area left unreduced will inevitably result in post-traumatic arthritis of the hip joint.

Unfortunately, the dome (roof) concept can be confusing, since it is really a 3D structure diagnosed on a 2D anteroposterior (AP) radiograph. On that view, the dome is represented by a line, but on the skeleton that line is only millimeters thin (Fig. 13.4E). The dome is best assessed on 3D CT (Fig. 13.12)

13.1.3 Mechanism of Injury

The pathological anatomy of the fracture depends on the position of the femoral head at the moment of impact (Fig. 13.5). The femoral head acts as a hammer against the acetabulum, producing the injury. There are two basic mechanisms of injury: first, those caused by a direct blow on the acetabulum and, second, the so-called dashboard injury, in which the flexed knee joint strikes the dashboard of a motor vehicle, driving the femur posteriorly on the acetabulum. A blow directly upon the greater trochanter usually causes a transverse-type acetabular fracture, depending on the degree of abduction and rotation of the femoral head, whereas the dashboard injury causes a posterior wall or posterior column fracture or fracture-dislocation of the hip joint.

In general, the externally rotated hip causes injuries to the anterior column, the internally rotated hip to the posterior column; the abducted hip causes a low transverse fracture, the adducted hip a high transverse fracture.

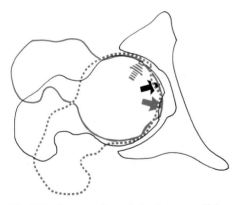

Fig. 13.5. The type of acetabular fracture will depend upon the position of the femoral head at the moment of impact. If externally rotated *(striped arrow)* the anterior column will be involved; if internally rotated *(red solid arrow)* the posterior column will be involved. (From Tile 1984)

13.2 Assessment

For logical decision making, a precise diagnosis is imperative, so careful assessment of the patient is essential.

13.2.1 Clinical Assessment

The general patient profile is of great importance in decision making. Older individuals have poor bone, reducing the holding power of screws and making anatomical open reduction much more difficult. Therefore, with severely comminuted fractures in older people, other options such as traction, followed by total hip arthroplasty, or even early total hip arthroplasty (Romness and Lewallen 1990) if necessary, are more advisable than for younger patients. Thus, the age and general medical state of the patient are important, as well as the assessment of other major injuries in the polytraumatized patient, especially those involving the affected limb, such as fractures of the femur or neurovascular injuries.

13.2.2 Radiological Assessment

Radiological assessment should include specific radiographic views of the pelvis and acetabulum and CT examination.

13.2.2.1 Special Radiographs of the Pelvis

Radiographic examination of the pelvis should include the anteroposterior view, the inlet view, and the outlet view (see p. 239). This will allow an overview of any other injuries in the pelvic ring.

13.2.2.2 Specific Acetabular Views

Anteroposterior View. It is essential that the surgeon treating these difficult fractures become completely familiar with the anatomical landmarks as seen on these particular views of the acetabulum. These landmarks include the iliopectineal line denoting the limits of the anterior column, the ilioischial line denoting the extent of the posterior column, the anterior lip of the acetabulum, the posterior lip of the acetabulum, and the line depicting the superior weight-bearing surface of the acetabulum, ending in the medial teardrop (Fig. 13.6 a, b). The anteroposterior view of the hip shows all of these landmarks clearly (Fig. 13.6 c).

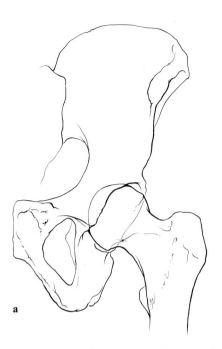

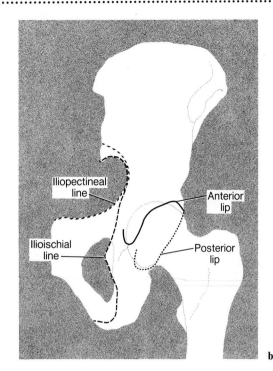

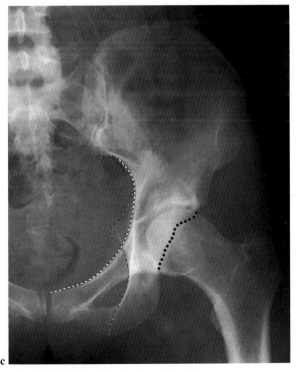

Fig. 13.6. a The anatomical landmarks seen on the anteroposterior radiograph. **b** The major landmarks by the various lines as follows: the iliopectineal line (anterior column, *short dashed line*); the ilioischial line (posterior column, *long dashed line*); the anterior lip of the acetabulum *(line)*; the posterior lip of the acetabulum *(dotted line)*. **c** Anteroposterior radiograph of the left hemipelvis with the major landmarks outlined. (From Tile 1984)

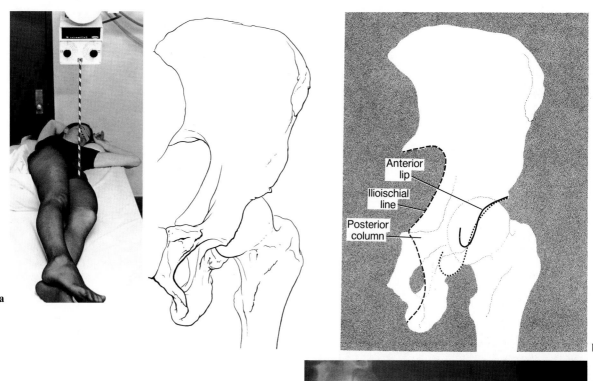

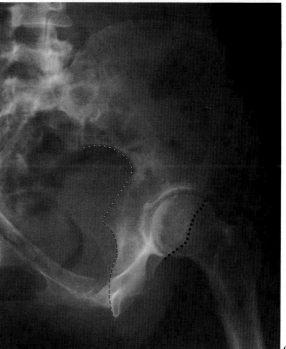

Fig. 13.7 a–c. Iliac oblique radiographic view. This view is taken by rotating the patient into 45° of external rotation by elevating the uninjured side on a wedge *(inset).* **a** The anatomical landmarks of the left hemipelvis on the iliac oblique view. **b** The various acetabular lines (for key, see Fig. 13.6 legend). **c** Iliac oblique radiographic view of the left hemipelvis with the superimposed lines. This view best demonstrates the posterior column of the acetabulum outlined by the ilioischial line as well as the iliac crest and the anterior lip of the acetabulum. (**a, b** adapted from Tile 1984)

Iliac Oblique View. The iliac oblique view is taken by externally rotating the affected hemipelvis. A foam wedge is inserted under the opposite hip of the patient, allowing external rotation of 45° (Fig. 13.7 a, inset). This view clearly shows the entire iliac crest and best depicts the extent of the posterior column and the anterior lip of the acetabulum (Fig. 13.7).

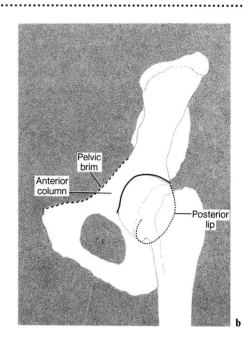

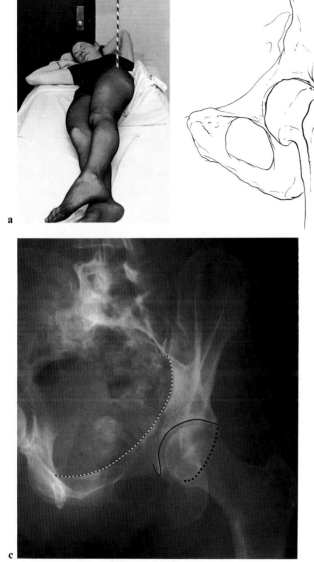

Fig. 13.8 a–c. Obturator oblique radiographic view. This view is taken by elevating the affected hip 45° to the horizontal by means of a wedge and directing the beam through the hip joint with a 15° upward tilt *(inset)*. **a** The anatomy of the pelvis on the obturator oblique view. **b** The important anatomical landmarks as indicated by various lines (for key, see Fig. 13.6 legend). **c** Obturator oblique radiograph of the left hemipelvis with the superimposed lines. In this view note particularly the pelvic brim, indicating the border of the anterior column and the posterior lip of the acetabulum (**a, b** Adapted from Tile 1984)

Obturator Oblique View. The obturator oblique view is obtained by internally rotating the affected hip 45° with the appropriate foam wedge under the affected hip (Fig. 13.8 a, inset). In this view, the iliac crest is seen perpendicular to its normal plane, so displacement of the iliac wing in the coronal plane is best noticed here. This view also best shows the anterior column and the posterior lip of the acetabulum (Fig. 13.8 b, c).

13.2.2.3 Tomography

Prior to CT, plain tomography gave much helpful information especially on the state of the acetabular dome (Fig. 13.9). It may still be helpful in select cases or when CT is not available.

13.2.2.4 Computed Tomography

CT has revolutionized our diagnostic abilities in the pelvis and acetabulum. Although the general acetabular pattern can be determined from the plain radiographs, CT gives much additional information regarding, for instance, impacted fractures of the acetabular wall, retained bone fragments in the joint, the degree of comminution, unrecognized dislocation (Fig. 13.10), and sacroiliac pathology (Fig. 13.11). Major advances in CT include the ability to reconstruct the pelvis into its ring form, allowing the overall pattern to be visualized (Fig. 13.11).

Fig. 13.10. a CT scan demonstrating a transverse fracture of the acetabulum; both the anterior column fracture and the large posterior wall fracture are clearly seen. The *arrow* points to a comminuted rotated bony fragment. **b** CT scan through the central portion of the acetabulum, showing a posterior dislocation of the hip with two large posterior wall fragments trapped within the joint, preventing reduction. The CT scan is most helpful in determining the presence and size of retained bony fragments in the joint. **c** CT scan through the central portion of the acetabulum. Note the large displaced posterior wall fracture on the *lower right*. The *arrow left* points to an impacted fracture of the articular surface. These depressed articular fractures are best seen on CT scanning. **d** CT scan showing the typical appearance of both-column (type C) acetabular fracture at the dome. The lateral area of the posterior aspect is the pathognomic spur sign. (From Tile 1984)

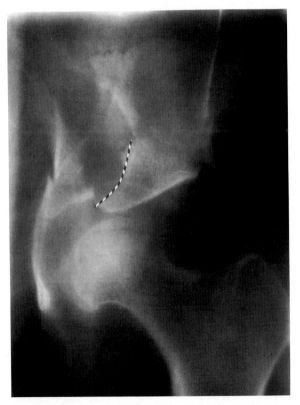

Fig. 13.9. Tomogram showing a dome fragment rotated 90°. This fragment remained unreduced in spite of an attempted closed reduction and traction. (From Tile 1984)

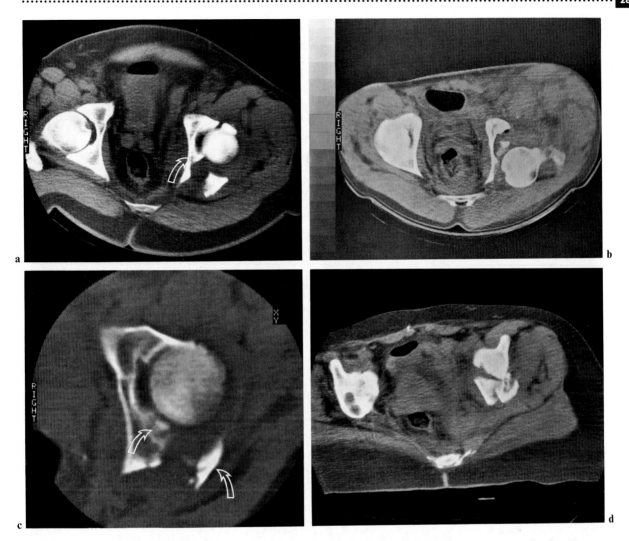

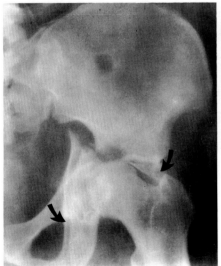

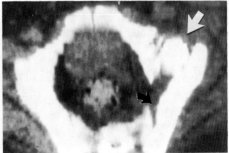

Fig. 13.11. a Anteroposterior radiograph of a comminuted transverse fracture of the acetabulum with a subluxated sacroiliac joint. Note the large fragment within the joint *(upper arrow)* and the split in the medial wall of the acetabulum *(lower arrow)*. **b** CT scan of the same patient with reconstruction of the pelvic ring. Note the marked displacement of the transverse fracture by the interposition of the femoral head *(upper arrow)*. Note also how clearly the sacroiliac opening is seen on the scan *(lower arrow)*

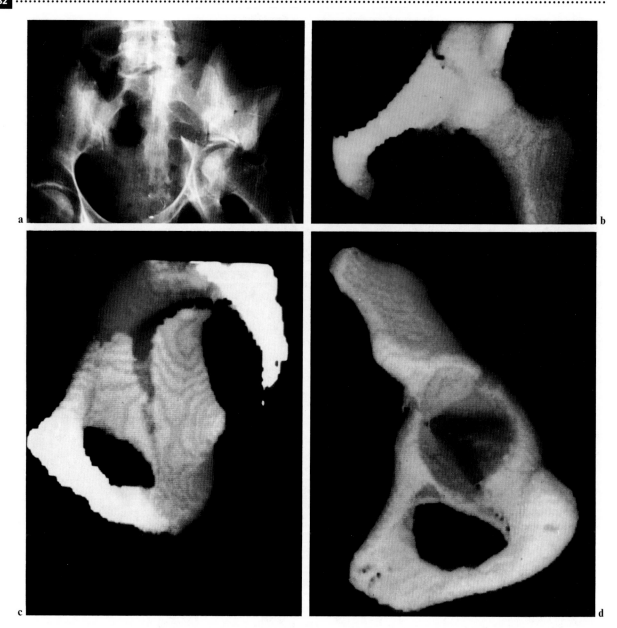

The newest development in CT is the 3D visual reconstruction of a fracture. This is truly an exciting advance which will greatly aid in decision making and at this time has achieved a surprising degree of sophistication and accuracy (Fig. 13.12 a–c). The femoral head may be subtracted by this technique and the articular surface of the acetabulum seen (Fig. 13.12 d).

The 3D CT allows the surgeon to visualize the pelvis and the fracture pattern of the acetabulum exactly. In my opinion, it is a major advance in understanding the injury and helping to plan the surgical approach.

Fig. 13.12 a–d. Three-dimensional CT. **a** Anteroposterior view of the pelvis showing a transverse fracture of the left acetabulum. **b** Three-dimensional reconstruction showing the transverse fracture. **c** Three-dimensional reconstruction showing the quadrilateral plate. **d** Subtraction of the femoral head showing the interior of the acetabulum

13.3 Classification

Classifications are useful in two areas: (a) in assisting the decision-making process for the individual case, and (b) in documenting case material for academic purposes.

For decision making, many factors must be built into any classification and no perfect classification exists. For this purpose, the degree of displacement, the amount of comminution, the presence or absence of a dislocation, and the state of the bone, whether osteopenic or normal, must be considered. For documentation, an anatomical classification is best which incorporates the parameters mentioned above.

Although several classifications exist in the literature, some simple facts should be examined first in order to remove the confusion that surrounds this subject. Basically, the acetabulum consists of four anatomical areas: an anterior and posterior column and an anterior and posterior wall of lip (Fig. 13.13). *All fracture types involve one or a combination of more than one of these.* Therefore, the following fracture types are possible: an isolated anterior column fracture or an isolated posterior column fracture, a combined anterior column fracture with an anterior lip fracture or a combined posterior column fracture with a posterior lip fracture.

If both columns are broken, we arbitrarily call that injury a *transverse fracture*, and if both columns are broken and separated from each other, it is called a *T fracture*. Either of those two main types, the transverse or T, may be associated with an anterior or posterior lip fracture as well. In this particular type (transverse) a portion of the acetabular dome is always attached to the intact ilium (Fig. 13.13 b).

This is contrasted to an unusual fracture of the acetabulum called the both-column fracture. The nomen-clature is confusing because in this pattern, both columns are fractured and separated from each other, but the fracture in the columns is proximal to the acetabulum in the ilium (Fig. 13.13 c). Therefore, this is really a true floating acetabulum, that is, no portion of the weight-bearing surface of the acetabulum remains attached to the axial skeleton. The fracture through the iliac wing separating off the dome is usually in the coronal plane.

Therefore, in decision making, the surgeon must examine the plain radiographs and the CT scans which are available, either plain or 3D, and draw the fracture lines on a dry skeleton. All cases have individual features and many defy classification. Hence, no attempt should be made to pigeonhole any particular case into a published classification for individual decision making. However, it is important to categorize a fracture for academic purposes, namely, clinical reviews. In these, more than just an anatomical classification is necessary.

In the Letournel and Judet classification (1981) all fractures are divided into simple and complex types. Our previously published classification according to the direction of displacement was an attempt to incorporate

Fig. 13.13 a–c. Classification of acetabular fractures. All fractures of the acetabulum are a combination of the major anatomical areas which may be fractured, such as the anterior or posterior lip (**a**) or the anterior or posterior column (**b**). Column fractures are commonly associated with fractures of the lip (or wall) when both columns are fractured through the acetabulum as noted in **b**. This is arbitrarily called a transverse fracture, and if the columns are separated from each other a T fracture. This leaves one major type, the so-called both-column fracture which is really a T-type fracture with a horizontal component of the T above the acetabulum, as noted in **c**. This fracture may also be associated with a fracture of the posterior wall

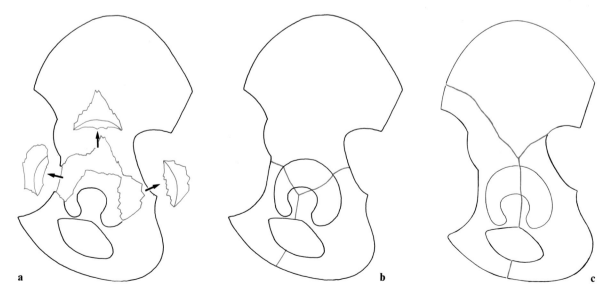

a   b   c

surgical decision making into the classification. Thus, fractures may be of the anterior, posterior, medial, or transverse type associated with anterior, posterior, or medial displacement.

A comprehensive classification has been developed in an attempt to standardize the nomenclature worldwide. This classification began with the AO group (Müller et al. 1990) and is based on Letournel's classic types. However, it also attempts to incorporate other important prognostic indicators, such as marginal impaction, comminution, and dislocation. With Helfet as facilitator, this classification is being used by SICOT and the OTA documentation committees.

The fracture types are anatomical and are grouped according to the AO–A,B,C, in order of increasing severity (Table 13.2). In the acetabulum, however, the type B fractures may be more difficult and severe than the type C fractures (Fig. 13.19).

Table 13.2. Comprehensive classification: fractures of the acetabulum (from Tile 1995)

Type A: *Partial articular* fractures, *one column* involved
    A1: Posterior wall fracture
    A2: Posterior column fracture
    A3: Anterior wall or anterior column fracture
Type B: *Partial articular* fractures (transverse or T-type
    fracture, both columns involved)
    B1: Transverse fracture
    B2: T-shaped fracture
    B3: Anterior column plus posterior hemitransverse
        fracture
Type C: *Complete articular* fracture (both-column fracture;
    floating acetabulum)
    C1: Both-column fracture, high variety
    C2: Both-column fracture, low variety
    C3: Both-column fracture involving the sacroiliac joint

Qualifiers
    α1) Femoral head subluxation, anterior
    α2) Femoral head subluxation, medial
    α3) Femoral head subluxation, posterior

    β1) Femoral head dislocation, anterior
    β2) Femoral head dislocation, medial
    β3) Femoral head dislocation, posterior

    γ1) Acetabular surface, chondral lesion
    γ2) Acetabular surface, impacted

    δ1) Femoral head, chondral lesion
    δ1) Femoral head, impacted
    δ1) Femoral head, osteochondral fracture

    ϵ1) Intra-articular fragment requiring surgical removal

    Φ1) Nondisplaced fracture of the acetabulum

Additional information can be documented concerning the condition of the articular surfaces, in order to further define the prognosis of the injury. The information should be, as aditional qualifiers, identified by Greek letters.

The type A fractures are a single wall or column, the type B fractures involve both columns – namely, transverse or T types with a portion of the dome still attached to the ilium – and the type C fractures in which both columns are fractured and are also separated from the axial skeleton, a true floating acetabulum. Several subtypes are described. Additional information is also recorded by the use of modifiers.

13.4 Management

Management must begin with a careful clinical and radiographic assessment to define the *personality of the injury*. As mentioned previously, this includes a careful assessment of the patient profile including age, general medical state, and the severity of other injuries. Assessment of the limb to include ipsilateral femoral fractures, knee injuries, or neurovascular injury is essential.

Specific radiographic examination of the fracture includes the degree of displacement, the amount of comminution, the presence or absence of a dislocation and, most importantly, the state of the bone, whether it be osteopenic or not. The precise anatomical features according to the classifications given above are also essential.

Also important is the expertise of the surgeon and the operative team.

13.4.1 Indications

The indications for operative treatment depend on fracture factors and patient factors.

13.4.1.1 Fracture Factors

The important factors are hip instability and/or incongruity. In general, nonoperative care is indicated when the joint is stable in all anatomical positions and congruity is acceptable. (Table 13.3). A fracture with *minimal*

Table 13.3. Nonoperative management: Fracture Factors (from Tile 1995)

Hip stable and congruous
Guidelines to be correlated to patient factors
    Undisplaced fractures (all Types)
    Minimally displaced fractures (low anterior
    column, low transverse)
    Fractures with secondary congruence
    (both-column C-Types)

---

displacement may be treated nonoperatively with the expectation of a good result, especially if congruity is retained in low anterior columns, low transverse or in both-column fractures.

Nonoperative Management

Displacement Less Than 2 mm. If a fracture is displaced less than 2 mm, no matter what the anatomical type, nonoperative treatment should yield good results. With minimal displacement, skeletal traction is not essential. If the surgeon is concerned about hidden instability, examination under image intensification will help to decide whether traction is necessary.

Distal Anterior Column Fractures. Prior to the advent of CT, the anterior column fracture was considered a rare acetabular injury. From examination by CT in our pelvic fracture population, we noted that fractures of the superior pubic ramus often entered the inferior portion of the acetabulum, violating the joint. Since these fractures are distal and do not involve the major weight-bearing portion, surgery is virtually never indicated and good results are usually obtained (Fig. 13.14).

Low Transverse Fractures. A transverse fracture occurring low on the acetabulum, that is, through the acetabular fossa area, (infratectal) may often be treated nonoperatively with skeletal traction with the expectation of good results. In the five cases so treated in our recent series, four achieved excellent results, the one poor result being from an unrelated problem in the patient. In these particular fracture types, the intact medial aspect of the acetabular wall acts as a buttress, preventing further displacement (Fig. 13.15 a, b).

Fig. 13.14 a–c. Fracture of the anterior column. **a** Diagram of a typical anterior column fracture dividing the anterior column just distal to the anterior inferior iliac spine. **b** The anteroposterior radiograph of the pelvis clearly demonstrates the fracture of the superior and inferior pubic rami *(arrows).* **c** The CT scan shows the comminution of the anterior column *(curved arrow)* and the intact posterior column *(straight arrow).* (From Tile 1984)

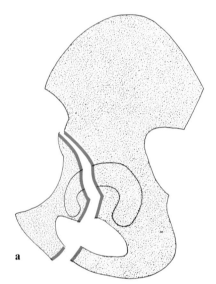

a

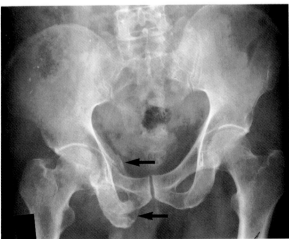

b

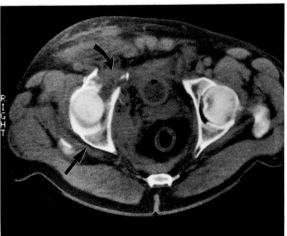

c

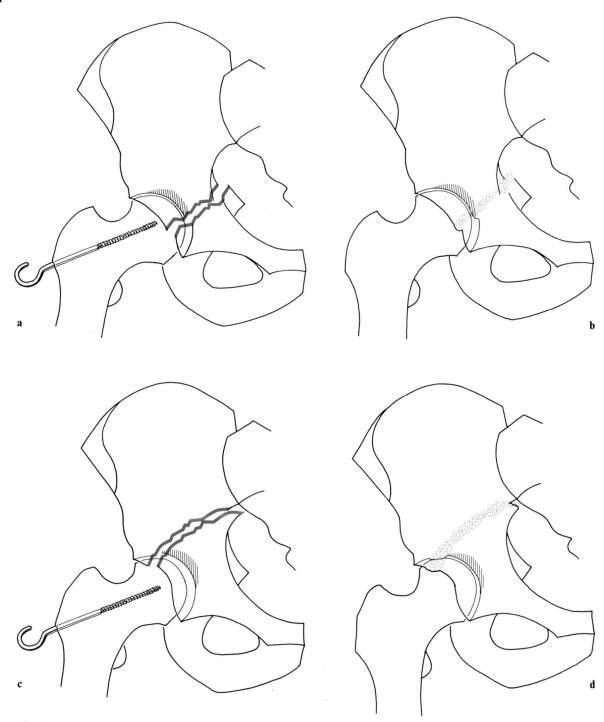

Fig. 13.15 a–d. Transverse fracture of the acetabulum. **a** Diagram indicating a low transverse fracture at the level of the acetabular fossa (infratectal). Closed reduction in this particular injury usually results in a congruous joint. Because the main portion of the weight-bearing dome is intact, as indicated by the *striped lines*, the medial portion of the dome acts as a buttress to the femoral head preventing redisplacement. **b** With healing, the femoral head retains its congruous relationship with the major weight-bearing portion of the acetabulum. **c** In this diagram a high transverse fracture (supratectal, transtectal) divides the mid portion of the superior weight-bearing dome. This shearing injury is difficult to manage with traction and usually results in incongruity because the medial fragment remains displaced and the femoral head is congruous with that portion rather than the dome portion (**d**).

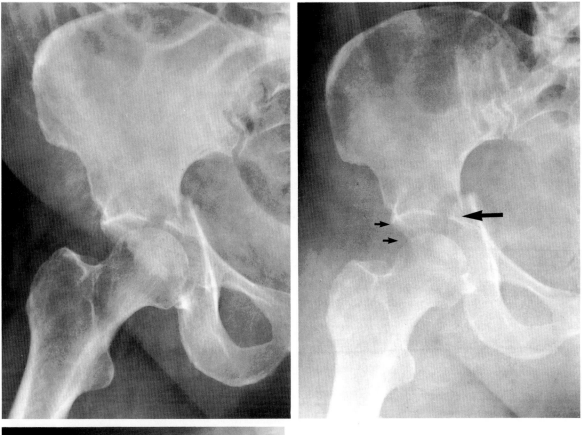

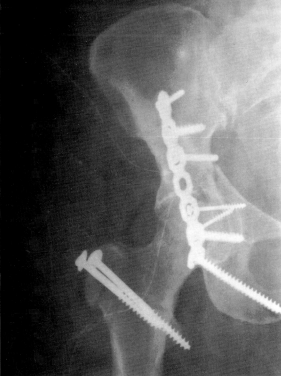

Fig. 13.15 e–g. e Anteroposterior radiograph of a patient with a transverse fracture of the acetabulum. Note that the femoral head is congruous to the medial fragment rather than to the dome. **f** Nine kilograms of traction were applied through a supracondylar pin *(small arrows)*, but the medial portion of the acetabulum did not reduce *(large arrow)*. Restoration of the joint anatomy was possible only with internal fixation (**g**). (From Tile 1984)

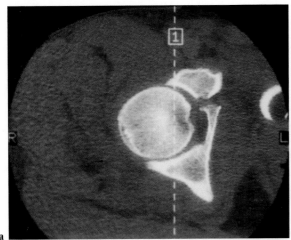

a

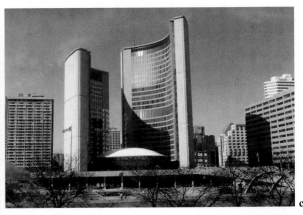

c

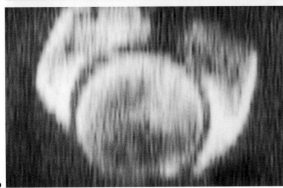

b

Fig. 13.16 a–c. Secondary congruence. The two columns anterior and posterior to the acetabular articular surface surround the femoral head, even though they may be separated by a gap. This is best seen on axial computed tomography (**a**) and the sagittal reconstruction (**b**). The way the two columns embrace the femoral head bears an uncanny resemblance to Toronto's City Hall, whose twin towers surround the round council chamber (**c**). (From Tile 1995)

Both-Column Fracture (Type C) Without Major Posterior Column Displacement. In this injury, both columns are fractured with no portion of the weight-bearing dome attached to the axial skeleton. Both columns are separated from each other; therefore, this is really a type T fracture with the horizontal limb above the acetabulum (resulting in a true floating acetabulum). This fracture occurs in the coronal plane. The transverse portion may be superior to or cephalic to the acetabulum and be truly extra-articular. If the posterior column is minimally displaced, skeletal traction may suffice as definitive treatment. Displacement of the posterior column is best seen on the iliac oblique radiograph which may show no displacement of the posterior column at the inferior pubic ramus. Also, these fractures may exhibit secondary congruence, a term coined by Letournel (1980), characterized by the two fractured columns surrounding the femoral head like peas in an open pod or like the Toronto City Council chamber surrounded by the administrative backup (Fig. 13.16). Secondary congruence in a patient with a both-column fracture (type C) may be managed nonoperatively (Fig. 13.17). The decision must be based on all the radiographic information, including CT and 3D CT where available.

Operative Management (Table 13.4)

Operative management is indicated for the unstable and/or incongruous hip joint.

Unstable Hip

Instability of the hip is most common in posterior types but may also be present with a large free fragment of the quadrilateral plate or in anterior types with anterior wall fracture.

Posterior Fracture Types with Hip Instability. If the posterior lip of the acetabulum is significantly displaced, allowing instability of the hip joint, open reduction and internal fixation are always indicated (Fig. 13.18). Posterior wall fractures may be isolated or they may be associated with posterior column, transverse, T, or double-column fractures. Since the posterior wall injury is usually caused by a blow on the flexed knee, the surgeon must look for knee injuries, including fractures of the patella, or posterior subluxation of the knee with posterior cruciate ligament tears. Also, with posterior dislocation of the hip, a high number of transient or permanent sciatic nerve palsies may be expected.

Table 13.4. Operative indications: Fracture Factors (from Tile 1995)

Hip unstable and/or incongruous
Guidelines to be correlated to patient factors
A. *Instability*: hip dislocation associated with
1. Posterior wall or column displacement
2. Anterior wall or column displacement
B. *Incongruity*
1. Fractures through the roof of the dome
a) Displaced dome fragment
b) Transverse or T types (transtectal)
c) Both-column types with incongruity
(displaced posterior column)
2. Retained bone fragments
3. Displaced fractures of femoral head
4. Soft tissue interposition

Central Instability

Central instability may occur when the quadrilateral plate is large enough to allow the femoral head to sublux centrally. In such cases, some form of medial buttress is essential, either a spring plate or cerclage wire. (Fig. 13.19).

Anterior Instability

Large anterior wall fragments, either in isolation with an associated anterior dislocation (A3) or with an anterior with posterior hemitransverse pattern (B3) may be large enough to allow anterior hip instability and require operative treatment.

Incongruity

The word incongruity comes from the Latin congruus – to fit exactly; therefore incongruity means lack of an exact fit. All major joints require congruity for good long-term function or secondary osteoarthritis will result. This is even more important with post-traumatic joints, since direct articular change is added to the incongruity. Congruity must be assessed on the plain radiographic views as well as by CT and 3D CT. Occasionally, incongruity can only be seen on one view and may be enhanced by CT.

Also unanswered is to what degree a joint can tolerate incongruity. Obviously, perfect anatomical reduction restoring normal anatomy is the ideal, but this may not be possible in all cases. Clinical significance of an incongruous fracture depends on many factors, including the location of the fracture, especially on the superior dome. Also, the size of the gap or more significantly, the size and location of the step is important. Gross instability is obvious (see Fig. 13.19) but more subtle types require careful evaluation (Fig. 13.20).

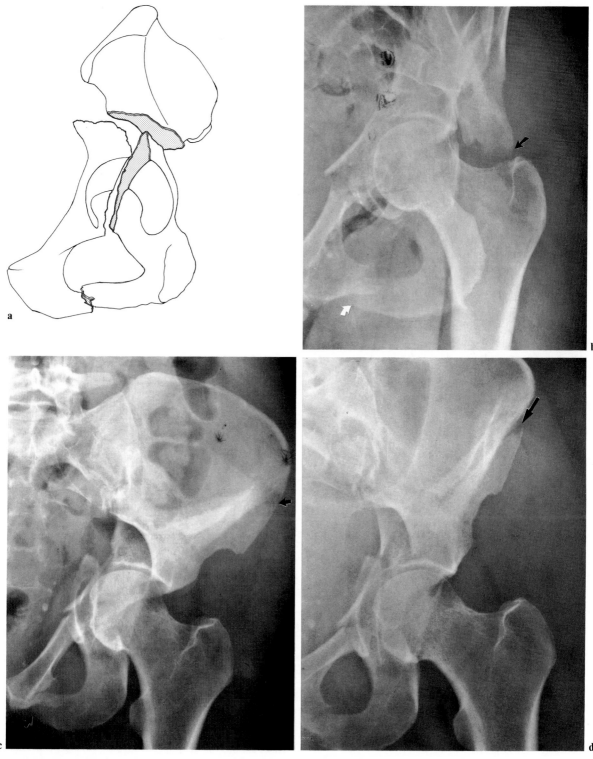

Fig 13.17 a–g. Both-column fracture (type C). **a** Diagram showing the typical appearance of a both-column fracture. The obturator oblique radiograph (**b**) shows the classic spur sign *(black arrow)* Note the split in the posterior column depicted by the fracture through the obturator foramen *(white arrow)* The iliac oblique (**c**) and anteroposterior (**d**) views show the fracture through the iliac crest *(arrows)*.

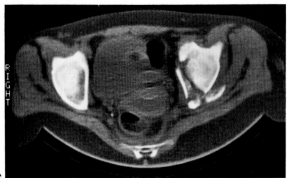

e

Fig 13.17 e–g. The computed tomography scan through the dome (**e**) shows the complex nature of the fracture, with a coronal split through the dome and a fracture in the posterior column. However, in this particular case, note that the femoral head is largely enclosed by the dome fragment. In this patient, a 49-year-old woman, traction was used as definitive treatment. At 2 years, the final result shows a congruous hip joint. The patient rated 90 on the Harris hip scale with only minimal discomfort from the partially united posterior column (**f, g**). (From Tile 1984)

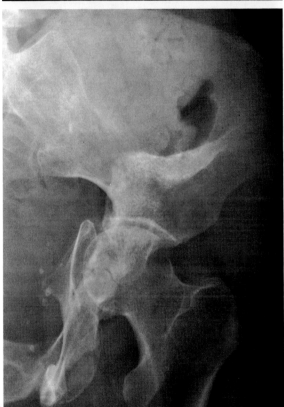

f

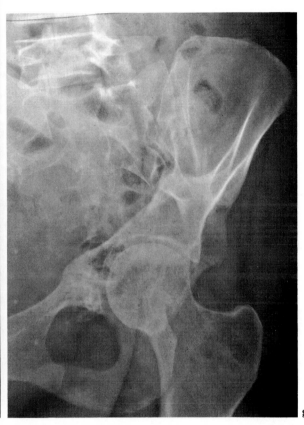

g

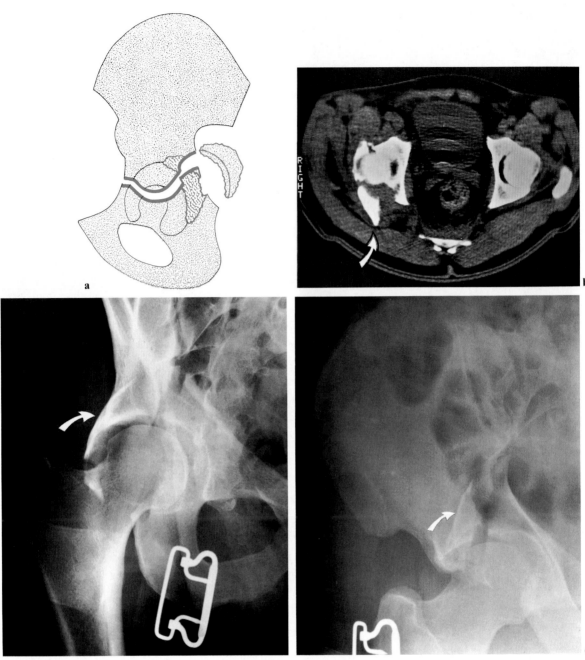

Fig. 13.18 a–d. Posterior fracture with instability. **a** Diagram of a transverse fracture associated with a posterior wall fracture. The computed tomography scan (**b**) shows gross displacement of the large posterior wall fragment through which the posterior dislocation of the hip had occurred. The hip was grossly unstable and the fracture dislocation required operative fixation. The obturator oblique view (**c**) and iliac oblique view (**d**) show the large posterior wall fragment *(white arrows)* and the transverse nature of the fracture. (From Tile 1984)

Fig. 13.19 a–f. Gross incongruity between the femoral head and the acetabulum. **a** Anteroposterior radiograph shows complete central protrusion of the femoral head within the pelvis. **b** On the night of admission, the patient was given a general anesthetic so that the femoral head could be reduced, to prevent articular cartilage pressure necrosis. Congruity was not restored in this T-type fracture. **c** Axial computed tomography (CT) shows the central dislocation of the head, the impingement on the lateral aspect of the head by the lateral fragment, and the classic nature of this T injury. **d,e** A three-dimensional CT image shows the classic appearance of a T fracture with a grossly unstable transverse component. **f** Open reduction and internal fixation using cerclage wires and lag screws achieved anatomical reduction. (From Tile 1995)

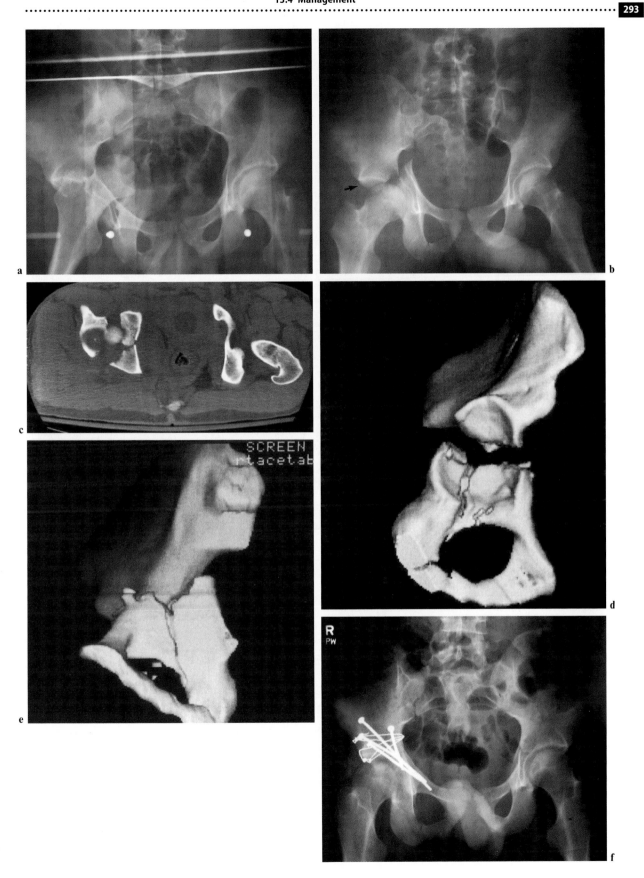

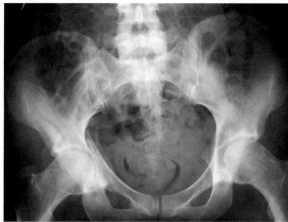

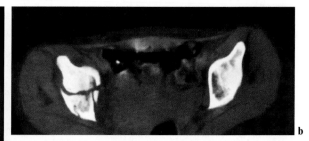

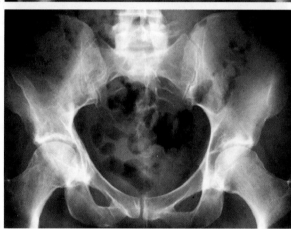

Fig. 13.20 a–c. How much incongruity? **a** Anteroposterior radiograph of a both-column fracture in a young woman injured while skiing. **b** Axial CT through the dome shows the coronal split and minimal incongruity. **c** Treatment consisted of traction without operative intervention. The result at 9 years is excellent congruity of the hip. The patient is functionally normal. (From Tile 1995)

Types of Incongruity (see Table 13.4)

Displacement of the Weight-Bearing Dome

Displaced Dome Fractures. Displacement of the acetabular dome may occur in several varieties of injury:

1. *Displaced triangular dome fragment.* A typical large triangular fragment involving the dome portion of articular cartilage may be displaced and even rotated 90°, as shown in Fig. 13.9. Open reduction and internal fixation are essential to restore the anatomical relationship of that fragment to the remainder of the hip joint.

2. *High transverse or T fractures.* These shearing type injuries involving the superior portion of the dome are extremely difficult to reduce by closed means. Often fragments of bone are interposed, making reduction impossible. In my opinion, these high-energy shearing injuries are extremely difficult to manage nonoperatively because anatomical reduction cannot be maintained and poor results will ensue (see Fig. 13.15 c–g).

3. *Displaced Both-Column Fracture (Type C)* (Fig. 13.21 a–c). In the both-column or floating acetabu-

Fig. 13.21 a–h. Typical type C both-column fracture. Internal ▶ fixation was performed through an anterior ilioinguinal approach. **a** The typical appearance of a type C both-column fracture (type C3) entering the sacroiliac joint *(white arrow),* which is markedly widened. **b** The obturator oblique view shows the pathogonomic spur sign associated with this injury *(black arrow).* **c** Iliac oblique view shows the displacement of the anterior column. **d** Axial computed tomography (CT) shows the widened sacroiliac joint and the fracture of the ilium. **e** The coronal nature of the split is noted, as is the spur sign on this axial CT *(black arrow).* In this case, reduction and fixation were performed through a modified ilioinguinal approach. **f** Fixation techniques used cerclage wire and an anteroposterior lag screw, as well as buttress plates and two anterior plates to fix the sacroiliac joint. **g** Anatomical reduction of the hip joint (**h**) was achieved. (From Tile 1995)

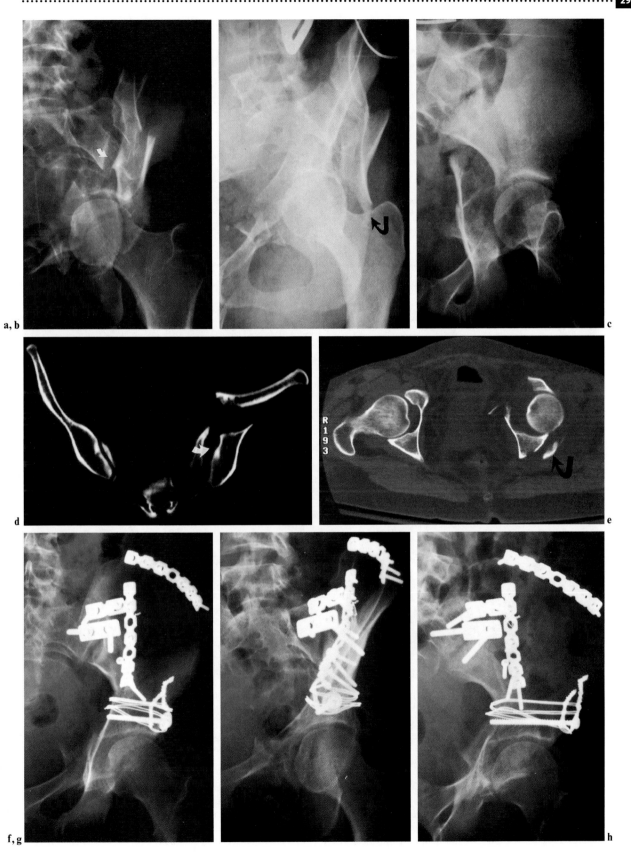

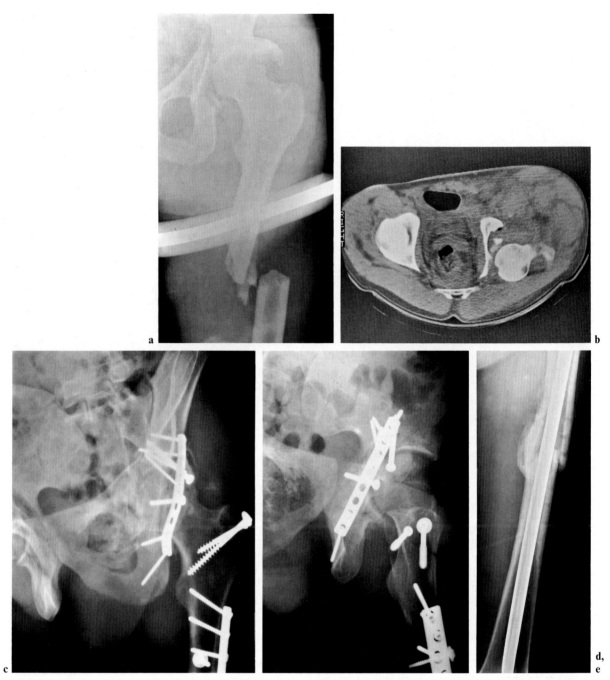

Fig. 13.22. a Anteroposterior radiograph showing a transverse fracture of the left acetabulum with a posterior wall fragment, associated with a comminuted fracture of the shaft of the femur. This patient also had severe involvement of his left sciatic nerve. The severe nature of this injury is best seen on the CT scan showing the posterior dislocation and the retained bony fragment (**b**). Because of his sciatic nerve lesion, his femoral and acetabular fractures were internally stabilized on the night of admission, the femur with a plate and interfragmental screws and the acetabulum through a transtrochanteric approach, using interfragmental screws for the posterior fragment and a neutralization 3.5-mm dynamic compression plate, as shown on the obturator oblique (**c**) and iliac oblique (**d**) radiographic views. Also, since we had planned to use the transtrochanteric approach to the hip, an intramedullary nail would have been technically difficult and undesirable. This patient had excellent restoration of congruity of his hip with an excellent clinical result. However, his femur failed to unite. Following a fracture through the plate at the site of the nonunion, an intramedullary nail was inserted (**e**), eventually resulting in sound union. The peroneal division of the sciatic nerve never recovered. In this situation, primary stable plating of the femur allowed full control of the femoral head without concern that the femoral fracture would redisplace. (From Tile 1984)

lum fracture, the coronal split of the ilium may extend directly into the joint with gross displacement visible in the coronal plane, best seen on the CT scan. Note the coronal split in the dome in Fig. 13.21 e, as compared to the split in the dome parallel to the quadrilateral plate, indicating a transverse type fracture. This type of both-column fracture is best managed by open reduction and internal fixation (Fig. 13.21 f–h).

Retained Bone Fragments. Large retained bone fragments within the acetabulum may act as a block to anatomical reduction or may prevent normal biomechanical function of the joint. These fragments are best seen on the CT scan (Fig. 13.22). They should be removed surgically as soon as possible following injury.

Occasionally, a small fragment of bone will be seen within the fovea on a CT scan (Fig. 13.23). This fragment often represents an avulsion of the pelvic attachment of the teres femoris ligament. Avulsion of a small fragment of bone from the femoral head may also be seen. Neither of these requires removal, since they do not interfere with joint function or joint congruity.

Fracture of the Femoral Head. With dislocation of the femoral head, large bone fragments may be avulsed, usually with an intact teres ligament. This type of injury may occur with a pure dislocation or with a concomitant acetabular fracture. If the head fragment is large enough to cause instability of the hip joint or is displaced enough to cause incongruity, it should be restored anatomically and fixed with screws (Fig. 13.24).

Soft Tissue Interposition. Occasionally, the posterior capsule may interpose between the femoral head and the acetabulum during reduction of a dislocation or may prevent reduction, both indications for operative care.

Other Operative Indications. These include:

1. The development of a sciatic or femoral nerve palsy after reduction of the acetabular fracture, indicating the possible entrapment of the nerve at reduction.
2. The presence of a femoral arterial injury associated with an anterior column fracture of the acetabulum. In this circumstance, the fracture should be fixed at the time of primary vascular repair.
3. Fracture of the ipsilateral femur, which makes closed treatment of the acetabulum virtually impossible; open reduction is therefore indicated for both the fractured femur and the acetabular fracture (see Fig. 13.22). The same is true for an ipsilateral knee disruption.

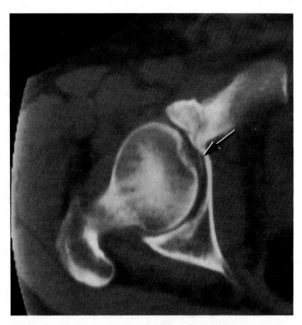

Fig. 13.23. Note the small avulsion fracture *(arrow)* located entirely within the fovea. This patient has a fracture through the anterior column and sustained a partial subluxation of the hip anteriorly. Upon reduction of the femoral head a small foveal avulsion is noticeable

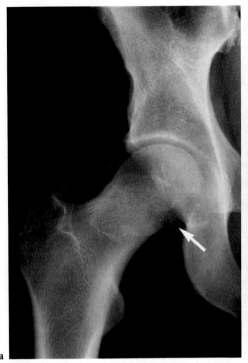
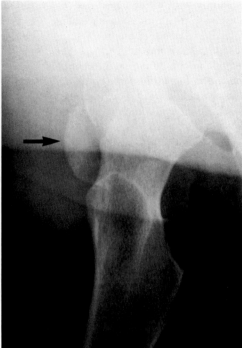

a

b

Fig. 13.24 a, b. Fracture of the femoral head. **a** Anteroposterior view of a 39-year-old man with a fracture of the femoral head secondary to a posterior dislocation. Note the large defect on the inferior aspect of the head *(arrow).* **b** On the lateral radiograph a large fragment is noted anterior to the femoral neck

Fig. 13.24 c–i This is clearly seen on the computed tomography (CT) scan (**c**; *arrow*). Note the posterior wall fracture on the CT scan cut through the dome (**d**; *arrow*). **e** The operative appearance of this fragment is indicated by the *arrow* and its size is readily appreciated following reduction (**f, g**). The fragment was fixed with two 4-mm cancellous screws (**h, i**). The final result at 4 years is excellent

13.4.2 Patient Factors

After full consideration of the fracture factors, the final decision regarding open vs closed treatment depends on the patient factors. These factors include the physiological age, the medical state, the associated injuries, and the type of trauma sustained.

Clearly, the younger the patient assuming an indication for operative care, the more the surgeon should strive for anatomical open reduction and internal fixation.

In older patients, the decision is often more difficult. These patients may have poor quality bone which will not hold a screw and severe comminution which may be impossible to reconstruct, so at the end of a 5- to 6-h difficult operative procedure, traction may still be required for 6–8 weeks. In these circumstances, it may be more prudent to use traction, restore some congruity, and wait and see. The results may be surprisingly good (Fig. 13.25 a, b). If osteoarthritis ensues, a total hip arthroplasty may be done. If in the older patient the surgery is simple, as in a posterior wall, and the indication

is strong, e.g., hip instability, then the benefits of open reduction are greater than the risks and should be performed. In rare instances, primary total hip arthroplasty may be done. (Romness 1990).

13.4.3 Decision Making Algorithm

After careful consideration of the *fracture personality*, including both fracture and patient factors, the treatment of the patient's acetabular injury will follow the algorithm shown in Fig. 13.26.

13.4.3.1 General Resuscitation

Since these patients are often severely injured or polytraumatized, aggressive early resuscitation is essential as previously outlined in Chap. 12 following the guidelines of The American College of Surgeons (Aprahamian et al. 1981).

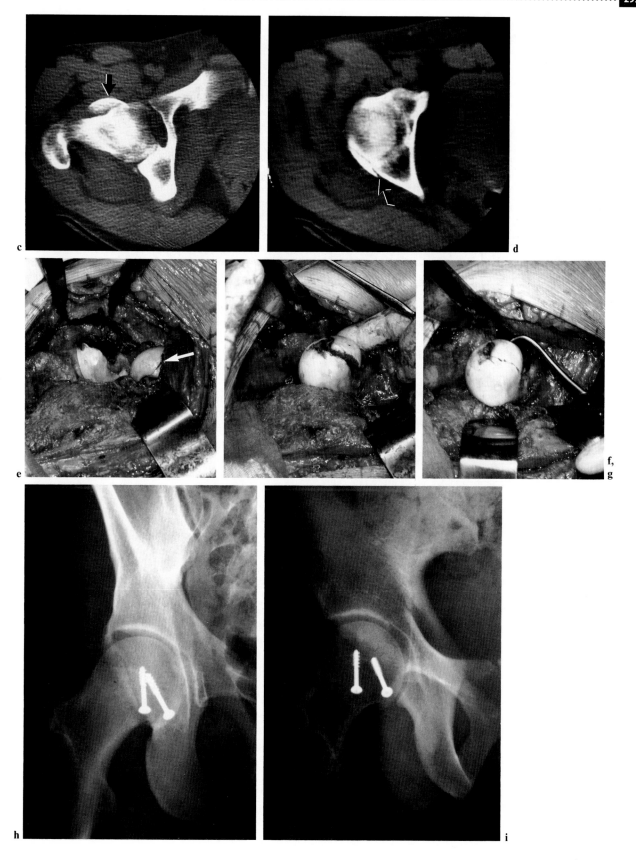

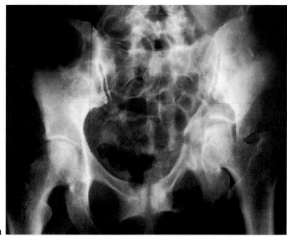

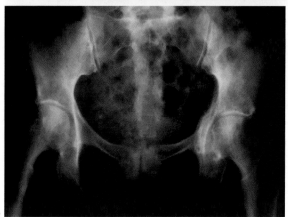

Fig. 13. 25. a Anteroposterior radiograph of a severely comminuted both-column fracture in an elderly woman. **b** Treatment in traction allowed reduction of the fracture and resulted in an excellent clinical and radiographic result. (From Tile 1995)

13.4.3.2 Fracture Personality Assessment

The guidelines for nonoperative care and the operative indications based on all factors have been detailed in the previous section (see Tables 13.3, 13.4). If the fracture is undisplaced or minimally displaced, retaining congruity and stability, nonoperative care with or without traction as necessary is advised.

13.4.3.3 Significant Displacement or Dislocation

If the patient has a *dislocation of the hip joint*, a general anesthetic should be administered to reduce the dislocation. During the same anesthetic, the stability of the fracture should be assessed under image intensification.

If the patient has *significant displacement* and traction fails to reduce it, this should also be reduced under general anesthesia. This is especially true for marked medial displacement of the femoral head, since failure to reduce the femoral head from the pelvis may cause early pressure necrosis of articular cartilage (Fig. 13.27), which may occur within 14 days of injury. Therefore, the femoral head should not be allowed to ride on the sharp lateral fragment of bone in these high transverse injuries. If the head can be easily reduced without an anesthetic, as will be indicated on image intensification or the plain radiograph, then a general anesthetic is not required.

Following reduction of the dislocation or the fracture under anesthesia or by traction without anesthesia, a skeletal traction pin is placed in the supracondylar area of the femur. *Do not insert a trochanteric pin at this stage, since the final method of treatment has not been determined.* If surgery is required and is delayed because of other factors, sepsis around that pin may jeopardize a surgical approach. Therefore, we feel that *there is no place for trochanteric traction in the immediate phase of fracture management.*

13.4.3.4 Urgent Open Reduction and Internal Fixation

Although most operative procedures on the acetabulum are delayed, there are indications for immediate or urgent surgery, including:
- An irreducible dislocation
- An unstable hip following reduction
- An increased neurological deficit following reduction or an increasing neurological deficit with CT evidence of pressure on the nerve
- An associated vascular injury
- An open fracture

13.4.3.5 Assessment of Congruity

Following closed reduction, and application of traction, usually using 30 lb (13.5 kg) two possibilities arise:
1. *Congruous reduction.* If the reduction of the acetabulum is congruous on the plain radiographs and CT scan, traction may be continued as the primary form of treatment. With anatomical restoration, a good result may be expected. We have already indicated those types of fracture which are most likely to result in a congruous reduction and those which are not. It is essential that the reduction is noted on all radiographic tests, including all plain views and CT.
2. *Incongruous reduction.* If the reduction is clearly incongruous, then further decision making is required. In most instances, incongruity may be suspected immediately and would be rarely altered by the appearance in traction.

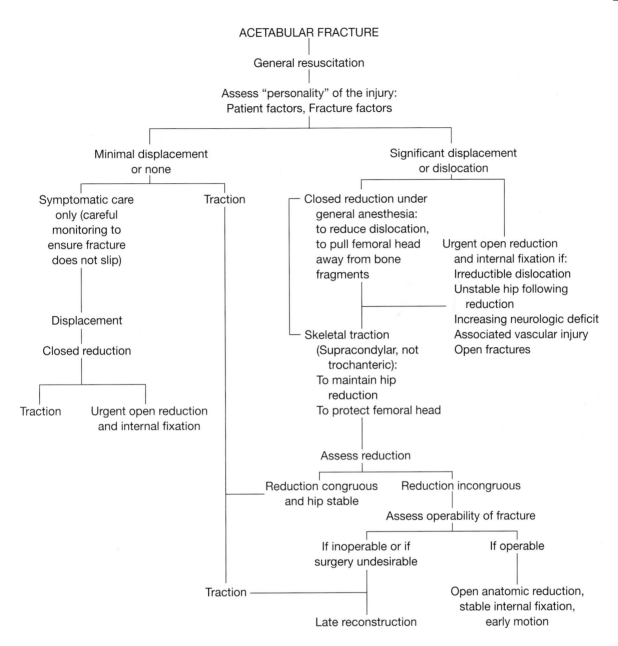

Fig. 13.26. Management algorithm. Application of indications to the individual patient. (From Tile 1995)

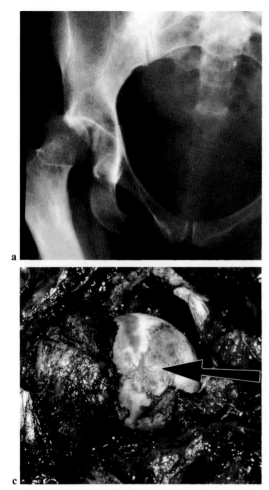

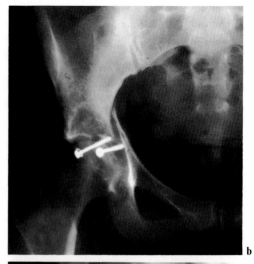

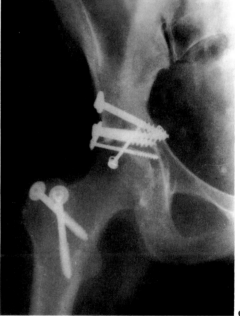

Fig. 13.27 a–d. Pressure necrosis of articular cartilage. **a** Anteroposterior radiograph of the right hip of a 48-year-old woman with a posterior fracture dislocation. **b** The postoperative radiograph at 6 weeks shows the fixation of the posterior wall fracture. The previously undisplaced transverse fracture of the acetabulum displaced in the 6-week period. **c** Intraoperative photograph showing the large zone of pressure necrosis of the articular cartilage on the femoral head *(arrow)*. **d** Postoperative radiograph showing the transverse fracture of the acetabulum fixed with four interfragmental screws. The reduction is anatomical. In spite of the large zone of pressure necrosis the patient has an excellent result at 2 years

13.4.3.6 Assessment of Operability

If the reduction is incongruous, the next step is to assess the *operability* of the fracture and any potential contra-indications to surgery. The important determinants concerning the operability of a fracture are the experience of the surgeon making the decision and the age and general state of the patient. Therefore the surgeon needs to ask the questions, is the fracture stable, and if so can I fix it or should I refer the patient? As one's experience grows, the number of one's seemingly inoperable cases become greatly reduced. In the case shown in Fig. 13.28, that of a 19-year-old male who jumped from a bridge, the surgeon recognized the difficulty involved but did not have the technical expertise to perform an adequate

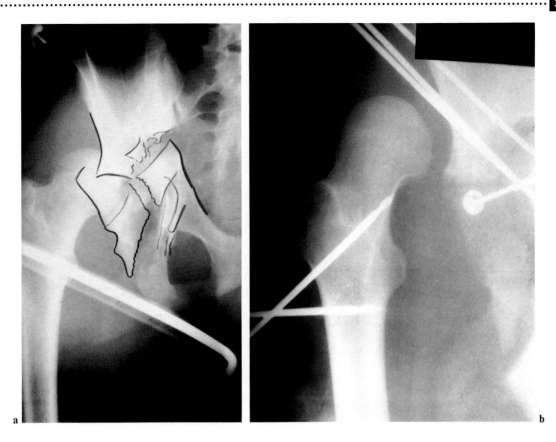

a   b

Fig. 13.28. a Anteroposterior radiograph of a 19-year-old man who jumped from a height, sustaining multiple injuries as well as a fracture dislocation of the right acetabulum. This fracture was severely comminuted. Fixation was attempted by a surgeon not versed in acetabular surgery. **b** The postoperative radiograph at 3 days. The fracture is not anatomically reduced, is inadequately fixed, and the femoral head is dislocated. (From Tile 1984)

open reduction and internal fixation, with disastrous results. The patient would have been far better managed in traction than by the method used. These types of injuries are best sent to centers where the volume of cases is sufficient to afford adequate experience with these difficult problems (Fig. 13.29). Therefore, if the patient's general state or age preclude surgery or the fracture cannot be technically fixed – and this latter contraindication is rare indeed – then traction should be continued and a late reconstructive procedure, namely, a total hip arthroplasty or arthrodesis anticipated.

Where the fracture is incongruously reduced but deemed technically operable, open reduction is indicated and the results will be improved if congruity is restored. The results will not be improved if surgery fails to achieve congruity (see Fig. 13.3); therefore, if surgery is performed at all, the surgeon must strive for anatomical reduction and stable fixation of all major components of

the fracture (Fig. 13.30). Early motion is then possible, allowing early rehabilitation of the hip joint.

At some centers (Romness 1990) where considerable experience in acetabular surgery has been gained early total hip arthroplasty is being recommended in patients in whom operative open fixation will yield poor results, such as the older patient with severe comminution especially with a fractured femoral head. The technical difficulties of securing good fixation of the acetabulum should not be underestimated and also requires considerable experience. Using the morselized femoral head as a bone graft and inserting an uncemented cup with screws is the present method of choice, but screw fixation may also be difficult in the porotic bone.

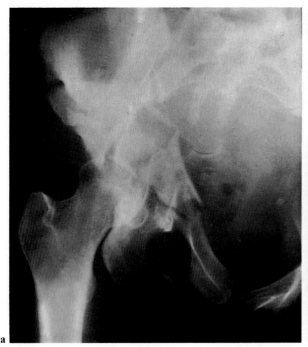
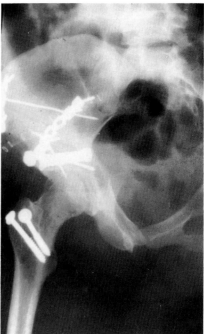

a   b

Fig. 13.29. a Severely comminuted both-column (C type) fracture of the right acetabulum. This fracture at first glance appears inoperable, but, with careful planning, surgical reconstruction was performed, resulting in an anatomical reduction and excellent internal fixation of this fracture (**b**). The result at 8 years is excellent

13.4.4 Surgical Considerations

13.4.4.1 General Considerations

Timing

We prefer to operate electively as early as is feasible following the traumatic incident, usually on the fourth to seventh day after trauma. The surgical procedures may be lengthy, often requiring 6 or more hours. Also, the best possible operating room team must be available. This is rarely possible at night.

There are indications for immediate open reduction (see Sect. 13.4.3.4 and Fig. 13.26), including entrapment of the sciatic nerve following closed reduction and rupture of the femoral artery, necessitating immediate vascular repair. In the latter instance, the incision should be carefully planned with the vascular surgeon to allow open reduction of the anterior column of the acetabulum, the usual offending bone, which penetrates the femoral artery and occasionally the femoral nerve. An irreducible dislocation is another indication for emergency surgery.

Antibiotics

Prophylactic intravenous antibiotics are given just prior to surgery and for 48 h following surgery.

Blood

Six to eight units of blood are usually required during the operative procedure. In rare instances, a previously ruptured and clotted superior gluteal artery may be manipulated, dislodging the clot. If the patient has had major blood transfusions preoperatively, bleeding may be profuse because of ineffective coagulation. In such cases, the area must be packed in the hope that clotting will ensue. If the artery cannot be visualized and bleeding continues, a safe procedure would be to close the wound, take the patient to the angiography department and use an arterial clot of Gelfoam (Upjohn Pharmaceutic Co., Kalamazoo, MI, USA) or other substance to stop the bleeding. If the patient is in extremis, a direct surgical approach in the pelvis is essential.

A cell saver is a very useful addition in these difficult cases.

Neurologic Monitoring. In most centers, neurological monitoring, either motor or sensory or both, is used almost routinely. Many studies indicate that early detection of nerve dysfunction intraoperatively will help to lower the incidence of permanent nerve damage postoperatively (Baumgaertner et al. 1993, unpublished; Vrahas et al. 1992; Helfet et al. 1991; Helfet and Schmeling 1992).

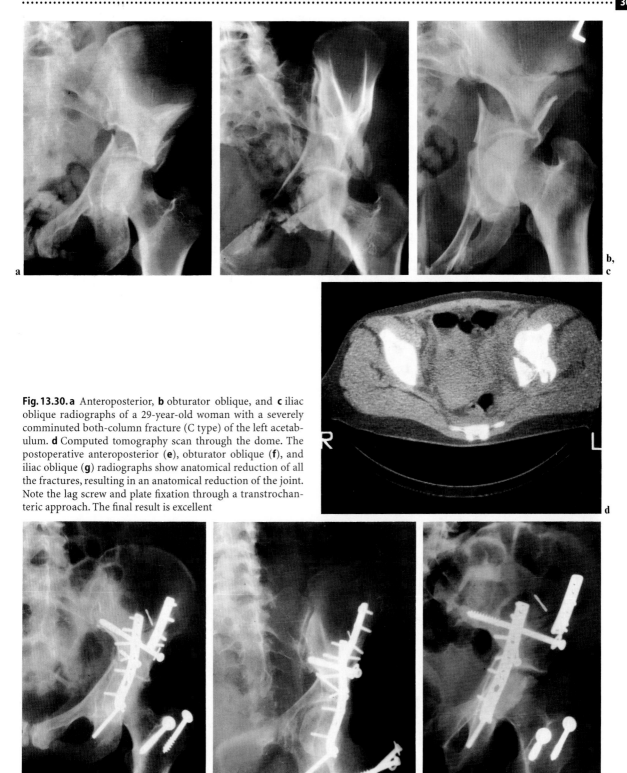

Fig. 13.30. a Anteroposterior, **b** obturator oblique, and **c** iliac oblique radiographs of a 29-year-old woman with a severely comminuted both-column fracture (C type) of the left acetabulum. **d** Computed tomography scan through the dome. The postoperative anteroposterior (**e**), obturator oblique (**f**), and iliac oblique (**g**) radiographs show anatomical reduction of all the fractures, resulting in an anatomical reduction of the joint. Note the lag screw and plate fixation through a transtrochanteric approach. The final result is excellent

13.4.4.2 Approaches

The choice of surgical approach is determined by the type of fracture. Several approaches are available to the surgeon and may be summarized as follows:

1. Anterior
   a. Iliofemoral
   b. Ilioinguinal

2. Posterior
   a. Posterior Kocher-Langenbeck
   b. Posterior transtrochanteric

3. Extensile
   a. Triradiate transtrochanteric
   b. Extended iliofemoral
   c. Combined approaches

We have found the guidelines given below helpful in determining the type of surgical approach we use (Table 13.5).

At this time, several trends as to selection of surgical approach have emerged. It is obvious that posterior wall fractures require posterior approaches and major anterior column displacements anterior approaches. However, there is some evidence and much perception that extensile approaches cause more complications than simple ones, and that anterior approaches are safer and less complicated than posterior. The trend is to use anterior approaches, where possible, and to fix the posterior column by retrograde techniques especially in both-column (type C) fractures (Helfet 1991). Also, a single approach rather than an extensile approach is advocated, again, using indirect fixation techniques under image intensification. Where necessary, a second approach (combined) done simultaneously is being advocated rather than the extensile approach (Winquist 1980).

The debate is not over, but the above are definite trends at this time. The extensile approaches are being used in difficult delayed reconstructions and also by some surgeons, as preferred.

Anterior Approach

Iliofemoral. For fractures of the *anterior column*, where the main displacement is superior to the hip joint, the iliofemoral approach will suffice (Fig. 13.31). With this incision, the surgeon cannot gain access to the anterior column distal to the iliopectoral eminence, but in many cases this is unnecessary. Increased exposure may be obtained by adduction and internal rotation of the hips. Through this approach, lag screw compression of the anterior joint fracture is possible, but a plate cannot be fixed to the anterior column distal to the joint. Proximal plates may be fixed to the ilium with ease. This approach has the advantage of relative simplicity and safety but its restricted exposure limits its use. Therefore, this approach is used for anterior column fractures (Fig. 13.32), anterior wall fractures, and anterior column with posterior hemitransverse fractures, since the posterior hemitransverse segment is often undisplaced.

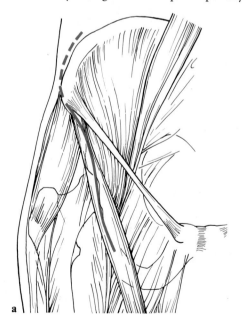

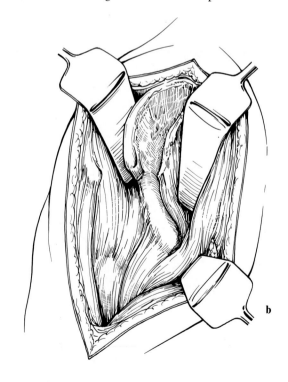

Fig. 13.31 a, b. Iliofemoral approach. **a** Skin incision. **b** Deep dissection by removal of muscles of inner and often outer surface of the pelvis

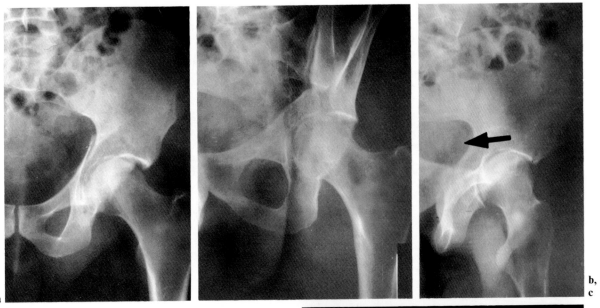

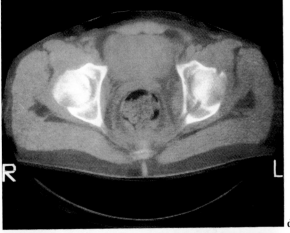

Fig. 13.32 a–f. Fixation of a high anterior column fracture. The anteroposterior radiograph (**a**) shows a high anterior column fracture of the left acetabulum. Note the medial displacement of the femoral head causing incongruity of the hip joint. This is more clearly seen on the obturator oblique view (**b**). The iliac oblique view (**c**) shows the posterior column to be intact *(arrow)* as does the computed tomography scan (**d**). The fracture was fixed through an anterior iliofemoral approach. Note the fixation by two interfragmental lag screws and a neutralization plate. The postoperative anteroposterior (**e**) and obturator oblique (**f**) radiographs show congruity restored to the hip joint. The result at 2 years is excellent

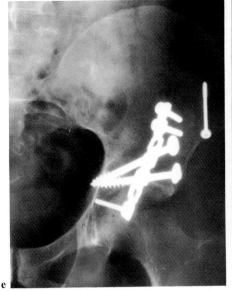

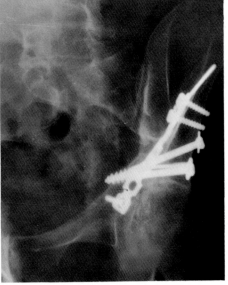

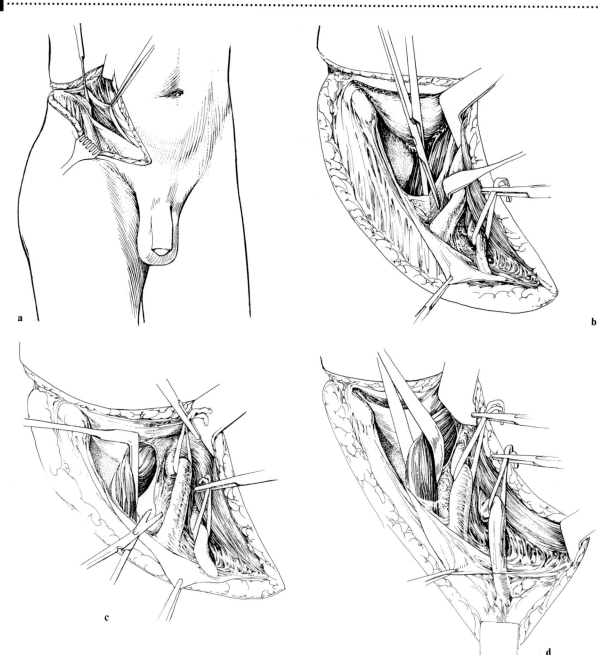

Fig. 13.33 a–d. Ilioinguinal approach. **a** The *inset* shows the incision, which begins along the lateral aspect of the iliac crest and extends forward over the anterior superior spine, then runs directly to the symphysis pubis. The periosteum on the iliac crest is divided to the anterior superior spine, and the iliacus muscle is dissected subperiosteally with an elevator from the interior aspect of the ilium. The sacroiliac joint can be exposed through this approach. The *dotted line* shows the incision through the external oblique aponeurosis. **b** The aponeurosis has been divided, exposing the spermatic cord and the underlying iliopsoas fascia. In the *inset*, the iliopsoas fascia is identified and is divided to the iliopectineal eminence. Note the retractor around the great vessels. **c** The position of the scissors has changed, and they now divide the iliopsoas fascia along the bony attachment in the region of the iliopectineal eminence. **d** Tapes have been placed around the spermatic cord, the femoral artery and vein, and the iliopsoas muscle, to allow access to the underlying bone. By retracting the iliopsoas medially, the iliac crest can be identified. By reflecting it laterally and the vessels medially, the quadrilateral plate can be reached.

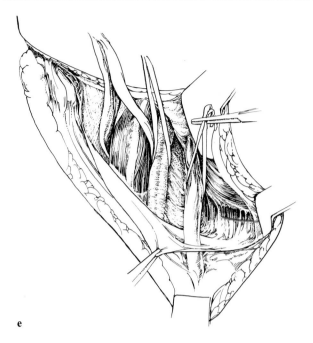

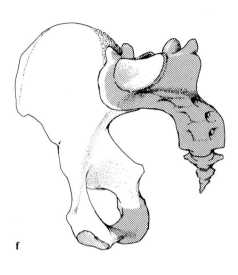

f

e

Fig. 13.33 e, f. e To reach the symphysis pubis, the rectoris abdominis sheath is divided and the muscle is removed from its insertion into the symphysis along the dotted line. **f** The *dotted area* reveals the access of the entire interior aspect of the pelvis, including the sacroiliac joint, which can be achieved through the ilioinguinal approach. (From Steinberg 1991)

Ilioinguinal. For difficult fractures with anterior displacement where access to the whole anterior column is essential, the ilioinguinal approach is ideal (Fig. 13.33). This approach allows access to the entire anterior column as far as the symphysis pubis, as well as to the quadrilateral plate. Some both-column fractures are also amenable to this approach, mainly those fractures with a large single fragment of posterior column. With these fractures, the posterior column may be approached anteriorly by exposing the quadrilateral plate. The posterior column forms the posterior portion of the quadrilateral plate and may be reduced and fixed by lag screws through this approach.

The Stoppa modification of the medial window of the ilioinguinal approach may allow more direct visualization of the posterior column and direct fixation with plates (Winquist 1980).

Because the original description of the ilioinguinal approach makes intra-articular visualization of the hip impossible, we often make a T extension of the incision just medial to the anterior superior spine to allow exposure of the hip joint anteriorly (Fig. 13.34). This is really the iliofemoral approach to the hip joint, exposing the articular surface of the joint which is so necessary in these intra-articular fractures (Gorczyca et al. 1994).

Table 13.5. Guidelines for choice of approach to acetabular fractures (from Tile 1995)

Type of fracture	Approach
Anterior	
Cephalad to iliopectineal eminence	Iliofemoral
Complex patterns requiring exposure to the symphysis and quadrilateral plate	Ilioinguinal
Posterior wall or posterior column	Posterior Kocher-Langenbeck
Transverse, with posterior lip involvement	Posterior Kocher-Langenbeck or transtrochanteric
Transverse, no posterior lip	Approach depends on the rotation of the fracture
T type	Approach depends on pattern: may be posterior, anterior extensile, or some combination
Both-column	Triradiate transtrochanteric, extended iliofemoral, ilioinguinal, modified ilioinguinal, or combined

The T extension extends between the tensor fasciae latae and the sartorius muscles, exposing the rectus femoris muscle. The lateral portion of the rectus femoris muscle is incised, exposing the anterior capsule of the hip joint which is incised medially approximately 2 mm beyond the acetabular labrum.

The anterior surface of the joint is now clearly visible. This approach allows the surgeon to see the anterior col-

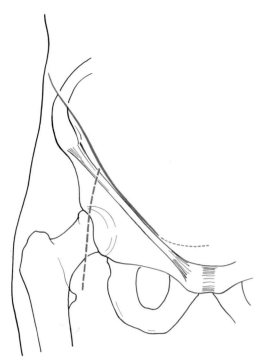

Fig. 13.34. Ilioinguinal approach with T extension to allow intra-articular visualization of hip joint

umn, the quadrilateral space, and the interior of the joint. It is extensile and allows fixation of the symphysis pubis if required. However, the approach requires considerable surgical expertise. It is recommended that it be done in the anatomy department or on a cadaver prior to its use in a patient. The approach is relatively safe, but care must be taken to protect the femoral nerve within the psoas sheath and the femoral vessels.

Posterior Approach

We have adopted the following philosophy where posterior approaches are indicated.

Kocher-Langenbeck. In *isolated posterior lip* injuries and in *posterior column* injuries, either isolated or associated with a posterior lip, a posterior Kocher-Langenbeck approach is employed (Fig. 13.35 a–c). The incision extends from a point distal to the posterior superior spine of the ilium obliquely to the greater trochanter and then distally down the shaft. The gluteus maximus muscle is split and the tensor fasciae latae muscle incised along the femoral shaft, exposing the greater trochanter and the short external rotators of the hip. The insertion of the piriformis tendon into the posterior aspect of the greater trochanter and the obturator internus tendon more distally into the greater trochanter are identified

and tagged. In most cases, the sciatic nerve exits the sciatic notch anterior to the piriformis muscle and posterior to the obturator internus muscle. The piriformis, the obturator internus, and the gemelli muscles are divided. The obturator internus protects the sciatic nerve and the underlying obturator bursa is the guide to the posterior column. In this manner, the greater and lesser sciatic notch and the ischial tuberosity can be identified. Interfragmental compression with screws and posterior plates can be applied in this area through this approach.

Posterior Transtrochanteric. For difficult injuries involving the dome of the acetabulum, such as the *transverse T types* with or without a *posterior lip* component, we use the same posterolateral Kocher-Langenbeck skin incision but remove the greater trochanter for increased visualization (Fig. 13.35 d,e). The approach through the gluteus maximus and tensor fasciae latae muscles is the same, and the piriformis muscle and external rotators are divided to expose the posterior column as previously described. However, we feel that removal of the greater trochanter greatly simplifies the operative procedure.

Prior to removal, the greater trochanter is predrilled with the 3.2-mm drill anteriorly and posteriorly to accept the 6.5-mm cancellous screws at the end of the operative procedure. Stable fixation of the trochanter is obtained by this method.

The trochanter is removed transversely and retracted superiorly. The plane between the hip joint capsule and the gluteus minimus muscle is developed, leading the surgeon to the superior aspect of the acetabulum as shown in Fig. 13.35 e. Excellent exposure of the dome and posterior column is obtained with this approach. Further exposure of the anterior aspect of the joint is made possible by dissection anteriorly to expose the anterior inferior spine and the rectus femoris muscle. Removal of the rectus femoris will allow the surgeon to examine the anterior column of the acetabulum. If necessary, fixation of the anterior column will require retrograde lag screws.

The hip joint capsule is often torn. Exposure of the femoral head should be made by dividing the capsule 2 mm beyond the acetabular labrum. Insertion of a corkscrew device into the femoral neck or a sharp hook over the trochanter will allow adequate distraction of the femoral head and excellent visualization of the articular surface (Fig. 13.35 e).

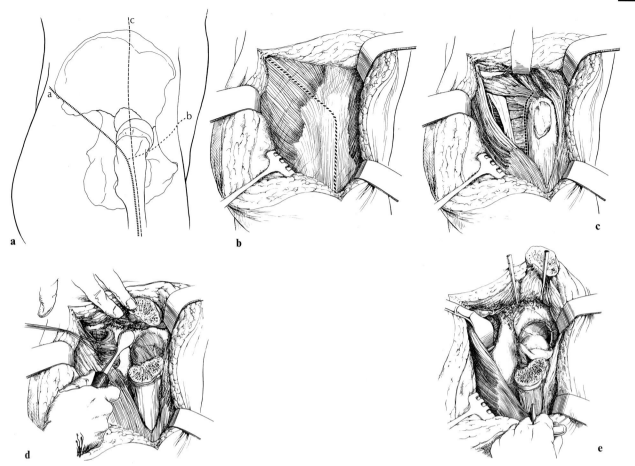

Fig. 13.35. a Diagram demonstrating the incisions for the posterior Kocher-Langenbeck approach *(a)*, a modified Ollier approach *(a+b)* or a straight lateral approach *(c)*. For posterior wall fractures the standard posterior approach *(a)* is routine. If the trochanter needs to be removed, it can be easily done through the same approach. **b** Following division of the skin and subcutaneous tissue the tensor fasciae latae and the gluteus maximus muscle are identified. These structures are divided by splitting the muscle fibers of the gluteus maximus and dividing the tensor fasciae latae longitudinally, as shown by the *striped line*. **c** Following division of the gluteus maximus and tensor fasciae latae, the posterior structures of the hip joint are identified. These include the piriformis, the short external rotators, the quadratus femoris, and the sciatic nerve. The tendons of the short external rotators and the piriformis are divided along the *checkered line*. Care should be taken to preserve the branch of the medial circumflex to the quadratus femoris since it also may supply the femoral head. **d** Elevation of the short external rotators will identify the obturator internus bursa and lead the

surgeon to the greater and lesser sciatic notch. The entire posterior column of the acetabulum is exposed. In order to expose the superior dome and allow access to the anterior column, the greater tuberosity is osteotomized, as shown. **e** Visualization of the posterior column, the superior dome, and the anterior column is excellent with proper exposure through the transtrochanteric approach. Note that the capsule has been opened just along the rim of the acetabular labrum, leaving enough capsular tissue to resuture following open reduction. Note also the superior gluteal vessels and nerve exiting the superior gluteal notch. By using a femoral head extractor inserted distal to the trochanteric osteotomy the femoral head can be pulled from the joint, visualizing the entire articular surface. This is essential if anatomical reduction is to be achieved. It is helpful to insert two Steinman pins under the abductor muscle mass for retraction. All fractures are stabilized provisionally with Kirschner wires and cerclage wires, and definitively with interfragmental screws, wherever possible. Finally, the fractures are stabilized with neutralization plates. (From Tile 1984)

Extensile Approach

Triradiate Transtrochanteric. Type C both-column fractures with major posterior displacement may be approached as previously indicated, that is, a posterolat-

eral incision is made, the same deep dissection carried out, and the trochanter removed. With this fracture, access to the iliac crest is essential, so the incision is carried anteriorly in a triradiate fashion to the anterior superior spine or just distal to it (Fig. 13.36). The tensor

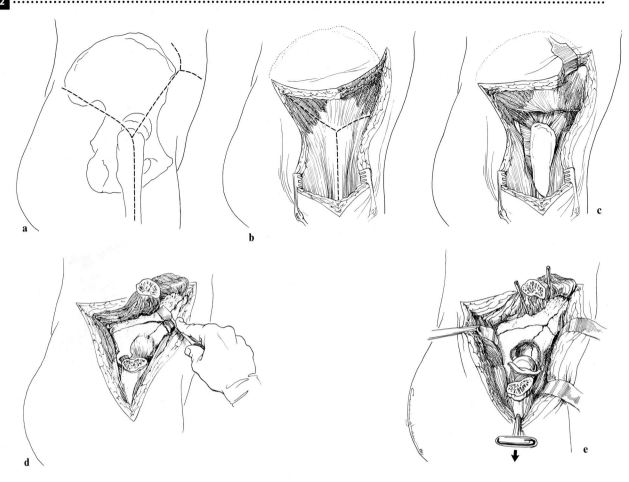

Fig. 13.36 a–e. Triradiate transtrochanteric approach. **a** Skin incision. No skin flaps must be raised: all dissection must be through fascial planes. **b** Exposure of the tensor fasciae latae muscle. **c** Division of the tensor fasciae latae and gluteus maximus muscles. **d** Removal of the greater trochanter and exposure of the lateral and posterior aspect of the pelvis. **e** Capsulorraphy of the hip capsule 2 mm from the pelvic attachment and insertion of a traction device into the femoral head facilitate access to the joint

fasciae latae muscle is divided, exposing the gluteus medius and minimus muscles which are dissected subperiosteally from the outer table of the ilium. The incision may be carried posteriorly along the iliac crest. The addition of the triradiate skin incision and the subperiosteal dissection posteriorly allows excellent visualization of the outer table of the ilium, so essential in the both-column fracture.

The triradiate approach may also expose the inner aspect of the pelvis by extending the anterior limb of the incision to the symphysis, converting it into an ilioinguinal approach. Therefore, this approach is truly extensile, since it allows exposure of both the outer and inner table of the ilium, including both columns.

A word of caution about the posterior approach: The *sciatic nerve* is in jeopardy in this approach and must be protected at all times by flexion of the knee and careful retraction using the muscle belly of the short external rotators for protection, otherwise there will be unacceptably frequent intraoperative damage to the nerve.

Injury to the *superior gluteal artery and nerve* must also be avoided. These can be visualized exiting the greater sciatic notch (Fig. 13.35 e); in this location, they can be easily injured when one is stripping the periosteum from the notch area. If injured, the artery may bleed massively and retract into the pelvis. Packing, embolization, or a direct surgical approach may then be necessary as described above.

Of equal importance is the superior gluteal nerve. This nerve supplies the major hip abductors and the gluteus medius and minimus muscles. Injury may be caused either by a periosteal elevator or by retraction of the abductor muscles superiorly in order to gain visualization of the superior aspect of the acetabulum. Removal of the greater trochanter diminishes this risk, but throughout the operative procedure one must be aware of the possibility of a traction injury to this nerve.

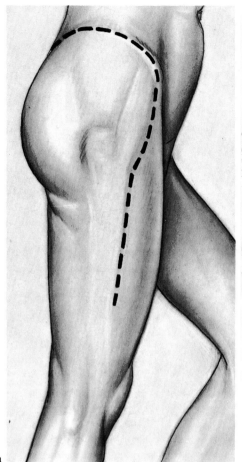

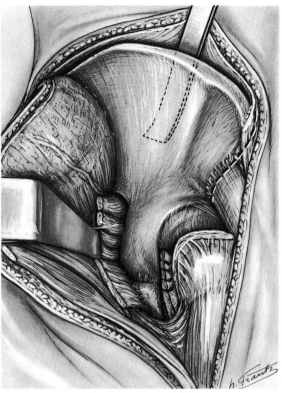

Fig. 13.37 a, b. Extended iliofemoral approach. **a** Skin incision. **b** Deep dissection showing the exposure of the lateral wall of the ilium and posterior column of the acetabulum. (From Letournel and Judet 1981)

Extended Iliofemoral. The extended iliofemoral approach gives excellent visualization of the outer table of the ilium, the superior dome, and the posterior column and may be further extended to include the inner wall of the ilium as well (Fig. 13.37). We have removed the trochanter in the usual fashion rather than divide the abductor muscles.

Heterotopic ossification is a major complication of this approach, as in all approaches which require removal of the abductor muscle mass from the outer table of the ilium. Although visualization is excellent, we have some concern about the vascularization of the very large abductor muscle flap. This abductor flap is based primarily on the superior gluteal artery and vein as they exit from the greater sciatic notch. Venous engorgement may occur, resulting in some vascular insufficiency to the outer end of the muscle and causing necrosis. For this reason, we tend to use the triradiate approach, which keeps a layer of skin intact over the iliac crest to ensure adequate skin healing.

Combined. A simultaneous combined anterior and posterior approach is possible with the patient in the "slop-

py" lateral position. The anterior approach is usually the iliofemoral, the posterior, the Kocher-Langenbeck. Usually the procedure is started using one approach, depending on the fracture type and the other approach used when it is obvious it will be required for anatomical reduction. This combined approach is most commonly used in type B transverse or T fractures to control rotation and is preferred by many surgeons because of the decreased complications and operative time. At this time, this is still debatable as the published results are still sparse (Ruedi et al. 1984); the question can only be finally answered by a large multicentered prospective series.

13.4.4.3 Reduction

Resources

Reduction may be the most difficult aspect of acetabular surgery even with a good exposure. In order to achieve an excellent reduction, the surgeon must have available the following human and material resources:

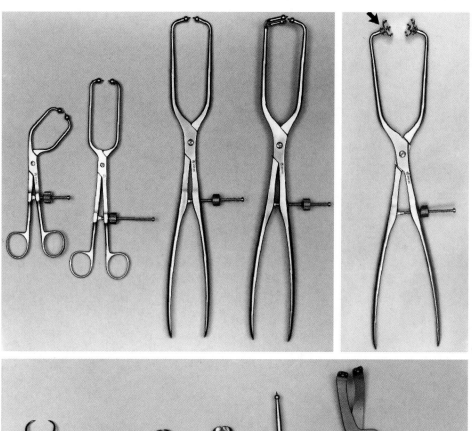

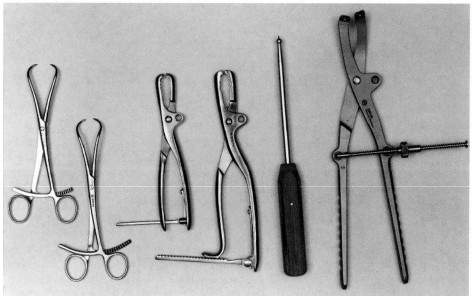

Fig. 13.38 a–c. Special clamps and the ball spike pusher to help with reduction in the acetabulum. **a, b** Clamps include the large and small offset clamp, the single-pronged and double-pronged clamp to fit over the iliac crest, pointed reduction clamps, Farabeuf clamps in two sizes, and pelvic reduction clamps. Note also the ball spike pusher, which is invaluable in reducing small fragments of the acetabular wall and for pushing on the iliac crest. **c.** All of these clamps and the ball spike pusher can be fitted with a spiked disc *(black arrow)* that fits over the ball to prevent the spike from sinking into osteoporotic bone

1. *Assistants.* At least two and occasionally three assistants are necessary for these operative procedures. Of even greater help than the number is the quality of the assistants, since the surgeon cannot continuously keep an eye on the vital structures, such as the sciatic nerve.
2. *Special instruments.* Essential instruments include pointed fracture forceps, fracture reduction clamps, fracture pushers, and other standard fracture clamps (Fig. 13.38). Special pelvic reduction clamps are also

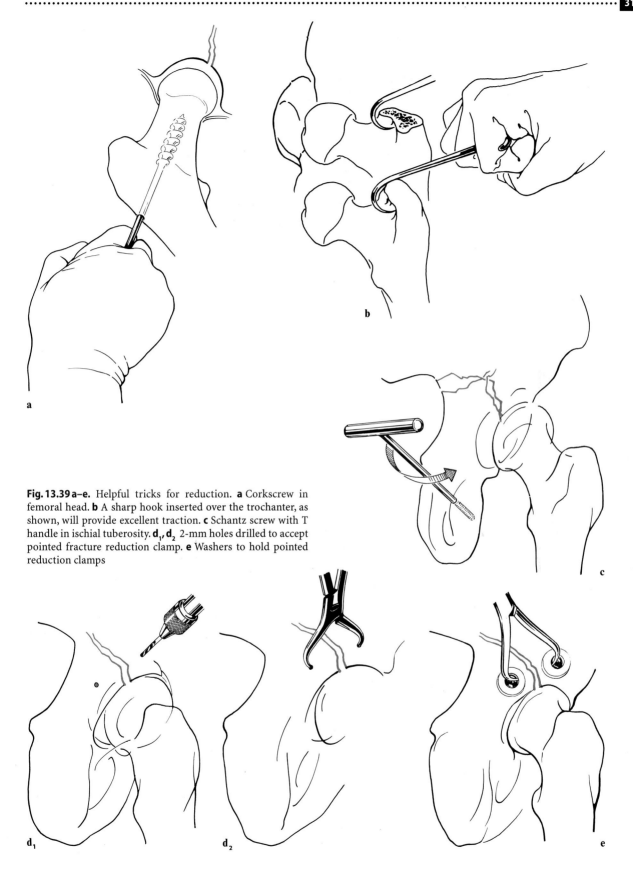

Fig. 13.39 a–e. Helpful tricks for reduction. **a** Corkscrew in femoral head. **b** A sharp hook inserted over the trochanter, as shown, will provide excellent traction. **c** Schantz screw with T handle in ischial tuberosity. **d₁, d₂** 2-mm holes drilled to accept pointed fracture reduction clamp. **e** Washers to hold pointed reduction clamps

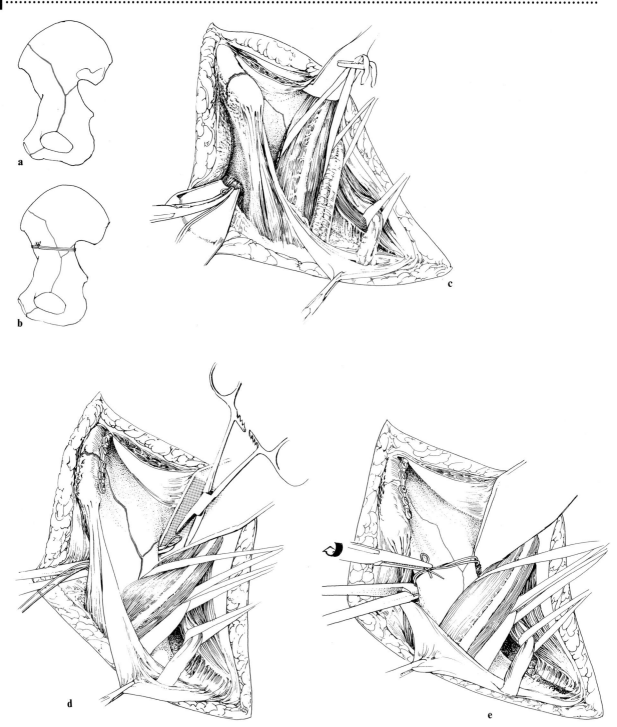

Fig. 13.40 a–e. Use of cerclage wires for reduction and temporary fixation. A both-column acetabular fracture (**a**) was reduced and fixed with a double-loop cerclage wire from the greater sciatic notch to a point just cephalad to the anterior inferior spine (**b**). The technique of insertion of the wires is as follows: (**c**) Both the medial and lateral aspects of the ilium are exposed to the greater sciatic notch. One exposure, usually the medial one, must be large; the opposite one may be small. Insertion of Rang refractors through the notch protects the sciatic nerve. The fracture must be reduced temporarily with clamps to safely pass the wire, in this case on a long, right-angled (Mixter) clamp. **d** The iliac fracture was previously fixed with a curved plate. The wire secures the posterior column. The approach in this case is the ilioinguinal one but modified to allow lateral exposure of the greater sciatic notch. **e** The final appearance of the wire in place through the first window of the ilioinguinal approach. (From Tile 1995)

available and are extremely helpful (Fig. 13.38). The pelvic reduction clamp is screwed directly to the bone using two 4.5-mm cortical screws or 6.5-mm cancellous screws. This clamp can be extremely helpful by applying direct forces to the fracture.

3. *Traction.* Traction on the femoral head is essential in obtaining a reduction. Traction may be obtained by the use of a traction table which must be adaptable, allowing the prone as well as the supine position. An unscrubbed surgeon or technician is needed to control the leg rotation. It is strongly recommended by Letournel (1993).

4. *Helpful Hints for Reduction.* The following tricks may be helpful during this stressful aspect of the surgery:

- The articular surface of the joint *must* be adequately visualized by a wide capsulorrhaphy in most cases. Only by direct visualization of the fracture lines within the joint can the adequacy of the reduction be confirmed (see Figs. 13.35, 13.36).

Most patients can be managed without a traction table, but direct traction on the femoral head is essential. This can be obtained by a corkscrew in the femoral neck to allow better retraction of the femoral head and visualization of the articular surface (Fig. 13.39 a); preferably, a sharp hook over the greater tuberosity can be used to give the same effect (Fig. 13.39 b).

- A 5- or 6-mm Schantz pin with a T handle should be inserted into the ischial tuberosity in high transverse or T type fractures to allow rotation of the posterior column, which in some instances cannot be reduced by any other method (Fig. 13.39 c).

- Holes should be drilled to accept the pointed forceps (Fig. 13.39 d).

- Washers with extensions have been developed for use with the pointed fracture forceps (Fig. 13.39 d,e).

- Work within the fracture. In visualizing impacted fragments from either an anterior or posterior approach, it is important to move the major fracture out of the way so that the impacted fragment can be visualized. This is akin to the tibial plateau fracture where the lateral fragment is retracted like a book to allow reduction of the impacted fragment. Therefore, work within the fracture where possible. Marginally impacted fractures must be reduced in this way.

5. *Cerclage wires* (Kang 1987; Schopfer et al. 1993). Cerclage wires inserted through the greater sciatic notch and around the anterior inferior iliac spine may greatly facilitate derotation and reduction of the columns, especially if either the posterior or anterior column is "high" on the greater sciatic notch (see Fig. 13.21 and Fig. 13.40).

13.4.4.4 Internal Fixation

Implants

Screws
- 6.5-mm cancellous lag screws
- 4.0-mm cancellous lag screws and 3.5 mm cortical screws (lengths up to 120 mm)
- 6.5-mm fully threaded cancellous screws

For lag screw interfragmental compression of the major fractures, we prefer the 6.5-mm cancellous screw. However, in some instances the 4.0-mm cancellous screw or the 3.5-mm cortical screws are essential, especially when fixing smaller fragments. These screws are available in lengths to 120 mm.

For fixation of the plate to the bone, fully threaded cancellous screws are desirable, the 6.5-mm screw for the large reconstruction plate (4.5-mm) and the 3.5-screw for the 3.5-mm reconstruction plate.

Cannulated screws may also be helpful.

Plates. A 3.5-mm reconstruction plate is the implant of choice for acetabular reconstruction. These plates can be molded in two planes and around the difficult areas such as the ischial tuberosity. Also, precurved 3.5-mm plates are available for anterior column fixation. These plates are fixed with the 3.5-mm cancellous screws. In large individuals, and in pelvic fixation, the 4.5-mm reconstruction plates are also useful, with fixation by the 6.5-mm fully threaded cancellous screws (Fig. 13.41); however, they are rarely used at this time.

- *Sites of application.* The plates may be applied to the anterior column from the inner table of the ilium to the symphysis pubis (Fig. 13.42 a). Plates may also be applied to the posterior column and the superior aspect of the acetabulum (Fig. 13.42 b). On the posterior column, the distal screw should be anchored in the ischial tuberosity. *Great care should be taken to ensure that screws in the central portion of the plate do not penetrate the articular cartilage of the acetabulum.* In most instances, no screws should be put into that danger area, but if screws are necessary for stable

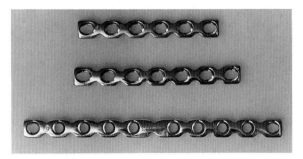

Fig. 13.41. The 3.5-mm and 4.5 mm reconstruction plates for pelvic fixation

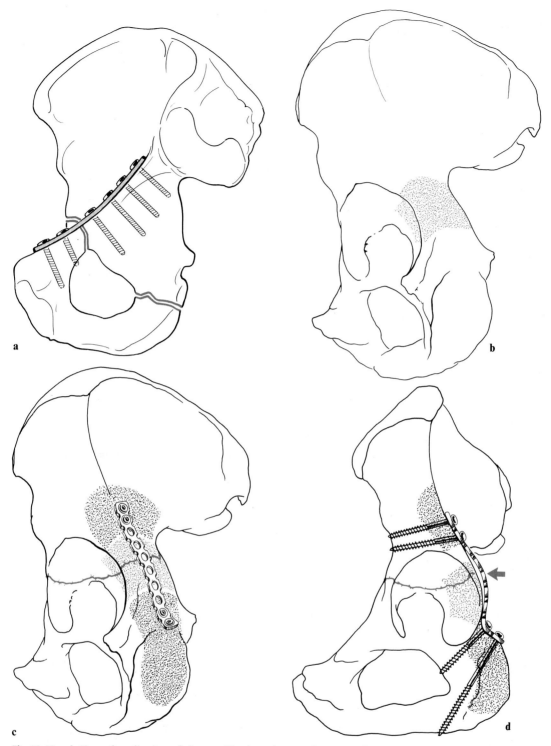

Fig. 13.42 a–d. Sites of application of plates. **a** Fixation of an anterior column fracture with an anteriorly placed plate. **b** Diagram indicating the danger zone for screw fixation in the midportion of the posterior column superior to the ischial spine, demonstrated by the red shading. The posterior column in this area is extremely thin and misdirected screws will commonly penetrate the hip joint. No screws should be placed in this area unless absolutely essential, and then only if directed away from the articular surface. **c** Diagram demonstrating the correct position of a plate placed on the posterior column of the acetabulum. Note that no screws are used in the central posterior portion of the acetabulum to avoid penetration of the articular surface. The most distally placed screw fixes the plate to the ischial tuberosity, best seen in **d**. (**b–d** From Tile 1995)

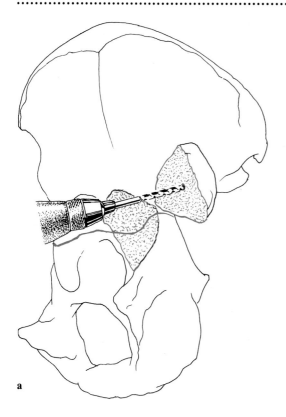
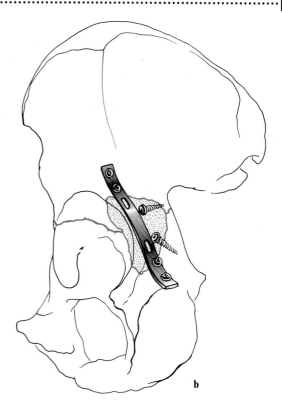

a   b

Fig. 13.43 a,b. Diagrams demonstrating the correct fixation of a posterior wall fracture. **a** The drill bit is positioned in a direction away from the joint so that the articular cartilage cannot be penetrated. After reduction of the fracture Kirschner wires are used for provisional fixation. This will allow the surgeon to carefully plan the position of the interfragmental screws and the neutralization plate along the posterior column (**b**). (**a** From Tile 1995)

fixation, they should be directed away from the joint (Fig. 13.43). Screws within the joint are a not uncommon cause of chondrolysis (Fig. 13.44).

Plates may be nested to buttress small fragments.

Methods of Stable Fixation

Internal Fixation. Stable fixation in the acetabulum, as in all areas, is best achieved by *interfragmental compression using lag screws.* Therefore, after provisional fixation of all fractures with Kirschner wires, or cerclage wires, screw fixation of the fractures is essential. The joint must be visualized at all times to ensure that anatomical reduction has been achieved and that no screw penetrates the articular cartilage. After fixation by interfragmental lag screws, plates may be used to neutralize the fracture. Plates may be placed either on

the anterior or posterior column, depending on the approach.

Adequate contouring of the plates is essential. Otherwise, displacement of the opposite column may occur (Fig. 13.45).

13.4.4 Postoperative Care

The postoperative care depends upon the ability of the surgeon to achieve stable internal fixation which, in turn, depends on the quality of the bone and the adequacy of the reduction. In general, we have maintained skeletal traction and continuous passive motion in the immediate postoperative period for 7 days, and then gradually wean the patient from the machine. If stability is deemed to be excellent, the traction may be removed and the patient ambulated. Weight bearing is not started until some signs of union are present, usually by the sixth postoperative week; however, the patients may be ambulatory with crutches during this period.

If there is concern about the quality of the bone, about gross comminution, especially of the medial wall of the acetabulum, or about inadequate stability, traction should be continued for 6 weeks until some healing of the fragments has occurred. Ambulation may then begin with crutches, followed by progressive weight bearing at approximately 12 weeks.

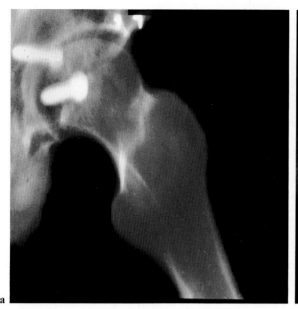 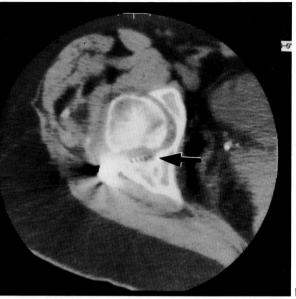

a   b

Fig. 13.44 a, b. Screw in the hip joint. **a** Fixation of a posterior wall fracture with two screws. The inferior screw has entered the hip joint and has eroded the femoral head. **b** Computed tomography scan showing the threads within the joint *(arrow)* and the posterior erosion of the femoral head

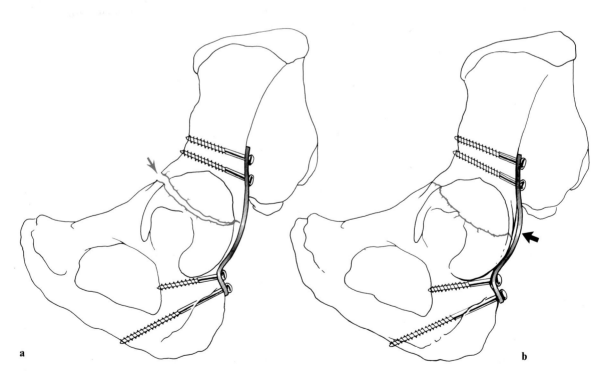

a   b

Fig. 13.45 a, b. Proper contouring of the plate is essential. If the plate is not contoured properly, a fracture which appears reduced posteriorly may in fact be malreduced anteriorly (**a**). Note the proper contour of the plate (**b**)

Indocid (25 mg tid) is used to prevent heterotopic ossification. Low-molecular-weight heparin or coumadin is used in addition to prevent thromboembolic disease.

13.5 Complications

Complications associated with acetabular fractures are common. As in all hip surgery, general complications include thromboembolic disease, wound necrosis, and sepsis. More specific complications include:

– Nerve injury
  1. *Sciatic Nerve.* The sciatic nerve may be injured at the time of trauma or during surgery. Most injuries occur with posterior type lesions or with posterior approaches to the hip. In our first 102 cases, there were 22 sciatic nerve lesions, 16 post-traumatic and six postoperative. All of the patients with postoperative lesions recovered, but the 16 with post-traumatic lesions, only four showed full recovery, while eight showed partial and four no recovery.
  2. *Femoral Nerve.* The femoral nerve may be injured by the spike of the anterior column or during surgery using an ilioinguinal approach. We have seen one patient with a post-traumatic femoral artery injury. A nerve cable graft was performed with poor results, that is, no quadriceps function was restored.
  3. *Superior Gluteal Nerve.* The superior gluteal nerve is situated in a vulnerable position in the greater sciatic notch, where it may be injured during trauma or during surgery, resulting in paralysis of the gluteus medius and minimus muscles.
  4. *Lateral Cutaneous Nerve of the Thigh.* The lateral cutaneous nerve of the thigh is commonly injured in iliofemoral or ilioinguinal approaches. The disability is well tolerated, but the complication is common.

– Heterotopic ossification is a major postoperative complication. In our series, there were 18 cases of significant heterotopic ossification, all associated with posterior approaches to the hip. At the moment, several authors have recommended indocid for the prevention of this complication, which is much higher in males, and in lateral extensile approaches of the hip which strip the gluteus medius from the lateral iliac crest. Moed and Maxey (1993); McLaren (1990) and others have reported on the efficacy although this has been disputed. (J.M. Matta, personal communication). In a recent report, Moed and Letournel (1993) have recommended indocid with one dose of postoperative radiation.

– Avascular necrosis of the femoral head is a devastating complication, developing in 6.6% of Letournel's 302 fractures (Letournel 1980). It was only seen in the posterior types in our series, and was 18% in that group.
Avascular necrosis of the acetabular segments may also occur, causing collapse of the joint.

– Chondrolysis following acetabular fractures can occur with or without surgical intervention. With surgical intervention, infection or metal within the joint must be suspected but it may occur with no apparent cause.

13.6 Conclusions

Our knowledge of acetabular trauma has advanced considerably since the first edition of this book. Our imaging methods especially 3D CT has made the pathoanatomy clear (Fig. 13.46 d,e) and we are reaching consensus of a comprehensive classification based on Letournel's types and using the AO suggested alphanumeric code. Also, most large metropolitan areas in the developed world have pelvic-acetabular referred centers with expert care available. The general orthopedic or trauma surgeon needs to resuscitate the patient with acute trauma and place the patient in traction. The surgeons must ask the question: Can I fix the fracture, can anybody? Straightforward fractures such as in a posterior wall or a posterior column fracture can be handled by most experienced surgeons. Unfortunately, these simple fractures may be complicated by marginal impaction or comminution and may lead to poor outcomes. If the fractures are comminuted, and complex (type B or C), referral to an expert center is desirable (Fig. 13.46 a–c). Referral should be prompt to allow early investigation and surgery to be performed, which will help with anatomical reduction. If the general orthopedic surgeon wishes to treat the more complex injuries, further courses and preferrably fellowship training are important.

In spite of our increased knowledge even in expert centers, the surgical outcomes may be disappointing (Johnson 1994). The prognosis depends on the original injury, which, as in all joint trauma, reflects the damage to the articular surface which has only limited regenerative powers. Furthermore, avascular necrosis and other complications may compromise the end result. Therefore, the surgeon who undertakes the operation must obtain an anatomical reduction and stable fixation for any chance of an improved result. The surgeon must also use all the described modalities to prevent the complications which occur frequently.

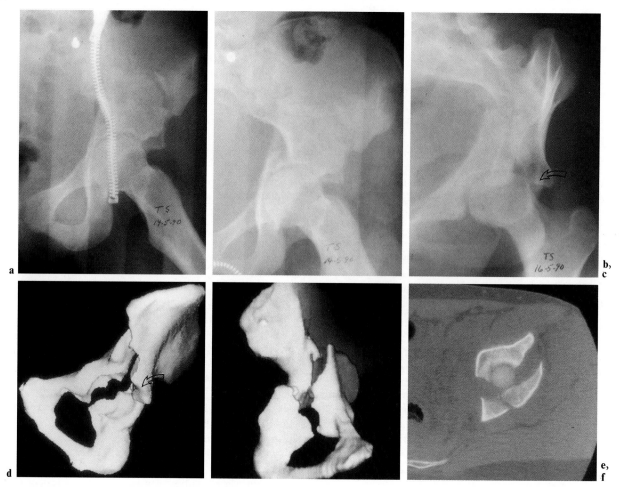

Fig. 13.46 a–f. Atypical T-shaped fracture was fixed through a combined anterior iliofemoral approach and posterior Kocher-Langenbeck approach. Anterposterior (**a**), iliac oblique (**b**), and obturator oblique (**c**) radiographs of an atypical T-shaped fracture of the left hip. Although there is a resemblance to a both-column fracture, a portion of the cartilage *(arrow)* is attached to the ilium. The pathoanatomy is best seen on the three-dimensional computed tomography (CT; **d, e**) and axial CT (**f**) views.

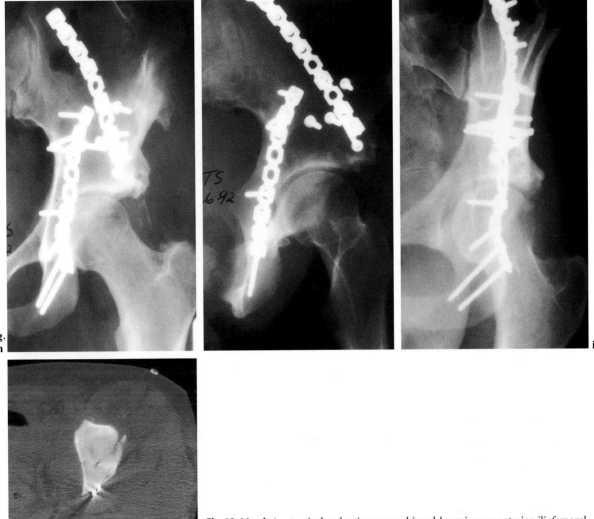

Fig. 13.46 g–j. Anatomical reduction was achieved by using an anterior iliofemoral approach and posterior Kocher-Langenbeck approach simultaneously with the patient in the lateral position. Fixation with intrafragmental screws and buttress plates is demonstrated in the anteroposterior (**g**), obturator oblique (**h**), and iliac oblique (**i**) radiographs. The excellent reduction is also noted on the axial CT (**j**), taken through the dome of the acetabulum. (From Tile 1995)

References

Aprahamian C, Carrico CJ, Collicott PE et al (1981) Advanced trauma life support course. Committee on Trauma, American College of Surgeons

Gorczyca J, Varga E, Woodside T, Hearn T, Powell J, Tile M (1994) The strength of iliosacral lag screws and transiliac bars in the fixation of vertically unstable pelvic ring injuries with sacral fractures. Presented at the Orthopaedic Trauma Meeting, Los Angeles, CA

Goulet JA, Bray TJ (1989) Complex acetabular fractures. Clin Orthop 240:9

Helfet DL, Schmeling GJ (1992) Somatosensory evoked potential monitoring in the surgical treatment of acute, displaced acetabular fractures: results of a prospective study. Orthop Trans 16:221

Helfet DL, Hissa EA, Sergay S, Mast JW (1991) Somatosensory evoked potential monitoring in the surgical management of acute acetabular fractures. J Orthop Trauma 5:161–166

Johnson K (1994) Acetabular fractures: long term follow up of open reduction and internal fixation. Presented at the Orthopaedic Trauma Association Meeting, Los Angeles, CA, September

Judet R, Judet J, Letournel E (1964) Fractures of the acetabulum: classification and surgical approaches for open reduction. J Bone Joint Surg 46A(8): 1615–1647

Kang CS (1987) A new fixation method of acetabular fractures. Presented at the SICOT meeting, Munich, Germany, 16–21 August

Letournel E (1980) Acetabular fractures: classification and management. Clin Orthop 151:81–106

Letournel E, Judet R (1981) Fractures of the acetabulum. Springer, Berlin Heidelberg New York

Letournel E, Judet R (1993) Fractures of the acetabulum, 2nd edn. Springer, Berlin Heidelberg New York

Matta JM, Mehne DK, Roffi T (1986) Fractures of the acetabulum. Ital J Orthop Trauma 13:27

McLaren AC (1990) Prophylaxis with Indomethacin for heterotopic bone. J Bone Joint Surg 72A: 245

Moed BR, Letournel E (1993) Combination low-dose radiation and indomethacin therapy for the prevention of hetertopic ossification following acetabular fracture surgery. Presented at the First International Symposium on the Surgical Treatment of Acetabular Fractures, Paris, France

Moed BR, Maxey JW (1993) The effect of indomethacin on heterotopic ossification following acetabular fracture surgery. J Orthop Trauma 7:33–38

Müller ME, Allgower M, Schneider R, Willeneger H (1990) Manual of internal fixation, 3rd edn. Springer, Berlin Heidelberg New York

Pantazopoulos T, Mousafiris C (1989) Surgical treatment of central acetabulum fractures. Clin Orthop 246:57

Pennal GF, Davidson J, Garside H, Plewes J et al (1980) Results of treatment of acetabular fractures. Clin Orthop 151:115–123

Powell JN, Bircher M, Joyce M (1988) Acetabular fractures: the results of treatment of 102 acetabular fractures by open and closed methods. Presented at the Orthopaedic Trauma Association Meeting, Dallas, TX

Romness DW, Lewallen DG (1990) Total hip arthroplasty of the acetabulum. J Bone Joint Surg 72B: 761

Rowe CR, Lowell JD (1961) Prognosis of fractures of the acetabulum. J Bone Joint Surg 43A(1):30–59

Ruedi T, von Hochstetter AHC, Schlumpf R (1984) Surgical approaches for internal fixation. Springer, Berlin Heidelberg New York

Schopfer A, Willett K, Powell J, Tile M (1993) Cerclage wiring in internal fixation of acetabular fractures. J Orthop Trauma 7:236

Steinberg M (1991) The hip and its disorders. Saunders, Philadelphia

Tile M (1984) Fractures of the pelvis and acetabulum. Williams and Wilkins, Baltimore

Tile M (1984) Fractures of the pelvis and acetabulum. Williams and Wilkins, Baltimore

Tile M (1995) Fractures of the pelvis and acetabulum, 2nd edn. Williams and Wilkins, Baltimore

Tile M, Joyce M, Kellam J (1984) Fractures of the acetabulum: classification, management protocol and early results of treatment. Orthopaedic Transactions of the J Bone Joint Surg. 8(3)

Vrahas M, Gordon RG, Mears DC, Krieger D (1992) Intraoperative somatosensory evoked potential monitoring of pelvic and acetabular fractures. J Orthop Trauma 6:50–58

Winquist R (1980) Fractures of the acetabulum. Presented at the American Academy of Orthopaedic Surgeons Annual Meeting, New Orleans, LA

Part IV Fractures of the Lower Extremity

14 Subcapital and Intertrochanteric Fractures

J. Schatzker

14.1 Anatomy and Blood Supply

14.1.1 Cross-Sectional Anatomy of the Head

The cross-sectional anatomy of a femoral head from an elderly adult shows that the trabecular bone is concentrated as a thin layer deep to the subchondral bone plate

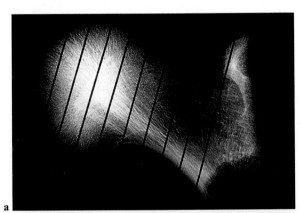

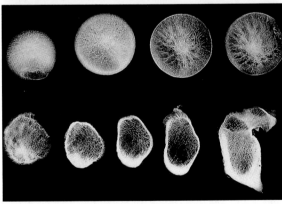

Fig. 14.1 a,b. Cross section of a femoral head of an elderly person. Note the concentreation of the trabeculae in the center of the head where the tension and the compression trabeculae intersect. The remainder of the head is filled sparsely with slender trabeculae which do not afford much purchase for fixation devices. Note also that as the neck approaches the shaft it changes in cross section from a circle to a rectangle

and in the center of the head where the tension and pressure trabecular network intersect (see Fig. 14.1). The surgeon should keep this in mind when considering points of purchase for internal fixation devices such as lag screws or angled blade plates.

14.1.1.1 Neck Shaft Angle

The normal neck shaft angle is between 125° and 135°. A value lower than that is considered a varus and any value higher than that is considered a valgus.

14.1.1.2 Greater Trochanter

The biomechanical functional varus and valgus is given by the relationship between the center of rotation of the head and the tip of the greater trochanter (see Fig. 14.2). Normally the tip of the greater trochanter is at or just above the center of rotation. When the center of rotation is higher than the tip of the greater trochanter, which is taken as the insertion of the abductor muscles, the hip is in functional valgus, and in any position lower, functional varus.

The distance from the center of the femoral head to the tip of the greater trochanter is normally two to two and a half times the radius of the femoral head.

These anatomical relationships determine the abductor lever arm and consequently the resultant of forces R about the hip and are important when the physician is faced with reattachment of the greater trochanter.

When the proximal femur is viewed from above, it can be seen that the greater trochanter is not centered on the neck but flares posteriorly some 30°–40°. Therefore, the more proximal the point of entry of a fixation device, the more anterior it must be in order to come into line with the axis of the neck. A 90° or 95° device must be inserted in the anterior half of the trochanter, and any device which is inserted through the shaft into the neck and head must be inserted into the middle of the lateral surface of the femur (Fig. 14.3). Any posterior placement along the lateral surface of the shaft results in the device entering the anterior half of the head, and any anterior insertion results in the device entering the posterior half

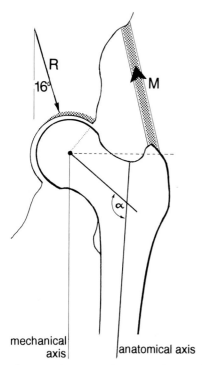

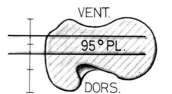

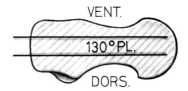

Fig. 14.3. Note that the trochanter is not centered on the neck but flares posteriorly some 30–40°

mechanical axis | anatomical axis

Fig. 14.2. The center of rotation of the head *C* is just below the tip of the greater trochanter. The neck shaft angle α is normally between 125° and 135°. The tip of the greater trochanter is 2-2$^1/_2$ times *r* the radius of the head from the center of rotation of the head. The anatomical axis is inclined at 9° to the midsagittal plane and at 5–7° to the mechanical axis. The resultant of the forces *R* is at 16° to the midsagittal plane. *M* is the direction of the abductor muscle pull

of the head. Such errors of insertion cannot be corrected by changing the angle of insertion of the device. The angle of insertion of a screw or of an angled device which is to traverse the neck and enter the head is also given by the anteversion of the neck. Such devices must be inserted parallel to the plane of anteversion.

14.1.2 Blood Supply

The specific configuration of the arterial blood supply of the head is responsible for its interruption in fractures of the neck. The posterior superior and the posterior inferior retinacular vessels arise from the medial femoral circumflex artery as it courses posteriorly along the intertrochanteric crest. They penetrate the capsule and run deep to the synovial retinaculum, which covers the femoral neck. Some of the retinacular vessels enter the neck. The majority enter the head close to its osseocartilagenous junction. The superior retinacular vessels give rise to the lateral superior epiphyseal vessels, which comprise the most important blood supply of the femo-

ral head. Vessels which enter the head via the ligamentum teres supply usually only a small portion of the head close to their site of entry. The lateral femoral circumflex artery runs along the base of the neck anteriorly. It gives rise to a few vessels which run along the anterior aspect of the neck. The anterior retinacular vessels enter the neck but do not contribute to the blood supply of the head (Fig. 14.4). This configuration of the vessels must be kept in mind whenever surgically approaching the neck and head of the femur and the surgeon must be very careful not to place retractors around the posterior aspect of the neck as this could seriously interfere with the blood supply of the head. A fracture disrupts the intraosseous blood supply to the head. If the retinacular circulation is disrupted the head will undergo avascular necrosis.

14.2 Classification

Fractures of the proximal femur are divided into *subcapital fractures*, which involve the neck, *trochanteric fractures,* which involve the trochanteric region, and *subtrochanteric fractures*. The latter are discussed in the next chapter. In this chapter we will limit the discussion to fractures of the neck and of the trochanteric region.

14.3 Subcapital Fractures

14.3.1 Classification

Pauwels classified fractures of the neck into three types on the basis of their mechanical stability (Pauwels 1965). Type I is a fracture at 90° to the resultant of forces *R*. As a result, the fracture is subjected to purely compressive

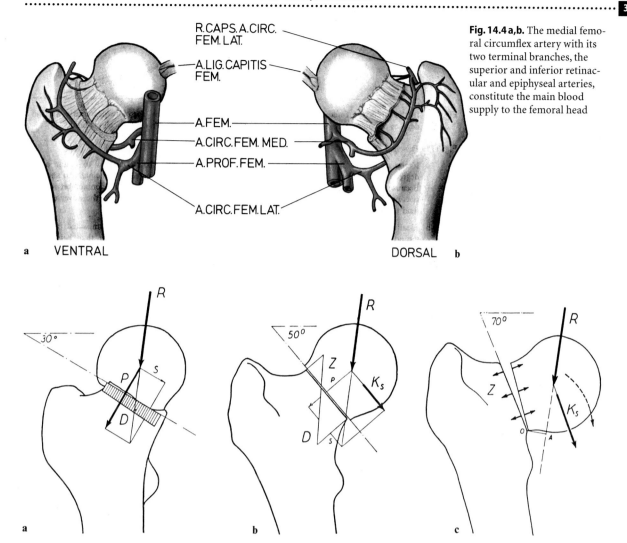

Fig. 14.4 a,b. The medial femoral circumflex artery with its two terminal branches, the superior and inferior retinacular and epiphyseal arteries, constitute the main blood supply to the femoral head

Fig. 14.5 a–c. Pauwels' (1965) classification of neck fractures is based on the angle which the fracture line subtends with the resultant of forces R

forces and is inherently stable. Type II is at 90° to the neck axis; it is subjected to shear and is therefore unstable. In type III, the fracture plane is almost in line with the anatomical axis of the femoral shaft. This fracture plane is subjected not only to shear, but also to forces which tend to distract the fracture. Thus, from a purely mechanical point of view, it is highly unstable (Fig. 14.5)

Garden (1964) classified subcapital fractures into four types. This classification is based on the degree of displacement and its influence on stability and incidence of avascular necrosis. He chose the relationship of the medial trabeculae (compression trabeculae) in the head and pelvis as an index of displacement (Fig. 14.6). Experience has shown that the biological behavior of the fractures separates them into two groups, undisplaced and dis-

placed. The fracture with the head impacted in valgus (Garden I) and the undisplaced fractures (Garden II) comprise one group with a low incidence of avascular necrosis. The partially displaced fractures (Garden III) and the completely displaced fractures (Garden IV) comprise the second group with a significantly higher incidence of avascular necrosis and a higher incidence of failure of fixation and nonunion (Müller et al. 1990, p. 126).

The Comprehensive Classification of fractures of the proximal femur divides the fractures into types according to the severity of the fracture. Thus type A are trochanteric fractures, type B are neck fractures, and type C are head fractures (Fig. 14.7).

The neck fractures are further subdivided into three groups, based on level of the fracture in the neck, stabil-

Garden 1964

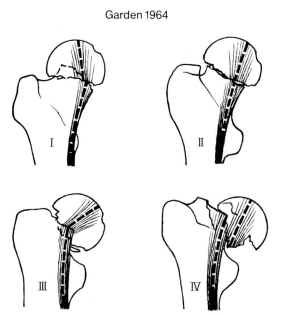

Fig. 14.6. Garden's classification is based on the relationship of the medial trabeculae (compression tabecuilae) in the head and pelvis

ity of the fracture, and its displacement. Thus BI are neck fractures, subcapital, with slight displacement; B2 are transcervical fractures; and B3 are subcapital fractures with marked displacement (Fig. 14.8).

We believe that the Comprehensive Classification of subcapital fractures in its detailed characterization of the fracture morphology is useful for research purposes. In clinical practice, for decision making and simple analysis of outcome, we rely on the classification of these fractures simply as undisplaced or displaced.

14.3.2 History and Physical Examination

Patients complaining of hip pain who have a shortened and externally rotated leg do not present a diagnostic challenge. The history is usually that of a simple fall at home or on the street. On physical examination, any attempt to move the leg is found to cause a great deal of pain. Similarly, patients who fall, are able to walk, but have pain, limp, and may need a cane are not too difficult to diagnose. The leg is not shortened or externally rotated, but manipulation of the hip and palpation over the groin produce pain. Such patients usually have an undisplaced or impacted subcapital fracture, which is easily seen on an X-ray and easily diagnosed. Patients complaining of pain after a fall whose physical examination and X-rays are inconclusive are the ones who tax the vigilance and diagnostic acumen of the surgeon. These

patients may have an undispaced fracture of the neck. If the diagnosis is not made and the fracture is missed, the next time these patients are seen the diagnosis is usually obvious because the fracture has displaced. A fracture with an excellent prognosis will have turned into a fracture with a much more serious outlook. The surgeon must be vigilant to prevent this from happening.

14.3.3 Imaging Techniques

14.3.3.1 X-Rays

A diagnostic examination of the hip consists of an anteroposterior (AP) projection of the pelvis and an AP and lateral projection of the involved hip. If the patient has a fracture, then the lateral projection has to be a cross-table lateral one because a broken hip cannot be abducted and externally rotated for the usual so-called frog lateral projection. If a fracture is suspected on clinical grounds and the X-rays fail to confirm the diagnosis, other forms of imaging have to be used.

14.3.3.2 Bone Scan

If an acute fracture is suspected, the technicium bone scan may not be positive until at least 3 days have passed since the injury. The increased uptake is a response to injury and takes time to develop. If the injury is more recent and a fracture is suspected but not evident on the X-ray, then tomography must be used.

14.3.3.3 Tomography

Tomography in two projections at 90° to each other will often disclose a crack in the cortex or a trabecular discontinuity not evident on plain X-rays.

14.3.3.4 Magnetic Resonance Imaging

We have not used magnetic resonance imaging (MRI) for the diagnosis of acute fractures.

14.3.4 Surgical Treatment

The choice of treatment when dealing with a subcapital fracture is between reduction and internal fixation or prosthetic replacement. We shall discuss how we evolve the rationale for one form of treatment or the other in the section on "Decision Making." In this section we will address the technical aspects of reduction and fixation.

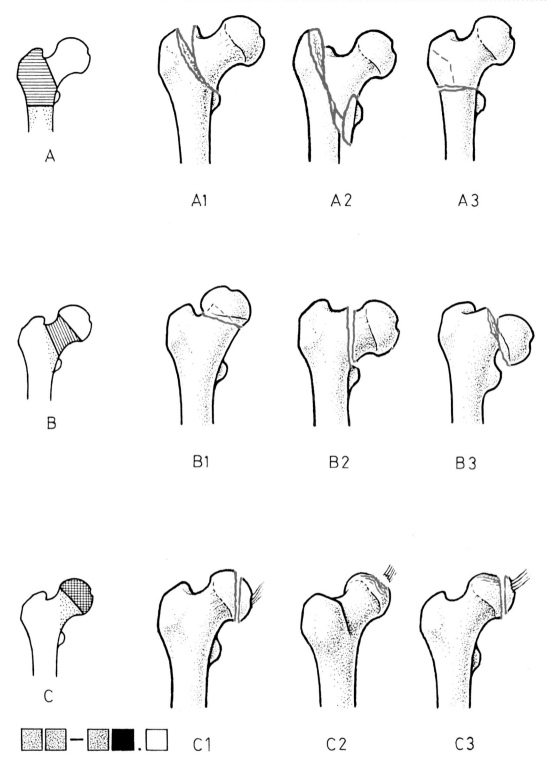

Fig. 14.7. The Comprehensive Classification (Müller et al 1990) of fractures of the proximal femur separates the fractures into head fractures type C, neck fractures type B, and trochanteric fractures type A. *A1*, trochanteric area fracture, pertrochanteric simple; *A2*, trochanteric area fracture, pertrochanteric multifragmentary; *A3*, trochanteric area fracture, intertrochanteric; *B1*, Neck fracture, subcapital, with slight displacement; *B2*, neck fracture, transcervical; *B3*, neck fracture, subcapital, with marked displacement; *C1*, head fracture, split; *C2*, head fracture, with depression; *C3*, head fracture, with neck fracture

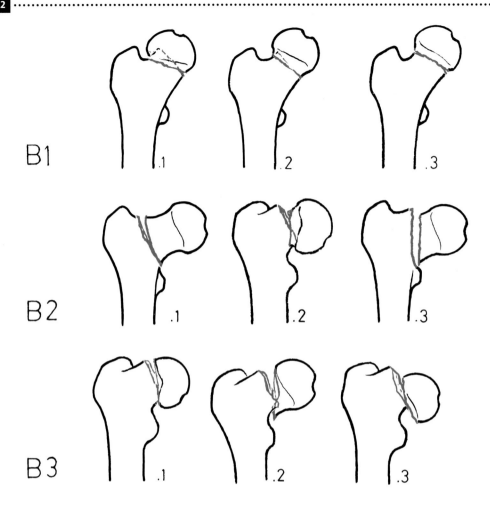

Fig. 14.8. The Comprehensive Classification (Müller et al 1990) of neck fractures. *B1*, neck fracture, subcapital, with slight displacement. *.1*, impacted in valgus ≥ 15°; 1) posterior tilt <15°; 2) posterior tilt >15°; *.2*, impacted in valgus <15°; 1) posterior tilt <15°; 2) posterior tilt >15°; *.3*, nonimpacted; *B2*, neck fracture, transcervical; *.1*, basicervical; *.2*, midcervical adduction; *.3*, midcervical shear; *B3*, neck fracture, subcapital, nonimpacted, displaced; *.1*, moderate displacement in varus and external rotation; *.2*, moderate displacement with vertical translation and external rotation; *.3*, marked displacement; 1) in varus; 2) with translation

14.3.4.1 Method of Reduction

a) Closed Reduction

Prior to any internal fixation, a displaced fracture of the femoral neck should be reduced. The surgeon must be extremely gentle in manipulating a subcapital fracture because any manipulation may put the blood supply at risk. In a subcapital fracture the intraosseous blood supply is interrupted. The only vessels which may be intact and providing a blood supply to the head are the poste-

rior superior and inferior retinacular vessels. These must never be put at risk.

The mechanism of displacement is simple. The femoral head displaces into varus and retroversion as the leg shortens and the femoral shaft externally rotates. The gentlest manipulation under anesthesia and full relaxation, which often brings about a reduction, consists of applying longitudinal traction and then gentle internal rotation. This is usually done with an image intensifier in place, which allows for an immediate check of the reduction obtained. The traction brings the head out of varus and the internal rotation corrects the retroversion. If this manoeuver fails, it can be repeated, but it must be remembered that any further manipulation increases the risk of rendering the head avascular. We are opposed to any other more vigorous attempts at reduction.

What is an adequate reduction? We aim for an anatomical reduction or one with the head in slight valgus and with the head in neutral version or minimally anteverted. We feel that any degree of residual varus or retroversion is unacceptable because it leads to an unacceptable incidence of failure as a result of loss of fixation and redisplacement. Therefore, proper reduction is one of the most essential factors for the successful treatment of neck fractures.

b) Open Reduction

If a closed reduction has failed and the decision has been made that the fracture should be managed by reduction and internal fixation in preference to an arthroplasty, then the next step is to proceed to an open reduction of the fracture.

In order to carry out an open reduction, the patient may be left on the fracture table, but the limb must be taken out of traction. After suitable preparation of the skin, the limb must be draped free to allow for manipulation as the reduction is being carried out. The skin incision is centered on the greater trochanter and is made as a straight line some 15 cm in length. The fascia lata is incised in line with the skin. This brings us to the lateral aspect of m. vastus lateralis, which is caudad, the greater trochanter with the m. gluteus medius, which is cephalad, and m. tensor fascia lata, which is anterior (see Fig. 14.9). The exposure of the capsule begins with the division of the most anterior fibers of the m. gluteus medius together with the tendon of m. gluteus minimus at their insertion on the anterior aspect of the greater trochanter. Once these two structures are cut, the surgeon goes on to develop the plane between the m. gluteus medius and the m. tensor fascia. Caution is needed concerning the vessels which run between the m. gluteus medius and the tensor. The set closest to the bone can be cauterized with impunity. The second, more anterior set of vessels, which is closer to the tensor should be protected because it usually contains the nerve to the tensor which runs forwards from the m. gluteus medius. The next step is to separate the iliopsoas fibers from the anteroinferior aspect of the capsule and pass a blunt Hohmann retractor below the inferior aspect of the capsule. An anterior Hohmann retractor is then passed in line with the axis of the neck and over the anterior aspect of the capsule. It is first passed with its tip facing anteriorly, and as it passes over the anterior lip of the acetabulum it is turned 180° so that its tip can be hooked over the anterior lip of the acetabulum. Great care is needed when passing a Hohmann retractor over the superior and cephalad aspect of the capsule, as this could damage the retinacular vessels. Instead it is better to retract the m. gluteus medius and minimus out of the way with a deep, right-angled retractor. These steps will expose the anterior aspect of the capsule. The exposure can be facilitated if a rolled sheet is placed under the thigh. This slight flexion of the hip releases the tension in the anterior soft tissues.

Once the capsule is exposed, an anterior capsulotomy is made in line with the long axis of the neck. The capsule is then cut at the base superiorly and inferiorly. This inverted T creates two flaps which can be retracted. The anterior Hohmann retractor should be removed and then reinserted by passing its tip from the inside of the hip joint through the overlying capsule. It should then be turned so that its tip faces down as it comes to rest over the anterior lip of the acetabulum. This manoeuvre lifts the capsule away from the neck and head and improves the exposure. A blunt-tipped Hohmann retractor can then be passed intracapsularly below the neck. Care is necessary in passing a Hohmann retractor above and around the neck as this could interfere with the blood supply of the head (Fig. 14.10). It is best to drive the tip of a Hohmann retractor into the superior aspect of the neck. The fracture is usually difficult to visualize because the leg is externally rotated, which brings the neck into the wound and obscures the head. To begin the reduction, the leg should be slightly adducted and flexed. A blunt hook should then be passed around the anteroinferior aspect of the neck. This allows the surgeon to apply lateral and distal traction. While maintaining lateral and longitudinal traction, the leg should then be abducted and internally rotated. This should be an extremely gentle manoeuvre; very little force is required

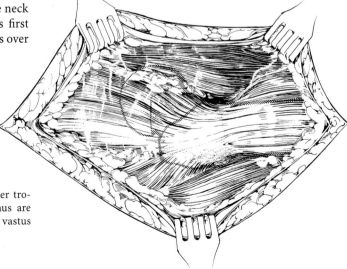

Fig. 14.9. The arrangement of muscles about the greater trochanter. Note that the m. gluteus medius and minimus are cephalad, the m. tensor fascia lata is anterior, and the m. vastus lateralis is caudad and posterior

to disengage the fragments and bring about the reduction of the head and neck. Occasionally, the head may move about and interfere with the reduction. If that should be the case, the head can be stabilized by driving a 2.5-mm Kirschner wire into the rim of the head. The Kirschenr wire can then be used as a joy stick to manipulate and steady the head. The reduction is done by manipulation of the leg. The surgeon should not try to manipulate the head onto the neck. The head is held stationary while the neck is manipulated into position. Once the reduction has been carried out, it should be checked with the image intensifier or an X-ray. We believe that an anatomical reduction should be aimed for. The head must not be in varus and the retroversion must be fully corrected. The version of the head is extremely difficult to judge during an open reduction. If an image intensifier or an X-ray is not available, then the only way that the reduction can be checked in both planes is to carry out a provisional fixation of the head with two 3-mm Steinmann pins passed along the neck into the head and then flexing the hip to 90°. At 90° of flexion an equal amount of head should be above and below the neck. If there is more head below the neck, the head is still in retroversion. If the reduction has failed, the steps are carefully repeated.

Some authors (Weber) have recommended a valgus reduction with the head in slight anteversion. Weber has likened this to hanging a hat on a hook. Slight valgus is certainly acceptable and increases the stability of the reduction, but the surgeon should guard agains excessive valgus because, as Garden has pointed out, this will lead to avascular necrosis of the head. Once an adequate reduction has been achieved, internal fixation can be performed.

14.3.4.2 Methods of Internal Fixation

Fractures of the neck of the femur are usually fixed with either multiple parallel lag screws or with an angled device which allows impaction and compression of the fracture (dynamic hip screw, DHS, Synthes; Fig. 14.11). Although the recent literature tends to favor parallel lag screws, the issue is far from settled. We tend to favor the DHS, but have embarked on a randomized blinded trial of the two methods with failure of union, displacement, and avascular necrosis as the end points in an effort to settle this controversy.

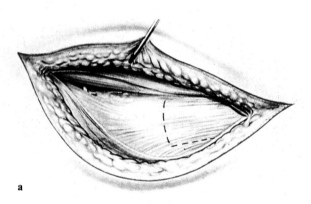

a

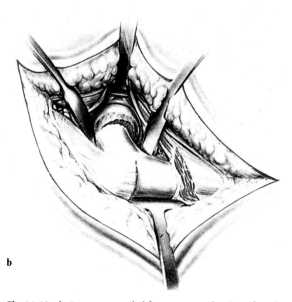

b

Fig. 14.10 a,b. Exposure needed for an open reduction of a subcapital fracture. (From Müller et al. 1970)

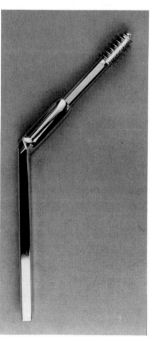

Fig.14.11. The Synthes DHS

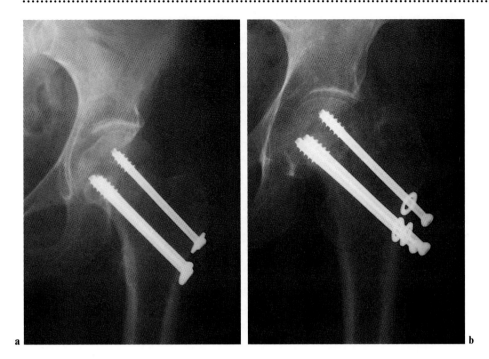

a   b

Fig. 14.12. a The cancellous screws used for fixation of a sub-capital fracture must be parallel to one another. **b** If the neck should resorb the screws must be able to back out. If the screws were not parallel they could penetrate through the head instead

a) Cannulated Screws

If lag screws are chosen for fixation, we usually use the large, 6.5-mm cancellous or the large, 7-mm cannulated cancellous screws. Since these are used as lag screws, in order to compress the fracture, it is usually necessary to use the screws with 16-mm thread to make certain that the threads do not cross the fracture. The screws should be inserted parallel to the axis of the neck and parallel to each other. They must be parallel to each other (Fig. 14.12 a,b) not only to act together as lag screws, but more importantly, if there is any resorption at the fracture, they must not block the head from settling down on the neck. If the screws are not parallel they can block the shortening, and instead of backing out they can advance through the head and perforate into the joint. The three screws are inserted at the apices of a triangle. We usually aim to have the base of the triangle cephalad, which means that we insert two screws cephalad to provide compression where there is a tendency for the fracture to distract. One screw is inserted inferiorly at the apex of the triangle. The exact orientation and placement of the apices of the triangle is not crucial. We are prepared to accept any random arrangement as long as the three screws are properly aligned. We aim to have the screws

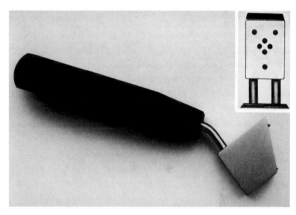

Fig. 14.13. The Synthes guide for the insertion of the cancellous screws

equidistant from the center of the head and not clustered. The threads of the screws should stop between 5 and 10 mm from the subchondral bone plate. The easiest way to insert the screws is to use the special guide (Synthes) available in the cannulated screw set (Fig. 14.13). If a guide wire is inserted through the center of the guide and if it comes to lie coaxial with the axis of the neck, the screws will have perfect placement. The first central guide wire must be inserted through the middle of the lateral surface of the shaft. If it is inserted too far anteriorly, the guide wire will be displaced into the posterior half of the head; if it is inserted too far posteriorly, which is the commoner mistake because of the internal rotation of the shaft, the guide wire will come to

336 ....

Chapter 14   **Subcapital and Intertrochanteric Fractures**

lie in the anterior half of the head. Changing the angle of the guide will not correct its placement in the head, as already explained. If malplacement occurs, the guide wire must be withdrawn and inserted through a new hole in the cortex. If it is inserted through a previously drilled hole in the cortex, it simply follows the old path every time. The surgeon must also pay attention to the level of the screws in relation to the level of the lesser trochanter. If any of the screws comes to lie below the level of the lesser trochanter, there is great danger of a subtrochanteric stress fracture through the screw hole. Thus we strongly advise against a low or steep placement of the screws. In our opinion the screws should be parallel to the axis of the neck. Impaction of the fracture is achieved by tightening of the lag screws. In order to prevent the screw heads from penetrating the cortex, we usually use washers.

b) Sliding Screw and Plate Method

A very popular sliding screw and plate system is the dynamic hip screw (Synthes; Fig. 14.11). It is an excellent device for the fixation of fractures of the neck. For fixation of neck fractures we use the compression screw with 16-mm thread and a two-hole side plate. As with the lag screws, the surgeon should aim to insert the compression screw in line with the axis of the neck. The angle of insertion is determined by the fixed angle of the plate. The plate which we use most commonly has an angle of 135°, but three other angles – 140°, 145°, and 150° – are available to accommodate the valgus neck. The tip of the compression screw should come to rest 5–10 mm from the subchondral bone plate, and its threads must not cross the fracture in order to allow for impaction. The screw itself should come to lie in the center of the head. Once again, the surgeon must pay attention to where the guide wire comes to lie. If it is in the anterior half of the head, it has been inserted too far posteriorly in the shaft and vice versa. As with the cancellous screws, changing the placement in the head requires not only a change in angulation with respect to the axis of the neck, but also very often a change of the insertion site through the cortex.

Stability of the reduction and of the fixation depends on the impaction of the fracture. This is as true for the cancellous lag screws as it is for the DHS. In order to impact the fracture in elderly patients with the DHS, we do not use the screw provided for this purpose. The bone within the femoral head of elderly patients is so sparse that instead of achieving compression of the fracture, the compression screw might be pulled out of the head. In order to impact the fracture, we insert the compression screw of the DHS into the head and then articulate the two-hole plate over the screw and secure it to the

shaft with two screws. Traction on the limb is then released, and we secure impaction with a few firm hammer blows delivered to the plate in the direction of the neck. We use the impactor with the plastic tip to prevent the scoring of the plate. We achieve excellent impaction in this manner.

14.3.4.3 Methods of Joint Replacement

For the elderly with a completely displaced subcapital fracture, for whom we have decided to carry out an arthroplasty, we usually choose a unipolar design such as the Moore or the Thompson prosthesis. We use the Thompson prosthesis if we cannot obtain rotational stability with the Moore prosthesis. Under these circumstances we cement the Thompson prosthesis. For elderly patients with a much younger physiologic than actual age who are healthy and very active and leading a fully independent life, we often carry out a total joint replacement. We have decreased the incidence of postoperative dislocation after a primary total hip replacement for fracture by using an anterior or a straight lateral approach. We also take great care to preserve and repair the capsule at the end of the procedure. We prefer to use a fixed acetabular cup rather than the bipolar prosthesis, because the outcome is uniformly better. We would consider the bipolar mobile cup if forced to replace the hip in a young patient or if we feel that there is reason to fear postoperative dislocation in elderly patients.

....

14.3.5 Decision Making

14.3.5.1 Undisplaced Fractures

All undisplaced subcapital fractures are stabilized either with parallel cancellous lag screws or the DHS. This is true for young as well as elderly patients. The undisplaced subcapital fracture (Garden II type) is inherently unstable and, if not stabilized surgically, will displace. The undisplaced subcapital fracture impacted in valgus with no retroversion (Garden type I), although inherently more stable than type II and capable of withstanding functional loading, can displace. If such a fracture displaces, the patient faces a far worse prognosis because of a much higher incidence of avascular necrosis. We feel, therefore, that it is an unjustifiable gamble not to stablize this fracture surgically unless there are definite reasons for not performing surgery.

14.3.5.2 Displaced Fractures

All displaced subcapital fractures require surgical treatment. The decision which the surgeon must make is whether to treat the fracture with reduction and internal fixation or whether to carry out a primary arthroplasty. Until the development of the Smith-Peterson nail, the subcapital fracture was an unsolved surgical problem. The development of a sound surgical method of internal fixation held out great promise. Shortly after the contribution of Smith-Peterson, Moore and Thompson each developed their unipolar replacement arthroplasty for the treatment of displaced subcapital fractures. One would think that after half a century the choice between reduction and fixation on the one hand and arthroplasty on the other would be a simple and straightforward issue based on clear guidelines. Nothing could be further from the truth. Despite the fact that the subcapital fracture is one of the commonest surgical problem which the orthopedic surgeon has to face, decisions are still based on personal prejudice or preference rather than fact. The problem is compounded by the lack of well-structured randomized clinical trials comparing the outcomes of treatment of internal fixation and of arthroplasty. If such trials were available, they would serve as appropriate guidelines for treatment. Our preferred method of treatment of the displaced subcapital fracture in the elderly is closed reduction and internal fixation. Our choice of treatment is modified by the factors discussed below.

a) Age

In setting guidelines for treatment based on the patient's age, we are faced with the difficulty of drawing a clear distinction between young and old. We have set 65 years of age as the arbitrary dividing line, but it is clear that this must be modified by such things as the patients physiologic age, general health, comorbid state, time of presentation for treatment, etc.

We believe that every effort must be made in young patients to save the femoral head. Thus all displaced subcapital fractures in young adults are treated as emergencies which cannot wait longer than 6 hours and are reduced and fixed internally. Although no clear data are available to indicate that a delay of several hours can prejudice the survival of the femoral head (because it is impossible for a number of reasons to conduct a randomized trial), we believe that persistent displacement could prejudice the circulation in the retinacular vessels. We do not aspirate the hemarthrosis prior to surgery, but we do not place the limb in traction. We feel that traction and extension of the hip will increase the intracapsular pressure of the hip in the presence of hemarthrosis. The limb is cradled on pillows in the position of maximum comfort until surgery. When the patient is fully anesthetized and relaxed, we attempt a gentle closed reduction. If this fails, we proceed to an open reduction. We feel that all forceful manipulations of the fracture must be avoided as they increase the risk of avascular necrosis. Once reduction has been achieved, fixation is carried out as already described.

b) Time of Presentation

Failure to recognize and treat a displaced subcapital fracture predisposes the head to avascular necrosis and adversely affects outcome. In the elderly, presence of displacement of 1 week or more is an indication for an arthroplasty. In younger patients in whom preservation of the head is important, neglected or unrecognized femoral neck fractures are regarded as nonunion. If the nonunion is mobile and a reduction is feasible, we carry out either a closed or an open reduction through the fracture. The reduced fracture is then stabilized internally either with cannulated screws or a DHS. If the deformity associated with the nonunion is fixed, we carry out an abduction osteotomy, as described by Pauwels (Fig. 14.14). Before carrying out a reconstruction of the neglected fracture, it is most important to establish the viability of the femoral head. Sclerosis on the head side of the nonunion is suggestive of viability because new bone formation requires the presence of a blood supply. A positive bone scan is also helpful. The most accurate assessment of viability is the MRI, which indicates not only whether circulation is present, but also whether there is a segmental deficiency. Knowledge of such factors enables the surgeon to predict outcome with much greater accuracy and thus be in a much better position to determine the course of treatment.

c) Additional General Risk Factors for Internal Fixation

The following factors are additional general risk factors for internal fixation:

1. *Hyperparathyroidism and renal failure.* Renal failure with or without hyperparathyroidism represents a contraindication to internal fixation because of the high incidence of delayed union and nonunion and a very high failure rate of fixation. These patients should have an arthroplasty.
2. *Previous stroke.* A previous stroke on the side of the fracture is a consideration only if the patient has been left with a significant neurological deficit. Spasticity, spasm, contactures, and paresis are a contraindication to internal fixation. Their presence will, of course, have an adverse effect on the outcome of an

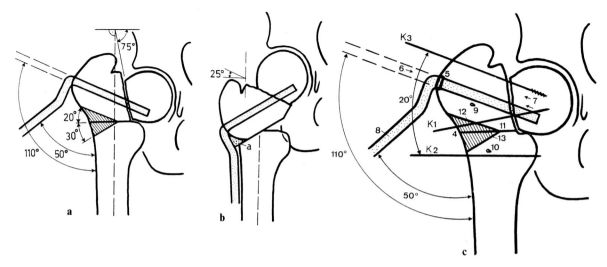

Fig. 14.14 a–c. Abduction osteotomy after Pauwels modified by Müller for the treatment of nonunion of the femoral neck. (From Schatzker 1984)

arthroplasty, but a positive outcome is more likely than with internal fixation.

3. *Parkinson's disease.* If associated with a serious tremor, rigidity, and deformity, Parkinson's disease is an indication for an arthroplasty.

4. *Rheumatoid arthritis.* The presence of rheumatoid arthritis alone is not a contraindication to internal fixation. However, if the joint is involved in the inflammatory arthritis, then an arthroplasy is indicated. If the joint is not involved by the rheumatoid process, treatment should be considered on the basis of general and local factors.

d) Local Risk Factors for Internal Fixation

Severe osteoporosis, comminution of the neck, preexistent local pathology, and the presence of degenerative arthritis are other very important risk factors associated with a high failure rate for internal fixation. In their presence we feel that elderly and most younger patients are better served by an arthroplasty.

e) Risk Factors for Arthroplasty

Before embarking on an arthroplasty, a number of important local factors representing risk factors for an arthroplasty must be ruled out. These include previous or ongoing sepsis, the presence of intact or broken pieces of internal fixation which may be blocking the medullary canal, bone deformity from trauma or disease, bone disease such as osteopetrosis, and degenerative disease involving the acetabulum. The latter is a contraindica-

tion for a unipolar arthoplasty as well as for reduction and fixation. In the presence of arthritis, a subcapital fracture is best treated by means of a total joint replacement.

14.3.5.3 Special Fracture Situations

a) Ipsilateral Neck and Shaft Fractures

Ipsilateral neck and shaft fractures are complex injuries. The treatment priorities are the preservation of the viability of the head and the accurate reduction and fixation of the neck fracture. If the neck fracture is undisplaced, we stabilize it provisionally with Kirschner wires and nail the femur, and then stabilize the neck fracture with cannulated screws. If the fracture of the neck is displaced, we feel that it is best to plate the femur first and then carry out a closed reduction and fixation of the neck. If the morphology of the shaft fracture is such that plating is deemed inadvisable because of the anticipated difficulties, a closed reduction of the neck should be tried first. If it succeeds, the neck should be stabilized provisionally and the femur nailed. If the closed reduction should fail, an open reduction of the neck should be carried out in order to reduce the neck and achieve its provisional fixation prior to nailing. Nailing of the femur can increase the displacement of the neck and jeopardize the blood supply to the head. A malreduction of the neck must not be accepted, because it will contribute to avascular necrosis and to mechanical malfunction of the hip. Once the neck is reduced, it should be provisionally fixed while the femur is nailed. Once the femur is nailed, the neck is fixed with cannulated cancellous screws. We feel that it can not be emphasized enough that the priority in treatment is the preservation of the blood supply to the femoral head and an accurate reduction of the neck. We also feel that an open fracture of the femur associated with a neck fracture is an absolute contraindication to nailing because of the risk of septic arthritis should the fracture become infected.

In carrying out internal fixation of this rare combined fracture, we have found that the second-generation reconstruction nails, such as the "Recon nail" (Smith Nephew Richards, Memphis, TN, USA), are difficult to use because they have to be inserted in such a way that they will accommodate not only the anteversion but also line up with the neck to afford fixation of the fracture with both screws. The new Synthes unreamed nail for the femur has very elegant proximal locking guides and jigs for the insertion of screws into the femoral neck. Although we have not had extensive experience with this device, it appears to be very promising in the treatment of these difficult combined lesions.

b) Fracture of the Neck and Dislocation of the Head

The presence of a fracture of the neck and dislocation of the head is almost an absolute guarantee of the complete disruption of the blood supply to the femoral head. Despite this, we feel that an open reduction and internal fixation of the fracture should be carried out in young patients. This belief is based on the fact that not every patient who develops an avascular necrosis requires further intervention and that the failure rate of arthroplasties is a time-dependent phenomenon and therefore not an ideal procedure for a young patient.

14.3.6 Postoperative Management

The central issue in the postoperative management of patients with fractures of the femoral neck is whether to allow them to bear weight or not. Younger patients should not bear weight for at least 8–12 weeks or at least until such time as it is certain that the fracture is uniting without complications. In the elderly, we allow full weight bearing as tolerated. This difference in regiment is based on the fact that the elderly patient cannot walk without taking weight on both lower extremities. We believe that early ambulation is essential in the rehabilitation of the elderly. We have followed this regiment without incurring a higher incidence of failure of internal fixation than that reported in the literature.

14.3.7 Complications

14.3.7.1 Nonunion

Non union in elderly patients is best treated by means of an arthroplasy. In younger patients, as already discussed above (see Sect. 14.3.5.2.2), every effort must be made to preserve the femoral head and the hip joint. We differentiate between mobile nonunions, in which the position of the fragments changes appreciably with traction, and those which are fixed. The mobile nonunion is usually a fracture which has either gone unrecognized for a number of weeks or been knowingly neglected. We are not referring to the long-standing untreated subcapital fracture where the head fragment has remained in the acetabulum and the shaft has drifted more proximally and laterally and the joint has functioned like a Girdlestone resection arthroplasty. This latter situation is a true nonunion with synovial-like tissue interposed between the fragments. What we are referring to is a delayed union with deformity. In these situations, as already mentioned, we carry out either a closed or an open reduction to achieve proper alignment of the fragments. In practice this has almost always meant an open reduction to achieve a slight valgus with full correction of retroversion. The fracture is then stablized either with cannulated screws or a DHS. We do not believe in carrying out the Judet or Meyers pedicle graft (Meyers et al. 1974) unless there is major bone loss on the posterior aspect of the neck. We believe that the function of the Judet or Meyers graft is largely supportive in securing union in the presence of significant bone loss. We do not believe that it plays any useful role in restoring the blood supply to the avascular femoral head.

In the established fixed nonunion, it is essential to determine the viability of the head before undertaking treatment. Sclerosis on the side of the head and a technicium bone scan showing uptake are suggestive of a preserved blood supply. We feel that MRI is not only the most sensitive technique, but also the most useful, because it will also reveal a segmental loss of perfusion. In young adults, if the femoral head is found to be avascular, this is not a contraindication to reconstruction. However, the knowledge that the head is avascular will enable the surgeon to give the patient a much more realistic picture of the proposed procedure, its complications, and the anticipated outcome. The reason that we feel that it is worthwhile to proceed to a reconstruction even if the femoral head is dead is that segmental avascular necrosis is compatible with function, and, although it is not perfect, it is preferable in young patients to an arthroplasty. The reconstructive procedure we favor is the abduction medial displacement repositioning osteotomy originally described by Pauwels and further popularized by Müller (Müller 1957; see Fig. 14.15 a,b).

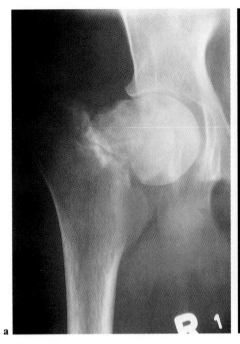
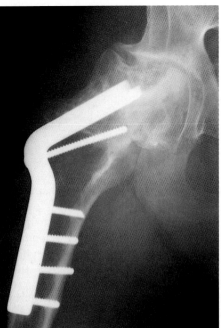

a   b

Fig. 14.15. a A subcapital nonunion in a 16-year-old girl 9 months following a missed fracture through the base of the neck. Magnetic resononance imaging indicated that the head and neck were completely avascular. **b** Eight years following an abduction repositioning osteotomy. The head and neck revascularized once the neck united and the head developed a segmental collapse. The patient has remained completely free of pain and able to walk up to 2 miles

14.3.7.2 Avascular Necrosis and Loss of Fixation

Avascular necrosis and loss of fixation are the two most commonly encountered complications. Loss of fixation in the elderly is treated with an arthroplasty. Since the introduction of the sliding screw plate and parallel cancellous screws, it is uncommon to see penetration of the femoral head by the fixation devices because of bone resorbtion at the fracture. This was a problem with the fixed-length devices such as the 130° blade plate which were used for the fixation of these fractures.

Avascular necrosis does not contribute to nonunion. As long as the fixation is stable, union will occur even if one fragment is avascular. Once union occurs, the femoral head will be gradually revascularized from the neck. Despite revascularization, the superolateral quadrant of the head frequently remains avascular and undergoes collapse. If the collapsed head leads to pain and disability, it is treated either by a unipolar or by a bipolar arthroplasty.

14.4 Intertrochanteric Fractures

14.4.1 Surgical Anatomy and Classification

Intertrochanteric fractures, more correctly referred to as pertrochanteric fractures, are fractures which occur in the region joining the greater and lesser trochanters. This is the insertion site of large muscle masses and is therefore a region with a very abundant blood supply. Nonunion of these fractures is rare, and if completely neglected these fractures usually heal with varus shortening and external rotation. Avascular necrosis of the femoral head is rare and occurs in less that 1 % of cases.

Most of the classifications of these fracture are based on the number of fragments and whether or not the lesser trochanter is split off as a separate fragment. Thus the two-part fracture is one where the fracture follows extracapsularly the course of the intertrochanteric crest. With further force the lesser trochanter and the greater trochanter can split off, creating the three- and four-part fracture. The lesser trochanter and surrounding bone are posteromedial. This is an area which is subjected to very large compressive stresses and is important to the load-bearing capacity of the femur. The presence of a fracture of the lesser trochanter and adjacent bone has led to the classification of these three- and four-part fractures as unstable and the two-part fracture as stable. This is the scheme followed in the classification of Kyle and Gustilo (Kyle et al. 1979). lt recognizes four types: type I, the stable nondisplaced fracture without commi-

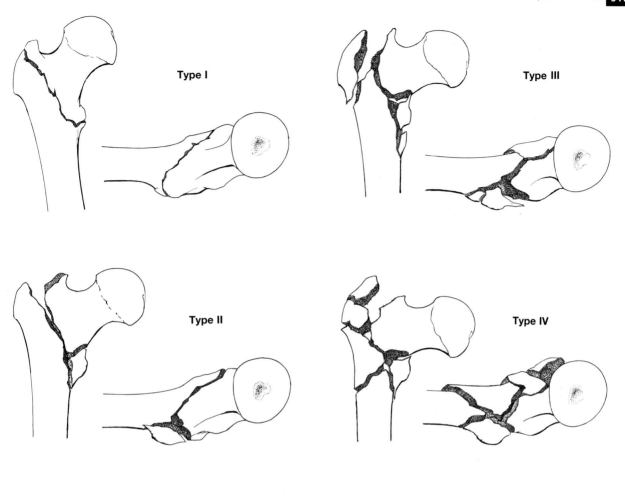

Fig. 14.16. The Kyle classification of intertrochanteric fractures (from Chapman 1993)

nution; type II, which is stable with minimal comminution; the type III, which is unstable and has a large posteromedial comminuted area; and type IV, which has a subtrochanteric extension and is highly unstable and difficult to treat (Fig. 14.16).

The Comprehensive Classification of fractures assigns the intertrochanteric fractures to type A fractures, which means that they are injuries of lesser severity than the subcapital fractures, which are type B. Group A1 (Fig. 14.17) corresponds to types I and II of the Kyle and Gustilo classification, and group A2 to types III and type IV. Group A3, the true intertrochanteric fractures, are singled out in this classification but not in the Kyle-Gustilo classification. We feel that for research purposes the Comprehensive Classification is superior, because the different fractures patterns are more completely represented (Fig. 14.17).

14.4.2 History and Physical Examination

These fractures are common in patients who are in their seventies or eighties and occur as a result of simple falls, but they can also occur in younger patients, usually as a result of high-velocity trauma. Elderly patients lying in the emergency department in pain, with one leg shortened and externally rotated, are an all too common sight. The diagnosis is simple. An X-ray is required, however, to differentiate between the intertrochanteric and the subcapital fracture. The radiological diagnosis is rarely a problem, but it is necessary to look out for undisplaced fissures, which are sometimes missed. Failure to diagnose an intertrochanteric fracture does not have the same dire consequence as the missed subcapital fracture. The displaced fracture can be reduced and the outcome will be the same as if the fracture were stabilized prior to displacement. Displacement of an intertrochanteric fracture has no bearing on the incidence of avascular necrosis.

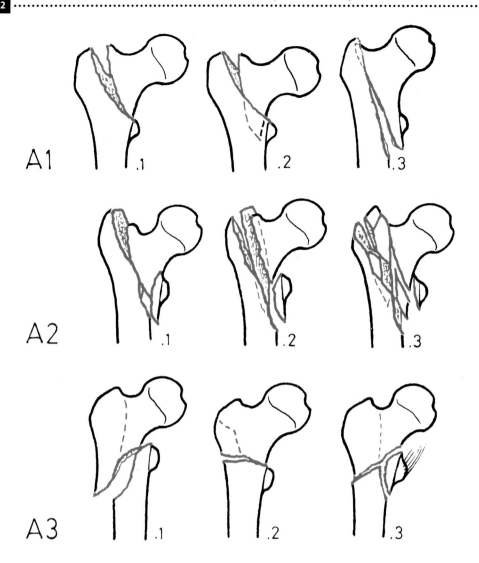

Fig. 14.17. The Comprehensive Classification (Müller et al 1990) of intertrochanteric fractures. Note the separation of the fractures into groups and subgroups. *A1*, trochanteric area fracture, pertrochanteric simple; *.1*, along the intertrochanteric line; *.2*, through the greater trochanter; 1), nonimpacted; 2) impacted; *.3*, below the lesser trochanter; 1) high variety; 2) low variety; *A2*, trochanteric area fracture, pertrochanteric multifragmentary; *.1*, with one intermediate fragment; *.2*, with several intermediate fragments; *.3*, extending more than 1 cm below the lesser trochanter; *A3*, trochanteric area fracture, intertrochanteric; *.1*, simple, oblique; *.2*, simple, transverse; *.3*, multifragmentary; 1), extending to the greater trochanter; 2), extending to the neck

14.4.3 Surgical Treatment

Classifying intertrochanteric fractures as either stable or unstable is misleading. For us a stable fracture is one which can withstand physiologic loading without displacement. Thus it is erroneous to speak of any intertrochanteric fracture as being stable, because the two-part or the three-part fractures are just as likely to displace under load. What led to the classification of stable and unstable was the observation that two-part fractures which were fixed with a fixed-angled device such as the 130° blade plate usually united without deformity. The three- or four-part fractures, on the other hand, often redisplaced into varus because the fixation device either bent or began to cut out. In the presence of internal fixation, the comminution of the buttress, the opposite cortex, has a major role in rendering the construct unstable under load. This observation led Dimon and Hughston to advocate medial displacement osteotomy (Dimon and Hughston 1967) and Sarmiento to advocate the valgus osteotomy (Sarmiento and Williams 1970). Both procedures were designed to overcome the deficiency of the medial buttress and hence restore stability and improve the results of treatment. At the same time,

Clawson and Massie both introduced sliding devices which allowed impaction of the fragments (Clawson 1964; Massie 1962.) These devices which allowed impaction of the fragments led to superior results over the fixed-length devices. These sliding devices have gained universal popularity as the fixation device for all intertrochanteric fractures. Thus today, although we still pay attention to the morphology of the fracture and recognize that the three- and four-part fractures are less stable and have a more guarded prognosis, the classification of the fractures into stable and instable or two- or four-part fractures does not guide the treatment. We treat stable and unstable fractures in the elderly exactly the same way. The fractures are reduced closed and stabilized with the same sliding screw plate device. Following surgery, all patients are encouraged to bear full weight. Despite this indiscriminate approach to weight bearing in our patient population, the failure rate, i.e., redisplacement into varus or failure of fixation, in "unstable" fractures is not higher than in stable fractures. We attribute this to the impaction of the major fragments which has become possible with the sliding screw devices such as the DHS (Synthes).

14.4.3.1 Reduction

a) Closed Reduction

The reduction of these fractures is carried out on the fracture table with the aid of image intensification. The limb is placed in traction and in slight abduction and internal rotation. This is usually sufficient to align the femoral head and neck fragment with the shaft and recreate the patients normal neck shaft angle. It is important to check on the lateral projection that the shaft has not sagged posteriorly. If this happens, it must be corrected. Frequently, this deformity cannot be corrected by simply externally rotating the limb, although this manoeuver will help to realign the fragments. Because the shaft has sagged, it must be lifted upwards and held there to secure reduction.

b) Open Reduction

Open reduction may sometimes be necessary. The surgical approach is very similar to that used for the neck and is through a straight lateral incision centered on the greater trochanter with a distal extension to accommodate the plate. The fascia lata is incised in line with the skin. To expose the femur, we prefer to reflect the m. vastus lateralis from the intermuscular septum and lift it forwards rather than splitting longitudinally the fibers of the muscle. This latter manoeuver denervates the posterior fibers and is often associated with greater bleeding from the branches of the perforating vessels. If the perforating vessels are encountered as the m. vastus lateralis is being reflected forwards, they should be ligated rather than cauterized. Cauterization causes the vessels to retract through the intermuscular septum. Once out of sight, they often cause troublesome bleeding which is very difficult to stop. Ligation of the perforators avoids this complication. If an open reduction is to be performed, the m. vastus lateralis should be detached with a periosteal elevator from the anterior surface of the femur. Anterior exposure of the neck is achieved by dissecting in the interval between the m.gluteus medius and tensor fascia lata as already described for subcapital fractures. Once the anterior aspect of the capsule is exposed, a Hohmann retractor can be passed over the anterior rim of the acetabulum. Great care must be taken to ensure that the tip of the Hohmann retractor does not enter the joint and damage the femoral head. The fracture must be disimpacted first by adduction of the limb and external rotation. Lateral traction on the shaft with a blunt hook will aid in the disimpaction. Once disimpacted, the distal fragment is abducted and internally rotated. The reduction is held by passing a Steinmann pin through the shaft fragment into the head and neck. An open reduction is rarely necessary in elderly patients in whom the surgeon is simply trying to secure a realignment of the shaft and head and neck fragment. In younger patients who sustain this injury in a high-velocity trauma, an anatomical reduction should be aimed for. If closed reduction fails to secure an anatomical realignment in younger patients, the surgeon should proceed to an open reduction, as described.

14.4.3.2 Internal Fixation

As already mentioned, the device we prefer for the fixation of intertrochanteric fractures is the DHS (Synthes), a fairly recent modification of the the sliding screw and plate fixation method. We have found this device ideal for the fixation of type I, type II, and type III fractures of the Kyle-Gustilo classification. Type IV fractures, intertrochanteric fractures with a subtrochanteric extension, and A3 fractures, true intertrochanteric fractures, are best handled with a 95° device such as the DCS (dynamic compression screw) or the condylar blade plate. The reasons for this are that the subtrochanteric extension of the intertrochanteric fracture makes it difficult, if not impossible, to secure adequate fixation in the proximal fragment with the DHS. The only purchase with the DHS in the head and neck fragments in such cases is with the compression screw. This leaves the proximal fragment free to rotate about the axis of the screw. The DCS and the condylar blade plate, on the other hand, allow the

Fig 14.18 a,b. The insertion of a screw through the plate into the calcar greatly increases the stability of the fixation of the device in the proximal fragment. (**a** From Müller 1979)

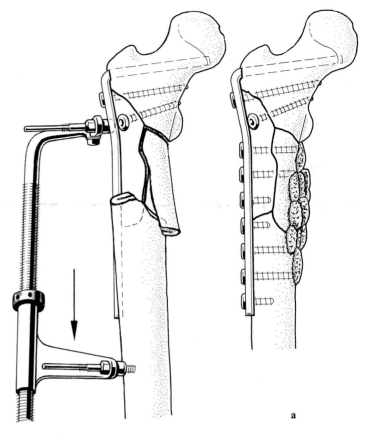

a

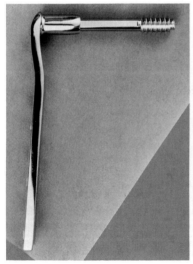

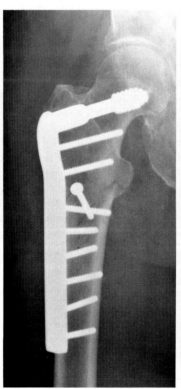

b

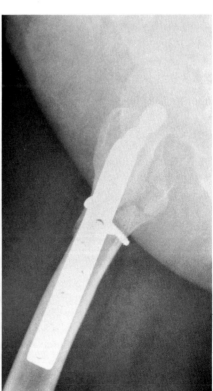

surgeon to insert a screw through the plate into the calcar, which greatly enhances the purchase and stability of the device in the proximal fragment (Fig. 14.18).

Intertrochanteric fractures with a subtrochanteric extension are reduced closed on the fracture table. This type of reduction is referred to as indirect reduction. It is preferred to a direct open reduction because it makes it possible to preserve the blood supply to all the intervening fragments. Once the fracture is reduced, the DCS is inserted into the proximal fragment and the plate is then fixed to the shaft distal to the subtrochanteric extension of the fracture, without any attempt being made to expose or fix any of the intervening fragments. This type of fixation is referred to as bridge plating. It is important not to attempt to visualize or fix any of the intervening fragments. As long as their blood supply is preserved, a bone graft is not necessary. In dealing with A3 fractures, i.e., true intertrochanteric fractures, it is possible to increase the stability of the fixation by placing the fracture under axial compression with the articulated tension device.

Type III fractures in young patients are reduced and internally fixed as described, but we make a further effort to secure fixation of the greater trochanter with a tension band wire, which is passed around the insertion of the abductors into the trochanter proximally and distally about a screw used to secure the plate.

Type IV intertrochanteric fractures with subtrochanteric extension can also be stabilized very well with the gamma nail (Howmedica Pfizer, New York, USA). We participated in an extensive trial of gamma nail fixation for intertrochanteric fractures and were very pleased with the results of fixation of type IV fractures. The gamma nail is introduced through the tip of the trochanter and tends to remain within the proximal fragment even if the fracture extends through the piriform fossa. Because of complications, such as shaft fractures through the distal-locking screws of the short gamma nail, we abandoned the device. The recently introduced long gamma nail (Howmedica, Pfizer, NY, USA) in all likelihood overcomes the problem of shaft fracture, but we have no personal experience with it. We have tried the Recon nail (Smith Nephew Richards). The intertrochanteric component of the fracture makes it very difficult to use this device because it tends to fall out of the proximal fragment. We have found the Recon nail to be technically very difficult to use in the fixation of type IV fractures and have found the failure rate in our hands to be unacceptably high. We feel that it is not a suitable device for the fixation of any femoral fracture which has an intertrochanteric extension. Thus the only device which we continue to use for the fixation of type IV fractures, and which has yielded consistently satisfactory results as long as the device was used as a bridge plate, is the DCS or the condylar blade plate.

14.4.4 Postoperative Management

As already indicated, we feel that elderly patients must be allowed immediate full weight bearing as tolerated. This is indeed the goal of surgery. The only exception which we make to this rule is in type IV fractures or in young patients in whom we have carried out an anatomical reduction.

14.4.5 Common Early and Late Postoperative Complications

The complication rate of treatment related to the fracture itself is below 10%. As indicated, avascular necrosis is very rare. The reason for the interruption of the blood supply is not clear. We have seen it in a patient with an undisplaced fracture (Fig. 14.19).

Shortening of the leg due to medialization of the shaft, because severe comminution, and because of shortening of the femoral neck due to resorption and collapse at the fracture is common, but is not a significant complication in the elderly. It is easily handled, if necessary, with an appropriate lift to equalize leg length.

In elderly patients, we do not attempt to fix the greater trochanter. It displaces upwards and posteriorly due to muscle pull and usually malunites in this position. The direction of the muscle pull is altered, as is the length of the lever arm. It undoubtly alters the biome-

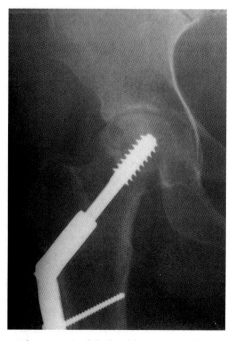

Fig. 14.19. Avascular necrosis of the head in a patient who had a minimally displaced two part intertrochanteric fracture

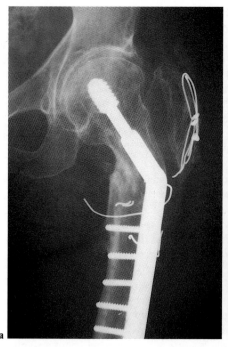 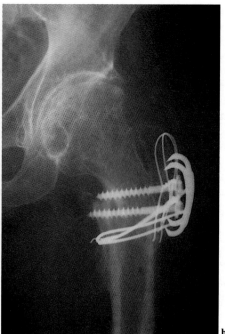

a   b

Fig. 14.20. a A nonunion of the greater trochanter following an intertrochanteric fracture. The patient complained of pain and walked with a marked lurch. **b** The trochanter united after stable internal fixation. The pain and lurch disappeared

chanics about the hip and contributes in some patients to a Trendelenburg lurch and in many patients to the need to use a walking stick. Occasionally, the trochanter reattaches only by means of fibrous tissue. In more active elderly patients, this may contribute to marked weakness of the abductor muscles and may interfere sufficiently with function to require surgical attention (Fig. 14.20 a,b). In younger patients in whom we carry out an anatomical reduction, the greater trochanter is secured with tension band wires. These are passed around the insertion of the abductor muscles into the greater trochanter proximally and distally around the most proximal screw passing through the plate.

Malunion results invariably in varus and in external rotation. This deformity is easily corrected in younger, more active patient by means of a valgus osteotomy (Fig. 14.21 a–d) In correcting this malunion, it is important to remember that carrying out the valgus correction requires lateralization of the shaft to preserve the normal distance of the anatomical axis of the femur from the midsagittal plane. Fixation devices such as the DHS, if used to secure the osteotomy, result in medialization of the shaft and in subsequent valgus overload at the knee. The exact fixation device has to be determined at the time of preoperative planning with the aid of the appropriate templates. We have found the 120° and the 130° repositioning blade plates to be the appropriate fixation devices, as they allow for lateralization of the shaft.

Nonunion may occur either after internal fixation or, rarely, as a result of neglect of the fracture. If a nonunion is recognized in an otherwise properly aligned reduction and maintained fixation of the fracture, it should be bone-grafted with autogenous cancellous bone before the fixation device fails. Once the fixation device fails, the surgeon is faced with a more formidable reconstructive problem. In younger patients, the hip should be preserved and an appropriate osteotomy be carried out to realign the fragments and attempt to place the nonunion as much as possible under compression by aligning it at 90° to the resultant forces R (Fig. 14.22 a,b). In elderly patients, a nonunion is best treated by means of a total hip replacement arthroplasty, particularly if the joint is damaged by the penetration of a fixation device (Fig. 14.23 a,b). One might argue in favor of either a unipolar arthroplasty, such as a Moore or a Thompson prosthesis, or a bicentric hip with a mobile cup when the acetabulum is normal. We prefer total hip replacement because it guarantees the patient a more normal hip function and better outcome.

Occasionally in severely osteoporotic patients, a four-hole side plate fixation may result in a fracture just below the plate. This complication is best handled by simply replacing the plate with at least an eight-hole side plate, placing the fracture under axial compression if possible, and adding an autogenous bone graft. In selecting the length of the side plate, it should be remembered that a longer plate with widely spaced screws will provide stronger fixation than a shorter plate with the same number but more closely spaced screws.

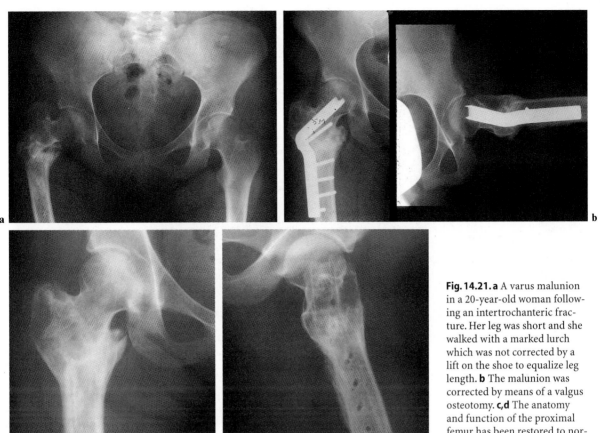

a   b

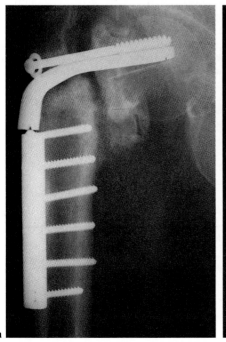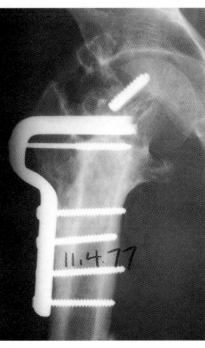

c, d

Fig. 14.21. a A varus malunion
in a 20-year-old woman following an intertrochanteric fracture. Her leg was short and she
walked with a marked lurch
which was not corrected by a
lift on the shoe to equalize leg
length. **b** The malunion was
corrected by means of a valgus
osteotomy. **c,d** The anatomy
and function of the proximal
femur has been restored to normal

Fig. 14.22. a An intertrochanteric nonunion in a middle-
aged man. **b** This was treated
by means of a valgus osteotomy

a   b

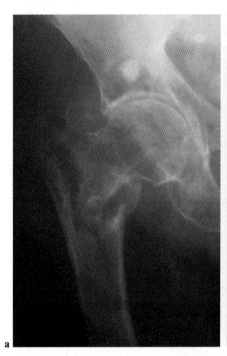
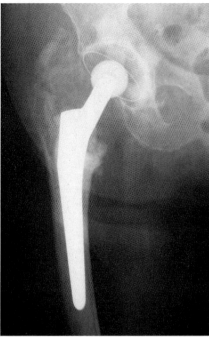

Fig. 14.23. a An intertrochanteric nonunion in an elderly patient. **b** This was treated by means of a total hip arthroplasty

a

b

References

Chapman M (ed) (1993) Operative orthopaedics, vol 1, 2 nd edn. Lippincott, Philadepelphia, pp 597–598

Clawson DK (1964) Trochanteric fractures treated by the sliding screw plate fixation method. J Trauma 4:737

Dimon JH, Hughston JS (1967) Unstable intertrochanteric fractures of the hip. J Bone Joint Surg 49A: 440

Garden RS (1964) Stability and union in subcapital fractures of the femur. J Bone Joint Surg 46B:630–647

Kyle RF, Gustilo RB, Premer RF (1979) Analysis of 622 intertrochanteric hip fractures: a retrospective and prospective study. J Bone Joint. Surg 61A:216

Lanz T, Wachsmuth W (1972) Bein und Statik, part 4, 2 nd edn. Springer, Berlin Heidelberg New York (Praktische Anatomie, vol 1)

Massie WK (1962) Extracapsular fractures of the hip treated by impaction using a sliding nail-plate fixation. Clin Orthop 22:180

Meyers MH, Harvey JP, Moore TM (1974) The muscle-pedicle bone graft in the treatment of displaced fractures of the femoral neck: indication, operative technique, and results. Orthop Clin North Am 5:779

Müller ME (1957) Zur Behandlung der Schenkelhalspseudarthorse. Z Unfallmed Berufskr 50:125

Müller ME, Allgöwer M, Willenegger H (1970) Manual of internal fixation, 1 st edn. Springer, Berlin Heidelberg New York

Müller ME, Allgöwer M, Schneider R, Willenegger H (1979) Manual of internal fixation, 2 nd edn. Springer, Berlin Heidelberg New York

Müller ME, Nazarian S, Koch P, Schatzker J (1990) The comprehensive classification of fractures of long bones. Springer, Berlin Heidelberg New York

Pauwels F (1965) Gesammelte Abhandlungen zur funktionellen Anatomie des Bewegungsapparates. Springer, Berlin Heidelberg New York, p 27

Sarmiento A, Williams EM (1970) The unstable intertrochanteric fracture: treatment with a valgus osteotomy and I-beam nail-plate – a preliminary report of 100 cases. J Bone Joint Surg 52A: 1309

Schatzker J (1984) The intertrochanteric osteotomy. Springer, Berlin Heidelberg New York

15 Subtrochanteric Fractures of the Femur

J. SCHATZKER

15.1 Biomechanical Considerations

15.1.1 Mechanical Forces

The subtrochanteric segment of the femur extends from the lesser trochanter to the junction of the proximal and middle thirds of the diaphysis. This segment of the femur is subjected not only to axial loads of weight bearing, but also to tremendous bending forces because of

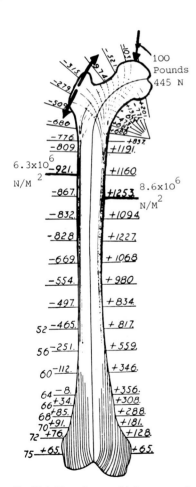

Fig. 15.1. Note the very high compressive stresses in the medial cortex and smaller tensile stresses in the lateral cortex. (From Cochran et al. 1980)

the eccentric load application to the femoral head (Fig. 15.1). Recent strain-gauge studies in vivo (Schatzker et al. 1980) have confirmed Pauwel's and the AO/ASIF contention that the bending forces cause the medial cortex to be loaded in compression and the lateral cortex in tension. Furthermore, they have shown that the compressive stresses in the medial cortex are significantly higher than tensile stresses in the lateral cortex. An appreciation of this asymmetrical loading pattern is important in determining the suitability of internal fixation devices for fixation of these fractures, in understanding the causes and the prevention of failure of these devices, and in appreciating the causes of nonunion or malunion. Factors important for the stability of a reduction and fixation, in order of importance, are the following:

1. Degree of comminution
2. Level of the fracture
3. Pattern of the fracture

15.1.2 Degree of Comminution

As we have emphasized elsewhere (see p. 382), the stability of a reduction depends on structural continuity. A simple fracture which is reduced anatomically and fixed with the aid of compression is stable and shows little tendency to redisplacement. Under load, the forces are conducted directly from one fragment to the other, with relatively little stress being borne by the internal fixation. In a comminuted fracture, on the other hand, where the cortex opposite the plate ("the medial buttress") is deficient or where a segment of bone is so shattered that structural stability and continuity cannot be restored, the forces of loading are borne almost entirely by the internal fixation. The reduction is unstable and the only factor preventing redisplacement is the internal fixation. Hence, failure is common. The internal fixation either pulls out of bone, breaks because of overload, or undergoes fatigue failure because of cyclic loading. Thus, irreconstructible medial cortical comminution (shattered medial buttress) and irreconstructible segmental comminution stand out as the most important causes of failure.

15.1.3 Level of the Fracture

Next in the order of importance in determining the prognosis of a subtrochanteric fracture is the level of the fracture. The significance of this factor will be appreciated if we consider the difference between two extreme situations, namely, a high fracture almost at the level of the lesser trochanter and a low fracture at the junction of the proximal and middle thirds of the femur. The closer the fracture to the lesser trochanter, the shorter the lever arm and the lower the bending moment. The involvement of the lesser and greater trochanter is of importance if we are considering an intramedullary nail as the mode of fixation. If the greater trochanter is involved as an extension of the subtrochanteric fracture, it is better to resort to an angled device for fixation. The trochanteric component of the fracture often makes it very difficult to keep the nail within the proximal fragment. The angled device permits relatively easy reduction and fixation of both fractures. Before the advent of the second-generation locking nails, involvement of the lesser trochanter in the subtrochanteric fracture was a contraindication for intramedullary nailing, because it was impossible to lock the nail in the proximal fragment. The advent of nails such as the "Reconstruction Nail" (Smith Nephew Richards Co., Memphis, TN, USA) or of the short and more recently of the long gamma nails (Howmedica Pfizer, New York, NY, USA), which lock

proximally within the femoral neck and head, have made it possible to nail subtrochanteric fractures in which the lesser trochanter is broken off.

15.1.4 Pattern of the Fracture

The pattern of the fracture is important in determining the mode of internal fixation if we are considering plating and only indirectly influences the outcome of treatment. In a transverse or short oblique fracture we rely on axial compression for stability. To achieve such compression we use a tension band plate. In a long oblique or spiral fracture, primary stability is obtained by interfragmental lag screw fixation, which is then protected by a neutralization plate. If we are dealing with a transverse or short oblique fracture with a long proximal fragment, we can also consider intramedullary fixation with a conventional or, preferably, with a locking nail.

15.1.5 Deformity

The proximal femur is surrounded by very large and powerful muscles. In the case of a fracture, their spatial arrangement, combined with their origin and insertion, results in a very characteristic deformity. The proximal fragment, as a result of contraction of the abductors, the external rotators, and the iliopsoas muscle, is flexed, abducted, and externally rotated. The adductors cause the shaft to be adducted and the force of gravity causes the distal fragment to fall into some external rotation. All the muscles which span the fracture combine to cause shortening. Thus, the resultant deformity is one of an anterior and lateral bowing of the proximal shaft, combined with considerable shortening and variable degrees of external rotation (Fig. 15.2).

15.2 Natural History

Nonoperative treatment of a subtrochanteric fracture is difficult and frequently unsatisfactory (Schatzker and Waddell 1980). All nonoperative forms of treatment involve the use of traction, exerted by either a supracondylar pin or a pin in the tibial tubercle. Longitudinal traction can correct the shortening, but it will not correct the deformity. The proximal fragment remains flexed, abducted, and externally rotated, and a large gap frequently remains between the fragments. In order to correct the deformity and close the gap, the distal fragment must be realigned with the proximal one. This involves traction in the so called 90/90 position, with the hip and knee flexed to 90°. This position is not only very difficult to maintain in adults, but also frequently fails to

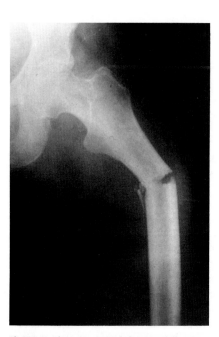

Fig. 15.2. Characteristic deformity following a subtrochanteric fracture. There is anterior and lateral bowing of the proximal shaft combined with external rotation and shortening

Fig. 15.3. a The varus bow of the shaft causes the tip of the greater trochanter to rise above the center of rotation of the femoral head. This causes a functional varus deformity of the hip and abductor insufficiency. **b** The deformity has been corrected by means of an osteotomy. A wedge with a lateral and anterior base had to be resected to achieve correction in two planes

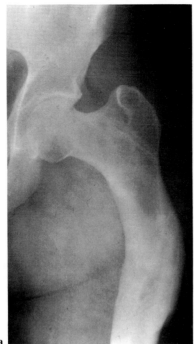
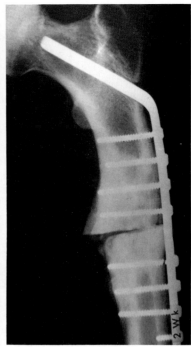

a

b

give a satisfactory reduction, and a significant degree of deformity often persists.

A malunion is not compatible with normal function. Patients with malunited subtrochanteric fractures walk with a Trendelenburg lurch and frequently complain of pain in the front of their thigh. A lift in the shoe to compensate for the leg length discrepancy neither stops the lurch nor abolishes the pain. The lurch and the pain are the result of the disturbed biomechanics about the proximal femur. The varus or lateral bow of the proximal femur causes the tip of the greater trochanter to rise above the center of rotation of the femoral head (Fig. 15.3 a). This brings about a functional varus deformity of the hip and laxity of the abductors. The laxity and inefficiency of the abductors is responsible for the Trendelenburg lurch. The anterior bowing is probably the cause of the anterior distal thigh pain. Both the pain and the lurch persist until the deformity is corrected surgically and the biomechanical relationships are restored to normal (Fig. 15.3 b).

15.3 Indications for Open Reduction and Internal Fixation

In our opinion, subtrochanteric fractures should be treated by open reduction and stable internal fixation, as this is the only form of treatment which ensures a high percentage of satisfactory results (Schatzker and Waddell 1980; AO Fracture Documentation, The AO Foundation, Davos, Switzerland). Nonoperative methods are not only fraught with all the serious complications of prolonged bed rest; in adults, as already indicated, they also frequently fail to reestablish acceptable alignment of the fragments.

Undoubtedly, the zeal of many surgeons is tempered by the unhappy memory of a frustrating surgical experience of trying to put together a badly comminuted subtrochanteric fracture. The inherent difficulties of a surgical procedure cannot, however, be used as an argument to justify nonoperative treatment, which, apart from the dangers of enforced and prolonged bed rest, frequently fails to yield satisfactory results because of malunion.

15.4 Surgical Techniques

15.4.1 Diagnosis

The precise diagnosis of a subtrochanteric fracture can only be made radiologically. The history, however, should not be neglected, because it yields valuable information on the manner of injury, on associated injuries, and on the patient's state of health and expectations of treatment.

In addition to anteroposterior and lateral radiographs of the involved femur, which must include the joints above and below, corresponding anteroposterior and lateral radiographs of the normal femur should be

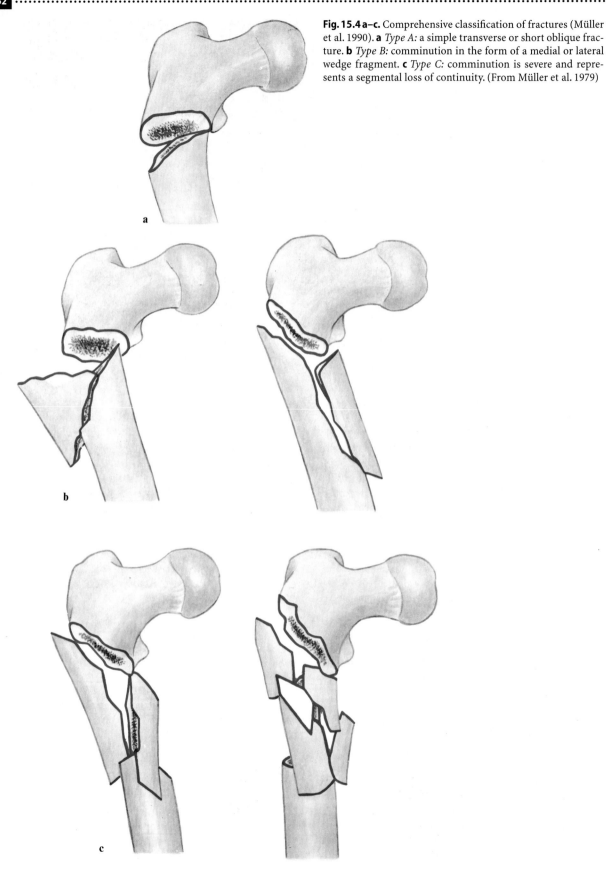

Fig. 15.4 a–c. Comprehensive classification of fractures (Müller et al. 1990). **a** *Type A:* a simple transverse or short oblique fracture. **b** *Type B:* comminution in the form of a medial or lateral wedge fragment. **c** *Type C:* comminution is severe and represents a segmental loss of continuity. (From Müller et al. 1979)

obtained; these will serve as a template for the reconstructive plan.

15.4.2 Classification

For a classification to be useful it must not only identify the fracture pattern, but also serve as a guide to treatment and therefore indicate prognosis.

As we have seen in the discussion of biomechanical factors, the most important factor determining the outcome of treatment in subtrochanteric fractures is the degree of comminution. We therefore favor the comprehensive classification of subtrochanteric fractures, because it identifies the fracture pattern and the inherent difficulty in treatment. Thus there are the simple "type A" fractures, which may be transverse, oblique, or spiral; the "type B" wedge fractures, which have either a medial or a lateral wedge, but which can still be reconstructed to yield a stable structural unit; and the "type C" fractures, which have as their hallmark comminution to such a degree that a stable unit cannot be achieved. This group includes fractures with such segmental comminution that it represents a segmental loss (Fig. 15.4). The comprehensive classification fails to indicate some features of the fracture pattern which are most important if we are considering locked intramedullary nailing as a form of stabilization. Thus it is important to know whether the fracture is below the lesser trochanter or whether the lesser trochanter is involved. Similarly, it is important to know whether the fracture pattern extends to involve the intertrochanteric area. This latter involvement should guide the surgeon away from intramedullary nailing.

15.4.3 Planning the Surgical Procedure

15.4.3.1 Implants

Once the diagnosis has been established and open reduction and internal fixation decided upon, it becomes necessary to formulate a careful plan of all the steps of the operative procedure. Let us begin with a discussion of the different methods of internal fixation available.

a) Intramedullary Nailing

Intramedullary nailing without interlocking has played a role in the stabilization of subtrochanteric fractures. As with fractures of the mid-diaphysis, only transverse and short oblique fractures could be considered ideally suited for this technique. Unfortunately, the majority of sub-trochanteric fractures are spiral and comminuted, and therefore only a relatively small number can be considered suitable for conventional intramedullary nailing.

The stability of the fixation provided by an intramedullary nail (see p. 374) depends on the length of contact and the degree of fit between the nail and bone on both sides of the fracture. The medullary canal of the subtrochanteric segment is very wide just below the lesser trochanter and narrows down like a cone toward the isthmus. The isthmus, or the narrowest portion of the medullary canal, is usually at the upper or midportion of the middle third of the diaphysis. Thus, a nail which snugly fits the isthmus obtains little fixation in the proximal fragment. Conventional intramedullary nailing of subtrochanteric fractures has been successful in teenagers and young adults, because in such patients the proximal femur is still filled with very dense cancellous bone, which gives the nail excellent purchase. In older individuals this cancellous bone becomes sparse. The nail fails to obtain purchase and the proximal fragment frequently drifts into varus. To overcome this complication, Küntscher devised a "Y-nail" (Küntscher 1967), which was later modified by Zickel (1976). Our experience with the Zickel nail has not been favorable. We were able to use it as the sole means of fixation only in transverse and short oblique fractures. Spiral and comminuted fractures required supplemental fixation, as described by Zickel (1976), which abolished the advantages of this technique. In addition, in some of the short oblique or transverse fractures the distal fragment demonstrated rotational instability, and rotational deformities were common. The difficulties of the technique and its complications have led us to the conclusion that, in comparison with other techniques, the Zickel nail has little to offer, and we have abandoned it in the treatment of subtrochanteric fractures.

Ender rekindled interest in the intramedullary mode of stabilization of these fractures with the introduction of his elastic nails (Ender 1970; Pankovich and Tarabishy 1980). Once again, we have found that this technique has considerable shortcomings. Stable subtrochanteric fractures, i.e., simple transverse or oblique fractures with little comminution, could be treated successfully with Ender's nailing. The "problem" subtrochanteric fractures, however – the ones with extensive comminution and segmental loss of continuity – fared badly. We were unable to maintain length or sufficient stability to keep the patients ambulant; patients with these unstable fractures treated with Ender's nailing had to be placed in skeletal traction for 3–6 weeks. In our opinion, an operative procedure which has to be combined with complete bed rest and traction is not justified. Long spiral fractures could be reduced and stabilized with cerclage wiring prior to the introduction of Ender's nailing. Such a combined mode of fixation is sufficiently strong to

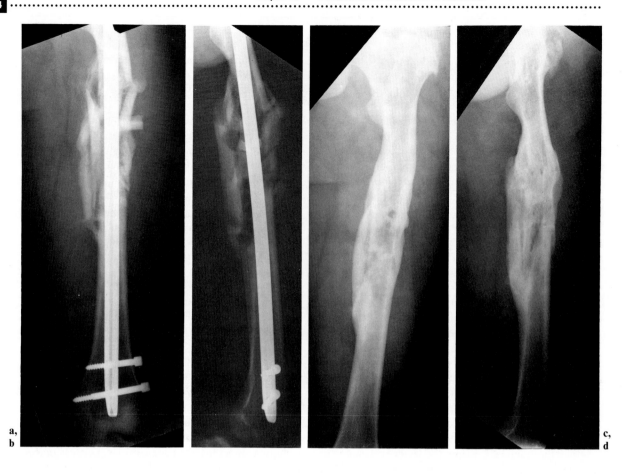

a,
b

c,
d

Fig. 15.5 a–d. A severely comminuted subtrochanteric fracture stabilized with a statically locked Grosse-Kempf intramedullary nail. **a** Anteroposterior radiograph. **b** Lateral radiograph. Note the abundant callus. **c, d** Radiographs taken after nail removal 2 years after fracture. Note the advanced degree of remodeling of the cortex

allow early ambulation, but the need for open exposure of the fracture defeats the biological advantages of the closed nailing, and we have abandoned the technique in preference to locked nailing.

The introduction of the locking intramedullary nailing system has greatly enlarged the scope of intramedullary nailing of subtrochanteric fractures (Kempf et al. 1985). We have found it an excellent technique for the treatment of subtrochanteric fractures. Locking the proximal fragment to the nail, which this system makes possible, has overcome the tendency of the proximal fragment to drift into varus, and locking the distal fragment to the nail has prevented shortening or rotation. The locking of the fragments has made supplemental internal fixation of the fragments, such as cerclage or lag screw fixation, superfluous. This allows us to take full biological advantage of intramedullary nailing. In addi-

tion, the development of "intramedullary bone grafting" (M. Chapman, personal communication) has permitted grafting of major defects while keeping the procedure closed. The fact that we do not have to interfere with the soft tissue envelope and the remaining blood supply of the bony fragments and soft tissues has resulted, in our hands, in a more rapid consolidation than with any other technique. The locking of the fragments provides exceptional rotational stability, which has also permitted us to deal with oblique or spiral fractures. Thus, we feel that of all the intramedullary devices, the locking intramedullary nail is the only device suitable for subtrochanteric fractures, as long as the proximal fragment is sufficiently long to permit stable locking (Fig. 15.5). Fractures with intertrochanteric extensions require a blade-plate or a compression screw and plate combination such as the dynamic condylar screw (Synthes, Paioli, PA, USA).

The difficulty in securing proximal locking with the first-generation locked intramedullary nails has led to classification of subtrochanteric fractures into those which involved the lesser trochanter and which were not suitable for locked intramedullary fixation and those which were below and which were suitable. The emergence of the second-generation locked intramedullary

All second-generation nails share two difficulties. The first is that the nail must be inserted in such a way as to accommodate the anteversion of the neck in order to make locking within the neck and head possible. The second is that if there is a fracture through the intertrochanteric area, the nail may fall out of the proximal fragment during insertion. In order to overcome this difficulty, we prefer to use an angled device of 95°, such as the angled blade plate or the DCS, whenever the subtrochanteric fracture extends to involve the intertrochanteric area. Whether or not the plate is used as a bridge plate depends on whether or not the subtrochanteric component is a complex fracture. Whatever the fracture pattern, indirect reduction techniques should be used to minimize the damage to the blood supply of bone.

b) Nail Plate

In a stable, strong internal fixation, an equal number of screws must traverse the plate and the bone on each side of the fracture. If the surgeon attempts to fix a subtrochanteric fracture with a straight plate, the fixation in the proximal fragment is frequently deficient. This is particularly true if the fracture line extends close to the lesser trochanter, because the femoral neck makes fixation in the proximal fragment with simple screws virtually impossible. This problem has been solved with a "nail plate" type of device; the introduction of the nail up the neck into the head greatly increases the fixation of the device in the proximal fragment.

Modern nail plate devices all have a fixed angle between the "nail" and the plate. They fall into two categories: those with sliding nail or screw assemblies and those with a fixed segment which is inserted into the proximal femur.

The best example of the "sliding" nail plate is the compression hip screw (Richards Surgical Ltd., Memphis, TN, USA) or the dynamic hip screw (Synthes). The design of this device is such that a large-diameter screw is screwed into the femoral head. The screw fits into a collar of the plate, which in turn is fixed to the femoral shaft. The two are so designed that the smooth shaft of the screw can slide within the collar of the plate and yet retain rotational stability. Thus, with these devices one can impact those fractures which are crossed by the sliding mechanisms.

The sliding nail principle with an angle of 125° or greater was developed for the impaction of subcapital and intertrochanteric fractures. It has a wide appeal to surgeons who, in surgery on the proximal femur, desire guidewire insertion with two-plane radiographic control as well as the use of the fracture table and traction (Fig. 15.7). What, then, about its use for the fixation of subtrochanteric fractures?

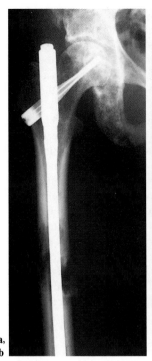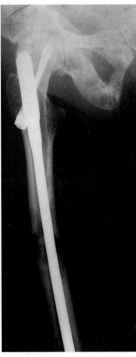

a, b

Fig. 15.6 a, b. Synthes second-generation nail, the unreamed intramedullary nail for the femur, locked proximally with the spiral blade (shown) and distally with screws (not shown)

nails has overcome this difficulty. These nails secure proximal locking within the femoral neck and head. The Russell Taylor Reconstruction Nail (Smith Nephew Richards Co.) secures the proximal locking by means of two screws which must enter the femoral neck and head. The AO/ASIF (Synthes) has recently introduced the unreamed nail for the femur, which has a very versatile array of proximal locking systems. One of these is the "spiral blade," which is inserted through the nail into the neck and head (see Fig. 15.6). The Howmedia Company popularized the short and more recently the long gamma nails, which are designed to overcome fractures of the femoral shaft associated with fractures of the lesser or greater trochanters. We were unhappy with the short gamma nail because of complications such as shaft fractures at the distal locking screw, and we have now abandoned the gamma nail system. Our recent experience with the new unreamed AO nail (Synthes) and its versatile proximal locking has been very favorable. We have had the most extensive experience with the "Recon nail" (Smith Nephew Richards Co.). Although technically challenging, it is an excellent device for the subtrochanteric fracture with involvement of the lesser trochanter. If the les-ser trochanter is intact we use the first-generation interlocking techniques.

356 ·

Chapter 15   **Subtrochanteric Fractures of the Femur**

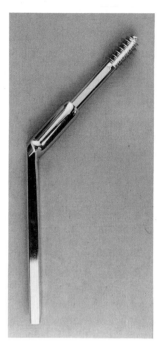

Fig. 15.7. A dynamic hip screw

    Its advocates have made claims that the device allows impaction of the subtrochanteric fracture and medialization of the shaft. They maintain that the medialization in turn reduces the bending moment and reduces the resultant of forces, which leads to a large varus moment and increases the stability of the fixation. This reasoning is unfortunately wrong. In order for the device to have secure fixation in the proximal fragment, it is essential to prevent secondary displacement in the frontal plane (varus) or in the sagittal plane due to rotation. Instability due to rotation of the proximal fragment about the screw can result in flexion or extension with consequent deformity and malunion (see Fig. 15.8). To prevent such rotation, the compression screw fixation must be supplemented with at least one screw inserted

through the plate into the proximal fragment. This is impossible to achieve in most high subtrochanteric fractures when a 130°-angled device is used for fixation. Furthermore, once a screw is inserted through the plate into the proximal fragment, the sliding mechanism is blocked, the fracture cannot be impacted, and the shaft cannot be medialized. Thus, the device is not ideal for use in high subtrochanteric fractures (Fig. 15.8). The only advantages to its use in lower subtrochanteric fractures are its strength and the fact that it can be inserted into the proximal fragment with the aid of guidewires and radiographic control. The only time the shaft can be medialized is when the fracture is at the level of the lesser trochanter, but even in such cases rotational instability of the proximal fragment and possible shortening of the extremity must still be considered.

    The 130° intertrochanteric and the 95° condylar angled plates and the DCS of the AO (Fig. 15.9) are useful devices for the treatment of subtrochanteric fractures. The 130°-angled plate, like the compression screw or the dynamic hip screw, is useful only in low subtrochanteric fractures, where fixation of the device in the proximal fragment can be supplemented by the insertion of one or two cortical screws. Thus, its use is limited, and when a 130°-angled device is to be used we prefer the dynamic hip screw because of its greater ease of insertion. The 95° condylar plate or the DCS is the one we prefer and commonly use, because its proximal extension usually makes

Fig. 15.8. a Malunion resulting from an improper choice of implant. A high subtrochanteric fracture cannot be stabilized with a 130°-angled device, as the fixation of the device in the proximal fragment must be supplemented with at least one screw, which in this case is impossible. The result is instability with varus deformity in the frontal plane and rotation about the axis of the blade in the sagittal plane. **b** A corrective osteotomy was fixed with the 95° condylar blade plate. This would also have been the better device for the initial fixation of the fracture

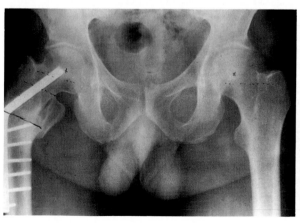
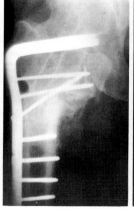
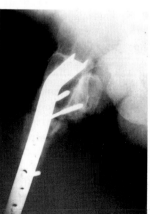

a   b

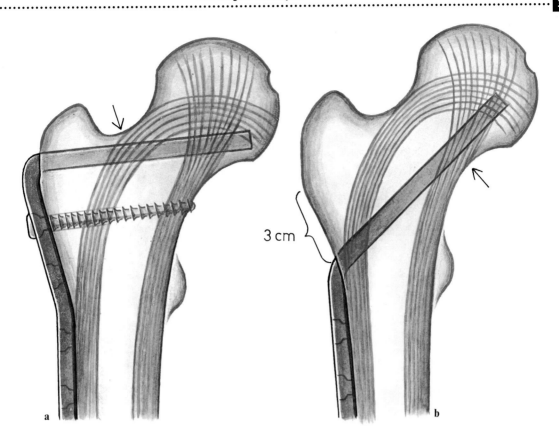

Fig. 15.9. a The condylar blade plate. **b** The 130°-angled blade plate. (From Müller et al. 1979)

it possible to insert two or more cortical screws through the plate into the calcar which greatly strengthens its hold in the proximal fragment and prevents varus or rotational deformities. Thus, the 95° devices can be used for the fixation not only of high subtrochanteric fractures, but also of those combined with intertrochanteric fractures. It can also be employed for lower subtrochanteric fractures, providing a sufficiently long plate is used. The greatest benefit of the 95° condylar plate or DCS is that they can be introduced into a short proximal fragment prior to the reduction of the subtrochanteric fracture (Fig. 15.10). This is a decided advantage when faced with a highly comminuted fracture in which reconstruction of the comminuted segment is impossible and in which locked nailing cannot be performed. When the 95° condylar plate is inserted into the femur, the anatomical landmarks of the proximal femur are used as a guide. If desired, the position of the guidewires can be checked radiologically prior to insertion of the blade. As will be clear from the discussion of the insertion technique (see Sect. 15.4.4.4), if a careful preoperative plan is executed and if the guidewires are carefully inserted under direct

visual control using the anatomical bony landmarks and templates as guides, accurate insertion of the blade becomes relatively easy. The radiograph is used not as a guide to insertion but rather as a check of its accuracy. The dynamic condylar screw (Fig. 15.10) like the condylar blade plate has a 95° angle; however, it is cannulated and uses a guidewire whose position can be checked radiologically. It is also easier to insert into bone because, like the dynamic hip screw, once proper positioning of the guidewire has been achieved the screw can be inserted with great ease. It can also be used in every situation in which a condylar blade plate would be indicated. Since we wrote the first edition of this book, we have had very extensive experience in the use of the DCS, which has completely replaced the condylar blade plate. The DCS has all the features of a blade plate, but it is easier and therefore safer to use.

15.4.3.2 Preoperative Planning

Preoperative planning is necessary whether one plans to nail or plate. For intramedullary nailing it is important to determine the type of nail, its diameter, length, and the mode of interlocking. If the surgeon should wish to plate the femur, then a more formal plan is required.

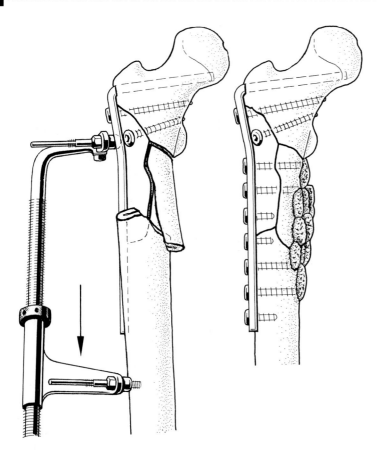

Fig. 15.10. Note that the condylar plate has been inserted into the proximal fragment prior to the reduction of the fracture. Indirect reduction techniques have made bone-grafting superfluous. (From Müller et al. 1979)

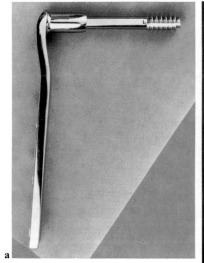

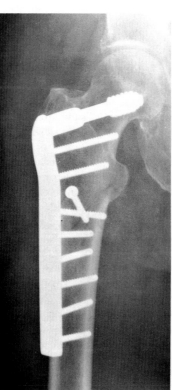

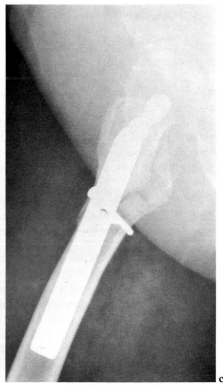

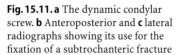

Fig. 15.11. a The dynamic condylar screw. **b** Anteroposterior and **c** lateral radiographs showing its use for the fixation of a subtrochanteric fracture

Once the diagnostic radiographs and those of the opposite, uninvolved extremity are available, a careful preoperative plan can be prepared (see Fig. 15.11 c). The radiograph of the normal proximal femur is reversed and the outline of the bone traced onto a sheet of tracing paper. If the fracture extends distally into the mid-diaphysis and is comminuted, so that identification and reduction of the fragments is difficult, the outline of the whole normal femur may have to be traced. The position of the proximal and distal fragments must be then marked on the tracing of the uninvolved femur and the gap between the main fragments measured. A further guide to length is to select the plate of correct length for the uninvolved femur and note at what point the distal fragment makes contact with the plate, i.e., how many screw holes of the plate are opposite the distal fragment. In this way correct length can be established intraoperatively. Where comminution is not so great, the most proximal and the most distal fracture lines are then carefully marked on the tracing of the proximal femur. It should be carefully noted where the fractures cross the medial and lateral cortices both proximally and distally. If the comminuted fragments are major and large, they are carefully drawn in. If the comminution is such that the outline and arrangement of the fragments is not identifiable, this is also noted. Any places where lag screws can be inserted between the fragments are marked. The surgeon should decide at this point and mark on the drawing which holes will be drilled first and in which order, as well as which will be gliding and which will be thread holes. The principle of converting a fracture with many fragments into one consisting of two major fragments no longer applies. It is better to leave the fragments with their blood supply preserved. In this way it can act as a living bone graft and lead to much more rapid consolidation than would a dead piece of cortex in its normal anatomical position.

Once the fragments are marked, a template is placed under the drawing, and the position of the plate and its length are carefully noted. In addition to the blade length and the length of the plate, the exact position of the entry of the blade into the lateral cortex of the greater trochanter must be carefully noted, since a window must be cut prior to the insertion of the seating chisel. The distance of the blade from the superior cortex of the neck is also noted, as is the position of the tip of the blade in relation to the center of the femoral head, where the tension and compression trabeculae intersect. These are all important landmarks. They can be identified at surgery and will give the surgeon the correct insertion of the blade into the proximal fragment, even when this is so small that the condylar guide cannot be employed intraoperatively as a check of the position of the seating chisel or the guidewire for the dynamic condylar screw. The position of the cortical window is best related to the rough line (easily identified intraoperatively) where the gluteus medius and vastus lateralis muscles meet. If comminution is present, the placement of the bone grafts, if they are to be used, should also be noted (Fig. 15.12).

The above is also true when a DCS is being used. The position of the window will determine the insertion site for the guidewire of the DCS. The relationship of the tip of the guidewire to the crossing of the tension and pressure trabeculae will indicate the direction of the guidewire in the frontal plane.

Locked intramedullary nailing is a closed procedure, and the reduction is achieved by closed manipulation and traction. Length cannot be judged intraoperatively; it must be carefully measured preoperatively. The most accurate method is to measure the sound extremity from the tip of the trochanter to the joint line and then subtract 2 cm. Next, a nail judged to be of the correct length or a ruler of suitable length is taped to the lateral side of the thigh in its midposition, and an anteroposterior radiograph of the femur is made. A more accurate assessment of length is obtained if the nail or ruler is taped to the lateral side of the thigh rather than placed on the table beside the leg. If the patient's thigh is large and the nail is taped to the X-ray cassette, there is a real danger of choosing a nail which is too long, because of X-ray magnification of the femur (the thicker the thigh, the longer the nail; Fig. 15.12). Once the correct length is confirmed radiologically, it gives the length of the nail to be used. All that is then necessary at surgery is to make certain that the tip of the nail is driven as far into the distal fragment as planned. When the femur is distracted and the nail is locked in its proper position, both proximally and distally, the correct length will have been achieved.

The above determination of nail length is necessary only when dealing with complex irregular fractures. When nailing simple or wedge fractures the nail length can be determined quite accurately once the fracture is reduced.

Rotational malalignment is a problem with closed intramedullary nailing. This cannot be avoided by any preoperative planning. Surgeons must be aware of this complication and remember to take the usual intraoperative measures to avoid it.

15.4.4 Surgery

15.4.4.1 The Operating Table

The techniques which we employ are greatly facilitated by intraoperative image intensifier or X-ray control. Although radiographs are not used as a guide for the insertion of the plates, we feel that once the implant is

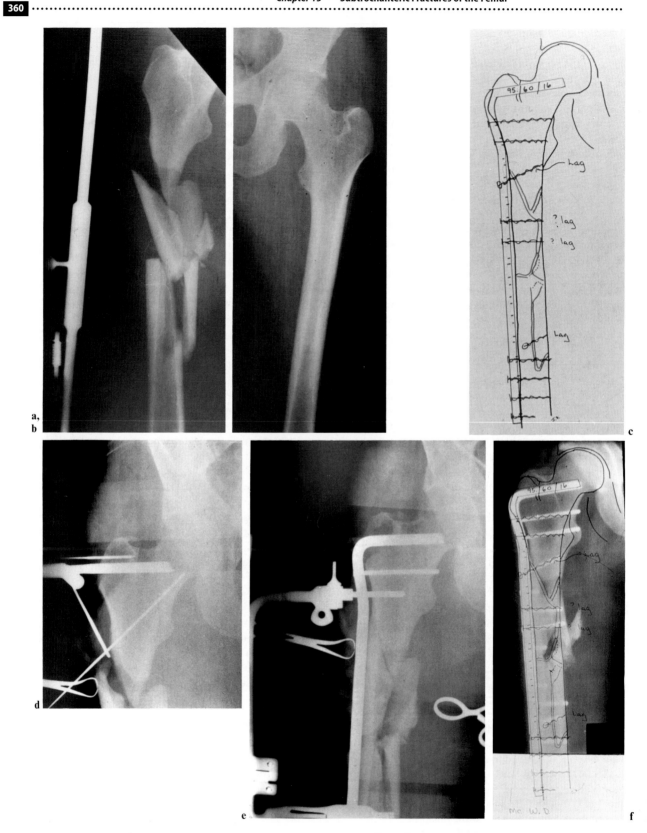

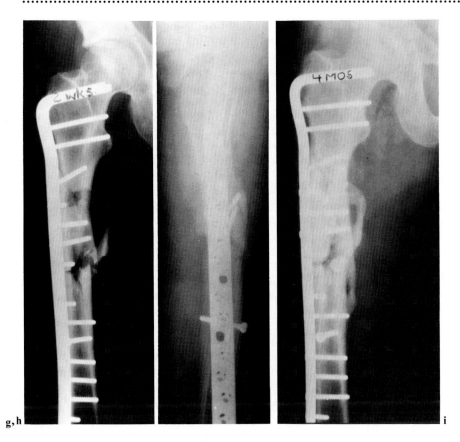

g, h   i

Fig. 15.12 a–i. Preoperative planning for open reduction and internal fixation of a subtrochanteric fracture. **a** A comminuted subtrochanteric fracture. **b** Radiograph of the opposite extremity. Reversed, it serves as a template. **c** Preoperative drawing of the planned internal fixation. **d** Intraoperative radiograph to check position of the seating chisel. **e** Intraoperative radiograph. Note the use of the distractor to achieve length and reduction of the comminuted fragments. **f** Internal fixation has been completed and a radiograph obtained in the recovery room. **g, h** Radiograph at 2 weeks after surgery. **i** At 4 months the fracture is solidly united. Note the formation of abundant callus in this "biological," internal fixation, where great care was exercised not to damage the blood supply to the comminuted fragments

inserted, anteroposterior and lateral radiographs should be obtained to make certain that the blade has not penetrated into the hip joint (see Fig. 15.12 d, e). Intraoperative traction is unnecessary – it may actually increase the difficulty of the surgery rather than ease the reduction. An AO distractor allows a more direct and accurate application of traction without tying down the extremity. For details on its use, please see Sect. 15.4.4.4 below.

For locked intramedullary nailing, either a special table designed for closed intramedullary nailing is employed, or the procedure is done on an ordinary operating table with a radiolucent extension.

Once the starting point is identified and the bone perforated at the insertion site, the guidewire or an unreamed nail are introduced and the fracture is reduced by traction. It is surprising how little traction is required to secure a reduction. The traction has to be maintained until the nail is inserted and locked. The advantage of operating on a radiolucent extension with the leg free and not in traction is that the patient can be positioned with the buttock supported on a sand bag. This provides greater freedom to access the starting point and greater freedom to manipulate the limb to secure a reduction. A further advantage is that the procedure progresses much more quickly because no time is lost in setting up the traction table or the patient in traction.

15.4.4.2 Positioning the Patient

For plating the patient should be placed in a supine position. We prefer to keep the pelvis level, and we do not use a roll to elevate the involved hip since this may lead to a rotational malreduction. The iliac crest and the anterior and lateral aspects of the hip and the leg are draped free.

This allows for full lateral access to the hip, it leaves the anterior iliac crest exposed as a donor site for bone-grafting, and it leaves the leg free to be manipulated as necessary during the reduction. In a badly comminuted fracture the only guide to correct rotational alignment is the range of hip motion. If the leg is in traction, or if it is draped in such a way that rotation of the hip is not possible, malreduction can easily occur. Furthermore, if the hip cannot be flexed to 90° it will become impossible to obtain a lateral radiograph of the hip during the procedure.

For *locked intramedullary nailing* we place the patient in a supine position, but elevate the hip on a sand bag to facilitate access to the entry point. This has to be kept in mind when checking the rotational alignment of the limb.

15.4.4.3 Surgical Approach for Plating

The surgical approach is through a straight lateral incision made in the skin along an imaginary line joining the greater trochanter with the lateral femoral condyle. It should extend from a point above the greater trochanter to approximately a hand's breadth below the fracture. The fascia lata is incised in line with the skin. As the next step, the surgeon should identify the interval between the tensor muscle of the fascia lata anteriorly, the anterior edge of the gluteus medius and gluteus minimus muscles cephalad, and the vastus lateralis muscle caudad. Once this interval is defined, the anterior and superior aspects of the hip joint capsule should be cleared and a Hohmann retractor inserted over the anterior pillar of the acetabulum (see Fig. 15.14).

In order to be able to insert an angled blade plate or a DCS into the femur without radiological control, an arthrotomy must be made to define the bony landmarks, such as the anteversion of the femur, the center of the femoral head, and the superior aspect of the neck. In order to carry out this arthrotomy, the exposed capsule is incised in line with the axis of the femoral neck and then a "T" is made at the base of the neck.

The fracture and the femoral shaft are exposed by reflecting the vastus lateralis muscle anteriorly. The femur should not be exposed through the substance of the vastus lateralis muscle, because such an exposure is often associated with unnecessary bleeding from the perforating branches of the profunda femoris artery and, after surgery, with considerable muscle scarring. The anterior arthrotomy incision is extended laterally just distal to the rough line on the lateral aspect of the greater trochanter. The rough line separates the fibers of the vastus lateralis muscle and those of the gluteus medius muscle. The incision is then carried distally through the fascia of the vastus lateralis muscle, just anterior to its posterior attachment, and the vastus lateralis muscle is freed with a periostial elevator from its attachment to the lateral intermuscular septum. The perforating branches of the profunda femoris artery should be cross-clamped and ligated. If cauterized and cut they may cause troublesome bleeding, since the posterior part may retract through the posterior intermuscular septum. Once retracted, a bleeding vessel is very difficult to find. In the region of the fracture the vastus lateralis muscle should not be detached from any loose comminuted fragments, since this completely devitalizes them. Proximally, in the region of the hip, the vastus lateralis muscle is reflected medially and distally, together with the inferior half of the hip joint capsule. In this way, full

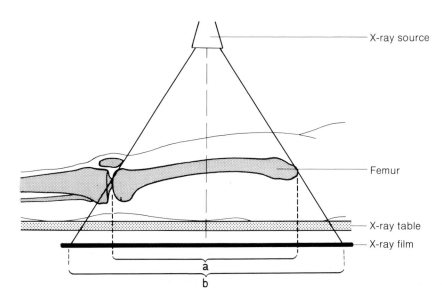

Fig. 15.13. The magnification factor: *a*, the actual length of the femur; *b*, the projected length. The thicker the thigh, the greater the distance between the femur and the X-ray cassette; thus, the greater the magnification

exposure is gained of the shaft, of the fracture, and of the hip joint (see Fig 15.13). The necessary Kirschner guide-wires can then be inserted and the open reduction and internal fixationperformed. To maintain the exposure we have found it useful to keep the muscle reflected with broad Hohmann retractors. The anterior exposure of the hip is maintained with the Hohmann retractor, which is passed over the anterior pillar of the acetabulum. The superior aspect of the neck is exposed by reflecting the cephalad flap of the hip capsule and driving the tip of a narrow Hohmann retractor into the middle of the super-ior cortex of the femoral neck. This prevents the tip of the retractor from slipping posterosuperiorly and pos-sibly damaging the retinacular vessels in their course to the femoral head. The inferior aspect of the neck and of the calcar is kept exposed by passing the tip of a retrac-tor below the neck (Fig. 15.14).

15.4.4.4 Technique of Open Reduction and Internal Fixation

Once the fracture is exposed, the surgeon must go back to the preoperative drawings and plan. Irrespective of the fracture type, it is best to introduce the angled blade plate or the screw of the DCS with the attached side plate into the proximal fragment prior to the reduction of the fracture. This is the key to securing an atraumatic reduc-tion with maximal preservation of the soft tissue attach-ment and minimal interference with the blood supply to the bony fragments.

The first Kirschner guidewire (*1* in Fig. 15.14) is placed inferiorly to mark the anteversion. The second guidewire (*2* in Fig. 15.14) will mark the direction of the seating chisel. Ideally, it should be inserted at 95° to the anatomical axis of the femur. In a comminuted femur which cannot be reduced, the anatomical axis cannot be determined from the bone at the time of surgery, and the surgeon has to consult the preoperative drawing in order to find the direction of this guidewire in relation to such identifiable bony landmarks as the superior cortex of the neck, the center of the femoral head, and the rough line of the greater trochanter. The preoperative drawing was made using the uninvolved side as the template for the femur. The plate was then fitted to the proximal femur using the template as a guide. The exact placement in bone and the exact direction of the seating chisel and the plate were therefore predetermined with accuracy. Kirschner wire 2 is now driven into the tip of the tro-chanter to be out of the way of the seating chisel (see Fig. 15.14). It is driven in parallel to Kirschner wire 1, which indicates the anteversion of the femoral neck, and in the same relationship to the superior cortex of the neck and the center of rotation of the femoral head as that marked on the preoperative drawing.

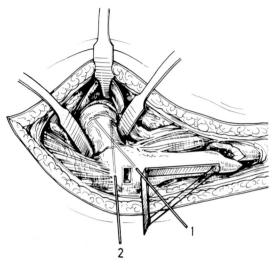

Fig. 15.14. Exposure of a subtrochanteric fracture. The vastus lateralis muscle is held retracted together with the inferior half of the joint capsule. The tip of the most anterior Hohmann retractor is passed through the capsule and then over the ante-rior pillar of the acetabulum. This ensures anterior exposure of the hip. Note the tip of a narrow Hohmann retractor driven into the cephalad superior aspects of the neck; this prevents the retractor from slipping and damaging the retinacular vessels posteriorly on the neck. Kirschner wire *1* indicates antiversion; Kirschner wire *2* indicates direction of seating chiseland is par-allel to *1*

Before the seating chisel can be inserted, a window in the lateral cortex of the greater trochanter must be cut. The correct placement of this window is very important. It bears different relationships to the midpoint of the lat-eral surface of the femur in the region of the greater tro-chanter and in the region of the shaft. If the femur is viewed end-on from above (see Fig. 15.15), it can be clearly seen that the neck is more anterior and not in line with the midpoint of the greater trochanter. Thus, for a blade to enter the middle of the neck when it is inserted through the greater trochanter, it must straddle the junc-tion between the anterior and middle thirds of the great-er trochanter (Fig. 15.15 a). If the window for the seating chisel is cut, in error, too far posteriorly, it is deflected anteriorly as it enters the neck, and the surgeon runs the danger of entering the hip joint anteriorly with the tip of the implant. Similarly, if the window is cut too far poste-riorly in the region of the shaft (Fig. 15.15 b) – which is easily done, particularly if the leg is in traction and the shaft internally rotated – the blade of a 130°-angled plate or the compression screw will be deflected anteriorly. The window in the trochanter for the condylar plate should be situated so that the seating chisel enters the neck 1 cm from the superior cortex of the neck. If the seating chisel is driven in too close to the superior cor-tex, it will be deflected downward, because the superior

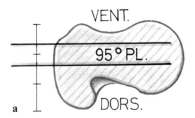

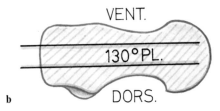

Fig. 15.15. a When viewed from above, the neck is more anterior and not in line with the midpoint of the greater trochanter. Thus, in order to enter the middle of the neck, a plate must be inserted through the junction between the anterior and the middle thirds of the trochanter. **b** In the region of the shaft (e.g., for a dynamic hip screw), the window must be cut in the middle of the lateral cortex. (From Müller et al. 1979)

curve of the neck will not accommodate the width of the chisel. If the window is made too far distally, the seating chisel will strike the calcar. This is not such a disaster in itself, but it may bring about two complications: if the proximal fragment is short, then the lower the blade lies within the proximal fragment, the less room the surgeon has to supplement the fixation with a screw through the plate into the calcar; furthermore, if the calculated length of the blade as determined in the preoperative drawing is used as a guide, the arrest of the seating chisel by the calcar might not be recognized, particularly if the latter is osteoporotic or the individual very young and the cancellous bone within the proximal femur very hard. Further blows of the mallet will drive the seating chisel into the calcar, which may shatter. In driving the seating chisel into bone, one further plane must be carefully observed. The flap of the seating chisel guide must be in line with the long axis to ensure that the proximal fragment will be neither flexed nor extended. Once the seat for the blade is cut, the seating chisel is withdrawn and the angled plate inserted. Once the plate is impacted into bone and is sitting flush against the cortex of the proximal fragment, it is secured in the proximal fragment by the insertion of a 4.5-mm cortical screw through the plate into the calcar. A 6.5-mm cancellous screw is too wide and may splinter the calcar; hence, its use in this position has been abandoned. The same considerations hold for the insertion of a guidewire for the compression screw of the DCS. The procedure is, however, very much easier. The surgeon does not have to cut a

window since the cortex will be opened up with the triple reamer. The position and insertion of the guidewire follows all the steps described for the seating chisel. Once the position of the guidewire is confirmed radiologically one proceeds to the insertion of the compression screw and to the mounting of the side plate. If the plate should not be parallel to the long axis of the shaft, the malalignment is easily corrected by twisting the compression screw in the right direction.

The reduction of the fracture can then proceed with relatively little effort. The shaft of the femur is lined up with the plate. Its rotation is adjusted and it is then held to the plate with a Verbrugge bone clamp (see Fig. 15.12e). No attempt is made to identify or reduce any of the comminuted fragments. The distractor is now inserted with one bolt through the second hole of the plate, and its second bolt is inserted into a predrilled 4.5-mm hole distal to the plate (see Fig. 15.10). The relationship of the most distal fracture line to the holes of the plate must be noted from the preoperative drawing. This helps to judge when the correct length of the femur is restored. The rotation should be restored as close to normal as possible prior to insertion of the distal bolt of the distractor, since only limited rotational correction can be achieved with the distractor in place.

The distractor is then used to distract the femur and gradually regain the correct length. The Verbrugge clamp may have to be loosened, but it should not be removed completely, since it guides the femoral shaft in the correct axial alignment as length is being regained. Once the correct length has been restored, the fracture should be viewed with the aid of the image intensifier. Occasionally the fracture may have to be overdistracted in order to aid the reduction of some major fragments. If at all possible, the surgeon should try not to expose and manipulate the fragments. If manipulation is essential, it should be done with a sharp instrument such as a dental pick in order to minimize the dissection.

Once reduction is achieved, the distractor is turned back until the correct length is regained. At this point we like to secure the position of the plate to the shaft with one screw distally and check the rotational alignment of the leg by flexing the hip and checking the degree of internal and external rotation. This is also a convenient moment to obtain anteroposterior and lateral radiographs of the hip (see Fig. 15.12e). Since we have chosen an operating table which facilitates anteroposterior radiographs, the anteroposterior radiograph is simple. In order to get a perfect lateral view of the femoral neck, the hip should be flexed to 90° and, while held flexed, abducted 20° in neutral rotation. A second anteroposterior exposure with the hip held in this position gives a perfect lateral projection of the femoral neck and head.

If the placement of the plate is correct, the internal fixation can then be completed. If there are major wedge fragments, these should have been noted on the preoperative drawing, as well as the possibility of securing these with lag screws (see Fig. 15.12 c) or to the plate. The lag screws are then inserted, together with the remaining screws, which secure the plate to the shaft. A plate used in this manner functions as a bridge plate and spans the zone of fragmentation. In applying it to the femur, as already emphasized, the fracture fragments should not be exposed and only as little of the distal fragment as is necessary to fix the plate should be exposed. The plate acts as an extramedullary splint, and union will occur by callus. This technique of reduction is referred to as indirect reduction. It serves to minimize the interference with the blood supply of the bone. In a simple fracture and in a wedge fracture, stable fixation should be obtained with the aid of axial compression and lag screws. These fractures cannot be simply bridged as a complex fracture can be, because the strain concentration at the fracture will be too great and the fracture will fail to unite.

15.4.4.5 Bone-Grafting

Multifragmentary fractures reduced atraumatically and fixed with a bridge plate do not require grafting. The fixation is only relatively stable as the plate acts as an extramedullary splint and healing will occur with the formation of callus. Bone-grafting is necessary in simple fractures and in wedge fractures which are plated and in open fractures with bone loss whether plated or nailed. The bone graft should be inserted through the fracture between the bone and the soft tissue prior to the reduction of the fracture. In this way we can avoid stripping the soft tissue, which invariably occurs when surgeons try to bone-graft after the reduction is complete. In fractures with stable fixation if there is a defect on the medial side, i.e., the side opposite the plate, the plate will be bent with loading of the femur, which may be no greater than that of simple muscular contraction. With unloading, because of its elasticity, the plate will spring back to its original shape. If allowed to continue unchecked, such cyclic loading will result in a fatigue fracture of the implant. In addition to the bending forces, there are also shearing forces, which contribute to the failure of the implant. Theoretically, the cyclic loading may be prevented by bridging the comminuted segments with a second plate applied to the medial side, but, apart from the technical difficulties of applying such a plate medially, a very heavy biological price would be incurred, i.e., the risk of rendering a segment of the femur next to the fracture totally avascular. This would delay healing and would increase the chance of nonunion and implant failure.

The autogenous cancellous bone is applied opposite the plate to bridge the defect. If it is successful, usually by the end of 6–8 weeks, it results in a radiologically visible bony bridge opposite the plate. Such a bridge is then ideally situated. The compressive stresses lead to its hypertrophy (Fig. 15.12 i). Because it is opposite the plate, it arrests all bending movements, brings all motion to a standstill, and protects the implant from failure. At this point, i.e., once a radiologically visible bridge appears, loading can be rapidly increased to full load without fear of implant failure. In fact, with increased stress the medial bridge is usually seen to hypertrophy and gain further strength.

Fractures treated with closed locked intramedullary nailing, with the exception of open fractures, do not require bone-grafting.

15.4.5 Postoperative Care

Patients recovering from surgery on the proximal femur do not require any special positioning or splinting. We believe that early ambulation is effective in preventing thrombophlebitis, but an anticoagulant regime is still necessary. All patients, if able, are up with crutches on the day after surgery. We discourage sitting, since in a patient with a swollen thigh and groin the sitting posture leads to compression of vessels in the groin and contributes to venous thrombosis. The amount of weight-bearing is determined by the stability of the reduction and of the internal fixation. Generally, in the type C fractures, weight-bearing is avoided until there is some evidence of osseous bridging medially, which usually takes up to 8 or 10 weeks to make its appearance. In stable fracture configurations, such as types A and B, partial weight-bearing of 10–15 kg is begun almost immediately. The above regimen applies to patients with plating or locked intramedullary nailing.

15.4.5.1 Signs of Instability

The surgeon must have a clear concept of the type of fixation attempted. Stable fixation such as is achieved with lag screws and a protection plate or with axial compression should result in union without the appearance of radiologically identifiable callus.

The absence of callus in the presence of stable fixation makes it difficult to judge the progress of healing. We must rely more on indirect evidence of union, such as the gradual disappearance of the fracture line, the absence of irritation callus, the absence of resorption around the screws and under the plate, the maintenance of the reduction without recurrence of deformity, and, clinically, on the absence of pain. Patients who either continue to have pain after an open reduction and stable fixation or develop pain after a period of painless mobilization must be considered to have either instability of the fixation or a deep-seated infection. In each instance the patient will have pain, local tenderness, and even redness with swelling. The latter applies more to the subcutaneous bones, such as the tibia, than to the femur. Usually, redness with swelling in the thigh signifies sepsis. Other confirmatory evidence, such as the patient's temperature, the white blood cell count, and the sedimentation rate, will aid in the diagnosis.

A multifragmentary fracture which has been splinted with a bridge plate will heal with callus. Thus it is necessary to know what type of fixation has been attempted in order to be able to judge whether the fracture is uniting satisfactorily or not.

15.4.5.2 Infection

If the diagnosis of a deep-seated infection is made, then, in addition to intravenous antibiotics, the patient must have the wound reopened and thoroughly débrided, and the wound packed open. Most infections are deep-seated and go right to the fracture. Superficial wound infections are rare and occur only in the immediate postoperative period. If redness, tenderness, and swelling appear a month or so after surgery, particularly in a case where prophylactic antibiotics were used during the surgery, it is almost certain that the patient has a deep-seated infection. A new course of antibiotic therapy may bring all the manifestations of the disaster under control, but only an inexperienced surgeon will take solace from this apparent cure: sepsis usually flares up a few weeks later. At this point the situation is usually more complex, because the smoldering infection has led to bone resorption, bone necrosis, and to some loss of stability. In addition to some periosteal bone formation at the ends of the plate, resorption of bone deep to the plate and a widening of the fracture line can usually be recognized radiologically. At this stage it is not enough to treat the infection aggressively with débridement and suction irrigation. It must be determined whether the internal fixation is stable. If stability has been lost because of loosening of the fixation, it must be revised. If stability exists or if the fixation has been revised, the fracture must be bonegrafted with autogenous cancellous bone to accelerate union and prevent failure of the implant. If the diagnosis is instability and failure of the fixation, then the situation must be treated aggressively, or fatigue fracture of the implant is certain.

References

Cochran GVB, Zickel RE, Fielding JW (1980) Stress analysis of subtrochanteric fractures: effect of muscle forces and internal fixation devices. In: Uhthoff HK (ed) Current concepts of internal fixation of fractures. Springer, Berlin Heidelberg New York

Ender SW (1970) Die Fixierung der Trochanterbrüche mit runden elastischen Kondylennägeln. Acta Chir Austriaca 1:40–42

Kempf I, Grosse A, Beck G (1985) Closed locked intramedullary nailing. J Bone Joint Surg 67A:709–720

Küntscher G (1967) Practice of intramedullary nailing. Thomas, Springfield, p 178

Müller ME, Allgöwer M, Schneider R, Willenegger H (1979) Manual of internal fixation, 2nd edn. Springer, Berlin Heidelberg New York

Müller ME, Nazarian S, Koch P, Schatzker J (1990) The comprehensive classification of fractures of long bones. Springer, Berlin Heidelberg New York

Pankovich AM, Tarabishy IE (1980) Ender nailing of intertrochanteric and subtrochanteric fractures. J Bone Joint Surg 62A:635–645

Schatzker J, Waddell JP (1980) Subtrochanteric fractures of the femur. Orthop Clin North Am 11(3):539–554

Schatzker J, Manley PA, Sumner-Smith G (1980) In vivo straingauge study of bone response to loading with and without internal fixation of fractures. Springer, Berlin Heidelberg New York, pp 306–314

Zickel RE (1976) An intramedullary fixation device for the proximal part of the femur. J Bone Joint Surg 58A:866–872

16 Fractures of the Femur

J. SCHATZKER

16.1 Introduction

The femur, the largest tubular bone in the body, is surrounded by the largest mass of muscles and is designed to withstand greater forces than any other bone. Fractures of the femur are almost always the result of great violence and are sometimes a threat to the patient's life, not only because of the immediate complications such as bleeding or associated injuries, but also because of subsequent complications related either to the treatment of the fracture, or to the complications of the associated injuries.

16.2 Factors Important in Evaluating the Mode of Treatment

Any fracture of the femoral shaft, if it goes beyond an undisplaced crack, is unstable and displaces further under the influence of physiological forces. The fragments always shorten, rotate, and angulate. Early systems for the immobilization of the femur frequently involved the immobilization of the whole patient as well as the immobilization of the leg, including the hip and knee joint. Immobilization of the fracture was recognized as essential for union. The development of splints, such as the Thomas splint, and the subsequent combinations of the splints with traction methods, either fixed or balanced, allowed for better control of the fracture. Patients nevertheless had to remain in traction for 3 months or longer before the fracture was sufficiently stable to allow ambulation. Even at this point, a number had to be protected in ischial-bearing long leg calipers to prevent refracture. A hip plaster spica could not be used as a successful method to treat fresh fractures because it did not allow control of angulation or shortening. It was recognized that an initial period of traction of 6–8 weeks was necessary before a fracture became sufficiently stable for the patient to be transferred into a hip spica. This freed the acute treatment bed, but did not influence the rate of union, nor did it improve the result of treatment.

Certain complications of prolonged traction, such as decubitus ulcers, can be overcome by better nursing, but the complications of prolonged bed rest such as bladder and bowel derangements, deep vein thrombosis, osteoporosis, and muscle wasting, to mention only a few, cannot be prevented. Furthermore, despite the most expert care, a disturbing number of patients end up with significant shortening of 2 cm or more, angulation of sufficient degree to effect the biomechanical function of their extremity, and, above all, knee joint stiffness. A return of 90° knee joint flexion was often considered as a most successful result of treatment, which could be achieved only at the end of a prolonged period of rehabilitation requiring many hours of hard work, not only from the patient, but also from the attending rehabilitative staff.

The resurgence of cast bracing (Sarmiento 1972; Sarmiento and Latta 1981) spurred many enthusiasts to apply this method to fractures of the femur. It was found, however, that it is not a method which can be used to treat fresh fractures. Initial reduction still has to be obtained and the limb has to be treated on a splint in traction until such time as callus renders the fracture sufficiently stable for the limb to be transferred into a cast brace. The average stay in hospital with this method is still between 6 and 8 weeks. Cast bracing, although suitable for fractures of the distal third of the femur, has been abandoned even by the enthusiasts of this technique for fractures of the mid and proximal third, because of complications of shortening and angulation.

Initial attempts at internal fixation of the femur were disastrous. The stability obtained with plates and screws was inadequate to nurse the extremity without the protection of splints, traction, or both. Despite the supplemental protection, failure of the internal fixation and resulting nonunion was common. Furthermore, the stiffness which resulted from surgery followed by immobilization was far greater than the stiffness from nonoperative methods alone. Thus, until the advent of the intramedullary nail, open reduction and internal fixation played a negligible role in the treatment of fractures of the femoral shaft. In 1940, Gerhard Küntscher introduced intramedullary nailing of the femur and revolutionized the treatment of femoral shaft fractures (Küntscher 1967). The stability obtained with his method of internal fixation was sufficient to render the patients pain-free, allow them early mobilization, and in certain cases, even allow early weight bearing. Later on,

Küntscher recognized that stability could be further increased by increasing the diameter of the medullary nail. In 1950, he introduced intramedullary reaming and further improved the results of his technique (Küntscher 1967). There remained, however, all the fractures not suitable for the intramedullary nailing technique, such as fractures of the proximal or distal third, long oblique and spiral fractures, and comminuted fractures with loss of segmental continuity.

The introduction of stable internal fixation with the aid of compression by the Swiss AO group in the early 1960s further revolutionized the surgical treatment of femoral shaft fractures (Müller et al. 1965). It now became possible, after a careful atraumatic anatomical reduction of the fracture, to achieve an absolute degree of stability by means of lag screws and tension band or neutralization plates. This rendered the extremity completely pain-free. The stability achieved was such that supplemental protection of splints or traction was no longer necessary. The patient could begin early active mobilization of the extremity, often with partial weight bearing. This led to a rapid recovery of the soft tissue envelope and to a rapid return of motion of the adjacent joints. Because of the absolute degree of stability achieved, union occurred in a very high percentage of the cases without loss of position and malunion or nonunion. Thus, the scope of internal fixation was greatly expanded and the indications for nonoperative treatment of the femur correspondingly reduced to a very small number.

The most recent advance in the treatment of femoral shaft fractures has been the development of the locking intramedullary nail (Kempf et al. 1985), which we describe in some detail later on in this chapter. This technique has made it possible to deal surgically with the most extreme degrees of comminution of the shaft which are completely beyond the scope of conventional intramedullary nailing or plating.

The techniques which we have described, conventional intramedullary nailing, the AO/ASIF methods of open reduction and internal fixation by means of screws and plates, and the most recent development of locking intramedullary nailing, are by no means devoid of complications, nor are they simple to execute. They comprise, however, together with external skeletal fixation, the best methods of treatment for femoral shaft fractures. Nonoperative means have a very small role to play as definitive methods of care for fractures of the femoral shaft. We must emphasize again and again that the decision to pursue a particular course of treatment must be based on the analysis of the personality of the fracture, that is, the nature of the fracture and of the patient: age, functional demands, etc. It must also be based on the environment where the care is being administered, and lastly on the skill of the surgeon with a particular technique. If a surgeon does not have the necessary skills to execute complex internal fixation, then it is clearly best to pursue nonoperative means. However, a surgeon who is going to treat fractures should acquire the skills to execute the forms of treatment generally accepted as the best, and recognize that nonoperative treatment for fractures of the femoral shaft should be viewed as nondefinitive and temporizing, and that the patient should be referred, if at all possible, to a center where appropriate treatment can be carried out safely and expertly.

16.3 Surgical Treatment

16.3.1 Timing of Surgery

Once the decision is made to pursue surgical treatment, the next important decision to be made is the timing of surgery. The decision as to when to operate must be based on a number of factors, the most important being the associated injuries.

16.3.1.1 Multiple System Injuries

The experience from trauma centers (Riska et al. 1976; Winquist et al. 1984; Sibel et al. 1985) indicates that immediate fixation of long bone fractures, particularly of the femur, has been instrumental in preventing or reversing progressive respiratory failure by allowing the chest to be nursed in a vertical position. Furthermore, these studies have demonstrated that there has been no increase in fat embolism as a result of immediate intramedullary nailing of femoral shaft fractures (Riska et al. 1976; Riska and Myllenen 1982; Winquist et al. 1984). By immediate, we mean as soon as possible after the general priorities such as airway, bleeding, and volume replacement, and cranial, abdominal, and thoracic priorities of patients with multiple injuries have been satisfied. Frequently, stabilization of long bone fractures can be begun while a general surgeon is dealing with injuries to chest or abdomen. If the position of the patient on the table renders internal fixation logistically not feasible, it should be executed under the same anesthetic as soon as the position can be changed. A previously healthy patient with multiple injuries will never be as fit for surgery as after the initial resuscitation and stabilization, while well oxygenated under endotracheal anesthesia, with fluid and electrolyte status under full control. This is true as long as there is no rise in the intracranial pressure or as long as no complications develop, such as ventilatory problems or coagulopathies.

Although the timing of long bone stabilization remains unchallenged, intramedullary nailing as the most appropriate form of stabilization has come under scrutiny (Pape 1993). Reaming has been recognized as contributing significantly to the damage of the blood supply to the cortex. Reaming has also been recognized to cause a marked increase in the intramedullary pressure of bone (Stürmer 1993) and in a marked rise in the associated embolization of marrow contents to the lung (Wenda 1993). These observations have resulted in the development of unreamed intramedullary nails for the tibia and femur. Although the unreamed nails are associated with less damage to the blood supply of the bone, they have not eliminated the events associated with manipulations of the medullary canal, and therefore, as expected, they have had little influence on the cardiopulmonary events. Thus the nailing of the long bone fractures of polytrauma patients with a high ISS, who had shock and who have concomitant injuries to the thoracic cage and lung contusion remains an unsettled issue. We feel that, until such time as this issue is clearly settled, these very ill patients should have their long bone fractures stabilized as early as possible if feasible with either a plate or an external fixator. Once their condition stabilizes the fixation of the fracture can be revised if indicated.

16.3.1.2 Head Injury

A head injury with unconsciousness was formerly considered a contraindication to any internal fixation. The nursing of unconscious patients with femoral shaft fractures was extremely difficult. They could not be nursed supine with limbs in traction. They demanded frequent turning to prevent respiratory complications, and their limbs could only be immobilized by propping them up and splinting them with pillows, with the traction adjusted as well as possible. The cardiorespiratory complications that ensued from the moving about of fractured femora and from the enforced supine position cannot be overemphasized. In addition, we have all witnessed the unnecessary lifelong crippling of accident victims whose skeletal injuries, such as dislocated hips, fractured hips, or fractured femora, were neglected because of their head injury and initial unconsciousness. Many such patients awoke 3–4 weeks after their injury with a clear sensorium and undamaged intellect, only to find their extremities permanently shortened and deformed. Neglect of skeletal injuries because of an associated head injury must be avoided.

An unconscious patient whose cerebral status is stable and who does not have an enlarging intracranial mass with rising intracranial pressure (these would be clear priorities in treatment) should have most of the significant musculoskeletal lesions treated definitively on an emergency basis, either operatively or nonoperatively. In the case of a fractured femur, the definitive treatment must be operative. This will not only prevent permanent deformities and disability, but will greatly enhance the ease and quality of the nursing care of such patients and greatly diminish morbidity. The advent of computed tomography and intracranial pressure monitoring has greatly eased the initial evaluation of intracranial injuries and has helped immeasurably in defining the fitness of patients for definitive care of their skeletal injuries.

16.3.1.3 Open Fractures

The débridement of an open wound should be carried out on an emergency basis. We believe that stable fixation of an open fracture is not only the single most important manoeuver after débridement in preventing sepsis, but also that it is the only manoeuver which will safeguard the optimal return of soft tissue function (Matter and Rittman 1978). How stability is achieved will depend upon the type of fracture. This will be discussed at length later in this chapter. However, at this point, it must be said that we believe that an open fracture must be stabilized at the time of surgical débridement, either by means of screws and plates, by an external fixator, or by means of an unreamed nail. As a rule, we prefer not to use intramedullary nailing in the IIIC open fractures.

16.3.1.4 Vascular Injury

Vascular injury clearly demands immediate intervention to safeguard the survival of the extremity. Although experience from the Vietnam war suggested that vascular reconstruction would not be jeopardized if the extremity were subsequently treated in traction, we feel that in the event of a vascular injury, immediate fixation of the femur should be carried out, either by means of internal or external skeletal fixation, but preferably by the former. To minimize the complications of ischemia, a temporary vascular shunt should be inserted before the internal fixation is undertaken.

16.3.1.5 Ipsilateral Neck Fracture or Dislocation of the Hip

Both injuries, but particularly the latter, create an emergency situation. The incidence of avascular necrosis is directly related to the time that the head remains out of the joint, to the degree of intra-articular hypertension, and to the displacement. If a closed reduction of the dislocation or of the neck fracture is to be attempted, then the shaft fracture must be first reduced and fixed. It is also best to stabilize the shaft fracture before the neck lest any manipulation of the shaft dislodge an internal fixation of the neck or trochanteric region. Also, it may be necessary for a number of reasons to do an open reduction of the dislocation. If so, the shaft fracture should be fixed at the same time and not treated in traction. Thus, if the neck fracture is undisplaced, we stabilize it provisionally with K-wires, nail the femur, and then stabilize the neck fracture with cannulated screws. If the fracture of the neck is displaced, then we feel that it is best to plate the femur first unless the fracture morphology of the shaft is such that plating would be inadvisable. Under these circumstances a closed reduction of the neck should be tried first. If it fails, one should carry out an open reduction of the neck in order to reduce the neck and achieve provisional fixation of the neck prior to the nailing. Nailing of the femur can increase the displacement of the neck and jeopardize the blood supply to the head. The priority in treatment is the preservation of the blood supply to the femoral head. We also feel that an open fracture of the femur associated with a neck fracture is an absolute contraindication to nailing because of the risk of septic arthritis. Similarly, an intertrochanteric fracture associated with a shaft fracture is best plated, because we have found that the second generation reconstruction nails are difficult to use in the presence of trochanteric fractures, particularly if the fracture should extend to involve the piriform fossa.

16.3.1.6 Ipsilateral Fracture of the Femoral Shaft and Ligamentous Disruption of the Knee

One cannot apply traction across a disrupted knee. Therefore, if for some reason surgery has to be delayed, skeletal traction should be applied through a supracondylar pin. Otherwise, it is best to proceed to an internal fixation of the fracture and to an immediate reconstruction of the disrupted ligaments.

16.3.1.7 Floating Knee Syndrome

Patients who sustain fractures of the ipsilateral femur and tibia have the so-called floating knee syndrome. This syndrome has recently received considerable attention. All who have concerned themselves with the care of these injuries agree that a proper evaluation of the knee is only possible once the knee and tibia have been stabilized by means of internal fixation, and that the best results of treatment of these and their associated ligamentous or intra-articular injuries are obtained if they are treated as soon as the general condition of the patient allows.

16.3.1.8 Isolated Fractures of the Femoral Shaft

After resuscitation of the patient with an isolated fracture of the femoral shaft, the surgeon has the option of either proceeding with definitive surgical treatment or delaying the treatment for a few days. Those who favor delay have frequently cited the difficulties encountered in attempting an immediate open reduction of a femoral shaft, particularly in athletic and muscular individuals. This can no longer be accepted as an indication for delaying treatment. The distractor (Fig. 16.1) will facilitate the early reduction out to length of even the most muscular thigh. Furthermore, immediate intramedullary nailing, except as indicated in the severely polytraumatized patients with chest trauma and pulmonary confusion, is not associated with an increased incidence of fat embolism syndrome (Riska et al. 1976; Riska and Myllenen 1982; Winquist et al. 1984; Schatzker to be published).

If surgery is to be delayed, the fracture must be properly splinted and the extremity placed in skeletal traction with the fragments in the best possible alignment. One should attempt to overdistract the fracture. This will ease subsequent reduction. Where circumstances dictate immediate intervention, an immediate internal fixation should be executed. The advent of locked intramedullary nailing has made it technically possible to stabilize even highly comminuted shaft fractures immediately, without running a higher risk of failure (see Fig. 16.12).

16.3.2 Surgical Technique

16.3.2.1 Positioning the Patient, Skin Preparation, and Draping

Open reduction and internal fixation of the femoral shaft fracture by means of screws and plates or open intramedullary nailing should not be attempted on the fracture table with the extremity in traction. The traction results in such tension of the soft tissue envelope that exposure and manipulation of the fragments is extremely difficult, if not impossible. Visualization is difficult, retraction of necessity is forceful, and unnecessary devitalization of the fragments is inevitable. An accurate anatomical reduction is almost impossible to obtain, and as a result, fixation is often not as stable as it should be.

We prefer to position the patient supine on a radiolucent table to permit intraoperative radiography.

During surgical scrubbing, the extremity must be elevated and kept in traction to prevent telescoping of the fragments which could lead to further soft tissue damage and further comminution of the fracture. Ipsilateral

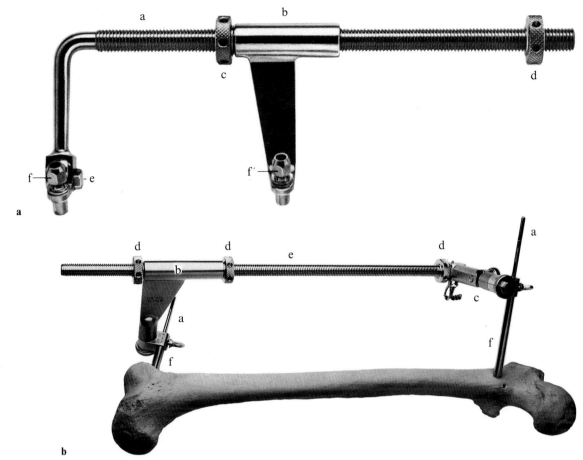

Fig. 16.1. a Distractor (large, simple model). *a* Threaded rod; *b* distal carriage; *c,d* locking nuts; *e* fixation nut; *f, f'* Schanz screw-holding sleeve. **b** Distractor (large, for three-dimensional application). *a* Proximal and distal Schanz screws are used for attaching the distractor to the fragments; *b* distal carriage and *c* proximal sleeve-holding bracket permit movement about several axes and in several planes; *d* locking nuts secure the parts, 14 mm inner diameter; *e* threaded rod; *f* Schanz screw-holding sleeve fixes the Schanz screws to the distractor. (From Müller et al. 1991, p.317)

posterior and anterior iliac crests should be included in the surgical scrub and should be subsequently draped free to serve as donor sites for bone grafting, should it prove necessary. The leg should be scrubbed almost to the ankle and, in draping, the knee should be left free so that it can be flexed as necessary during the procedure. If a Steinmann pin has been used for preoperative traction, it should be draped out of the field and left in until the internal fixation is complete. Sometimes, despite the best of intentions, the limb may have to be placed in traction again. It is best not to use pillows, but to rely on sterile folded sheets which are placed under the scrubbed leg. These can then be rearranged as necessary during the reduction to support the bone and prevent redisplacement.

A tourniquet is not used. Even if a sterile tourniquet were used, it would get in the way of the incision. If vascular reconstruction has to be carried out at the same time as the internal fixation, then it is best to place the patient supine on the table to provide free access to the groin and medial aspect of the popliteal fossa.

16.3.2.2 Surgical Approach

The standard approach to the whole femoral shaft is through a straight lateral incision, which is made along an imaginary line joining the greater trochanter with the lateral femoral condyle (Fig. 16.2). The fascia lata is incised in line with the skin. One should not approach the bone through the substance of the vastus lateralis muscle, even if the latter has been pierced by bone. The vastus lateralis should be carefully dissected with a sharp periostial elevator from its attachment to the intermuscular septum and should be lifted forward and medially to expose the shaft (Fig. 16.3). The perforating

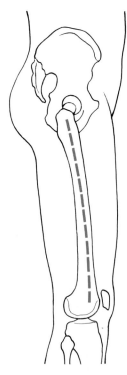

Fig. 16.2. The standard approach to the whole femoral shaft is through a straight lateral incision which is made along an imaginary line joining the greater trochanter with the lateral femoral condyle

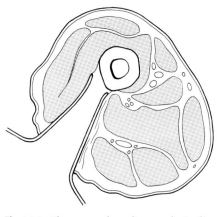

Fig. 16.3. The vastus lateralis muscle is dissected from its attachment to the intermuscular septum and is lifted forward and medially to expose the shaft

vessels which are found within the substance of the vastus lateralis 4–8 mm from the bone should be cross-clamped and ligated. If they are cauterized and cut, the posterior portion of the vessel may retract through the intermuscular septum and begin to bleed. Bleeding from it during surgery is a nuisance because it is difficult to find the vessel and to stop the bleeding. It may also begin to bleed after closure and result in a large, troublesome hematoma.

16.3.2.3 Technique of Open Reduction

Whenever an open reduction of a fracture is being carried out, one should make an extreme effort to be "atraumatic." This means that one should be extremely gentle in handling the soft tissue and make every effort not to strip muscle from bone as this greatly interferes with the blood supply of the cortex. If one is forced to carry out a direct reduction, as might be necessary in a fracture which has been neglected and allowed to remain shortened for days, one should not expose the comminuted fragments. The main fragments should be gripped with a reduction clamp with narrow jaws (Fig. 16.4). This keeps the devitalization to a minimum. In manipulating the fragments, care must be taken not to squeeze the handles of the reduction clamps as this could result in crushing of the bone and in extensive comminution.

The trick in reducing a comminuted fracture with one or two large wedge fragments is to reduce the wedge fragments and fix them with lag screws to one or both fragments. In this way, the comminuted fracture is converted to a simple fracture. This greatly eases the final reduction (Fig. 16.5). It is very difficult to regain length by longitudinal traction. If possible, the main fragments should be grasped and angulated through the fracture until the cortices can be hooked on. Length is then reestablished by simple realignment of the bones while the cortices are maintained engaged. If this is impossible to achieve because of the obliquity of the fracture or because of comminution, then the simplest and safest

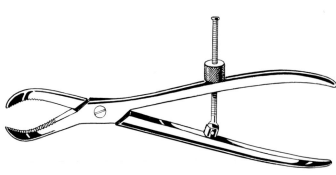

Fig. 16.4. Special reduction clamps with narrow jaws. They keep devitalization of fragments to a minimum

Fig. 16.5. In a comminuted fracture, the fragments are fixed with lag screws to each other and to the main fragments where possible. This converts a comminuted fracture into a simple fracture. (From Müller et al. 1979.) Do not strip the muscle from the fragments. This devitalizes them and greatly prolongs the time to union. It is more important to preserve the blood supply than to secure fixation of small fragments

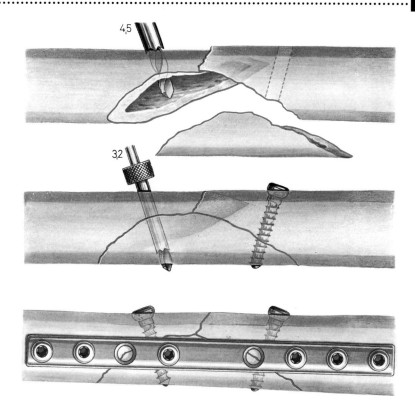

way to achieve length and reduction is to use the distractor (see Fig. 16.1). If reduction is going to be difficult because the fracture was allowed to foreshorten, then preliminary overdistraction with the distractor should be executed before any reduction is attempted. The distraction must be carried out very slowly to allow the soft tissues to stretch without tearing.

We have come to rely on the distractor more and more, even for simple fractures, as it ensures reduction with the least amount of soft tissue trauma. It is invaluable in dealing with multifragment fractures. In these, length can be easily restored by slight overdistraction. As the soft tissue envelope is stretched, the comminuted fragments frequently reduce spontaneously or require only minimal manipulation to be fitted in place. The larger fragments can then be lagged together with the least damage to their blood supply.

We have described in the preceding paragraphs the technique of direct reduction because this is at times unavoidable. The preferred technique of reduction is the indirect technique whereby traction is used to achieve reduction without any direct manipulation or lag screw fixations. The direct manipulation of the main fragments is kept to a minimum. This technique is fully described in the chapter on the general aspects of internal fixation. Indirect reduction of a multifragmentary fracture does not automatically mean no fixation of the intervening fragments. The shape of the fragments must be carefully assessed in order to decide whether axial

prestress is possible after reduction without this resulting in shortening. If so, axial compression should be carried out, as well as any lag screw fixation between the large fragments because this greatly increases the strength of the fixation.

16.3.2.4 Technique of Fracture Fixation

There are three methods available for fixation of the femur. These are intramedullary nailing, internal fixation by means of screws and plates, and external skeletal fixation.

a) External Skeletal Fixation

External skeletal fixation of the femur is used chiefly to stabilize severe open fractures and infected pseudoarthroses, or in emergency situations where temporary stability is required but the patient's condition does not allow a complex intervention. The large muscle mass, the proximity of the other leg near the groin, and the medial course of the femoral artery and the posterior course of the sciatic nerve present specific problems to be dealt with when erecting an external skeletal fixation frame. For stability to be achieved in the femur, one would ideally require three-plane fixation. In the proximal femur, however, the pins cannot exit medially because of

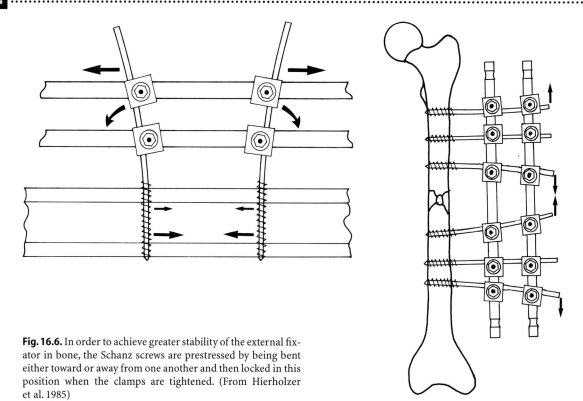

Fig. 16.6. In order to achieve greater stability of the external fixator in bone, the Schanz screws are prestressed by being bent either toward or away from one another and then locked in this position when the clamps are tightened. (From Hierholzer et al. 1985)

the proximity of the other leg and the perineum. Thus, in the proximal third, only a half-frame can be erected laterally.

If one wishes to insert transfixing pins through the shaft, this must be done under direct vision from the medial side with identification of the femoral artery in order to prevent its damage with the pins. Transfixing pins can be inserted safely only through the condyles and through the immediate supracondylar area. Transfixing pins cannot be inserted in the anteroposterior plane because of the sciatic nerve which is directly behind the femur. Hence, only an anterior half-frame can be erected, with the pins stopping just at the point of exit through the posterior cortex. The difficulty with all the pins (except those in the frontal plane in the condylar area) is that they penetrate large muscle bellies; this frequently gives rise to pin track sepsis. The anterior half-frame transfixes the quadriceps muscle mechanism and blocks any knee movement. Therefore, it can be used only if knee motion must be sacrificed or if it is already absent, as in an infected pseudoarthrosis or if the fixation is temporary. Half-frame systems, such as the Wagner leg lengthening device, the Judet external fixator, or a unilateral AO tubular frame, do not provide a high degree of stability if used on fresh fractures. The Wagner device provides a greater degree of stability if used for leg lengthening because it is pulling against the

resistance of tight soft tissues. Such soft tissue tension is absent in fresh fractures. Stability is further influenced by the question of comminution and whether axial compression can be exerted or not. In order to achieve greater stability, the fragments should be compressed, or, if this is impossible because of comminution, then the pins should be prestressed against one another (Fig. 16.6). This is possible to achieve with such devices as the AO tubular external fixator system, but not with the Wagner leg-lengthening device. The stability of the system can be further increased by erecting the system in such a way that the pins transfix the bone close to the fracture. Our current practice whenever indicated is to use a lateral half frame for temporary fixation of closed fractures or open fractures. We convert the external fixation to intramedullary nailing as soon as possible. If this has to be delayed for more than a week or if any purulent drainage appears around the pins, we convert the fixation to a plate since conversion to a nail might carry the risk of sepsis.

b) Intramedullary Nailing

Gerhard Küntscher is credited with the development of modern intramedullary nailing (Küntscher 1967). He reasoned that if one were to introduce into the rigid

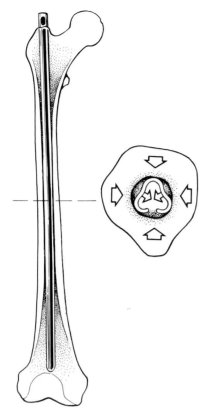

Fig. 16.7. According to Küntscher, an elastic deformable nail, when inserted into a slightly smaller medullary canal, will be deformed. Its elastic recoil results in the nail gripping the bone which provides fixation for the fragments. (Adapted from Küntscher 1967)

displacement corresponding to the distance between the nail and the endosteum at each end (Fig. 16.8). In the young, the metaphyseal areas are filled with dense cancellous bone which resists this angular displacement, but in the elderly the metaphyses are filled with sparse, weak trabeculae which offer virtually no resistance. Intramedullary reaming enlarges longitudinally the area of contact between the nail and the bone (Fig. 16.8). In clinical practice, we aim for at least 5 cm contact on each side of the fracture. Therefore, the exact diameter of the nail can best be determined only at the time of surgery, although one can arrive at an approximation from preoperative measurement of the endosteal diameter.

Resistance to rotation of the bone about the nail depends on the degree of friction between the two surfaces. The greater the surface area of contact, the greater the friction. The concept of the bone squeezing the elastic, deformable nail which in its elastic recoil grips the bone is not entirely correct. Viewed under high magnification, the channel cut by the reamers is seen to be a series of peaks and valleys. The fixation is in reality an interference fit between the nail and the bone. As the

bone of the medullary canal an elastic, deformable nail somewhat larger than the medullary canal, the nail would be squeezed and its elastic recoil would result in the nail gripping the bone along its endosteal surface (Fig. 16.7). The initial nail was V-shaped in profile. It was subsequently changed to the familiar cloverleaf configuration. It was elastic and slit along its full length to make it compressible. It was bowed anteriorly to correspond to the physiological curvature of the femur with its slit coming posteriorly.

Studies have shown that the holding power of the nail depends on a combination of a number of factors. If we think of the nail as a tube within a tube of bone, several of the biomechanical properties of this type of fixation become obvious. A nail has to overcome the forces of bending, rotation, and shortening. The resistance to bending depends on the length of intimate contact between the two tubes. Thus, a nail introduced without reaming would have contact only over a short area at the isthmus and, theoretically, bending could occur, with the fulcrum at the isthmus and the amplitude of

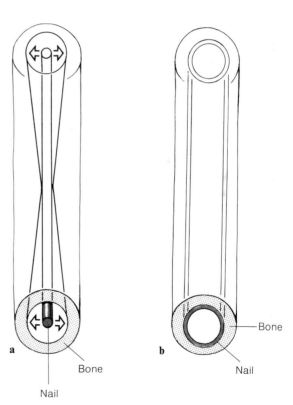

Fig. 16.8. a A nail introduced without reaming has contact only along the narrowest segment of the medullary canal. Bending can occur at either end. **b** After reaming, the length of contact of the "tube within a tube" is significantly increased, as is stability

contours of the nail and bone do not correspond exactly, there are areas of greater pressure where the bone is forcing the nail to follow its contour. Where the reduction is such that the fracture fragments are in contact, rotational control is achieved by the interdigitation of the fragments, and not by friction. Axial muscle force keeps the fragments in opposition. This applies to short oblique and transverse fractures. Longer oblique and spiral fractures lack rotational stability for two reasons. The first is that a long split decreases the available areas of bone for contact and thus decreases rotational control, and the second is that the long spiral fracture can open. This not only interferes with rotational stability, but also with longitudinal stability.

Intramedullary reaming not only enhances the resistance to bending and rotation, but also allows one to use a thicker nail, which will be able to withstand the physiological forces of bending. A nail, because of its special orientation in relationship to the mass of the femur, is in a much more advantageous position than a plate to withstand deformation. Because of this, it can be used as a load-sharing device and permit much earlier weight bearing.

The nail has to substitute for the bone while the bone is uniting; therefore, it must be just as strong. The bending strength of a nail is related to its cross-sectional configuration and to the orientation of this configuration. Thus, for example, in a diamond-shaped nail, the larger diameter affords a greater resistance to bending than the smaller diameter. The spatial distribution of the material is also important: a tube has greater bending resistance than a solid rod.

The bending strength is also related to the diameter of the nail. The nail should extend from the piriform fossa almost to the subchondral bone of the distal metaphysis. It should not be allowed to jut out into the abductors because it often causes pain, lurching, or both, and may result in heterotopic calcification and/or ossification, which may result in permanent malfunction of the abductors. The slit in the nail weakens its torsional resistance.

Longitudinal stability depends on the ability of the bone to withstand axial compression. Thus, it is dependent on the fracture pattern, as already mentioned, and on the degree of contact between the main fragments. The ideal fracture pattern for axial stability is the trans-

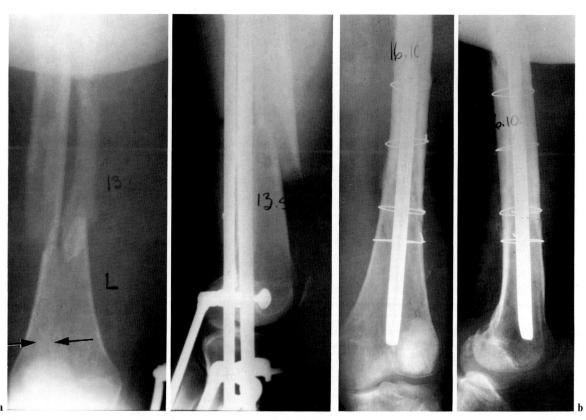

Fig. 16.9 a, b. Severely comminuted fracture of the femoral shaft. Longitudinal stability was restored by reduction and cerclage wiring of the fragments prior to nailing. Note that all the fragments are large. Today this case would be an ideal indication for a "locked" intramedullary nailing

verse fracture, but even here the degree of stability is a function of the degree of contact. If there is comminution, the less the circumferential contact between the main fragments, the less the stability. If the contact falls below 50 %, then the likelihood of collapse increases significantly unless the comminuted fragments can be reduced and kept in place by supplemental fixation such as cerclage wiring. This applies, of course, only to open nailing. In closed nailing where supplemental fixation cannot be carried out, one must carefully assess the degree of contact between the main fragments in order to assess accurately the degree of stability and the applicability of the technique.

Loss of reduction of long or spiral fractures can be prevented either by cerclage wires or by the insertion of lag screws between the main fragments (Fig. 16.9). Longitudinal splits can be prevented by cerclage if the comminution is not too extensive and the fragments not too small. If the segmental loss of contact cannot be restored by an open reduction and internal fixation, then, once the femur is nailed with the main fragments out to length, shortening can be prevented by bridging the zone of comminution with a narrow plate. The medullary canal is anterior to a thick ridge of bone which represents the linea aspera. Thus, a plate can be screwed to the posterolateral aspect of the femur with the screws passing posterior to the nail. If a zone of comminution is bridged by a plate, then only the main fragments are reamed prior to the reduction, in order to keep the devitalization of the comminuted segment to a minimum (Figs. 16.10, 16.11). The fixation of oblique spiral fractures, the fixation of comminuted segments, and the bridging of defects implies open intramedullary nailing with exposure of the fracture. If closed intramedullary nailing is chosen, then reduction of the unstable fracture must be maintained either by traction or in a hip spica.

From the foregoing, it should be evident why conventional intramedullary nailing is suitable as a method of internal fixation only for fractures of the middle third of the femur and ideally only for transverse and short oblique fractures. Its use for other fracture patterns is an extension of the technique beyond the ideal indications and, if employed, often requires combination with cerclage, lag screws, or plates.

The limitations imposed on the conventional nail by the location of a fracture and its pattern have given rise to the development of the interlocking nail (Kempf et al. 1985). Locked intramedullary nailing has greatly increased the indications for closed intramedullary nailing of femoral fractures not only of the middle third, but also of the proximal and distal thirds (Fig. 16.12). The advantage and biological prerequisite of this technique is that the nailing must be done closed. This preserves any remaining soft tissue attachment and viability of the comminuted fragments, which greatly accelerates the formation of callus and stability. The reamings add some bone grafting effects but are less important.

The locking feature of the nail is achieved by the insertion of bolts through the bone and nail which lock the two together. Thus, if a bolt is inserted proximally and distally, a femur, even with extreme comminution of the diaphysis, can be kept out to length and rotationally stable. Similarly, fractures of the proximal and distal femur can be stabilized by the insertion of the corresponding bolts proximally or distally. While the bolts are in place, the nail acts as a distracting device; thus, instead of being a weight-sharing device, it becomes a weight-bearing device. Once callus begins to form, weight bearing can begin. Removal of the bolts is not necessary.

The first generation interlocked nails greatly extended the indications of intramedullary nailing to fractures of the proximal and distal part of the diaphyseal segment of the femur and tibia. Certain fractures of the proximal femur, such as subtrochanteric fractures involving the lesser trochanter or associated with intertrochanteric fractures, could not be stabilized with the first generation nails. This stimulated the development of the second generation nails such as the reconstruction nail (Smith Newphew Richards, Memphis, TN, USA) or the short and long gamma nail (Howmedica Pfizer, New York, NY, USA). This type of locking has made it possible not only to stabilize fractures of the proximal and distal third of the diaphysis, but also to treat subtrochanteric fractures with involvement of the lesser trochanter and ipsilateral fractures of the shaft and neck of the femur (Kyle 1994).

For many years intramedullary reaming was considered an essential component of modern intramedullary nailing techniques because it not only improved the stability of the fixation, but more importantly it allowed surgeons to use larger nails which overcame the complications of nail bending, and breakage. A number of studies (Rhinelander 1973; Perren 1991) demonstrated that reaming produces extensive damage to the endosteal blood supply of bone. The desire to use intramedullary nailing for the fixation of open fractures and the recognition that further dead bone from the reaming could result in further infection led to the development of unreamed nails. Metallurgical and technical advances have overcome many of the early problems with small diameter nails. The recent experimental evidence that hollow nails appear to support infection has given rise to the development of solid unreamed nails for the femur and for the tibia (Synthes). The unreamed solid nail for the femur (Synthes) is a second generation implant which embodies a number of very elegant proximal locking techniques.

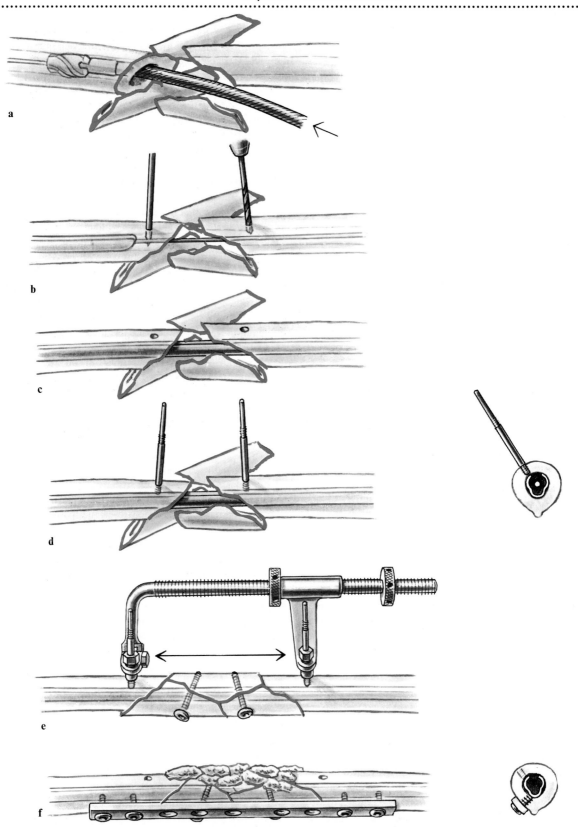

Fig. 16.10 a–f. Schematic representation of **a** reaming, **b–d** nailing, **e** reducing with the aid of a distractor, and **f** finally, with the aid of screws and a narrow plate, securing fixation of a severely comminuted fracture of a femur. (From Müller et al. 1991.) Note the bone graft. In this type of "locked" open intramedullary nailing a bone graft is a must

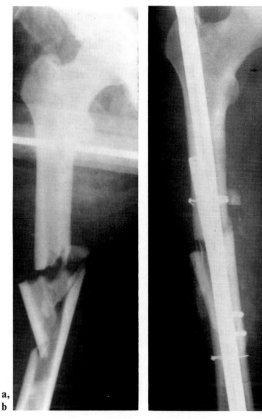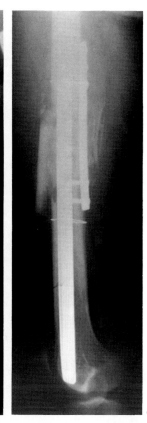

a,
b

c

Fig. 16.11. a A severely comminuted fracture of the middle third of the femoral shaft. Some of the fragments are too small for cerclage wiring. **b** The fixation has been achieved with a combination of an intramedullary nail, cerclage wiring, and a plate. The main function of the plate is to maintain length and rotational stability. **c** Note the extreme posterior position of the plate, just in front of the linea aspera. Note also the bone graft in **b**

c) Plate Fixation

Locked intramedullary nailing is the preferred method of internal fixation of long bones. However, there are situations when intramedullary nailing is contraindicated, such as previous infection, deformity of the bone, or the presence of a total hip, to name a few, and plating cannot be avoided. Thus plating techniques of the femur, despite their greater technical demands, continue to be important.

Absolutely Stable Internal Fixation of the Femur

As already discussed, plates can be used to achieve absolute stability or relative stability.

Absolutely stable fixation is indicated for simple fractures and for wedge fractures. In order to achieve absolute stability plates are used either in combination with lag screws as protection plates, or alone as compression or tension band plates. Whenever plates are used to bridge zones of fragmentation, they are referred to as bridge plates and are used as splints. Splinting is only relatively stable and union is by callus. Bridge plating cannot be used to stabilize simple or wedge fractures because the strain generated in the fracture gap becomes too great. The excessive strain inhibits bone formation. The fracture fails to unite and failure is the usual outcome. Thus, whenever plating is chosen as the technique of internal fixation, the surgeon must decide on the basis of fracture morphology at the outset of the procedure, on the type of fixation and the degree of stability which must be achieved.

The forces acting on the femur are much greater than those acting on any other bone. The surgeon must thus not only observe all biomechanical considerations in carrying out absolutely stable fixation of the femur, but also remember that, whenever absolute stability is aimed for, autogenous cancellous bone grafting must be carried out in order to prevent failure.

The femur is an eccentrically loaded bone. In vivo strain gauge work has demonstrated that in vivo the lateral cortex is loaded in tension and the medial in com-

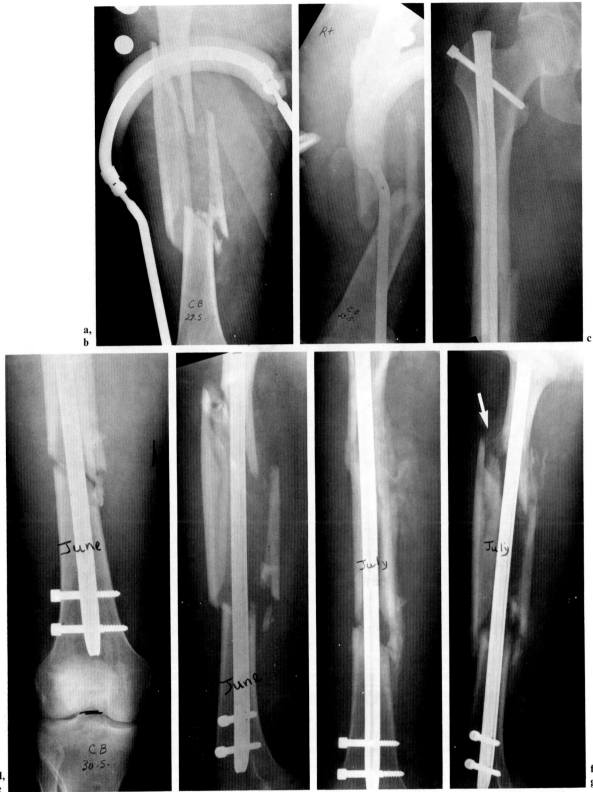

a,
b

c

d,
e

f,
g

spiral fractures are stabilized first by means of lag screw fixation, which assures interfragmental compression. The primary fixation with lag screws, as elsewhere, is then protected by means of plates which are fixed to the main fragments (Fig. 16.15). These plates are referred to as neutralization plates. If axial continuity of bone exists under the plate, then, even when primary lag screw fixation of the fragments has been obtained, the neutralization plate should be placed under tension. In this way, it acts as a neutralization and as a tension band plate.

An attempt should be made, if at all possible, to insert at least one lag screw through the plate and across the fracture. This greatly enhances the rotational and bending stability of the fixation.

The femur must be fixed with broad plates. The length chosen should be such that the cortex is traversed by screws in at least seven places on each side of the fracture. This rule applies to young individuals with strong cortical bone. In osteoporotic bone, the plate should be correspondingly longer to permit the use of a greater number of screws to compensate for the decreased holding power of screws in osteoporotic bone. It should be remembered that increasing the distance between the individual screws when plating increases the strength of the fixation of the plate to bone; thus when the length of the plate is increased, the screws should be staggered, resulting in a lower relative number of screws (Tornkvist 1994). Two plates should not be used for the fixation of a normal diaphysis. The interference with the blood supply of the cortex that the two plates bring about is so great that a segment of bone so plated undergoes intense osteoporosis as a result of revascularization and is greatly weakened. At one time, it was thought that two-plate fixation would be the answer to all difficult problems of internal fixation of the femur. Experience has shown, however, that double-plating is associated with a much higher failure rate. It should be recognized that this applies to the diaphysis only. In metaphyseal areas where the cortex is thin and filled with a network of trabecular bone instead of a medullary canal, two plates may be used and, indeed, at times comprise the only possible means to stable internal fixation. If the metaphysis is double plated, it must be bone grafted. Under exceptional circumstances where the cortex of a diaphysis is very much thickened, such as in a hypertrophic pseudarthrosis (Fig. 16.16), two plates may be employed as necessary. One should be shorter than the other to allow for a more gradual transition between the rigid double-plated segment and the remainder of the bone. The posterolateral side of the femur just in front of the linea aspera is the ideal site for plate application. If two plates are used, they should be inserted at 90° to one another.

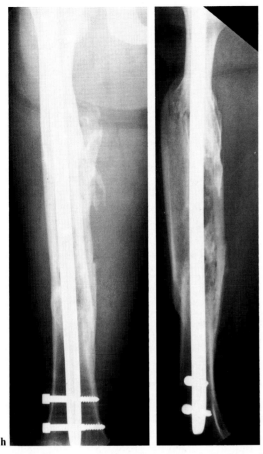

Fig. 16.12 a–i. A comminuted fracture of the femoral shaft treated with a locking intramedullary nail. **a, b** Note the severe comminution and displacement of the diaphyseal fragments. Such displacement and comminution usually denote a high-velocity injury. **c, d** Anteroposterior and **e** lateral views of the proximal and distal fragments. Note the proximal and distal locking screws which traverse the bone and the nail. **f** Anteroposterior and **g** lateral views of the same femur 6 weeks after surgery. Note the rapid formation of callus, which is a biological advantage of closed intramedullary nailing. **h** Anteroposterior and **i** lateral views at 2 years after surgery. The proximal screw was removed at 3 months to dynamize the nail. Usually the distal screws are removed at the same time. Note at this time just prior to nail removal the advanced remodeling of the cortex and the full incorporation of severely displaced fragments

pression (Schatzker et al. 1980; Fig. 16.13). The femur is therefore suitable for tension band fixation with plates (compression plates). In this bone, the integrity of the medial buttress for stable tension band fixation is more important than in any other bone because of the enormous bending forces. In order to achieve stable fixation, the reduction must be anatomical to regain structural continuity (Fig. 16.14). Stability of fixation is secured as elsewhere by means of compression. All oblique and

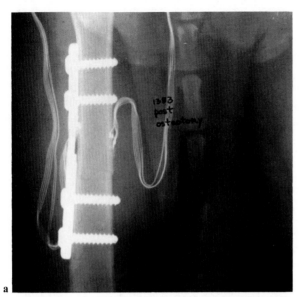

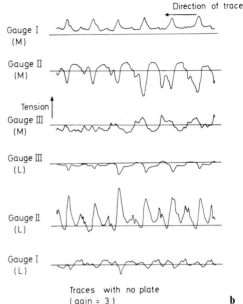

Fig. 16.13 a, b. An in vivo study by means of strain gauges or the bone response to loading in the dog. **a** One rosette of strain gauges was placed on the medial cortex and one on the lateral cortex just under the milled-out portion of the plate. **b** A trac-

ing of the deflections produced as the dog walked about; note gauge II (*M*, medial and *L*, lateral). The principal medial strain is compression and the principal lateral strain is tension

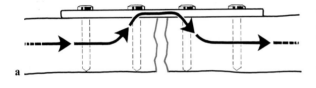

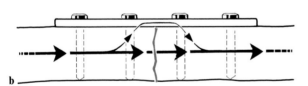

Fig. 16.14. a A fracture has been fixed with a plate, but the reduction is incomplete: a gap has been left between the fragments and there is no structural continuity. Under load, the whole force must be transmitted by the plate from one fragment to the other. **b** The fracture has been reduced anatomically. There is structural continuity and no gap between the fragments. Under load, the force is transmitted from bone fragment to bone fragment and only partially through the plate

Relatively Stable Internal Fixation of the Femur

Bridge plating is indicated whenever one attempts to plate a complex fracture. Under these circumstances one should always resort to indirect reduction techniques in order to preserve the blood supply to all fragments. Once

all the fragments have been realigned by traction, one must assess the configuration of the different fragments to see if there is continuity of bone under the plate, or if it is possible to secure fixation between some fragments with lag screws or to secure fixation of these fragments to the plate. All these manoeuvers increase the strength of the fixation. Axial preloading of the bone by axial compression greatly increases the strength of the internal fixation and should be attempted whenever possible, but not at the expense of length. Prerequisite for this is the continuity of the cortex under the plate. If a gap is present, axial compression would result in shortening. Although bridge plating is only relatively stable and relies for union on the formation of callus, increasing the stability of the construct will only add to the safety margin of the fixation and not interfere with union. It is the piecemeal reduction of the fragments and the individual lag screw fixation which render the fragments avascular and prevents them from participating in union by the formation of callus. Avascular fragments require absolute stability for their revascularization. Generally, if the technique is done properly, union will be by callus and bone grafting is not necessary. This is not true if one chooses bridge plating for the fixation of an open fracture. These must always be bone grafted at a later date because their propensity to union is much lower for a number of reasons.

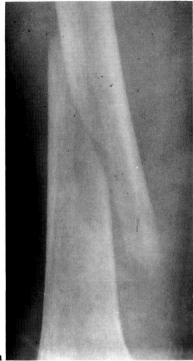
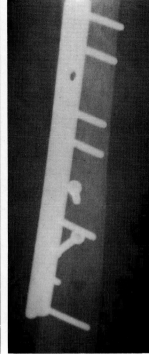
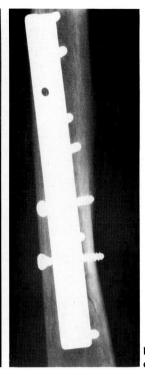

Fig. 16.15. a A spiral fracture of the femur. **b, c** Lag screws used to secure interfragmental compression between the fragments. A plate is used to neutralize the forces of bending, shear, and torque, and to protect the lag screw fixation

16.3.2.5 Bone Grafting

Whenever a femur is plated to achieve absolute stability, no matter how perfect the internal fixation, it should be bone grafted to diminish the incidence of failure. In intramedullary nailing, bone grafting should be carried out whenever a delayed union is foreseen, such as would occur in open fractures particularly whenever there is loss of bone. In bridge plating of closed fractures, a graft is not necessary but would be indicated in open fractures.

16.3.2.6 Wound Closure

In elective incisions for closed fractures, wound closure is rarely a problem. If tension should exist and threaten the survival of the wound edges, then the wound should be left open. Because the plate is under the cover of the vastus lateralis muscle, it is not exposed if the wound is left open. The muscle is usually rapidly covered by granulation tissue. If a secondary closure cannot be achieved within the first week, then the wound can either be left open to re-epithelialize slowly or be skin grafted.

16.3.3 Postoperative Care

Because the object of the open reduction and internal fixation is the rapid return to function of the soft tissue envelope and adjacent joints, the details of postoperative care are as important as those of the operative procedure. Compressive dressings should not be used in an effort to prevent wound hematomas; suction drainage is much more efficient. The drains should be withdrawn 24–36 h after surgery. One should beware of compartment syndrome following the reduction of femoral fractures. This is almost never seen following plating because the open reduction decompresses the compartments. A compartment syndrome can develop, however, following closed intramedullary nailing of the femur. Its development is likely due to the decrease in the volume of the compartments produced by the lengthening of the leg rather than due to the reaming.

Following any surgery on the shaft of the femur, the knee should be immobilized for the first 2–3 days, in 90° of flexion. This will prevent postoperative knee stiffness and greatly reduce the time spent on postoperative rehabilitation. With flexion of the knee, the vastus lateralis muscle descends 3–4 cm. If the reflected vastus lateralis is allowed to fall back into place at the end of a procedure

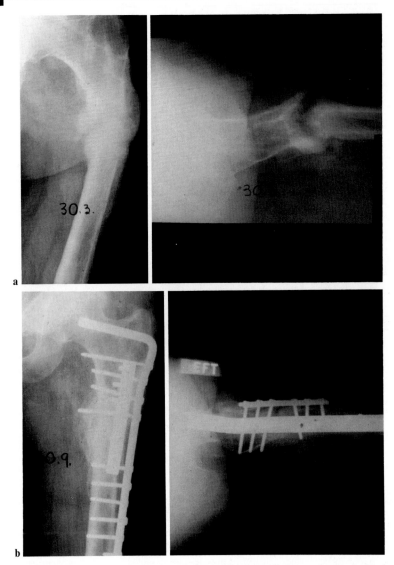

Fig. 16.16. a A hypertrophic pseudarthrosis of the femur. **b** Two plates have been used for fixation. The cortex is flared and hypertrophied and stress shielding will not result in any significant weakening of the bone

and the knee is then kept extended for 5 days or more, the muscle fibers reattach rapidly in the preshortened position. Any effort at flexion pulls on these muscle fibers and stretches the joint capsule. Both give rise to pain which results in protective splinting. This sets up a vicious circle which takes many weeks to be reversed. If, however, the knee is kept flexed, the capsule is kept stretched, and the muscle fibers attach more distally. Once the splint is removed, the patient is usually able to regain full extension within 30–60 min. Extensor lag or a flexion deformity has never been seen; patients can usually maintain the 90° of flexion and continue to regain further flexion in the ensuing days. If one considers that, in patients treated in traction on a Thomas splint and Pearson knee piece, a 90° range of flexion achieved at the end of a rehabilitative period was considered an excellent result, then a method which at the start of the rehabilitative period guarantees 90° of flexion must be considered superior.

It is best to support the knee in 90° of flexion in a very well padded, light cast which leaves the foot free. To facilitate drainage, the extremity can be supported on a special splint or pillows, but the patient must be cautioned not to roll the leg into external rotation, lest this lead to compression of the peroneal nerve. We like to leave the foot free so that the patient can exercise the ankle and in this way activate the venous pump. We prefer the padded cast to a padded splint because the patient is not immobilized and can stand up with crutches or be sat up. This is very important if the chest is to be kept upright and respiratory insufficiency prevented. The time of mobilization cannot be governed by the calendar alone. If wound healing is not progressing satisfactorily, then knee mobilization may have to be postponed for a day or two. We use the 90° position also for closed intramedullary nailing.

16.4 Special Considerations: Open Fractures of the Femur

We cannot emphasize enough that the most important goal in the treatment of an open fracture is the prevention of infection. Stability of the bone fragments is, next to the débridement of the wound, the most important prophylactic maneuver in preventing infection. In addition to preventing infection, stability of the bone fragments allows early mobilization of the damaged soft tissue envelope, which promotes the optimal recovery of soft tissue function.

The grade II open fracture of the femur rarely presents a serious problem in management (see classification of open fractures, Chapt. 3). If the fracture is received early for treatment and its contamination is relatively minor, then the open wound is débrided and is left open. The fracture is then treated as if it were a closed injury. Initially, we felt that one should not carry out intramedullary nailing of open fractures because of the increased risk of sepsis. Thus, isolated fractures of the femur with minimal soft tissue damage, if considered best suited for intramedullary nailing, were first thoroughly débrided and then kept in skeletal traction for 7–10 days; they were nailed only if one could be certain that infection had been prevented. The other fracture patterns were either stabilized immediately by means of plates and screws or, if too comminuted and definitely beyond the scope of internal fixation, initially stabilized in an external fixator. Recent experience with immediate intramedullary nailing of grade IIIA and, at times, even of grade IIIB open fractures in patients with multiple injuries, particularly with the use of unreamed nails, would indicate that fears of an increased occurrence of sepsis with immediate intramedullary nailing of the femur were exaggerated. We feel, however, that caution must be exercised because an infected intramedullary nailing is the most difficult type of infection to eradicate.

We feel that the safest approach to the severe grade IIIC open fracture is to provide skeletal stability by means of one of the modern external fixators. This may become the definitive form of fixation, but more often we lean towards revision to either a plate or even an ureamed nail if the state of the wound justifies such a form of fixation.

Difficulties invariably arise when surgeons seek to complete the care of an open fracture in one operation.

We consider the surgical care of an open fracture as a series of surgical procedures timed and executed as directed by preceding events and by the progress of the fracture and the wound. Thus, after the débridement and stabilization of the bone, the wound is left open. Within the first 48–72 h the patient returns to the operating room, the dressing is removed, and the wound is inspected. If further débridement is necessary, this is carried out. Once the wound is clean and beginning to granulate, a cancellous bone graft may be added and a secondary closure is executed as far as possible. The remaining open wound is left to granulate in or a split-thickness skin graft is applied. Once closure is achieved and infection prevented, the next decision to bone graft is usually made 4–6 weeks after fracture.

If it has been decided to use the external fixator as the definitive fixation, the fracture must be bone grafted. If the fracture is bone grafted, and no complications arise, the external fixation can be continued until union occurs. Usually, if union has not occurred by the end of the third month and evidence exists that a delayed union or nonunion is developing, it is best to intervene and convert the fixation to one with a plate and screws. If a large gap still exists which has to be bridged, it may be of advantage to use the modified broad AO plates which Wagner has developed for use in leg lengthening. Because these plates have no holes in their mid zone, they are stronger and fail less readily when subjected to bending.

If complications arise early in the course of treatment with an external fixator, then, as soon as one can be certain that infection has been prevented, one should convert the external fixation to internal fixation as outlined already. If the knee has stiffened, it may be manipulated at the time of the conversion to internal fixation in order to regain a useful range of flexion.

We have had limited experience with the Ilizarov technique in the treatment of open fractures of the femur. We have found it to be a very labour intensive device which tends to be quite painful for the patient but capable of producing spectacular results. We have reserved its use for cases with major bone loss which otherwise could only be managed with a free bone pedicle graft.

References

Charnley J, Guindy A (1961) Delayed operation in the open reduction of the fractures of long bones. J Bone Joint Surg 43B:664–671

Hierholzer G, Allgöwer M, Rüedi T (1985) Fixateur-externe-Osteosynthese. Springer, Berlin Heidelberg New York Tokyo

Kempf I, Grosse A, Beck G (1985) Closed locked intramedullary nailing. J Bone Joint Surg 67A:709–720

Küntscher G (1967) Practice of intramedullary nailing. Thomas, Springfield, p 34

Kyle RF (1994) Fractures of the proximal part of the femur. J Bone Joint Surg 76A:924–950

Lam SJ (1964) The place of delayed internal fixation in the treatment of fractures of the long bones. J Bone Joint Surg 46B:393–397

Matter P, Rittman WW (1978) The open fracture. Huber, Bern

Müller ME, Allgöwer M, Willenegger H (1965) Technique of internal fixation of fractures. Springer, Berlin Heidelberg New York

Müller ME, Allgöwer M, Schneider R, Willenegger H (1979) Manual of internal fixation, 2nd edn. Springer, Berlin Heidelberg New York

Müller ME, Allgöwer M, Schneider R, Willenegger H (1991) Manual of internal fixation, 3rd edn. Springer, Berlin Heidelberg New York

Pape H-C, Regel G, Dwenger A, Sturm JA, Tscherne H (1993) Influence of thoracic trauma and primary femoral intramedullary nailing on the incidence of ARDS in multiple trauma patients. Injury 24 (Suppl 3):82–103

Perren SM (1991) The concept of biological plating using the limited contact-dynamic compression plate (LC-DCP). Scientific background, design and application. Injury 22 (Suppl 1):5

Rhinelander FW (1973) Effects of medullary nailing on the normal blood supply of diaphyseal cortex. A.A.O.S. Instructional course lectures. Mosby, St. Louis, pp 161–187

Riska EB, Myllenen P (1982) Fat embolism in patients with multiple injuries. J Trauma 22:891–894

Riska EB, von Bonsdorff H, Hakkinen S, Jaroma H, Kiviluoto O, Paavilainen T (1976) Prevention of fat embolism by early internal fixation of fractures in patients with multiple injuries. Injury 8:110–116

Sarmiento A (1972) Functional bracing of tibial and femoral shaft fractures. Clin Orthop 82:2–13

Sarmiento A, Latta LL (1981) Closed functional treatment of fractures. Springer, Berlin Heidelberg New York

Schatzker J (to be published) The Toronto experience with fractures of the femur

Schatzker J, Manley PA, Sumner-Smith G (1980) In vivo strain-gauge study of bone response to loading with and without internal fixation. In: Uhthoff HK (ed) Current concepts of internal fixation of fractures. Springer, Berlin Heidelberg New York, pp 306–314

Sibel R, Laduca J, Hassett J, Babikian G, Mills B, Border D, Border J (1985) Blunt multiple trauma (ISS36) femur traction and the pulmonary failure-septic state. Ann Surg 202:283–295

Smith JEM (1964) The results of early and delayed internal fixation of fractures of the shaft of the femur. J Bone Joint Surg 46B:28–31

Stürmer KM (1993) Measurements of intramedullary pressure in an animal experiment and propositions to reduce the pressure increase. Injury 24 (Suppl 3):7–21

Tornkvist H, Hearn T, Schatzker J (1994) Unpublished data

Trentz O (1994) Personal communication

Wenda K, Runkel M, Degreif J, Ritter G (1993) Pathogenesis and clinical relevance of bone marrow embolism in medullary nailing – demonstrated by intraoperative echocardiography. Injury 24 (Suppl 3):73–81

Winquist RA, Hansen ST, Clawson DK (1984) Closed intramedullary nailing of femoral fractures. J Bone Joint Surg 66A:529–539

17 Supracondylar Fractures of the Femur (33-A, B, and C)

J. Schatzker

17.1 Introduction

A supracondylar fracture of the femur (Fig. 17.1) is a grave injury which for years represented an unsolved problem in trauma and was considered to result almost always in varying degrees of permanent disability. It was felt that the fate of the joint was determined by the injury rather than by its treatment. Closed procedures were almost always used in treatment and consisted principally of splinting and traction. The traction was applied either through a two-pin system, one through the supracondylar fragment and one through the tibial tuberosity, or through a single pin through the tibial tuberosity. The reduction was accomplished by traction or, if necessary, under general anesthesia. The extremity was then immobilized on a splint. Padding, flexion of the knee, and skeletal traction were used to maintain reduction. The difficulties with these methods were, first and foremost, an inability to control displaced intra-articular fragments which did not reduce with manipulation or traction, and, secondly, that occasionally the supracondylar fragments displaced posteriorly. Further major drawbacks consisted of knee stiffness and the necessity for prolonged hospitalization and bed rest in the supine position which often exceeded 6–8 weeks.

Open reduction and internal fixation was attempted from time to time, but the results were largely unsatisfactory, because the techniques of internal fixation and the devices available did not allow stable fixation which would allow early motion without deformity and nonunion. Stewart et al. and Neer et al. gave good summaries of the state of the art as it was in the mid 1960s. In 1966, Marcus Stewart et al. published a review of 442 patients who were treated over a period of 20 years. The purpose of his review was to compare methods of treatment. Some 213 patients were closely analyzed and followed. Of the 114 patients treated by closed methods, 67% had an excellent or good result, whereas of the 69 patients treated by open reduction with internal metallic fixation or some type of bone graft, only 54% had an excellent or good result. Patients treated with skeletal traction stayed an average of 62 days in hospital, whereas patients who had surgery had an average stay of 33 days. The ten nonunions and ten delayed unions were

all in the operated group. The authors concluded that "the additional trauma of surgery and the proximity of metallic implants to the joint predispose to excessive reaction and subsequent adhesions. Even though one obtains an excellent roentgenographic result with solid union, final function may be quite poor. No doubt, a few surgeons have mastered the technique of operative correction and internal fixation..., but they are in the minority.... Conservatism should be taught and practiced more universally."

In 1967, Charles Neer et al. reviewed a series of 110 unselected supracondylar fractures in order to analyze the results of internal fixations compared with those of closed methods of treatment. Only 52% of those treated by open means obtained a satisfactory result, whereas closed treatment yielded satisfactory results in 90% of patients. It must be noted, however, that in this review, patients were satisfied if they could flex the knee 70°! Thus, a patient whose knee flexed only 80° lost only 40% in the numerical rating used to assess function. This considerably boosted the seeming excellence of nonoperative treatment.

It must be noted that the patients who were included in the reviews of Stewart and Neer et al. were treated at a time when the techniques of internal fixation and the implants used were very limited. If accurate reduction was achieved, it was very difficult to maintain. The stability achieved was never sufficient to render the extremity painless. Thus, active motion was inhibited by pain and further complicated by frequent loss of position of the fragments, which led to malunion or nonunion with further loss of function.

In conclusion, Neer et al. felt that "no category of fracture at this level seemed well suited for internal fixation, and sufficient fixation to eliminate the need for external support or to shorten convalescence was rarely attained." They felt that surgery should be limited only to open fractures or to the internal fixation of a fracture associated with an arterial injury or some other unusual problem.

In 1970, the AO group published its first review of 112 patients with supracondylar fractures who were treated according to the principles of accurate anatomical reduction, stable internal fixation, and early motion (Wenzl et al. 1970). Of these patients, 73.5% achieved a

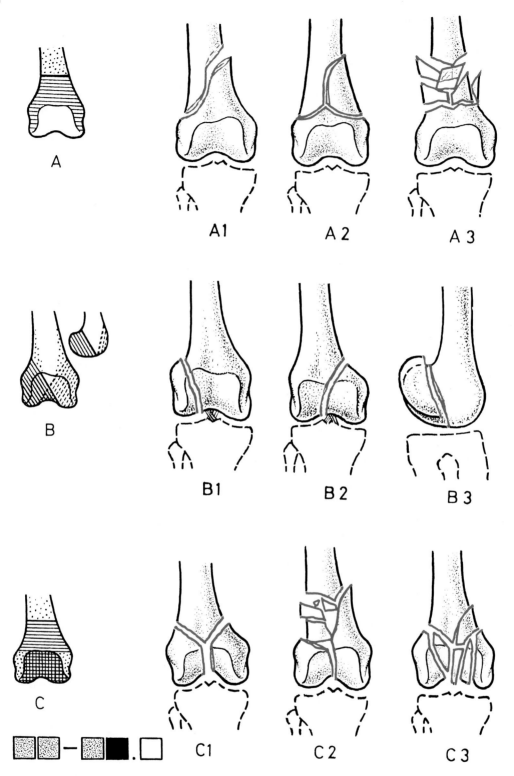

Fig. 17.1. Femur distal: the groups. *A1*, extra-articular fracture, simple; *A2*, extra-articular fracture, metaphyseal wedge; *A3*, extra-articular fracture, metaphyseal complex; *B1*, partial articular fracture, lateral condyle, sagittal; *B2*, partial articular fracture, medial condyle, sagittal; *B3*, partial articular fracture, frontal; *C1*, complete articular fracture, articular simple, metaphyseal simple; *C2*, complete articular fracture, articular simple, metaphyseal multifragmentary; *C3*, complete articular fracture multifragmentary

good to excellent result. This result was certainly better than any previously published results of open treatment. Surgeons steeped in the older methods advanced arguments against this new surgical method. They felt that these AO results were obtained by master surgeons who were the innovators of their technique and that the results in the hands of other surgeons would be no better than those previously published.

In 1974, Schatzker et al. published a review of the Toronto experience with supracondylar fractures from 1966 to 1972. Patients whose fractures were treated in accordance with the AO principles obtained 75% good to excellent results, which contrasted sharply with the 32% of good to excellent results of patients who were treated nonoperatively. The study clearly demonstrated the superiority of the AO method not only as a surgical technique but as a method of treatment, because the Toronto surgeons were not members of the Swiss AO group and were considered very skilled in the nonoperative methods of treatment of the supracondylar fracture.

In 1979, Schatzker and Lambert published the results of the surgical treatment of a further 35 patients. Of the 17 patients who were treated in accordance with the AO principles, 71% achieved good to excellent results. In 18 patients, the surgeons employed the AO implants, but failed to achieve anatomical reduction and stable internal fixation. The results in this group of patients were very poor, with only 21% having good to excellent results. When this second group of patients was further analyzed, it became evident that elderly patients with severe osteoporosis were in the majority. The failure on the part of the surgeon to treat these patients in accordance with AO principles was not always due to neglect of the principles. The comminution frequently associated with osteoporosis and the poor holding power of osteoporotic bone presented a challenge which could not be met with any consistency. The study also clearly outlined the dictum that stable internal fixation is not achieved automatically by carrying out an open reduction and by the insertion of the AO implants. In those patients in whom the goals of surgery were realized (that is, in whom an accurate anatomical reduction was achieved, the internal fixation was absolutely stable, and early unencumbered mobilization was possible), the results continued to be excellent. This study further illustrated that, despite the excellence of the treatment, the results were tempered by the severity of the trauma, the type of fracture, and by osteoporosis. An analysis of the age incidence as related to the type of trauma revealed two groupings of patients. The younger patients in their twenties and thirties had sustained high-velocity trauma, which often results in a more severe fracture with greater intra-articular disruption or segmental comminution. Severe comminution, particu-

larly of the joint, had an adverse effect on the final result. Other factors which tended to temper the excellence of the final outcome were the presence of an open wound and soft tissue injuries or other fractures, such as fractures of the ipsilateral tibial plateau or tibia or of the contralateral femur, and the presence of major ligamentous disruptions. More recent studies (Silisky 1989) have confirmed our earlier observations. The presence of an open fracture leads to a higher incidence of infection, but in the presence of stable fixation infection and open fracture are still compatible with a good outcome (Schemitsch 1991). The most significant factor affecting the outcome of treatment of both closed and open fractures is the severity of the soft tissue lesion and in the elderly patient the severity of osteoporosis (J. Schatzker, unpublished data).

The older patients often sustained their fractures in a low-velocity injury, such as might result from a simple fall. Because of severe osteoporosis, despite the low-velocity nature of their injury, the comminution of the fracture was occasionally quite marked. The advent of cast bracing has improved the results of nonoperative treatment because patients can be mobilized earlier. Cast bracing, however, has had no beneficial effect on residual joint disorganization or on fractures which could not be controlled in traction.

17.2 Guides to Treatment and Indications for Surgery

In evaluating the criteria for surgery in the supracondylar fracture, the surgeon must carefully weigh the results achieved by nonoperative and operative treatment and the factors which adversely affect the results in each group. The experience in Toronto between 1966 and 1972 with nonoperative treatment, where only 32% of patients achieved a good to excellent result, serves to emphasize that if the same strict criteria are applied in evaluating the final result, it becomes evident that conservatism as advocated by Stewart et al. (1966) and Neer et al. (1967) is not a panacea for the supracondylar fracture and can be undertaken only with great reservations. If surgery is to be undertaken, however, the surgeon must be certain that the objectives of treatment, namely, accurate anatomical reduction, stable fixation, and early motion, will be achieved, for failure to achieve these might lead to results worse than those achieved by closed means. Therefore, the surgeon must carefully assess the nature of the fracture, which includes the patient's age, level of activity, and functional demands, the severity of the trauma, whether it was caused by high- or low-velocity impact, the individual fracture pattern, and the type and severity of associated injuries. The surgeon must also honestly evaluate his or her own skill and environment. The evidence from clinical stud-

390 ·

Chapter 17   **Supracondylar Fractures of the Femur (33-A, B, and C)**

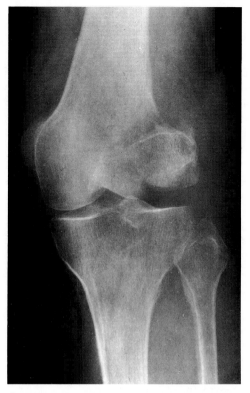

Fig. 17.2. Unicondylar fracture of the femur

ies as well as from the experimental investigations of Mitchell and Shepard (1980) on the effects of anatomical reduction and stable fixation on cartilage regeneration, and of Salter and Harris (1979) on the effects of rest and continuous passive motion on cartilage regeneration indicates irrefutably that the goals in the treatment of all intra-articular fractures should be:

1. Accurate anatomical reduction of the joint surface
2. Atraumatic reduction of the metaphyseal component of the fracture with restoration of normal axial alignment and length
3. Stable internal fixation of the articular surface
4. Buttressing of the metaphysis
5. Early motion

In the majority of fractures, these goals are attainable only by surgical means. Indications for surgical treatment are either absolute or relative. The absolute indications relate to fractures which have to be treated surgically because nonsurgical methods are certain to lead to poor results.

· ·

17.2.1 Absolute Indications

17.2.1.1 Intra-articular Fractures in Which Adequate Joint Congruity Cannot Be Restored by Manipulation

Under this heading, we would like to single out particular fractures as given below.

a) Unicondylar Fracture (33-B)

In our experience, unicondylar fractures, if treated in a cast brace, traction, or plaster, frequently displace with joint incongruity and axial nonalignment (Fig. 17.2).

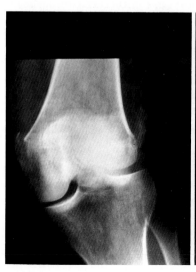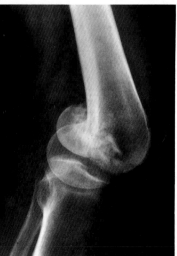

Fig. 17.3. Bicondylar fracture of the femur in the coronal plane (Hoffa fracture)

Fig. 17.4. Supracondylar and intracondylar fracture C2. Note the rotation of the condylar fragments. Their fracture surface faces posteriorly

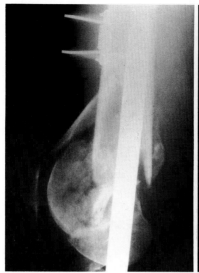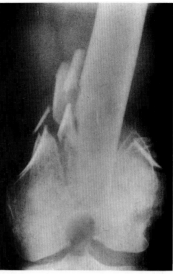

b) Bicondylar Fracture in the Coronal Plane (33-B)

This intra-articular fracture (the Hoffa fracture) cannot be reduced by closed means because the only soft tissue attachment (if any) is the synovial reflection and posterior capsule of the joint. Thus, traction has little effect on the position of the fragment (Fig. 17.3).

c) The T or Y Bicondylar Fracture with Rotational Displacement of the Condyles (33-C1)

The classic displacement of the supracondylar fragments is posterior angulation (rotation about the knee joint axis) due to the pull of the gastrocnemius muscle and anterior displacement of the shaft due to shortening (Fig. 17.4). If the displacement cannot be corrected by flexion of the knee and traction, then only an open operation can effect a reduction. This is particularly true if treatment is delayed for 1 week or longer.

A more important displacement is the rotation of one condyle with respect to the other. Manipulation and traction cannot effect a reduction and, if left, this displacement results in permanent joint incongruity.

d) A Supracondylar Fracture Above a Total Knee Replacement (33-A)

The function and long-term survival of a total knee replacement depends on accurate axial alignment of the components. A supracondylar fracture above a total knee replacement, if displaced, cannot be realigned by closed means. Some degree of malalignment is almost

certain. The malalignment will seriously compromise the function or the survival of the total knee replacement.

17.2.1.2 Open Intra-articular Fractures

In any open fracture, the main cause of permanent disability is sepsis, because it leads to scarring of the soft tissue envelope and to joint stiffness. In the treatment of an open fracture, therefore, all efforts must be directed to the prevention of sepsis. Mounting clinical evidence, as well as experimental work (Rittman and Perren 1974), indicates that after thorough surgical débridement, the next most important factor in the prevention of sepsis is absolute stability of the bony fragments. Therefore, after débridement, the surgeon should carry out an internal fixation of the fracture in order to achieve stability to prevent infection. Recent evidence disputes the conclusion of Stewart et al. (1966) that the proximity of metal to joints increases the likelihood of sepsis and stiffness (Olerud 1972).

17.2.1.3 Associated Neurovascular Injuries

Stability of the skeleton is most useful in the protection of any neurovascular repair.

17.2.1.4 Ipsilateral Fracture of the Tibial Plateau

The presence of two separate fractures on opposite sides of the same joint makes an open operation mandatory in order to reduce displaced fragments.

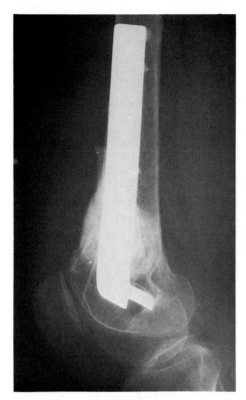

Fig. 17.5. Pathological supracondylar fracture through a large metastatic deposit from a breast carcinoma. Methyl methacrylate was used to fill the eroded portion of the bone. Note that at 18 months the posterior cortex has united

17.2.1.5 Ipsilateral Fracture of the Tibia (The Floating Knee)

In the presence of these two fractures, control of the knee by closed means is impossible and, in order to preserve function, an open reduction and internal fixation is necessary.

17.2.1.6 Multiple Injuries

In a patient with multiple injuries, the stabilization of the fracture may be desirable for reasons other than the fracture itself.

17.2.1.7 Pathological Fractures

Pathological fractures cannot be treated successfully by immobilization in plaster, because of the bone destruction caused by the presence of tumor. An open reduction with the evacuation of the tumor and a composite type of internal fixation which employs methyl methacrylate and metal is necessary (Fig. 17.5).

17.2.2 Relative Indications

As we have already indicated, we believe that a major intra-articular or periarticular fracture is best treated by open reduction and stable internal fixation because it is the most certain way of preserving the best possible function of the joint. We must caution, however, that these are technically very difficult fractures and that the first attempt of the surgeon in operating on these fractures should not be a badly comminuted intra-articular fracture, as these are far too demanding.

17.3 Surgical Treatment

17.3.1 Timing of Surgery

A major intra-articular or periarticular fracture is a difficult surgical undertaking which should not be executed in the middle of the night without a very careful evaluation of the fracture and without the necessary help. Clearly, the condition of the patient with multiple injuries may dictate that surgery be carried out at a less than optimal time, maybe even as an emergency operation if the fracture is open or if there is an associated vascular injury. If circumstances permit, however, a short delay, during which proper preparations are made, is time well spent and will often be an important factor in effecting a favorable outcome of surgery. The delay should not be protracted. We have reconstructed supracondylar fractures at 3–4 weeks from the time of the injury, but the longer the delay, the more difficult the reconstruction. The limb shortens and the fragments become embedded and covered by soft tissue and new granulations. An even greater difficulty is the healing of the compacted cancellous bone, which obliterates the fracture lines and makes their definition as well as the reduction very difficult.

The limb should be splinted while the patient awaits surgery. If surgery is to be delayed for more than a few hours, then we prefer to splint the extremity on the Thomas splint in skin traction to maintain some length and immobilization. If surgery has to be delayed for a few days, then we feel the extremity should be splinted on a Thomas splint with a Pearson knee piece with the knee in 20°–30° of flexion. Instead of skin traction, we use skeletal traction through the tibial tubercle, which should be sufficiently strong to pull the limb out to length and even overdistract the fracture. This greatly eases the subsequent open reduction. Care must be taken to insert the Steinmann pin a handbreadth or so below the projected lowermost point of the skin incision so as to avoid the risk of contamination and sepsis from the pin tract. Another very useful technique for temporary preservation of length and immobilization of the fracture is external fixation. For temporary immobilization we prefer an anterior unilateral half frame with two anterior pins in the femur and two anterior pins in the tibia. The knee is locked in slight degree of flexion. Over a short period of time the transfixing pins will not lead to sepsis or scarring of the muscle.

17.3.2 History and Physical Examination

It is important that a careful history be taken to determine whether the injury is a high- or low-velocity injury. Physical examination is the most readily available and the simplest method to determine whether there is an associated nerve or vascular injury.

17.3.3 Radiological Examination

A radiological examination, however, is necessary to obtain a detailed view of the fracture. We begin this examination by obtaining an anteroposterior, a lateral, and two oblique roentgenograms of the injured side as well as an anteroposterior and lateral view of the uninjured side which serve as a template for the surgical reconstruction of the fracture. If necessary, anteroposterior and lateral tomograms of the fracture are obtained. These are invaluable in evaluating the intra-articular components and the extent of the supracondylar comminution. In complex fractures computed tomographic (CT) scanning is almost a must. This portrays the distal femur in cross section, which is particularly helpful in identifying fracture lines in the frontal plane. Three-dimensional (3D) reconstruction has been useful in the planning of osteotomies for the correction of intra-articular malunions; however, it is not necessary for the radiological evaluation of acute fractures.

17.3.4 Classification

We rely on the comprehensive classification of supracondylar fractures because this classification defines the fracture, indicates its prognosis, and helps one decide which is the best type of internal fixation to use. Thus, the fractures are divided into type A, which are extra-articular, type B, which are partial articular fractures with part of the articular surface intact and in contact with the diaphysis, and type C, the complete articular fractures in which the articular surfaces are not only fractured but have also lost continuity with the diaphysis (see Fig. 17.1). These major types are further subdivided into subtypes in ascending order of complexity. Thus, the C_3 supracondylar fracture is one with extensive

intra-articular and extra-articular comminution and, as such, is the most difficult to stabilize and has the worst prognosis.

17.3.5 Planning the Surgical Procedure

Once a detailed radiographic assessment is available and all associated injuries and the soft tissues have been evaluated, it is possible to make an accurate diagnosis of the fracture and plan its treatment. The surgical treatment begins with a careful preoperative plan of the procedure. Tracing paper is used together with the radiograph of the patient's normal extremity. The anteroposterior radiograph is turned over to give the outline of the opposite side (Fig. 17.6).

An outline of the distal femur is then drawn on the tracing paper and the radiographs and tomograms of the fracture used to carefully draw in all the fracture lines as well as any bony defect present. A similar drawing is made of the lateral projection. Then the surgeonis ready to plan the internal fixation. In the properly executed plan of the surgical procedure, every step must be drawn in and numbered.

Thus, drawings a_1 and a_2 show the outline of the bone in the anteroposterior and lateral projection with all the fracture lines drawn in. Drawings b_1 and b_2 are copies of a_1 and a_2, respectively, on which the position of the window for the condylar plate or dynamic condylar screw (DCS) has been marked in as step I. Step II shows the position of the lag screws used to secure fixation of the condyles. Step III shows the position of any gliding holes or thread holes which should be drilled prior to the reduction of the fracture.

Drawings c_1 and c_2 are copies of b_1 and b_2, respectively. They are the definitive drawings on which one marks in the internal fixation. The plate is drawn in with the aid of a transparent template (obtainable from Synthes on request: Synthes USA, Paioli, PA, USA, or Synthes AG, Chur, Switzerland). This helps the surgeon to judge the length of the blade or screw required as well as the length of the plate and the number of screws. If lag screws are to be used, they are then drawn in and numbered in the order in which they will be inserted. To complete the drawing, the remainder of the screws are sketched in and also numbered in the order in which they will be inserted.

Such careful preoperative planning helps the surgeon with every step of the operative procedure. We are critical of the surgeon who thinks that the fixation can be planned properly only after the fracture has been exposed. Often, much less can be seen at surgery than on the preoperative radiographs. If the type and size of the implant has not already been determined, it may not be available when required. Furthermore, at the time of

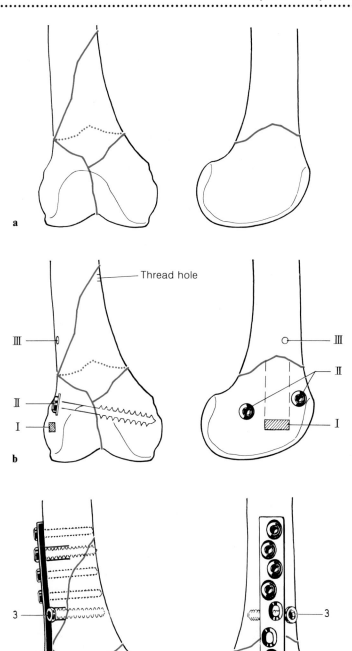

Fig. 17.6. a Anteroposterior *(left)* and lateral *(right)* outlines of the distal femur drawn with the aid of an anteroposterior and lateral radiograph of the opposite femur. Note that the fracture lines have been drawn in. **b** Copies of a left and right views. Step *I*: the position of the window for seating chisel is marked; step *II*: lag screws used to secure fixation of the condyles; step *III*: note the position of any gliding holes or thread holes which should be predrilled prior to reduction of fragments. **c** Copies of **b** left and right views on which the plate has been drawn in with the aid of a template and the screws numbered in order of insertion

surgery, one is rushed to keep the wound open for as short a time as possible in order to keep down the infection rate and the time required to plan the surgical procedure in detail cannot be afforded.

17.3.6 Surgical Anatomy of the Distal Femur

The anatomical axis of the knee joint does not coincide with the weight-bearing axis. The latter crosses the center of the femoral head and the center of the knee. The anatomical axis is in valgus and subtends an angle of 81° with the knee joint axis (Fig. 17.7).

Viewing the femur from one side (Fig. 17.8) and projecting the posterior cortex distally on a line, it can be noted that the posterior positions of the condyles appear as if they were tacked onto the posterior cortex of the shaft, with the anterior position of the condyles appearing as a continuation of the shaft. The application of this anatomical fact is illustrated in Fig. 17.8: the blade of the condylar plate or the screw of a DCS must be inserted into the anterior part of the condyles which is the distal projection of the shaft, or the plate will not fit the femur.

The distal femur, when viewed in cross section, is seen to be a trapezoid (Fig. 17.9). The anterior articular surface is not parallel to a line joining the posterior cortices of the condyles. Furthermore, the distance anteriorly between the medial and lateral wall is less than the distance posteriorly because the medial and lateral walls are inclined toward one another. The medial wall has the greater slope of the two and is inclined at 25° to the vertical. These facts are important to remember when

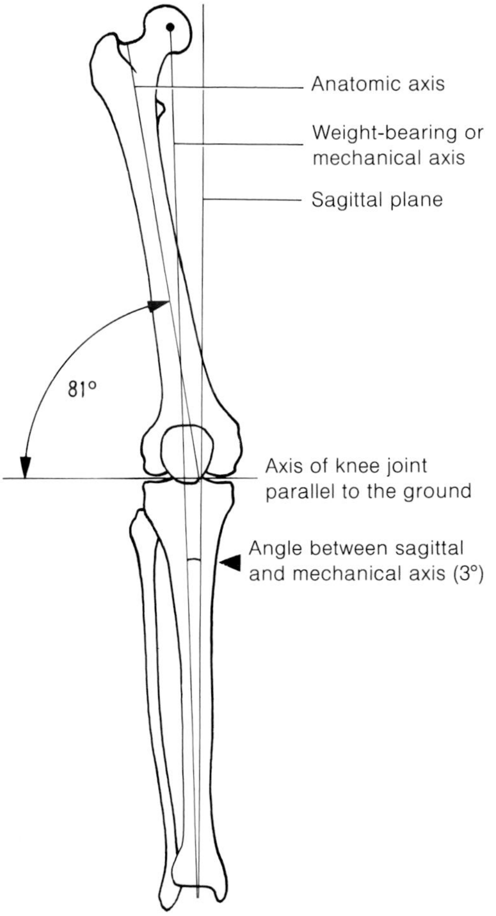

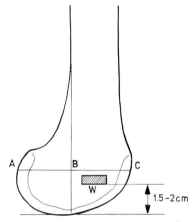

Fig. 17.8. When the posterior cortex of the shaft is projected distally as a line, it divides the epiphysis into an anterior and posterior half. The condyles appear as if they were tacked on posteriorly to the shaft. Note that the longest diameter *AC* is at 90° to the axis of the shaft. The window *W* for the condylar plate or a DCS is in the middle of the anterior half *BC* and 1.5–2 cm from the distal end of the femur

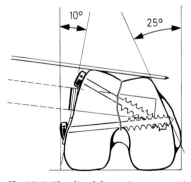

Fig. 17.9. The distal femur in cross section is a trapezoid. Note that the anterior and posterior surfaces are not parallel and that both the medial and lateral walls are inclined. This results in the anterior diameter being smaller than the posterior diameter. (Adapted from Müller et al. 1979)

Fig. 17.7. The mechanical axis is a line projected through the center of the femoral head, knee joint, and ankle joint. It subtends an angle of 3° with the sagittal plane and an angle of 6° with the anatomical axis of the femur. The knee joint is parallel to the ground. The anatomical axis subtends an angle of 81° (79°–82°) with the knee joint axis

Labels in Fig. 17.7:
- Anatomic axis
- Weight-bearing or mechanical axis
- Sagittal plane
- 81°
- Axis of knee joint parallel to the ground
- Angle between sagittal and mechanical axis (3°)

selecting the length of the blade of the condylar plate or the length of the compression screw. The projected width of the femur on a radiograph is the maximum width and represents the most posterior distance between the medial and lateral wall and not the distance in the anterior half where the blade must come to lie. Therefore, a blade which would correspond in length to the posterior cortex would be too long and would jut out through the bone intra-articularly just deep to the anterior fibers of the medial collateral ligament. The blade or the screw should stop 8–10 mm from the projected medial wall.

17.3.7 Positioning and Draping the Patient

We prefer to carry out the surgery with the patient supine on a radiolucent table. The leg should not be put in traction on a fracture table, as traction only tightens the soft tissue envelope and makes the visualization and manipulation of fragments almost impossible: thus, instead of making the reduction easier, it makes it more difficult. We like to cleanse the skin to the umbilicus above and to the ankle below. This permits us to drape the limb in such a fashion that the anterior iliac crest is left exposed should it be necessary to obtain a bone graft during the procedure. We expose at least half of the leg and drape the leg free. In this way, if we wish, we can extend the incision. The leg has to be free so that the knee can be flexed over one or two rolled-up, sterile sheets. This greatly facilitates the exposure and the reduction. We do not use a tourniquet, even if a sterile one is available, because bleeding can be readily controlled if the perforating vessels, when encountered, are clamped and ligated and all other vessels cauterized.

17.3.8 Surgical Exposure

17.3.8.1 Lateral Exposure

For a lateral exposure the skin is incised along an imaginary line joining the greater tro3hanter with the midpoint of the lateral condyle. The incision is then curved forward, aiming for a point just distal to the tibial tuberosity. The length of the skin incision depends on the type of fracture. With a type A fracture the incision often stops at the joint line, whereas in type C fractures it is often curved to a point distal to the tibial tuberosity. The fascia lata is incised in line with the skin just anterior to the iliotibial tract (Fig. 17.10a). Distally, the incision is extended through the lateral quadriceps retinaculum capsule and synovium. Even in type A fractures it is necessary to expose the joint so that the guide wires for the insertion of the angled device can be positioned.

Proximally, the femur is exposed by reflecting the vastus lateralis muscle from the lateral intermuscular septum. The perforating vessels are usually encountered close to the femur, but not directly over the bone. They should be cross-clamped, divided, and ligated (Fig. 17.10b). When one is dealing with type C_3 fractures, which have severe and complex intra-articular and supracondylar comminution, it becomes necessary to increase the intra-articular exposure so that the distal femur can be viewed from directly in front (Müller et al. 1979). To achieve this we extend the skin incision distally and medially, expose the tibial tubercle, and osteotomize it in such a way that the infrapatellar tendon can be lifted with a piece of bone. Once the fat pad is detached from the tibia and the synovium divided in the supracondylar region, the whole quadriceps muscle can be folded over upwards and medially, which exposes not only the whole joint but also the medial side of the shaft (Mize et al. 1982). The surgeon can then work unobstructedly on the whole joint surface, and also, if necessary, fix a second plate to the medial side of the femur without having to make a second incision.

17.3.8.2 Anterior Exposure

In recent years we have used the exposure employed for total knee arthroplasty in preference to the osteotomy of the tibial tubercle for the C_3 fractures which do not have major extensions into the diaphysis. The total knee exposure involves a midline skin incision which is centered on the patella and which is then extended distally just past the tibial tubercle and proximally as far as dictated by the fracture. A medial parapatellar arthrotomy is then made which is extended proximally through the tendons of the rectus femoris and vastus intermedius muscles. The patella with the lateral half of the quadriceps is then reflected laterally and the knee is flexed. It is best to support the flexed knee over two or three rolled-up sheets. The flexion of the knee exposes fully the articular surfaces (Fig. 17.11).

The great advantage of this approach for multifragmentary articular fractures is that the surgeon is facing the articular surface with full medial and lateral access for the insertion of fixation devices. This greatly facilitates the reduction and fixation of the articular fragments. A further advantage is that the exposure does not lead to any additional devitalization of the bony fragments and that it leaves the distal insertion of the quadriceps undisturbed.

Once the articular surface is reconstructed, fixation of the metaphyseal component can be performed. If using either the condylar blade plate or the DCS, the seat for the blade can be precut or the compression screw of the DCS inserted while the knee is still flexed. In order to

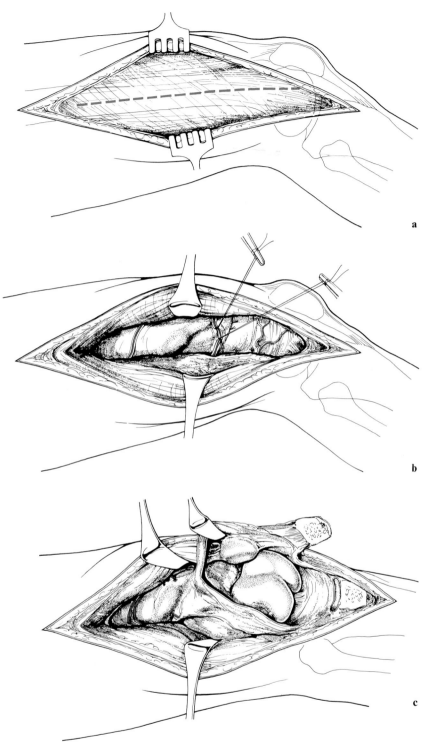

Fig. 17.10. a The skin incision is along an imaginary line joining the greater trochanter with the lateral condyle. The incision is aimed distally for a point just past the tibial tubercle. The fascia lata is incised in line with the skin incision. **b** The vastus lateralis muscle is reflected from the intermuscular septum. The perforating vessels should be clamped, divided, and ligated. **c** An extensile exposure of the distal femur. The insertion of the infrapatellar tendon is osteotomized and the quadriceps muscle insertion is reflected upward. The release of the vastus lateralis muscle from the septum allows full exposure of the distal femur and of the medial side of the shaft which is sufficient to permit the fixation of a plate to the medial side. A medial counterincision is unnecessary

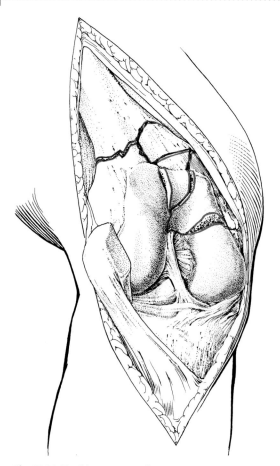

Fig. 17.11. Total knee approach

insert the plate and reduce the fracture the knee is extended and the plate is fixed to the distal fragment with the most distal screw if possible. An indirect reduction is then carried out either with the aid of the articulated tension device or a distractor. If using the femoral condylar buttress plate the plate should be fixed to the distal fragment once the knee is extended. It is best to fix it first with only one or two screws until it is certain that the plate is at 90° to the line AC (see Fig. 17.8). Once the plate is fixed to the distal fragment an indirect reduction can be carried out as before either with the aid of the articulated tension device or the femoral distractor. The choice of the distraction device is made on the basis of the fragmentation of the metaphyseal component and on the distance that one has to distract the fracture. Distraction can be achieved, of course, by simply pulling on the leg. The advantage of the mechanical devices, however, is that they are much less traumatic since the distraction is controlled because of the fixation of the devices to the bone and because of the mechanical leverage of the distracting devices. To put the leg under traction an assistant must be available to pull on the extremity. Manual traction cannot be as controlled, it is never as

strong, it robs one of an assistant, and it begins to fail once the assistant fatigues.

A further advantage of the total knee approach is that if the femoral condylar buttress plate is being used and if there is loss of cortical continuity medially, the inevitable varus deformity can be prevented by inserting a second plate anteromedially. This can be done without having to extend the exposure or add to the devitalization. We have found the lateral tibial condylar plate (see Fig. 17.12) to be very useful for this purpose. Its contour fits the femur well on the medial side, and the holes in the distal portion of the plate allow excellent fixation with multiple screws into the distal fragment (see also Fig. 17.27 a+b).

17.3.9 Techniques of Reduction and Internal Fixation

The techniques of reduction and subsequent stable internal fixation of supracondylar fractures of the femur pose many problems. At times, the reduction and subsequent internal fixation may be so difficult that it will tax to the limit the surgical judgment and technical expertise of the most skilled surgeon. We feel, therefore, that it is most worthwhile to discuss each fracture type in considerable detail.

17.3.9.1 Type A Fractures

Types A1, A2, and A3

A1, A2, and A3 are supracondylar fractures without an intra-articular extension. The difference between these three is the degree of metaphyseal fragmentation (see Fig. 17.1). The surgical exposure is (as already described for a supracondylar fracture) through a lateral incision

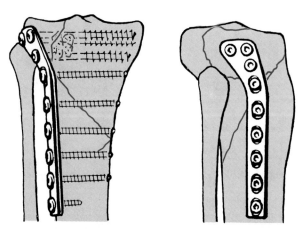

Fig. 17.12. The different buttress plates for plateau fractures. Lateral tibial head plate applied

Fig. 17.13. On **a** the lateral and **b** the antero-posterior drawing of the distal femur note the position of the three Kirschner wires *a, b,* and *c*. Guide wire *a* indicates the plane of the patellofemoral joint. Guide wire *b* indicates the plane of the knee joint axis. Guide wire *c* is the final guide wire, denoting the direction of the seating chisel and of the blade of the condylar plate or the position of the screw of the DCS. It is parallel to *a* and *b*

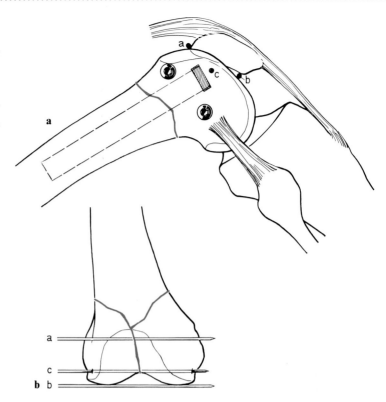

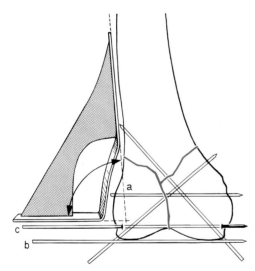

Fig. 17.14. In simple fractures such as A2 or C1 the reduction can be provisionally held with crossed Kirschner wires. The position of guide wire *c* can be checked with the condylar guide

with an opening into the joint to permit the visualization of the articular surface and the insertion of two guide wires (Fig. 17.13 a, b). The first guide wire to be inserted *(a)* guides the inclination of the anterior articular surface of the femur, that is, of the patellofemoral joint (Figs. 17.9, 17.13). The second guide wire to be inserted

(b) denotes the axis of the knee joint and is parallel to the distal articular surface of the femoral condyles (Fig. 17.13). The third guide wire *c* must be parallel to *a* in the coronal plane and to *b* in the frontal plane (Fig. 17.13). Guide wire *c* is the definitive guide wire for the insertion of the seating chisel or the DCS. The design of the 95° condylar plate or of the DCS is such that, as long as its blade or screw is inserted parallel to the knee joint axis (that is, to guide wire *c*), the normal anatomical axis of the femur will automatically be restored when the shaft is screwed to the plate.

Inexperienced surgeons and those who have some difficulty with conceptualization and visualization in three dimensions may find it hard to grasp how one wire *(c)* can be parallel to two other wires *(a* and *b)* which are not parallel to one another. They forget that guide wires *a* and *b* are in different planes, the one coronal (cross section) and the other frontal or anteroposterior.

In simple fractures, such as type A without comminution, where the main fragments can be held together provisionally with crossed Kirschner wires, the direction of guide wire *c* in the coronal or frontal plane can be further checked with the condylar guide (Fig. 17.14). Once the fracture is reduced and the guide wires inserted, all that remains is to insert the seating chisel and then the condylar plate. The condylar blade plate has to be inserted into the anterior half of the femoral condyles, which are the distal continuation of the femoral shaft (see Fig. 17.8). The same holds true for the DCS.

The simplest and most reliable way of determining the anterior half of the lateral femoral condyle is to palpate the most posterior margin of the lateral femoral condyle, then determine the direction of the longest diameter of the condyle, and divide that distance in two. The anterior half of this line denotes the anterior half of the lateral condyle. The condylar plate or the condylar screw was designed to be inserted 1.5–2 cm proximally to the distal articular surface of the femoral condyle. If we now take the midpoint of the anterior half of the lateral femoral condyle at a point 1.5–2 cm from the distal articular margin, we will have determined accurately the center of the window to be cut for the insertion of the seating chisel and subsequently of the condylar blade plate (see Fig. 17.8) or the insertion point of the compression screw of the DCS.

The insertion of the seating chisel in very young people can be difficult because their distal femoral epiphysis is filled with very dense, hard cancellous bone. The difficulty is not only the resistance the bone offers to the insertion of the seating chisel, but also the fact that dense cancellous bone does not yield as the seating chisel is hammered in and it can explode. In order to ease the insertion of the seating chisel and prevent this serious complication of splitting the supracondylar fragment, one should predrill the slot for the seating chisel with the 3.2-mm drill bit. It is enough to make three or four holes parallel to the guide wire *c* and drill the central one of these all the way through the opposite medial cortex. With a depth gauge, one can then determine the depth of this hole and in this way check exactly the width of the femur at this point against the preoperative drawing; any necessary adjustment in the selection of the implant should be made at this time.

Because of the difficulties encountered with the insertion of the condylar plate, the AO/ASIF has developed a "dynamic condylar screw" (DCS). In its design and conception it is identical to the dynamic hip screw (Synthes). The difference is that instead of "hammering in" a seating chisel, if a DCS *is being used,* all that has to be done is to insert the reaming guide wire in the center of the area where the window for the seating chisel would have been cut and make it parallel to guide wire *c* (its position can be verified radiologically at this point if desired). The seat for the DCS screw–plate combination is then precut with a special triple reamer and a tap. The insertion of the implant into bone has thus been greatly simplified. The DCS has one further advantage: the sagittal plane is not as critical as it is for the condylar plate. Any malalignment of the DCS in the sagittal plane is simply corrected by sliding off the plate and turning the screw the desired amount to achieve correction of the

malalignment. Apart from the differences mentioned, the DCS is identical to the condylar plate in indications and use. Because the DCS is so much simpler and safer to insert we have almost completely abandoned the use of the condylar blade plate. We have not encountered any problems related to the size of the hole left in the condyles by the compression screw.

One of the most common errors inexperienced surgeons make when they are using the condylar blade plate is to make the window for the insertion of the seating chisel much too small. This makes the insertion of the seating chisel difficult and can lead to the explosion of the lateral cortex of the distal fragments. The holding power of the condylar blade plate is not dependent on the tightness of its fit in the lateral cortex. Furthermore, the holding power is not interfered with by the predrilling in hard bone of the slot to be cut by the seating chisel because the plate does not rely on a tight fit for its holding power. The strength of the fixation of the plate in the distal fragment is determined first, by the pressure between the broad surface of its blade and the bone as compression is generated, and, secondly, by one or preferably two cancellous screws which must be inserted through the plate into the distal fragment. These screws are essential to give the implant rotational stability, and in those fractures where, because of comminution, no axial compression is used, they are the only fixation of the implant in the distal fragment. These two screws are also needed when the DCS is used.

Once the window is precut and the slot for the seating chisel predrilled, the seating chisel is hammered in. The flap of the seating chisel guide is used to determine the sagittal plane. As long as it is parallel to the long axis of the femur as viewed from the side, the condylar plate will fit the femur when hammered in, and its plate will not point either forward or backward.

If the slot is not cut in the anterior half, but in error is cut at the midpoint of the lateral condyle or further back, then it becomes impossible to align the shaft with the plate. A gap of 1 cm or so between the plate and the reduced shaft always arises (Fig. 17.15). One must not destroy the cortex above the blade in order to drive the blade or the screw deeper. This will gravely weaken the supracondylar fragment, decrease the holding power of the device in the distal fragment, and drive the tip of the blade or screw out through the medial cortex. Similarly, the shaft must not be lateralized to fit the plate because this destroys the stability of the reduction and functionally medializes the distal fragments, which may have subsequent adverse biomechanical consequences on the function of the knee joint. A further problem with the posterior insertion of either the condylar blade plate or the DCS is that the blade or the screw can enter the intercondylar notch and transect one or both cruciate ligaments (Fig. 17.16 a,b).

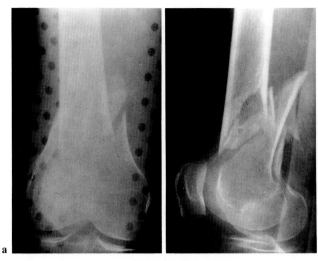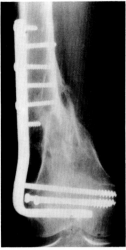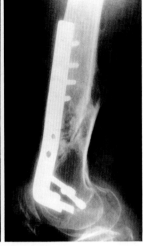

a   b

Fig. 17.15. a A3 fracture before reduction. **b** Same fracture after reduction and insertion of the condylar plate. The plate was not inserted into the anterior half of the condyles, but more posteriorly. Note the resultant malreduction and medial translocation of the distal fragmen

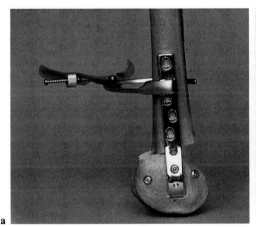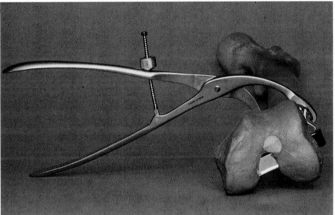

a   b

Fig. 17.16. a Posterior insertion of the angled device. **b** Note the danger to the cruciate ligaments in the intercondylar notch

Once the condylar plate is inserted and the fracture reduced, the fracture should be placed under axial compression, either with the aid of a tension device or, if the reduction is anatomical and there are no gaps in the fracture, by means of the self-compressing principle of the DC plate. This also applies for the DCS. The surgeon should strive, if at all possible, to cross the supracondylar fracture line with a lag screw which should be inserted through the plate. This greatly increases the stability of the fixation (Fig. 17.17).

If the supracondylar fracture is very low and the supracondylar fragment small, then it may be impossible to use the condylar plate or DCS because it may be impossible to fix the distal fragment to the plate with at least one cancellous screw. If that should be the case, then fixation should be carried out with the condylar buttress plate (Fig. 17.18). Once the distal portion of the plate is fixed to the supracondylar fragment with screws, the fixation proceeds in exactly the same manner as with a condylar plate or the DCS. This buttress plate can be placed under tension with the tension device, and thus axial compression can be achieved.

The reduction and fixation of an A3 or C3.3 fracture is very much more difficult because the supracondylar fragmentation. The problems which face the surgeon are: (a) correct insertion of the fixation device into the distal fragment prior to reduction of the supracondylar fracture; and (b) subsequent reduction of the femur out to length and in proper rotational alignment. The exposure of an A3 fracture is similar to an A1 or A2 fracture, although the incision may have to be extended distally and proximally.

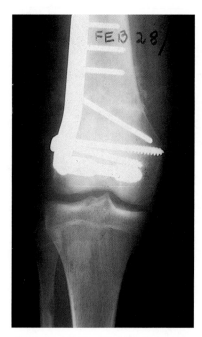

Fig. 17.17. Note the DCS fixation of this C1 fracture and the lag screw which is crossing the fracture. This greatly increases the stability of the fixation

The first difficulty which the surgeon will encounter is the proper orientation of the distal fragment. This fragment frequently rotates about its axis because of the pull of the gastrocnemius muscles so that, when exposed, the distal articular surface is actually pointing anteriorly (see Fig. 17.4).

The best guide to the orientation of this fragment is the long diameter of the lateral condyle. The outline of the lateral femoral condyle must be carefully palpated

and parts of it exposed as necessary to determine the orientation of its long diameter. Once the orientation of the long diameter is determined, one should mark its direction and its midpoint on the bone with methylene blue. Through the midpoint, one should drop a line which is at 90° to the long diameter. This blue line indicates the direction of the long axis of the femur (see Fig. 17.8). Next, with methylene blue, one should mark in the position of the window in the anterior half of the lateral condyle. The Kirschner guide wires *a*, *b*, and *c* should now be inserted. The surgeon must be extremely careful at this step because the alignment in the frontal plane of the guide wire *c* cannot be double-checked with the condylar guide. Any error will result in either a valgus or varus misalignment of the distal fragment.

The window in the lateral cortex of the condyle is then cut and the slot in the supracondylar fragment predrilled with the 3.2-mm drill bit, as already described. The next crucial step is the insertion of the seating chisel into the supracondylar fragment. It must be very carefully inserted parallel to the guide wire *c* with the flap of its guide parallel to the line drawn at 90° to the long diameter of the lateral femoral condyle. Once inserted, it is carefully withdrawn, and the condylar plate is inserted and fixed with one cancellous screw to the distal fragment.

Fig. 17.18. a The condylar buttress plate is used either when the distal fragment is too small for the insertion of the condylar plate or when the fracture lines are in the frontal plane, as in a C3 fracture, in which the blade of the condylar plate would interfere with the lag screws which must be inserted from front to back. **b** A Hoffa fracture fixed with a T plate. A condylar buttress plate could also have been used

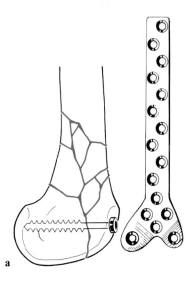

a

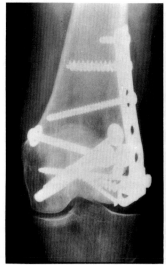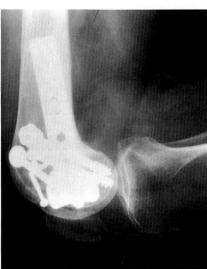

b

The length of the condylar plate will have been previously determined from the preoperative drawing and checked with the depth gauge. The length chosen should be such that, depending on the quality of the bone, there are at least four holes above the zone of comminution through which screws will be inserted to fix the plate to the proximal main fragment.

The same considerations apply for the insertion of the DCS. The exception is that it is much easier to change the direction of the reaming guide wire of the DCS or the alignment of the plate in the saggital plane which is done simply by twisting the compression screw clockwise or counterclockwise as indicated.

The plate in the distal fragment is now aligned with the shaft, the rotational alignment is checked, and the plate is fixed to the femur with a Verbrugge clamp. The supracondylar fracture with a segmental bone loss because of comminution is difficult to reduce. Length is determined from the preoperative plan by noting where the proximal fragment stops in relation to the screw holes in the plate. Simple traction on the leg is rarely sufficient to regain length. The mechanical advantage can be increased and traction applied by flexing the knee over a rest which is raised up from the table. This is more efficient than simple traction, but is awkward and also rarely adequate. The best, least traumatic, and most efficient way to restore length to the femur is to correct rotational alignment and then use the AO distractor (Fig. 17.19). One of the bolts of the distractor is inserted into the proximal shaft above the plate, and the second is inserted through the first hole or, if a screw has already been inserted, through the second hole of the plate into the distal fragment. With the distractor, one can gradually pull the femur out to length. It is often advantageous to overdistract slightly. This permits rearrangement of some of the comminuted fragments and improves the reduction which occurred spontaneously as traction was applied. The distraction is eased off until normal length is attained. Occasionally, if there is continuity of the lateral cortex between the fragments, one can compress axially with the distractor and increase stability. The plate can then be fixed to the shaft with one screw and the rotational alignment checked clinically by testing the internal and external rotation of the hip and comparing it with the normal range of the uninjured extremity, which has to be determined preoperatively. At this point, one should also obtain a radiograph to check the alignment of the extremity and assess the reduction. If all is well, the internal fixation is completed. Where possible, the comminuted fragments are then fixed to one another with lag screws as well as to the plate, and the plate is fixed to the proximal and distal fragments by inserting the remainder of the screws.

This type of reduction of the metaphyseal component of the fracture, after the insertion of the device into the

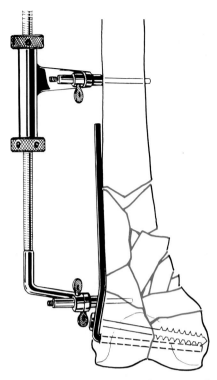

Fig. 17.19. The distractor makes the reduction of comminuted fractures relatively easy

distal fragment, is referred to as indirect reduction. We have been practicing this type of reduction for over 15 years and have become very convinced of the great advantages of indirect reduction. The main advantage is that one does not interfere with the soft tissue attachments to the comminuted fragments. This preserves their blood supply, which makes bone grafting most often unnecessary.

Once the metaphyseal and diaphyseal components of the fracture are restored to length and alignment, the internal fixation is completed by fixing the plate to the proximal fragment. In the femur seven cortices are required to secure the plate to the proximal fragment. One can increase the strength of the fixation by simply increasing the length of the plate. As the length of the plate is increased, fewer screws are required for fixation (Tornkvist 1994). The screws must be spaced apart with one as close to the fracture as possible and one through the end of the plate. This fact is of great importance when securing a plate to osteoporotic bone. In wedge fractures the wedge is either lagged to the main fragments or to the plate or it is simply left as a viable bone graft. What is done depends on the size of the wedge. In either case one can usually achieve stable fixation. If the fracture is complex, the fragments are simply bridged with the plate. If used in this way the plate functions as a splint and is referred to as a bridge plate. Such fixation is only relatively stable and union is by callus. This will occur only as long as the intermediate fragments have retained their blood supply. The reduction must therefore be atraumatic and must be carried out by indirect methods with as little manipulation of the intervening fragments as possible.

17.3.9.2 Type B Fractures

The reduction and internal fixation of partial articular fractures such as 33-B1 or 33-B2 fractures is relatively simple. The surgical approach can be through either a lateral or medial incision, depending on the side of the fracture, or through a midline approach as used for a total knee replacement. An anatomical reduction of the articular fracture is essential. The internal fixation is principally with lag screws. Buttressing is essential to prevent displacement under axial load. A buttress plate does need not to be very strong. We have used either the narrow 4.5 plates or the T plates for this purpose. It is important to remember that the buttress plate must be carefully contoured to the shape of the femur or a deformity can result. The the partial articular unicondylar posterior or Hoffa fracture (33-B3) is more difficult. In young patients with strong bone lag screw fixation with large cancellous screws from in front will suffice. These must be inserted if at all possible outside the articular surface. If a screw has to be inserted through the articular surface, its head must be well countersunk below the articular surface. In an older patient the fixation of the condyle has to be buttressed. The approach for a Hoffa fracture should be made either medially or laterally, depending on the side of the fracture. Once the sheared portion of the condyle is reduced and fixed with lag screws it must be buttressed with a plate which must be posterior to prevent displacement of the fragment under axial load.

17.3.9.3 Type C Fractures

The reduction and internal fixation of type C fractures is further complicated by one or more fractures of the epiphysis splitting the femoral condyles. The first step in the open reduction of any intra-articular fracture is the careful reconstruction of the joint. Thus, in C1 and C2 fractures, the vertical component of the supracondylar fracture must be reduced and fixed. C1 and C2 correspond in their supracondylar components to A1, A2, and A3. The steps in the open reduction and internal fixation are identical once the supracondylar fragment is reduced and stabilized.

In simple intra-articular fractures, e.g., C1 and C2, in order to visualize the articular surface, leave the supra-condylar fracture unreduced. The shortening of the leg slackens the quadriceps which usually allows all the retraction necessary to expose the articular surface and permit an accurate reconstruction.

As the first step in the reconstruction, one should assess the lateral condyle and mark in with methylene blue the position of the window for the seating chisel as well as the position of the plate. This step is important because one must know exactly where the condylar plate or DCS is going to be before any of the cancellous lag screws are inserted; otherwise, the one may be in the way of the other (see Fig. 17.13).

Once the condyles are anatomically reduced, they are fixed with two cancellous lag screws, which should be inserted over washers to prevent their heads from sinking through the cortex as the screws are tightened. One should take particular care with the insertion of the anterior lag screw and washer. Unless it is inserted as far anteriorly as possible, usually at the osteocartilagenous junction, it will interfere with the placement of the plate and displace it further posteriorly with the consequences already described. If necessary it can be left out and the fragments lagged through the plate.

The window is then prepared by first drilling three 4.5-mm holes in the lateral cortex. These are then enlarged and joined with a router. A bevel is cut with an osteotome proximally in the lateral cortex to make room for the bend in the plate. The three guide wires a, b, and c are now inserted as described on p. 399.

The condyles which have been reduced and fixed with the cancellous screws can be easily driven apart by the seating chisel, particularly if the patient is young and the cancellous bone dense, offering resistance to the advancement of the seating chisel. How to avoid this complication has been described on p. 399. An assistant should also apply counterpressure as the seating chisel is being driven in. The seating chisel must be parallel in both planes to the definitive guide wire c, and the flap of the seating chisel guide must be parallel to the line drawn at 90° to the long diameter of the femoral condyle, which represents the long axis of the femur. Once the seating chisel is introduced to the predetermined depth for the blade, it is removed, and the condylar plate is inserted. One is now ready for the reduction and fixation of the supracondylar fracture. As already stated, because of these difficulties which one can encounter with the insertion of the seating chisel we have switched over almost entirely to the DCS.

If the fracture is simple, as in C1, the reduction usually follows without difficulty. The more severe the supracondylar comminution, the more difficult is the reduction. The steps to be followed are those described in the reduction and fixation of A1, A2, and A3 fractures and use the AO distractor to regain length.

The most difficult fracture type is C3. In order to be able to reduce the joint and subsequently fix the shaft with two plates, which is often the case, one is frequently forced to free and reflect the quadriceps mechanism by detaching the patellar tendon from its insertion together with a surrounding block of bone as described in Sect. 17.3.8 (see Fig. 17.10 c) or one uses the approach as for a total knee replacement. In recent years we have used only this approach for the C3 fractures and have almost abandoned the distal detachment of the quadriceps patellar mechanism.

The joint reconstruction begins by careful reduction of all articular fragments and their provisional fixation with Kirschner wires. The definitive fixation of these articular fragments is secured with lag screws which are inserted wherever possible through nonarticular portions of the joint. Occasionally, it may be necessary to insert a screw through articular cartilage. Such a screw must be countersunk below the articular level and must not be inserted through weight-bearing surfaces. Wherever possible, one should endeavor to use a condylar plate or a DCS for the fixation of C3 fractures. Because of the fixed angle, once properly inserted the plate ensures, the normal axial alignment of the femur. At times, the fracture pattern of the condyles and the path of screws necessary for the fixation of the fracture are such that a condylar plate cannot be used. In these instances, we use the condylar buttress plate which, instead of a blade portion, relies on screws for its fixation to the distal femur (see Fig. 17.18). With this plate, it is more difficult to achieve the correct axial alignment of the femur because one lacks the constant relationship of a fixed angle device to the joint axis. Therefore, before such a plate is securely fixed to the supracondylar fragment, one should check its position radiographically. This applies to the anteroposterior or frontal plane because the axial alignment in the sagittal plane is the same as for a condylar plate, namely, at 90° to the long diameter of the lateral condyle. The buttress plate, like the condylar plate, must be fixed to the anterior half of the lateral condyle. If it is fixed more posteriorly, not only will it fail to fit the shaft, but there is also the great danger that the posterior screw will damage the lateral collateral ligament of the knee.

Whenever the condylar buttress plate is used as a bridge plate a second plate must be used on the medial side to prevent a varus deformity (Fig. 17.20). This varus deformity occurs because the screws which traverse the plate are not fixed to it and can move in the screw holes. Under load, an angular deformity results. If a second plate is used it will inevitably interfere with the blood supply of the intervening fragments. To ensure and to accelerate union the fracture should be bone grafted (see Fig. 17.21).

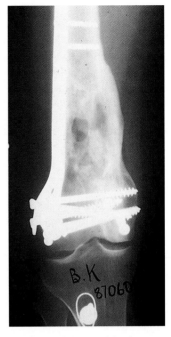

Fig. 17.20. Note the varus deformity. If the condylar buttress plate is used as a bridge plate a second plate must be used medially to prevent the angular deformity from occurring

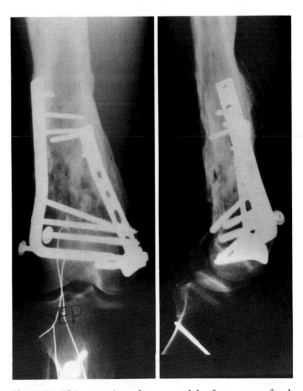

Fig. 17.21. This comminuted supracondylar fracture was fixed with a condylar plate laterally and with a T plate medially. The two plates were necessary to secure fixation of a severely comminuted segment which had resulted in loss of continuity between the shaft and the distal fragment

Similarly, if there is actual major loss of bone, as may occur in an open fracture, two plates may have to be used to achieve the desired stability. We have found the T plate or the tibial condylar buttress plate to be most useful as the medial plate, although any plate, if properly contoured, can serve this purpose (Fig. 17.21). One must take great care, of course, not to damage the femoral artery and accompanying veins as they pass through the adductor canal. The lateral plate is applied first and the medial plate second, with the comminuted fragments of bone or bone graft between them.

17.3.9.4 Supracondylar Fractures Above a Total Knee Replacement

Supracondylar fractures are an absolute indication to open reduction and internal fixation because anatomical reduction and normal axial alignment cannot be restored by closed means. They occur in elderly people whose extremity has been already compromised to some degree by the underlying disease and its treatment. The bone is almost always osteoporotic and the fragment attached to the femoral component of the knee invariably small. A revision cannot be comtemplated because an attempt to separate the femoral component from the residual bone would result in total destruction of the bone. We have found two procedures to be useful in coping with this problem.

If the fracture is either a simple or a wedge fracture, we have been successful in securing its fixation with two plates. The knee is reexplored through the original approach, which is extended more proximally. A condylar buttress plate is secured to the distal fragment on the lateral side and a T plate is fixed to the distal fragment on

the medial side. The fracture is then reduced and the plates fixed to the proximal fragment. Methyl methacrylate as described in Sect. 17.3.11 later on in this chapter is used to supplement the fixation of the screws, particularly in the distal fragment (Fig. 17.22).

If the fracture is complex and extends into the diaphysis it should be secured with a nail developed for the fixation of supracondylar fractures (Smith Nephew Richards, Memphis, TN, USA). We do not like to use this device for the treatment of fresh fractures because it must be inserted transarticularly. In a total knee replacement, as long as the femoral component has no stem, it can be inserted with relative ease through the intercondylar notch of the component. Great care must be taken to restore the normal length, rotation, and valgus alignment. We have found it helpful to insert the nail through the distal fragment into the medullary canal of the proximal fragment prior to the restoration of length or alignment. Once the nail is in place, the leg is pulled out to length over the nail until the end of the nail is flush with the intercondylar notch. At this point axial and rotational alignment must be restored and maintained while the nail is locked first distally and then proximally (Fig. 17.23). With either technique the knee is splinted for the first 2–3 days after surgery and then mobilized. Weight bearing is protected until there is evidence of union.

Fig. 17.22. a,b Note this simple supracondylar fracture above a total knee replacement. **c,d** This fracture has been fixed with two plates. The lateral plate is a condylar buttress plate and the medial a T plate

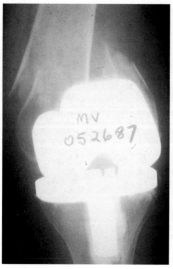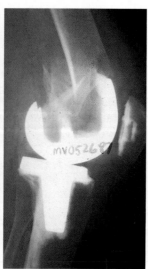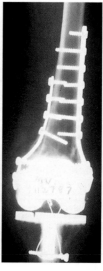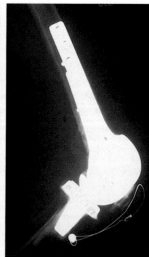

a-d

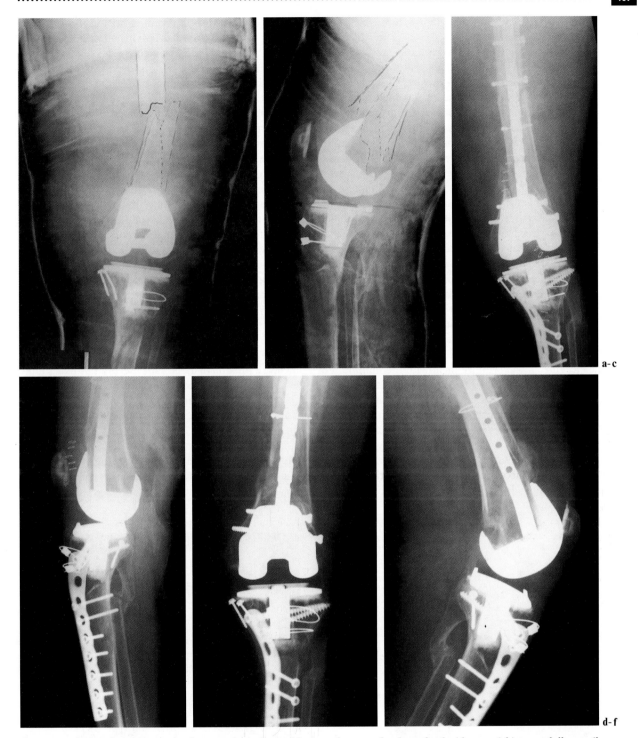

Fig. 17.23 a–f. Note that this complex fracture above the total knee replacement has been fixed with a special intramedullary nail (Sect. 17.3.9.4)

17.3.9.5 The Open Supracondylar Fracture

The principles governing the treatment of open joint fractures are very similar to those governing the treatment of open fractures of the diaphyseal segment. The emergency care, the initial assessment, and the débridement are the same. However, major avascular joint fragments, which are covered by articular cartilage and which are essential to the mechanical integrity of the joint area, should be preserved even though this courts sepsis. A diaphyseal defect can be reconstructed at a later date. A joint defect is permanent. Although this is a gamble which may result in infection and subsequent removal of the fragment, we feel it is justifiable.

Stability is important in preventing sepsis. In dealing with the articular fragments one cannot resort to temporary splinting of the joint by means of an external fixateur and delay the articular reconstruction. The articular fragments are supported by cancellous bone which unites rapidly. The longer one delays the articular reconstruction, the more difficult it becomes to achieve. It is for this reason that at the time of the initial surgery one should carry out an anatomical reduction of the articular fragments and stabilize them with the minimum of internal fixation. It is best to use lag screws as these provide the best stability and can be left as the definitive means of fixation (Fig. 17.24).

Once the epiphysis is reconstructed the surgeon must decide whether to reconstruct the metaphysis or delay its reconstruction until a stable soft tissue envelope has been achieved. The timing of the metaphyseal reconstruction depends entirely on the damage to the soft tis-

sue envelope. If there is any doubt as to the integrity of the soft tissue envelope it is best to delay the reconstruction of the metaphysis. The metaphysis is either bridged by a plate (Fig. 17.25) or is bridged with an external fixateur. This means bridging across the knee joint as already described. The choice of technique depends on the state of the soft tissue envelope. The metaphyseal reconstruction is then delayed until a stable and healed soft tissue envelope has been achieved and infection has been prevented (Fig. 26).

If there is good soft tissue cover, good tissue viability, low contamination and no segmental defect, one can carry out a primary reconstruction of the metaphysis. If the metaphyseal fracture is simple, it is reduced and fixed. If the fracture is multifragmentary, it should be reduced by indirect means to minimize on the devitalization of the fragments and then bridged by a plate. Any ensuing bone defects are bone grafted at a later date.

All open fractures are left open, but in articular fractures one should cover articular cartilage to prevent its desiccation and damage. Therefore, the synovium and capsule should be closed if possible, but the wound should be left open for subsequent closure which may involve a rotation or a free flap if necessary. Metal should not be left exposed if at all possible. Thus, if a flap is necessary to achieve coverage, fixation of the metaphysis is delayed and the fracture is kept out to length in an external fixateur.

Early motion is important but motion of the knee should not be started until one can be certain that it will not compromise wound healing and result in sepsis. The delay rarely needs to exceed a few days. Once a

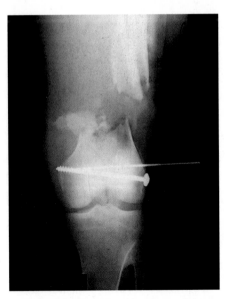

Fig. 17.24. The articular component of this open C2 fracture has been stabilized with lag screws

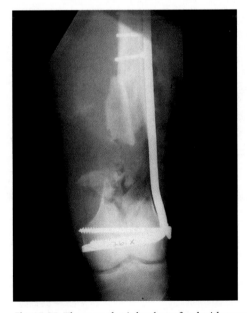

Fig. 17.25. The metaphysis has been fixed with a condylar plate

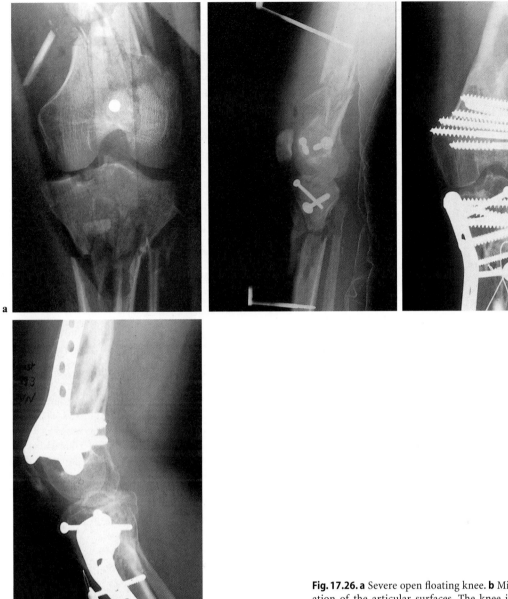

Fig. 17.26. a Severe open floating knee. **b** Minimal internal fixation of the articular surfaces. The knee is bridged with an external fixator. **c, d** The fractures definitively reconstructed and united

stable soft tissue cover has been achieved and the fracture is stabilized, vigorous mobilization of the joint can commence.

Open fractures require bone grafting. The more severe the open fracture, the less likely it is to unite. In addition, open fractures are frequently associated with bone loss. The bone grafting is usually carried out at 5–6 weeks once a stable soft tissue envelope has been achieved and infection has been prevented. If a major bone defect has been left in the metaphysis for subsequent reconstruction by delayed bone grafting, we have

found it best to fill this defect with methyl methacrylate antibiotic impregnated beads (Fig. 17.27). This not only helps in controlling sepsis but it keeps the soft tissues out of the gap. At the time of bone grafting when the beads are removed, healthy bleeding granulation tissue is left as a bed for the bone graft which facilitates its revascularization.

The outcome of treatment of an open fracture is determined by the severity of the open wound. Recent experience with the severe type C open supracondylar fractures has resulted in 80% of satisfactory results

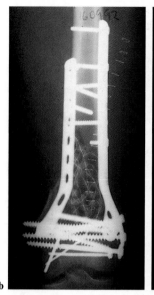
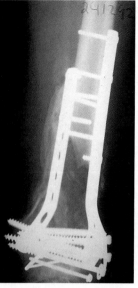

a, b

Fig. 17.27. a Note the defect in the metaphysis has been filled with methyl methacrylate antibiotic impregnated beads in the interval before bone grafting. **b** Fracture bone grafted and united. Note the use of the tibial condylar plate on the medial side

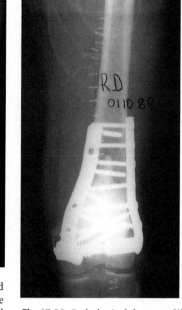

Fig. 17.28. Pathological fracture filled with methyl methacrylate

despite serious soft tissue problems and even sepsis (E. Schemitsch, personal communication; Silisky et al. 1989).

17.3.10 Bone Grafting

The intra-articular epiphyseal portion of a supracondylar fracture runs through well-vascularized cancellous bone and usually goes on the heal, even if inaccurately reduced and not well fixed. This is not true, however, of fracture lines which are subjected to a major shear stress, such as the B type fractures of the condyles.

The supracondylar extra-articular portion of the fracture involves the expanded portion of the diaphysis where, particularly in the older patient, the cancellous bone filling the medullary canal is very sparse and the cortex thin and brittle. Internal fixation in this area is difficult and if comminution exists, stability may be difficult to obtain. We feel, therefore, that any supracondylar segment with bone loss should be bone grafted with autogenous corticocancellous and cancellous bone. This will accelerate union and will protect the internal fixation from failure. Bone grafting in the presence of comminution is determined by the blood supply of the comminuted fragments. If an indirect reduction was performed and the fragments are presumed to have retained their soft tissue attachment, a bone graft is not necessary. If direct manipulation of the fragments took

place, one should consider a bone graft if there is any question about the viability of the fragments. The bone graft should be inserted opposite the plate to form a biological bridge and protect the plate from failure. In order to insert the bone graft opposite the plate one often causes further stripping and devitalization. Therefore, if one can anticipate that a bone graft will be necessary, the bone should be inserted through the fracture to the medial side prior to reduction and fixation.

17.3.11 Methyl Methacrylate

Occasionally, it may be necessary to carry out an open reduction and internal fixation in a patient whose bone is extremely osteoporotic. Such bone offers very poor holding power for the screws and, as a result, stability may be obtained despite an accurate reduction and proper position and insertion of the implant. Under these circumstances, we have made use of methyl methacrylate to increase the holding power of the screws. In order to retard the setting time of the cement, both the powder and the liquid should be cooled in the deep freeze. The internal fixation is then carried out. The crucial screws, the holding power of which has to be supplemented, are withdrawn, and the hole in the near cortex is overdrilled with a 4.5-mm drill bit. The tip of a 20-ml disposable plastic syringe is drilled out with a 3.5-mm drill bit. This enlarges the hole and eases the injection of the cement. The precooled cement is now mixed, and as soon as it reaches a uniform liquid phase, it is poured into the syringe and injected into the screw holes. This creates a cement plug which spreads out in the medulla and extends through both cortices. The screws are then inserted into their corresponding holes, and once the cement polymerizes, they are retightened. An amazing degree of purchase for the screws is usually obtained with this technique. Methyl methacrylate is also used for the fixation of pathological fractures. After evacuation of the tumor and internal fixation of the bone, the defect left is filled with methyl methacrylate. It should be inserted while still viscous to ensure full distribution around the fixation devices and throughout the bony defect (Fig. 17.28).

17.4 Postoperative Care

At the end of the surgical procedure, it is necessary to splint the joint to prevent a contracture which would result in a loss of movement and function. The knee joint has been traditionally splinted in full extension in the so-called position of function to ensure that if stiffness were to ensue, at least the extremity would be in a position in which it could function to some degree. The AO group recommended immobilization of the knee in 90° flexion for 3–4 days following surgery (Müller et al. 1979). We adopted this unorthodox position at first with some reservations, but we have since become very strong advocates of it. We have not had one instance which could be attributed to positioning where a patient failed to regain full, active extension after a period of immobilization in flexion. The decided advantage of this position is the rapid return of flexion. This is the arc of motion which has been repeatedly noted by previous authors to be the range frequently lost and the range responsible for permanent disability (Stewart et al. 1966; Neer et al. 1967). When the flexion splint is removed, patients are instructed to begin active flexion and extension exercises. Usually within the first hours, the patients regain full extension, but more important is the fact that all patients maintain the 90° flexion and most go on to increase their range of flexion from that position. In recent years, we have employed continuous passive motion machines in the immediate postoperative period and for the first 4–7 days and have found them extremely helpful in the rehabilitation of patients with intra-articular fractures.

Not all patients can begin unprotected active exercises. A ruptured lateral collateral ligament must be repaired at the time of the open reduction and internal fixation, and such repairs are never sufficiently strong to withstand unprotected active movement. After the initial period of splinting and rest or continuous passive

motion, we have transferred patients with this injury into a cast brace with polycentric hinges without blocks. This has allowed early, active mobilization of the knee with full protection from the undesirable valgus/varus forces.

Ruptured cruciate ligaments should be repaired only if they have been avulsed with a piece of bone which can be securely fixed either with a tension band wire or a lag screw. Such fixation is usually sufficiently secure to permit early motion. An in-substance tear or an avulsion without bone is best ignored and treated later if cruciate insufficiency becomes a problem. We have adopted this attitude because experience has taught us that in dealing with intra-articular fractures following an open reduction and internal fixation, the immediate goal must be motion. Early motion will not only ensure a useful range of movement, but also aids articular cartilage regeneration.

This also applies to unstable internal fixation. At the end of an open reduction and internal fixation, the surgeon must judge the stability of the internal fixation. Only the surgeon knows how many screws stripped at the time of insertion, how strong the bone really was, and how good its holding power. If, at the end of an internal fixation, the surgeon judges that the internal fixation is not stable, then once again early motion must be begun to ensure return of joint motion, but external protection must be employed to prevent overload which could result in loss of fixation and malunion or nonunion. It is very important to judge the degree of instability correctly. Very unstable fixation is best protected in skeletal traction. Other fractures which are more stable can be protected in a cast brace. Unstable and insecure fixation must be bone grafted and revised quickly if at all possible.

17.5 Complications

An analysis of the patients whose results of surgery were less than satisfactory revealed that the most common errors responsible for failure were technical, and therefore preventable (Schatzker and Lambert 1979). The most common error of all was incomplete reduction. Inaccurate reduction of joints results in incongruency of joint surfaces and rapid development of post-traumatic osteoarthritis. This is often accelerated by concomitant axial deformity with overload. Axial varus or valgus deformities are often the result of malreduction, but at times are also the result of error in insertion of the implant. The development of bridge plating has resulted in some confusion. If the plate is used as a splint to maintain the metaphyseal and diaphyseal fragments of a complex fracture out to length and in proper rotational alignment, and if these fragments have retained their

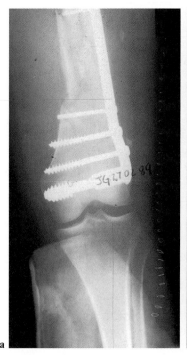
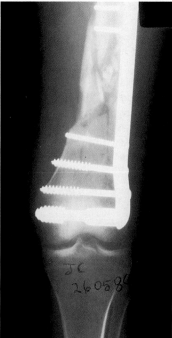
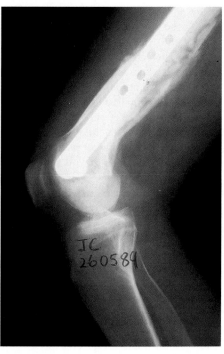

a   b, c

blood supply, then an anatomical reduction is not necessary. The fracture will heal with the formation of callus (Fig. 17.29). Simple fractures cannot be treated with a bridge plate. The resultant strain concentration in the fracture gap will be too great and union will not take place and the plate will eventually fatigue and break. Indirect reduction and bridge plating does not mean that stable fixation is no longer necessary. Each have their indications and limits which must be observed.

The second most common error found was failure to achieve interfragmental compression with lag screws or to apply axial compression where possible to increase the stability of the fixation.

The third most common error found was improper selection and insertion of the condylar plate. Blades which are too long penetrate the medial cortex, irritate the joint, cause synovitis, and come to lie deep in the medial collateral ligament where they cause pain and lead to joint stiffness. Furthermore, the blade plates were sometimes inserted without observance of the three planes of reference, which resulted in deformity with subsequent failure.

Fig. 17.29. a A C2 fracture which has been fixed with a DCS used as a bridge plate. **b,c** Note the absence of lag screws between the small fragments and the healing with callus. Bridge plating is only relatively stable

17.6 Conclusions

The supracondylar fracture is a difficult problem. The modern techniques of open reduction and stable internal fixation, however, if properly executed, can ensure the majority of patients an excellent result (Olerud 1972; Schatzker et al. 1974; Schatzker and Lambert 1979; Mize et al. 1982; Silisky et al. 1989). The only patients in whom a poor result can be accepted are those with C3 fractures in which the articular portion of the fracture is not reconstructible, or patients with severe soft tissue lesions associated with open fractures whose ultimate function is prejudiced by the soft tissue component of the injury despite excellent reconstruction of the fracture.

References

Mitchell N, Shepard N (1980) Healing of articular cartilage in intra-articular fractures in rabbits. J Bone Joint Surg 62A:628–634

Mize RD, Bucholz RW, Grogan DP (1982) Surgical treatment of displaced comminuted fractures of the distal end of the femur. J Bone Joint Surg 64A:871–879

Müller ME, Allgöwer M, Schneider R, Willenegger H (1979) Manual of internal fixation, 2nd edn. Springer, Berlin Heidelberg New York

Neer CS, Grantham S, Shelton L (1967) Supracondylar fracture of the adult femur. J Bone Joint Surg 49A:591–613

Olerud S (1972) Operative treatment of supracondylar-condylar fractures of the femur. Technique and results in fifteen cases. J Bone Joint Surg 54A:1015–1032

Rittmann WW, Perren SM (1974) Cortical bone healing after internal fixation and infection. Springer, Berlin Heidelberg New York

Salter RB, Harris DJ (1979) The healing of intra-articular fractures with continuous passive motion. Am Acad Orthop Surg Lect Ser 28:102–117

Schatzker J, Lambert DC (1979) Supracondylar fractures of the femur. Clin Orthop 138:77–83

Schatzker J, Horne G, Waddell J (1974) The Toronto experience with the supracondylar fracture of the femur 1966–1972. Injury 6:113–128

Silisky JM, Mahring H, Hofer HP (1989) Supracondylar intercondylar fractures of the femur. J Bone Joint Surg 71A:95–104

Stewart MJ, Sisk TD, Wallace SH Jr (1966) Fractures of the distal third of the femur. A comparison of methods of treatment. J Bone Joint Surg 48A:784–807

Tornkvist H, Hearn T, Schatzker J (1994) Annual OTA meeting. Los Angeles

Wenzl H, Casey PA, Hébert P, Belin J (1970) Die operative Behandlung der distalen Femurfraktur. AO Bulletin, December

18 Fractures of the Patella

J. Schatzker

18.1 Introduction

The patella is a sesamoid bone which develops within the tendon of the quadriceps muscle. Any fracture which results in displacement of the fragments in the longitudinal axis represents a disruption of the quadriceps mechanism.

18.2 Methods of Evaluation and Guides to Treatment

Just as one cannot expect a return of function in the hand without repair of a ruptured flexor tendon, one cannot expect a return of function of the quadriceps mechanism if the displaced fracture of the patella is left unreduced. Loss of quadriceps function means loss of active extension of the knee and loss of the ability to lock the knee in extension. Individuals with such lesions can neither walk on the level without the knee being unstable and buckling, nor can they walk upstairs or downstairs or on inclined planes. The disability is profound. Thus, the indication for open reduction and internal fixation of the patella is any fracture which leaves the quadriceps mechanism disrupted. The patella is intimately bound to the quadriceps tendon proximally, to the infrapatellar tendon distally, and on either side to the retinacular expansions which are adherent to the capsule. We have come to differentiate three groups of fractures of the patella, each requiring different treatment.

18.3 Classification

18.3.1 Osteochondral Fractures

Osteochondral fractures of the patella (Fig. 18.1), which usually involve varying portions of the medial facet and subjacent bone, are the result of patellar dislocation. Surgery is required to remove the intra-articular loose body and repair the quadriceps mechanism to prevent recurrences of the dislocation. In this injury, the extensor mechanism as such is not interfered with. This fracture may only be visualized in the "skyline" radiographic projection of the knee as on computed tomography

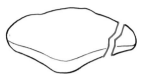

Fig. 18.1. Osteochondral fracture of the medial facet sustained in a lateral dislocation of the patella. This fracture is usually not visible on an anteroposterior or lateral radiograph of the knee and must be looked for on a "skyline" view of the patella

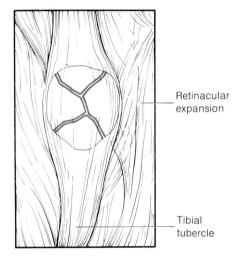

Retinacular expansion

Tibial tubercle

Fig. 18.2. In a vertical or stellate fracture of the patella, the retinacular expansions remain intact. The patient is able to execute straight leg raising against gravity

and therefore is frequently missed in routine radiographs of the knee.

18.3.2 Stellate Fractures

A stellate, undisplaced fracture of the patella (Fig. 18.2), or a vertical fracture, is usually the result of a direct blow to the patella. The continuity of the quadriceps mechanism is undisturbed and the retinacula are not torn. The fracture is stable and will not displace under the normal physiologic stresses of active motion. Surgery is unnecessary.

18.3.3 Transverse Fractures

A sudden, violent contraction of the quadriceps muscle, such as might occur when an individual stumbles and tries to stop the fall, may disrupt the quadriceps mechanism. Thus, there may be an avulsion of the quadriceps tendon, or of the infrapatellar tendon, or there may be a transverse fracture of the patella, together with a tear into the retinacular expansion (Fig. 18.3).

18.4 Surgical Treatment

We shall concern ourselves here only with disruptions of the extensor mechanism.

18.4.1 Undisplaced Fractures

A transverse, undisplaced fracture of the patella is an avulsion fracture. The function of the quadriceps mechanism is not disrupted and the patient is able to maintain the knee extended because the retinacula on either side of the patella are not torn. The fracture is, however, potentially hazardous because, with further sudden strong contractions of the quadriceps, the retinacular expansions might tear. The fracture will displace and the quadriceps function will be disrupted. The knee requires simple protection. Excellent results have been achieved either by allowing motion, but keeping the patient on crutches, or by immobilizing the knee in a cylinder cast and allowing weight bearing.

18.4.2 Displaced Fractures

A transverse fracture, either simple or comminuted, has, as an integral part, an associated disruption of the quadriceps retinacula (see Fig. 18.3). Thus, the quadriceps function is lost and surgical repair is necessary.

18.4.2.1 Surgical Approaches

We prefer to expose the patella through a transverse incision made directly over the defect. The transverse incision does not pull apart when the knee is flexed and it heals with the least noticeable scar. It can also be readily extended if greater exposure is needed to visualize the retinacular tears. These must be exposed so that the articular surface is visible as the patella is being reduced and fixed.

18.4.2.2 Biomechanical Considerations

Fractures of the patella and fractures of the olecranon are the two ideal indications for tension band fixation with wire (Müller et al. 1979). If the patella is reduced and held together with a cerclage wire passed circumferentially, reduction is maintained as long as the knee is not flexed or the quadriceps muscle is not contracted. The moment the knee is flexed, the fracture gapes anteriorly, the contour of the patella is changed, and congruency is lost (Fig. 18.4). This will also happen as the result of a strong quadriceps contraction, even if the knee is immobilized in extension in a plaster cylin-

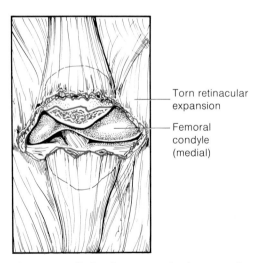

Fig. 18.3. In a displaced transverse simple or comminuted fracture of the patella, the retinacular expansions are torn and the patient loses the ability to extend the knee against gravity

Torn retinacular expansion

Femoral condyle (medial)

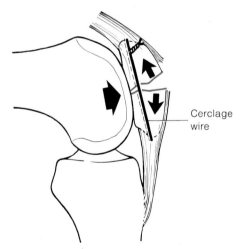

Cerclage wire

Fig. 18.4. Circumferential cerclage wiring of the patella is unable to neutralize the pull of the quadriceps and infrapatellar tendons. Under load, such as flexion of the knee, the fracture gapes anteriorly and stability of the fracture and congruity of the patella are lost

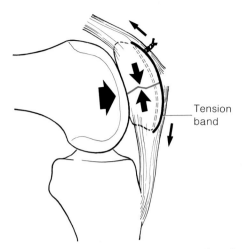

Fig. 18.5. A tension band wire applied to the anterior surface of the patella absorbs the distracting forces. In flexion, the patella is pulled against the intercondylar groove and the fracture closes with the fragments under axial compression. This is an example of dynamic compression

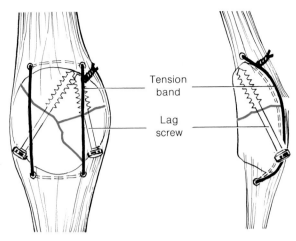

Fig. 18.7. Major comminuted fragments of the patella can be lagged together. This is best for vertical or oblique fracture lines because a tension band applied about the quadriceps and infrapatellar tendons will not compress a vertical fracture line. The remaining fracture lines are fixed with a tension band. Note the double twist

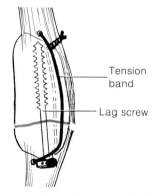

Fig. 18.6. Small fragments of the patella, such as an avulsed inferior pole or a lateral fragment, are best fixed to the remainder of the patella with a lag screw. This fixation must be further protected with a tension band wire

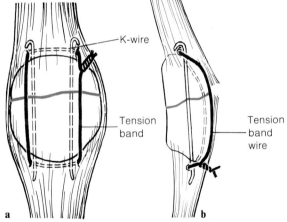

Fig. 18.8 a, b. Kirschner wires provide rotational and lateral stability. If used, they must be inserted parallel or they will block interfragmental compression of the tension band. The K-wires should be bent over on one side only to facilitate removal. Note the two twists in the tension band, which ensure uniform compression on both sides of the fracture

der. With tension band fixation, flexion of the knee results in an increase of compression across the fracture (Fig. 18.5), and contraction of the quadriceps if the knee is extended will not cause the fragments to gape.

18.4.2.3 Techniques of Internal Fixation

The tension band wire is passed through the quadriceps and patellar tendons before it is tied over the anterior surface of the patella. We do not like the figure of eight configuration for the tension band wire. Crossing the wires removes their ability to control

rotation of the fragments about the long axis of the patella. One wire is ususally enough, although in large individuals two should be used to increase the strength of the fixation. The wire should be tied on both sides to ensure uniform compression of the fracture. We like to use a large-bore needle (gauge 12–14) to guide the wire through the tendons. This ensures its accurate placement and allows its passage through the substance of the tendon. The fracture must be reduced and the knee extended before the wire is tied under tension. We like

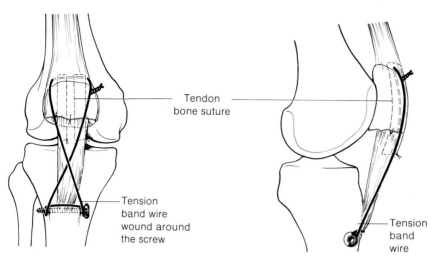

Fig. 18.9. If the inferior half of the patella is sacrificed because of severe comminution, the infrapatellar tendon is sutured to the remaining bony fragment. The suture line is protected with a tension band wire, which allows early mobilization of the knee

to observe the fracture as the wire is tightened, and we tighten the wire until a slight overcorrection occurs and the articular fissure begins to gape. The knee is then flexed to beyond 90°. This maneuver places the whole fracture surface under compression, impacts the fragments, and closes the articular fissure without an anterior gap or distortion of the patella. Compression can also be achieved with lag screws, a technique which is particularly necessary with fractures of the distal pole because if only tension band wiring is used, the small distal fragment displaces and tilts into the joint (Fig. 18.6). The tension band wire is applied once the lag screw is tightened. It serves to protect the lag screw fixation. Similarly, if there are major comminuted fragments, we like to reduce and fix them in place with lag screws (Fig. 18.7). If Kirschner wires are used to secure fixation of the fragments, they must not be crossed; otherwise impaction and compression of the fragments will not occur. If the tension band is placed around the Kirschner wires rather than through the tendon, there is great danger of pulling the Kirschner wires forward, deforming them, and having the tension band wire slip off (Fig. 18.8). We use Kirschner wires only if the patella is grossly comminuted and the wires are necessary for stability. We feel that the patella should be preserved at all cost and that a primary patellectomy should be performed only if the fracture is such that it is impossible to save even a portion of the patella. If a portion of the patella is retained, the suture of the tendon to bone is protected with a tension band wire (Fig. 18.9).

18.5 Postoperative Care

The joint is immobilized in 40°–60° flexion for 2–3 days and the extremity is kept elevated on a Böhler–Braun splint. On the second or third day, if we judge that the wound is healing satisfactorily, we instruct the patient to begin active flexion and extension exercises, but we allow only partial weight bearing for the first 6 weeks. We do not splint the knee in extension. It is wrong to immobilize the knee after open reduction and internal fixation of an articular fracture. Not only is motion required to enhance the healing of the articular cartilage, but also in a patellar fracture knee flexion is necessary to enhance the stabilizing effect of dynamic compression on the fracture interface, and this is exerted only when the knee is flexed. Thus, we do not use cylinder casts to protect the internal fixation. Usually, in 6 weeks or so the fracture will have consolidated and the patient will have regained a good range of movement. At this point, the patient can begin full weight bearing. Some protection is advisable until full quadriceps strength has been regained. We use CPM only in patients who have difficulty regaining a range of motion.

Reference

Müller ME, Allgöwer M, Schneider R, Willenegger H (1979) Manual of internal fixation, 2nd edn. Springer, Berlin Heidelberg New York, pp 42–47

19 Fractures of the Tibial Plateau

J. SCHATZKER

19.1 Introduction

A survey of the literature indicates that many authors report only slightly better than 50 % satisfactory results with either closed or operative methods of treatment of fractures of the tibial plateau. The failures of treatment are usually due to residual pain, stiffness, instability, deformity, recurrent effusions, and giving way. Our own review of over 140 of these fractures treated by both closed and operative methods has shed considerable light on the reason for the failures (Schatzker et al. 1979).

Fractures of the tibial plateau are intra-articular fractures of a major weight-bearing joint. They occur as a result of a combination of vertical thrust and bending (Kennedy and Bailey 1968). This mechanism of fracture usually leads to varying degrees of articular surface depression and axial malalignment. When part of the articular surface becomes depressed, the articular surface becomes incongruous and a smaller portion of the joint comes to bear all the weight, which increases the stress borne by the articular cartilage. If, in addition,

there is an axial malalignment, the weight-bearing axis is shifted to the side of the depression (Fig. 19.1). These two mechanisms of overload alone can give rise to post-traumatic osteoarthritis. If this destructive mechanism is combined with traumatic damage to the articular cartilage, the destruction of the joint will progress more rapidly. Occasionally, at the time of fracture, the deforming force may be such that, in addition to the fracture, the corresponding collateral ligament and even the cruciate ligament may rupture (Roberts 1968; Rasmussen 1973; Hohl and Hopp 1976; Schatzker et al. 1979; Hohl and Moore 1983). This results in joint instability. Instability may also be present as a result of joint depression and incongruity without ligamentous disruption (Hohl and Moore 1983). From whatever cause, the instability interferes with normal joint function because of insecurity and the concomitant axial malalignment and overload. Thus, joint incongruity, axial malalignment, and instability will act in concert or alone to produce post-traumatic osteoarthritis. Thus, to be successful, treatment of a tibial plateau fracture must ensure that the joint remains stable, that the articular surfaces

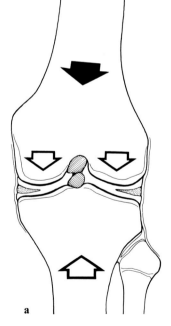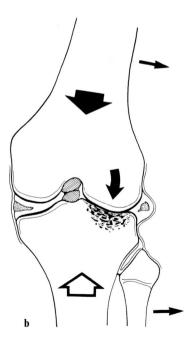

Fig. 19.1. a In a normal knee, the articular surfaces are congruous and, when weight-bearing, the medial and lateral compartments share the load almost equally, the medial taking slightly more than the lateral. **b** When fractured and partially depressed, the articular surface becomes incongruous and a smaller portion of the joint carries the full load. The load can be further increased by axial malalignment

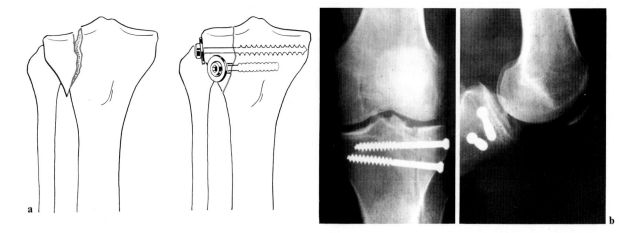

Fig. 19.2. a Wedge fracture of the tibial plateau. **b** In young people, the proximal tibia is filled with strong cancellous bone. Lag screws alone suffice for fixation

remain congruous, that the joint is painless, and that it retains a satisfactory range of motion.

Our experience with the tibial plateau fractures has led us to the conclusion that it is wrong to speak of these fractures collectively, because they differ not only in their pattern of fracture and required therapeutic approach, but also in their prognosis. Thus, we have developed a classification which groups the fractures into six types (Schatzker et al. 1979). Each type represents a group of fractures which are similar in pathogenesis and pattern, pose similar problems in their treatment, and have a similar prognosis.

··

19.2 Classification and Guides to Treatment

··

19.2.1 Type I (41-B1)

The type I fracture is a wedge fracture of the lateral tibial plateau, which occurs as a result of bending and shearing (Fig. 19.2). It occurs mostly in young people, since the dense cancellous bone of the lateral plateau resists depression. If undisplaced, these fractures require early motion and protection from weight-bearing because, under stress, displacement may occur. There are three basic patterns of displacement. The lateral wedge fragment is either spread apart from the metaphysis, which results in a broadening of the joint surface, or it is depressed, or it may be both spread and depressed. In our experience, all of these fractures, if significantly displaced, have had the lateral meniscus trapped in the fracture. Thus, we believe that, when displaced, these fractures should be operated upon, because if the lateral meniscus is trapped in the fracture line, it prevents any manipulative reduction. Furthermore, if trapped and

displaced, the meniscus will give rise to a major intra-articular derangement, which will grossly interfere with future joint function. Clearly, the effect of the widening of the lateral plateau depends on the degree to which it occurs. If minimal, the split is partially covered by the lateral meniscus and is of no consequence. If major, not only may the meniscus be trapped in the fracture line, but the spread may also result in joint incongruity and in varying degrees of instability. Both the incongruity and instability are incompatible with normal function. As this fracture type occurs most commonly in young people under 30 years, we must strive for the best possible result of treatment. Thus, for displaced fractures, we feel that open reduction and internal fixation are justified because of the potential internal derangement, joint incongruity, instability, and axial overload. If the displacement is minor and the indications for surgery not clear-cut, then the surgeon should at least examine the joint with an arthroscope to make certain that the meniscus is not trapped in the fracture. Excellent function was obtained in all patients who had this joint carefully reconstructed.

··

19.2.2 Type II (41-B3.1)

The mechanism of injury for type II fractures is the same as for type I, but the patients are older (average age is over 50 years) and frequently have some osteoporosis.

In this type, the lateral wedge is combined with varying degrees of depression of the adjacent remaining weight-bearing portion of the lateral tibial plateau (Fig. 19.3). The depressed segment may be anterior, central, posterior, or a combination of all three. Similarly, the wedge may vary from being simply a rim fracture to one involving almost one third of the articular surface. The displacement of this fracture consists of a widening of the joint with spreading apart of the wedge, in combination with a depression of the lateral plateau. We have

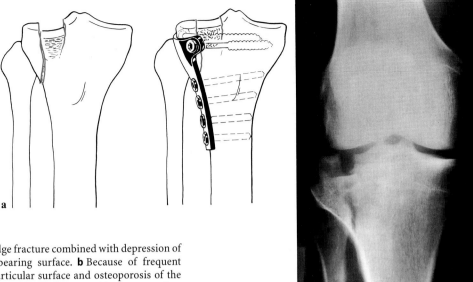

Fig. 19.3. a Type II wedge fracture combined with depression of the adjacent weight-bearing surface. **b** Because of frequent comminution of the articular surface and osteoporosis of the condyles, it is best to combine the fixation with a buttress plate

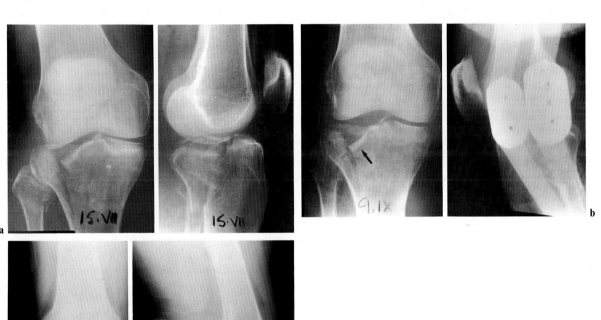

Fig. 19.4. a Type II fracture in a 56-year-old woman prior to reduction. **b** After an initial period of traction, the patient was transferred to a cast brace. Note the failure of reduction of the depressed portion of the articular surface. **c** Some 2 years after fracture, the patient shows signs of post-traumatic osteoarthritis. Note, in flexion, the subluxation of the femoral condyle into the depressed posterior portion of the articular surface, which was left unreduced

graded the depression by measuring the vertical distance between the lowest recognizable point on the medial plateau and the lowest depressed fragment of the lateral plateau. We have found that a depression greater than 4 mm was significant and, if left unreduced, it resulted in joint incongruity, valgus deformity, and a sense of instability. The degree of these defects was proportional to the degree of joint widening and the central depression.

All poor results of open or closed treatment could be related to residual joint depression, incongruity, and joint instability, either because it was accepted in the first place, or because the reduction was not perfect, or because redisplacement occurred in the postoperative period.

Closed manipulative reduction combined with traction, or traction alone, was associated with varying degrees of success. The displaced lateral wedge sometimes reduced surprisingly well; however, the anterior or posterior wedge fragments remained relatively unaffected. Furthermore, depressed articular fragments which were impacted into the metaphysis could never be dislodged by closed means (Fig. 19.4). If the depression of the fragments was significant and was responsible for joint instability, this instability remained and was present at the end of conservative treatment. The joint depression did not fill in with fibrocartilage, but remained as a permanent negative articular defect. Plaster immobilization of these intra-articular fractures, even of short duration such as 3–4 weeks, resulted in marked irreversible stiffness. The advantage of traction, even if it failed to yield an acceptable reduction, consisted in the relief of pain and in the ability of the patient to start early motion while in traction. If a disruption of a collateral ligament was coexistent with a fracture, it was repaired. After surgery, immobilization of the joint in plaster even for a few days frequently resulted in a serious permanent loss of motion. Therefore, we have made immediate use of the cast brace to protect the ligamentous repair. We have also found the cast brace to be an ideal method of external splintage of unstable internal fixation and a very satisfactory method of protection of undisplaced fractures in unreliable and noncompliant patients. Certain displaced fractures which were not operated upon but which were treated in traction were transferred into the cast brace once they became "sticky." The cast brace maintained axial alignment of these unstable fractures

with joint depression, but the malalignment frequently recurred once the brace was removed because the joint depression responsible for the instability did not fill in with fibrocartilage. The cast brace could not be used as a method of reduction, but it served as an excellent method of functional treatment once reduction was obtained, allowing motion while unloading the damaged portion of the articulation.

We feel, therefore, that displaced lateral wedge fragments associated with significant depression greater than 4 mm should be treated by open reduction, elevation of the depressed fragments, bone grafting, stable fixation, and early motion. If the patient is elderly or if there are contraindications to surgery, then the patient should be treated by closed manipulative reduction, skeletal traction, and early motion and should be transferred into a cast brace as soon as the fracture is no longer displaceable, even though it may be still deformable. At no time should the fracture be immobilized in plaster, as such treatment frequently results in significant degrees of joint stiffness. If at the end of closed treatment joint instability and/or deformity persist, secondary reconstructive procedures become necessary.

19.2.3 Type III (41-B.2)

Type III represents a depression of the articular surface of the lateral plateau without an associated lateral wedge fracture (Fig. 19.5). It is usually the result of a smaller force exerting its effect on weaker bone. Indeed, it commonly affects a somewhat older age-group (55–60 years)

Fig. 19.5. a Type III fracture. There is depression of the articular surface, but no associated wedge fracture. **b** In this patient, the whole plateau was depressed, the joint was unstable, and an open reduction was necessary

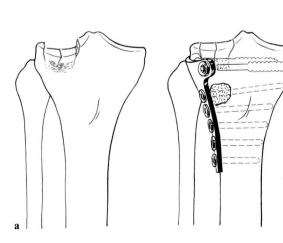

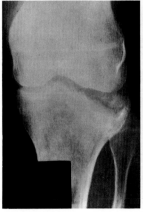

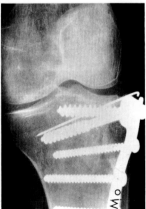

a

b

than type II fractures and one in which osteoporosis is more marked. This fracture pattern is the least serious of all the tibial plateau fractures. The stability of the joint is rarely affected and excellent function without joint incongruity is the usual outcome. The degree of joint involvement may vary, however, from a small central plateau depression to one involving the whole plateau (Fig. 19.5 b). The depression is usually lateral and central, but it may involve any part of the articular surface. Lateral and posterior depressions are usually associated with a greater degree of instability. Thus, it is important when evaluating this fracture to examine the knee under anesthesia in full extension and in different degrees of flexion. If no instability is found, it is safe to treat such a fracture with early motion without weight-bearing. If instability is demonstrated, then, depending on the degree of instability and other factors (patient's age, expectations, etc.), open reduction and internal fixation should be performed.

In our experience, this fracture pattern was the most common. The few patients who required an open reduction and internal fixation did well as long as their reduction and joint congruity was maintained. Patients whose joints were stable when examined under anesthesia and who were treated by early motion did well.

19.2.4 Type IV (41-B1, 41-B2, and 41-B3)

This is a fracture of the medial tibial plateau (Fig. 19.6). It occurs either as a result of a high-velocity injury or as a result of a rather trivial varus force in the elderly and carries the worst prognosis of all the tibial plateau fractures, for the following reasons. If the fracture occurs as a result of a rather trivial low-velocity injury, it usually occurs in an elderly person with grossly osteoporotic bone in whom the medial tibial plateau simply crumbles into an irreconstructible mass of fragments. The poor prognosis is that of a fracture which is technically

beyond reconstruction. Traction rarely results in a reasonable alignment of the medial condyle and of the articular surface, and the poor result is due to joint incongruity and instability. The medial plateau is more difficult to overload and fracture than the lateral; therefore, the force which gives rise to a fracture of the medial plateau is of higher magnitude. If this fracture is the result of a high-velocity injury, it usually involves a younger individual. The medial plateau splits as a relatively simple wedge, similar to the wedge fracture of the lateral plateau, but there is often an associated fracture of the intercondylar eminence and adjacent bone with the attached cruciate ligaments. Furthermore, there is frequently a concomitant disruption of the lateral collateral ligamentous complex (which may be through the substance of the ligament or be an avulsion of bone, such as the proximal fibula) and a stretching or rupture of the peroneal nerve as a result of traction. In some cases there may also be damage to the popliteal vessels. A disruption of this magnitude represents a subluxation or a dislocation of the knee which has been realigned. Thus, in younger patients the poor prognosis of this injury is not the result of the fracture, but the result of the associated injuries and other complications such as compartment syndrome, Volkmann's ischemia necrosis, or foot drop.

If undisplaced and not associated with significant soft tissue lesions, type IV fractures can be treated successfully by closed means as long as motion is begun early and axial malalignment is prevented. If displaced and/or associated with ligamentous or neurovascular lesions, these fractures must be treated open with repair of the ligamentous components of the injury and stable internal fixation of the fracture. Some of the fractures are also associated with a posterior split wedge of the medial pla-

Fig. 19.6 a, b. Type IV fracture of the medial tibial plateau. Note the associated fracture of the intercondylar eminence

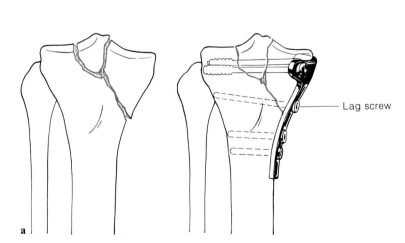

Lag screw

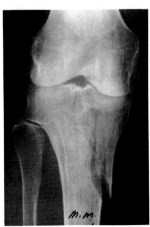

a

b

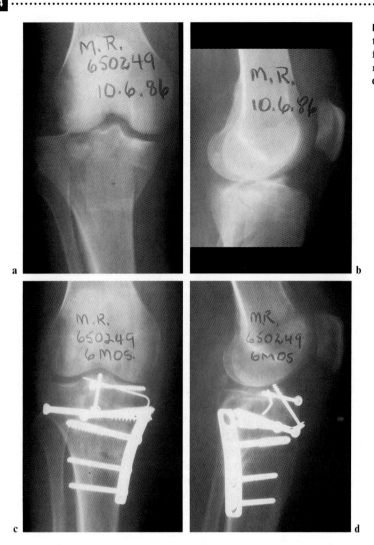

a   b

c   d

Fig. 19.7 a–d. Posterior split in addition to the fracture of the medial tibial plateau. Note that in **b** the femoral condyles follow the posterior split, which results in a subluxation of the joint. Note also in **d** the posteriomedial buttress plate

teau (see Fig. 19.7). This fracture causes the femoral condyle to subluxate posteriorly on flexion and greatly increases the instability of the joint. This fragment must be reduced and securely fixed to stabilize the joint.

19.2.5 Type V (41-C1)

Type V is a bicondylar fracture which consists of a wedge fracture of the medial and lateral plateaux (Fig. 19.8). It results from an equal axial thrust on both plateaux. There is usually no associated depression of the articular surface, although this may occur. The prognosis depends whether the fracture involves the articular surfaces or whether it begins extraarticularly in the intercondylar eminence. Because of the soft tissue attachment to the split wedge fragments, traction frequently results in an acceptable reduction and, once the fracture

has become "sticky," it is easily managed in a cast brace. Although the cast brace can maintain alignment, it cannot prevent minor degrees of shortening. As a result, once transferred to a cast brace, many of these fractures tend to telescope, with some spreading of the tibial condyles (Fig. 19.8 b, c). This leads to a relative lengthening of the collateral soft tissue hinges, which results in minor varus/valgus instability. In an individual without athletic aspirations, this minor varus/valgus instability is of no consequence. In younger, athletically inclined individuals, however, the varus/valgus rocking can constitute a significant disability. Thus, in younger individuals, if the fracture is displaced, we prefer to carry out open reduction and internal fixation. The same would apply, of course, to older individuals in whom traction had failed to yield an acceptable reduction (Fig. 19.8 d). If the articular surfaces are involved, the fracture requires an open reduction and stable fixation.

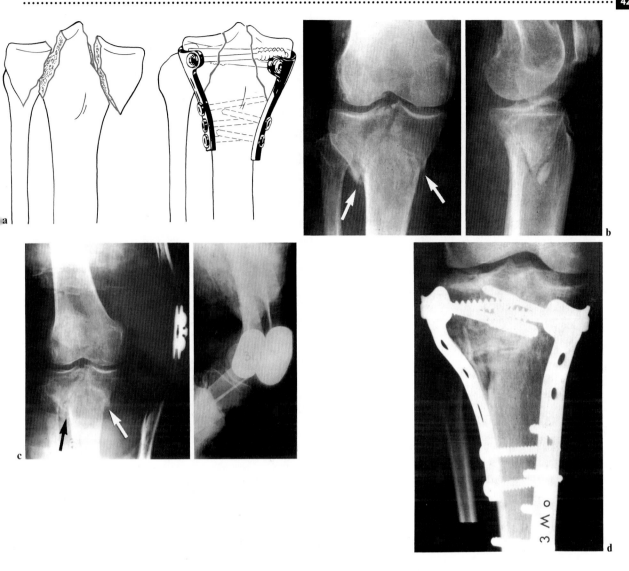

Fig. 19.8. a Type V fracture. Note that the fracture lines begin close to the intercondylar eminence. There is frequently no depression of the articular cartilage. **b** A bicondylar fracture in traction. Note the slight overriding of the cortices, indicating shortening. **c** The position of the fragments and alignment is maintained in a cast brace. **d** Two buttress plates are necessary in addition to lag screws to maintain a stable fixation

19.2.6 Type VI

Type VI fractures are the most complex tibial plateau fractures. Their hallmark is a fracture which separates the metaphysis from the diaphysis (Fig. 19.9). The significance of this is that traction tends to separate the diaphysis from the metaphysis without any reduction of the metaphysis or of the impacted articular components (see Fig. 19.9 c). This makes this fracture less amenable to nonoperative treatment. The fracture pattern of the articular component is variable and can involve one or both tibial condyles and articular surfaces. Because the medial condyle is stronger it usually survives as a large single split fragment. The fracture is almost always the result of a high-velocity injury and therefore is often associated with marked displacement and depression of the articular fragments. Such articular disorganization can be corrected only through direct surgical intervention.

A word of caution is in order. These fractures may be so comminuted as to defy even the most skilled surgeon and must therefore be very carefully evaluated. If there is doubt about whether an open reduction can be successfully performed, it is best to treat such a fracture by nonoperative means, despite its limitations. *The result of a failed open reduction and internal fixation is always*

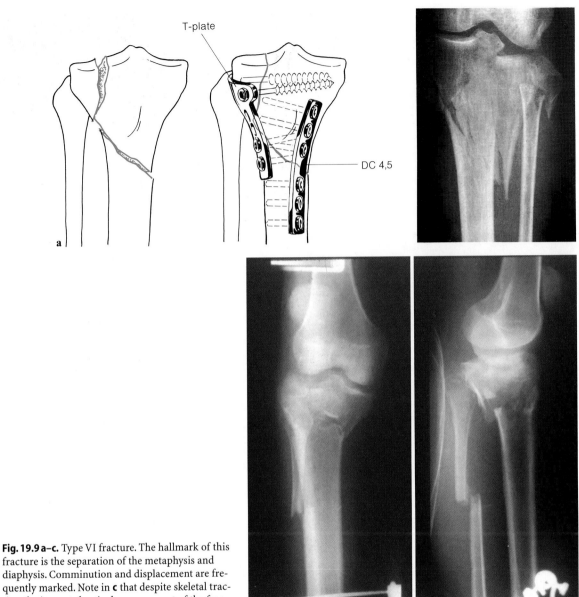

Fig. 19.9 a–c. Type VI fracture. The hallmark of this fracture is the separation of the metaphysis and diaphysis. Comminution and displacement are frequently marked. Note in **c** that despite skeletal traction the impacted articular component of the fracture remains unreduced

worse than the result of a failed closed treatment. Despite the severity of this injury, 80 % of the patients who came to surgery ended up with a most satisfactory result (Schatzker et al. 1979).

··········

19.2.7 Relationship of the Comprehensive Classification to the Six Fracture Types

If we consider only the partial and complete articular fractures and exclude type A, the metaphyseal fractures, then there are only six groups in the Comprehensive Classification, just as there are six types in Schatzker's classification. Unfortunately, there is no one-to-one relationship. The B group, the partial articular fractures, correspond to the Schatzker types I, II, III, and IV. The C group, the complete articular fractures, corresponds to the Schatzker types V and VI. The C1 group corresponds to the Schatzker type V. The C1 fractures, including the subgroups C1.1, C1.2, and C1.3, are all extraarticular and therefore have a better prognosis then some of the type B partial articular fractures involving the medial side of the plateau. Note also that the medial plateau fracture – the type IV of the Schatzker classification– is found in the Comprehensive Classification (Müller et al. 1990) as subgroups B1.2, B1.3, B2.3, B3.2, and B3.3 (see Fig. 19.10).

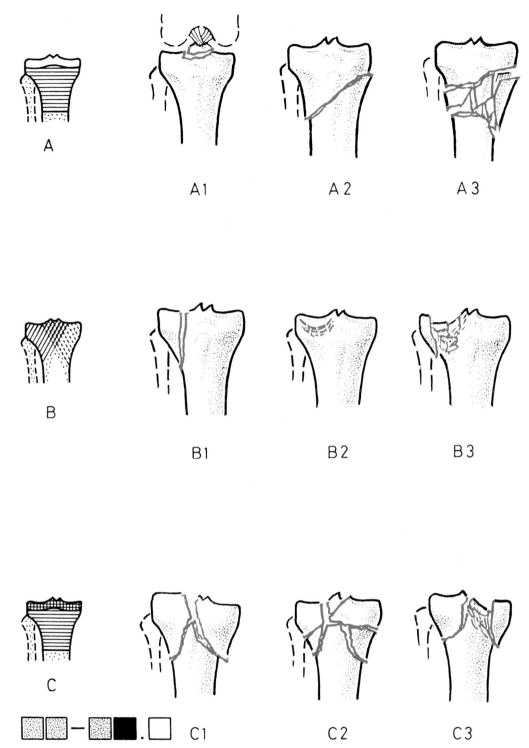

Fig. 19.10. Tibia/fibula proximal. *A*, extra-articular fracture (*A1*, avulsion; *A2*, metaphyseal simple; *A3*, metaphyseal multiframentary); *B*, partial articular fracture (*B1*, pure split; *B2*, pure depression; *B3*, split–depression); *C*, complete articular fracture (*C1*, articular simple, metaphyseal simple; *C2*, articular simple, metaphyseal multifragmentary; *C3*, multifragmentary). Note the grouping of all partial articular fractures together as type B regardless of the severity, in contrast to the Schatzker type IV

As already mentioned the fracture of the medial plateau is a very serious lesion which deserves more recognition than simply as a subgroup member. These are the shortcomings of the Comprehensive Classification, which attempts to order all fractures in accordance with a unified approach to all segments. A regionally based classification, such as Schatzker's classification, is able to address more accurately the regional idiosyncrasies, although the Comprehensive Classification allows for a more detailed description of the fracture morphology.

19.2.8 Absolute Indications for Surgery

In considering the therapeutic approach required to ensure the best possible result, certain situations must be isolated and added to what has just been said above. Because of their nature or potential effects, these injuries demand operative rather than closed treatment and can be considered to comprise absolute indications for operative intervention.

19.2.8.1 Open Fractures

As stability is the mainstay of prophylaxis against sepsis, in addition to débridement, stable internal fixation of an open intra-articular fracture is a necessity.

19.2.8.2 Acute Compartment Syndrome

Occasionally, while contemplating whether a fracture should be treated open or closed, the surgeon's hand is forced by the development of an acute compartment syndrome. Once a compartment is decompressed and a previously closed fracture converted to an open one, we feel that stable internal fixation of the fracture is the most advisable course, because the same considerations then apply as in an open fracture.

19.2.8.3 Associated Vascular or Neurological Injury

Vascular injury is most often associated with type IV tibial plateau fractures. They usually represent fracture dislocations (Hohl and Moore 1983). The popliteal vessels must be repaired. The fracture should then be stabilized and the associated ligamentous tears repaired.

19.3 Methods of Assessment

Before we are able to classify a tibial plateau fracture and thus arrive at a plan of treatment, the patient and the fracture must be carefully assessed. We cannot overemphasize the importance of an accurate diagnosis: it identifies all the components of the injury, facilitates the therapeutic approach, and effects a better recovery from the injuries in the patient.

19.3.1 History

A case history is important because it allows us to determine whether the injury was caused by low- or high-velocity force. Although the patient is rarely able to relate the exact mechanism of the injury, it is usually possible to determine the direction of the force as well as the deformity produced. These are important clues. A history also allows us to evaluate the patient's expectations and level of function.

19.3.2 Physical Examination

Physical examination is the only accurate method of evaluating the state of the soft tissue cover. Tenderness elicited on physical examination is often the only clue available to indicate a concomitant disruption of a collateral ligament. Examination for any neurological or vascular deficits as well as for the presence of a compartment syndrome is also very important.

19.3.3 Radiological Examination

A radiological assessment of the injury is indispensable, because this is the only means available which leads to an accurate evaluation of the fracture pattern and its severity. Anteroposterior and lateral radiographs alone are inadequate: they must be supplemented with at least an internal and an external oblique view. The degree and location of the articular surface depression are best seen on the oblique projection (Fig. 19.11). Frequently, the four standard exposures are inadequate and it is necessary to resort to tomography in order to be able to evaluate accurately all fracture lines in their extent and position, determine the degree of comminution of the fracture and thus judge its operability, and determine the presence and extent of articular depression. It is important to ensure that both anteroposterior and lateral tomographic cuts are obtained. These complement one another and permit the surgeon to get a much more accurate three-dimensional concept of the fracture (Fig. 19.12).

Computed tomography is much more useful than tomography, and we use it routinely in the evaluation of all complex fractures of the proximal tibia. Its frontal and sagittal reconstructions give all the information that can be gleaned from tomography. In addition, it shows

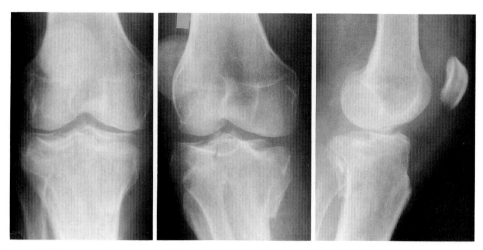

Fig. 19.11. Internal and external oblique X-rays are necessary for a complete visualization of the tibial plateau

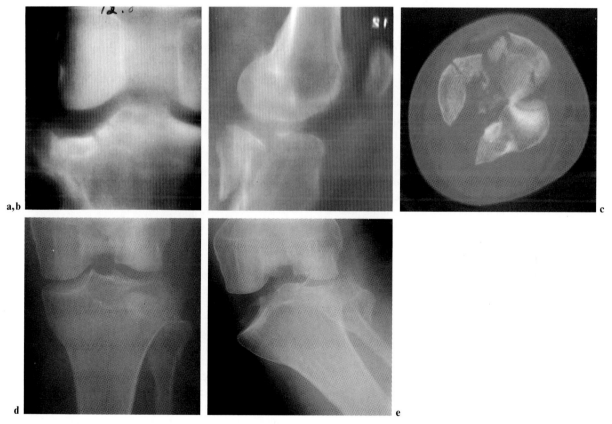

Fig. 19.12. Note the information obtained from the anteroposterior (**a**) and lateral (**b**) tomogram of a knee injury. Frequently, plain radiographs fail to reveal important fracture lines, the number of fragments, and their depression. Note the posterior subluxation of the femoral condyles. **c** Note the advantage of computed tomography (CT) in providing the cross-sectional anatomy of the fracture. **d, e** Note the information one can obtain from a gentle-stress X-ray. The medial collateral ligament is completely torn

the surgeon the cross-sectional anatomy of the fracture, indicates clearly the planes of the fracture lines, and often discloses unsuspected fracture lines. Thus it is an indispensable tool in preoperative planning and in classification of the fracture. It is also very useful if the surgeon is planning to insert some of the fixation screws percutaneously.

An arteriogram should be considered whenever there is concern about the possibility of an arterial lesion. An intimal tear may be present without a clinically detectable deficit. At surgery an intimal tear can lead to occlusive thrombosis and endanger the survival of the extremity. The fracture pattern most commonly associated with an arterial injury is the Schatzker type IV, the fracture of the medial tibial plateau, but the surgeon must remember that any fracture dislocation of the knee may have an associated arterial injury.

A gentle-stress X-ray can be very useful in patients in whom a tear of a collateral ligament is suspected (see Fig. 19.12 d, e).

19.4 Surgical Treatment

19.4.1 Planning the Surgical Procedure

Having carefully evaluated the patient and the radiographs, the surgeon is now able to decide on the best plan for treatment. If an open surgical approach is chosen, the surgical procedure must be carefully planned. This involves a reasoned choice of the approach, a detailed drawing of the fracture pattern, a careful plan of all the steps necessary in the open reduction, and a plan of the internal fixation. The latter must include a detailed position of all the screws and their function, together with the appropriate implant and its position.

19.4.2 Approaches

The essence of a good surgical approach is maximum visualization combined with minimum devitalization and the preservation of all vital structures. Initially, we employed the exposures as recommended in the second edition of the *AO Manual* (Müller et al. 1979). We changed the shape of the skin incisions, and their placement, as we became aware of certain difficulties which an improper skin incision may pose if the surgical procedure fails and some years later a total joint arthroplasty becomes necessary. Thus, we have abandoned the triradiate "Mercedes" incision recommended by the AO group for complex tibial plateau fractures (Müller et al. 1979) and prefer all approaches to be as straight and as close to the midline as possible (Fig. 19.13). It should also be remembered that the skin incisions must be

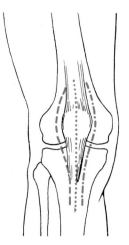

Fig. 19.13. The incisions should be straight. Increase in exposure is gained by extension of the incision proximally and distally

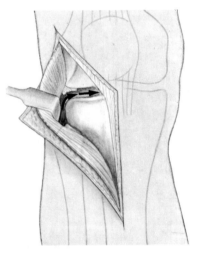

Fig. 19.14. The arthrotomy should be made by incising the capsule transversely below the meniscus. (From Müller et al. 1979)

planned in such a way that they do not come directly over an implant. The flaps which are raised must be of full thickness, consisting of the subcutaneous fat down to the fascia lata and the quadriceps retinacular expansions. This will ensure the survival of the flaps and prevent wound edge necrosis or partial loss of the flap due to ischemia.

We have also come to appreciate the importance of the meniscus in safeguarding subsequent joint function. The meniscus appears to share in weight transmission and distributes the weight over a broader surface area (Schrive 1974; Walker and Erkman 1975). This cushioning effect protects the elevated articular cartilage fragments and enhances cartilage healing. We therefore feel that the meniscus must be preserved in the execution of a surgical exposure; it should *never* be excised to facilitate exposure. We believe that the capsule should be incised horizontally below the meniscus. This allows the surgeon to pull up on the meniscus together with the capsule to which it remains peripherally attached, thus achieving an unobstructed view of the articular surface (Fig. 19.14). (If the arthrotomy is made above the meniscus, the meniscus will keep most of the articular surface hidden from view and will interfere with the attempts to execute an accurate open reduction.) If a peripheral detachment of the meniscus is encountered, or even a tear in the meniscal body, this should be meticulously repaired at the end of the procedure. Every effort should be made to preserve the meniscus (Wirth 1981; Hohl and Moore 1983).

Fig. 19.15. The best exposure of the depressed fragments is gained by opening the fracture. The lateral wedge is pulled to the side like the cover of a book. In order to achieve exposure of bilateral tibial plateau fracture lines, it is best to divide the infrapatellar tendon in a Z fashion and divide the medial and lateral capsule across below the menisci. The capsule, the attached menisci, and patella are then lifted up to give unlimited exposure of the whole proximal tibia. If osteotomy of the tibial tubercle reaches the main fracture lines, subsequent fixation becomes very difficult

In order to gain exposure of the depressed articular fragments, the surgeon should make use of the fracture. Thus, if there is a peripheral wedge fragment, regardless of its size, it should be hinged back on its soft tissue attachment, like the cover of a book. This allows perfect visualization of the joint depression (Fig. 19.15). The soft tissue attachment preserves the blood supply to the wedge fragment.

In carrying out the exposure, we have found it helpful to incise to the deep investing fascia and to develop full-thickness flaps. At this point the knee is flexed to 90°, which causes the iliotibial band to course more posteriorly. Thus as the capsule is cut horizontally, the iliotibial band escapes. If necessary, the surgeon can cut horizontally across the iliotibial band at the level of the joint to facilitate exposure. The lateral collateral ligament must be preserved. At the end of the procedure, the iliotibial band should be resutured with a nonabsorbable suture. We have done this many times with complete impunity and have not encountered a single instance of varus instability as a result.

We prefer to incise the coronary ligament of the meniscus together with the capsule. Then, with upward retraction, we gain exposure of the underlying cartilage. Some surgeons have recommended the detachment of the anterior horn of the meniscus to gain similar expo-

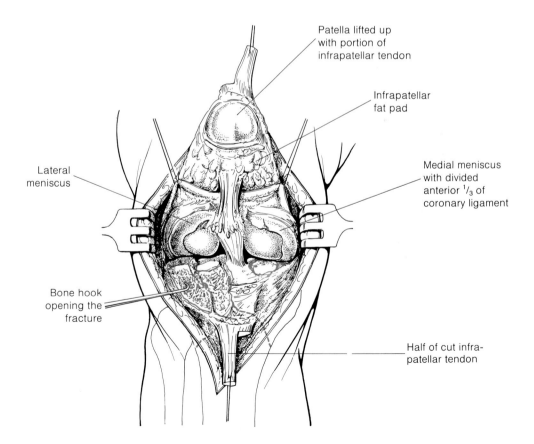

Patella lifted up with portion of infrapatellar tendon

Infrapatellar fat pad

Lateral meniscus

Medial meniscus with divided anterior 1/3 of coronary ligament

Bone hook opening the fracture

Half of cut infra-patellar tendon

sure. We have found this to be more limiting, and we have also had greater difficulty reattaching the anterior horn than simply resuturing the capsule. Thus we continue to recommend the exposure below the meniscus as described.

Occasionally, in the very severe fractures which involve both tibial plateaux, it may become necessary to reflect the quadriceps mechanism upward so that, as the knee is flexed, both sides of the joint are simultaneously exposed. The infrapatellar tendon should not be detached from the tibia together with its surrounding bone. In the severe fractures, the tibial tubercle and adjacent cortex may be the only intact anterior cortex. If destroyed, the reduction is made considerably more difficult and it may prove impossible to reattach the tubercle, particularly if the posterior cortex is also comminuted. If necessary for exposure, we have found it best to cut the infrapatellar tendon in a Z fashion (Fig. 19.14). At the end of the procedure, we have resutured the tendon together with the horizontally incised quadriceps retinacula and capsule. In order to secure the resuture, the repair can be protected with a tension band wire which is passed through the quadriceps tendon just above the patella, crossed over the front to form a figure-of-eight, and then passed either through bone or through a transverse cannulated screw inserted through the anterior cortex, just below the tibial tubercle. We have had no complications with this approach and have had no secondary ruptures of the tendon or any extensor lags (Fig. 19.15). A posterior split wedge fracture requires a posteriomedial counterincision to facilitate the reduction and fixation of the fracture (Hohl and Moore 1983).

The posterior wedge fracture can be reduced and secured with lag screws through an anterior approach. If the fragment is large, however, a posterior buttress plate must be inserted to prevent redisplacement of the wedge due to axial forces. This can be done through the anterior incision, but it requires the raising of a large flap in order to gain the posterior surface of the tibial. In order not to undermine such a large flap, we prefer to insert the buttress plate through a second posteromedial incision.

19.4.3 Positioning the Patient

The patient should be positioned supine on the operating table in such a way that the table can be flexed during the procedure and the knee flexed. Flexion of the knee improves visualization of the joint. If the table is tilted to induce a slightly inclined Trendelenburg position, the patient will not slide forward. The dependent position of the leg applies traction, obviates the need for an assistant to hold the leg, and allows the surgeon to apply a varus or valgus force by simply pushing on the foot in the desired direction.

19.4.4 Timing the Surgical Procedure

There are only three situations in which a tibial plateau fracture has to be treated as an emergency. These are an open fracture, an acute compartment syndrome, and a fracture associated with a vascular injury. The guide to the timing of the surgical procedure in all other cases is provided by the state of the patient, the state of any associated injuries, the state of the limb, and, finally, the state of the soft tissue envelope. In some cases, the initial swelling or contusion of the soft tissue envelope may be so severe as to preclude an early surgical repair. If there are no contraindications, the simple plateau fracture may be dealt with immediately. In the more complex fracture patterns, particularly if the comminution is severe, we prefer to perform the repair on an elective basis after a careful evaluation of the fracture with all the necessary ancillary studies completed. If a delay of more than 1–2 days is necessary, then the leg should not be immobilized in a long-leg plaster or other type of splint because this does not prevent shortening, which will result in further displacement and telescoping of fragments. It is best to place the leg in skeletal traction until such time as the surgical procedure can be executed (Apley 1979). The positioning of the Steinmann pin for traction is very important. If placed too high, it will either be in the fracture or will interfere with the safety of subsequent surgical repair. It should be inserted a hand-breadth below the most distal discernible fracture line.

Another way to maintain the leg reduced to length and the fracture partially reduced is to bridge the knee with an external fixator.

19.4.5 Methods of Open Reduction and Internal Fixation

Before discussing the open reduction and internal fixation of each type in detail, we would like to point out certain generalities which are important. The lateral plateau is convex from front to back and side to side, whereas the medial one is concave. The lateral plateau is higher than the medial one. Both the medial and lateral plateaux slope approximately 10° from front to back. Therefore, in a standard anteroposterior radiograph of the knee, the plateaux appear elliptical in shape, and the posterior joint edge is represented by the lower of the two lines (Moore and Harvey 1974).

The medial plateau is usually much less comminuted than the lateral; hence, if both plateaux are fractured, better purchase can usually be obtained with screws in the medial one. Because the lateral plateau is higher, care has to be taken when inserting the proximal screws medially from the lateral side so as not to enter the medi-

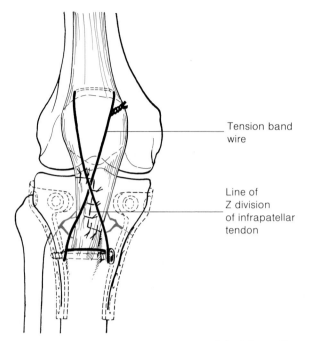

Tension band wire

Line of Z division of infrapatellar tendon

Fig. 19.16. The resuture of the Z division of the infrapatellar tendon is protected by means of a tension band wire. This allows immediate mobilization of the knee

al joint space and damage the medial plateau. In a bicondylar fracture the reconstruction should begin with the simple fracture, which is usually the medial of the two.

We have already described the positioning of the patient and the flexion of the knee which facilitates reduction. Another very useful maneuver is to use the distractor on one or both sides of the plateau, depending on the configuration of the fracture. One Schanz screw of the distractor is inserted into the femur and the other into the tibia (see Fig. 19.16). Distraction causes the fracture fragments to reduce by ligamentotaxis. This type of reduction is referred to as indirect reduction. Its great advantage that it is atraumatic and that it keeps devitalization of the bony fragments to a minimum.

Furthermore, it is sparing to the soft tissue envelope. If reduced by ligamentotaxis, some larger fragments can then simply be stabilized without exposure by means of percutaneous lag screws. These considerations are particularly important in the complex fractures such as types V and VI, in which there is usually considerable contusion and swelling of the soft tissue envelope.

In elevating the depressed articular cartilage fragments, it is best to elevate them "en masse" from below. If surgeons attempt to lift up the fragments through the joint, they are usually left with a number of totally devitalized loose articular fragments which cannot be successfully put back and fitted together. When the articular fragments are driven into supporting cancellous bone of the metaphysis, the cancellous bone compacts and holds the fragments together. When the fragments are elevated together with the compacted cancellous bone, they do not fall apart, but behave as if they were held together by skin. Thus, to initiate the elevation, a periosteal elevator should be pushed deep into the compacted metaphysis. With upward pressure, the whole segment is gradually dislodged. A broad bone punch is then introduced from below and the fragments are gradually tapped back into place until they are slightly overreduced.

In certain fracture types, such as types I, II, and III, an arthroscope can be used to advantage to visualize the articular surfaces while a reduction is being carried out of the depressed fragments from below. In the more complex types, we have found the arthroscope of little value. Because of the complex morphology of the fracture, direct exposure, even if limited, is almost always essential. Therefore, little is accomplished with the arthroscope which cannot be accomplished more expediently under direct vision. Furthermore, in complex fractures, because of their connection with the diaphysis, there is the danger of inducing a compartment syndrome with the fluid used to achieve joint distention and irrigation.

Once the fragments are elevated, the surgeon is obviously then faced with the problem of how to keep them from falling back. There are two maneuvers which are helpful. The first is to insert a massive bone graft below the fragments into the hole in the metaphysis which is created when the fragments are elevated. The second is to compress them circumferentially by means of the remaining intact portion of the plateau. This is accomplished with lag screws which, when tightened, tend to squeeze and narrow the proximal tibia. Some authors have suggested the use of cortical slabs to hold up the elevated fragments. Cancellous bone allograft stored appropriately has also been used successfully in these areas with good healing and incorporation of the grafted bone (A. Gross, 1983, personal communication). We prefer pure cancellous bone autograft such as can be obtained either from the iliac crest or the greater trochanter. The cancellous bone adapts better to the shape of the hole and, when compacted, provides excellent support for the articular fragments, strong enough to permit early movement but not early weight-bearing.

Some authors have also recommended passing screws or Kirschner wires close to the subchondral bone plate of the elevated fragment to prevent its collapse. We feel that screws close to the subchondral plate cause the plate to become abnormally stiff, which can result in chondrolysis (Manley 1982). Such chondrolysis and subsequently fragmentation of bone has been erroneously blamed on avascular necrosis of the fragments. Fixation devices should be at least 5 mm from the subchondral bone plate.

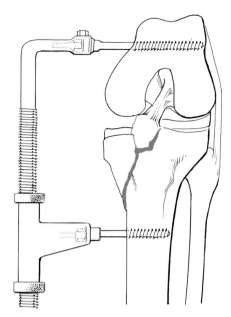

Fig. 19.17. By means of ligamentotaxis, the distractor brings about indirect reduction of all major fragments which have soft tissue attachment. Impacted articular fragments remain unreduced. In fractures involving both condyles two distractors can be used

The plates which are used to support the cortex of a metaphysis from crumbling or displacing under axial thrust fulfill the function of buttressing and are called buttress plates (see Fig. 19.3 b). Any plate, if it is carefully contoured to the shape of the metaphysis, can be made to function as a buttress plate. Because metaphyses in different areas of the body have specific contours, the AO/ASIF, to save the surgeon time in contouring, have made available several precontoured plates for use. Thus, for the proximal tibia, we have the regular T plate, which best fits the medial side. For the lateral side, we have the precontoured T buttress plate and the L buttress plate, which are available in a right and a left version (Fig. 19.17), or the tibial condylar buttress plates.

A buttress plate must be accurately contoured to the cortex it is supposed to buttress. Even the precontoured plates must be adjusted to fit, for if a buttress plate were to be accidentally placed under tension, it could lead to the very displacement it is trying to prevent. Therefore, whenever a buttress plate is fixed to the bone, the first screws should be inserted through the distal end of the plate and the remainder inserted in orderly fashion one after another approaching the joint. If the two ends of the plate are fixed to bone first and there is a gap between the plate and bone, as the remaining screws are inserted, the plate is brought under tension, which instead of buttressing would result in displacement and deformity.

On the medial side, as already stated, the plate is applied to the anteromedial face of the proximal metaphysis deep to the pes anserinus and the anterior fibers of the medial collateral ligament. On the lateral side, because of the proximal fibula, the plate has to be fixed slightly obliquely with its distal end flush with the anterior tibial crest and its proximal end as far posterolaterally as is necessary. The L plate allows more lateral buttressing without getting in the way of the proximal fibula. We have usually found it best, as already stated, to fix the plate first distally and then advance proximally with the screws as the plate is fixed. The proximal lag screws are usually inserted through the most proximal holes at the very end or above or beside the plate. Their position is governed by the configuration of the fracture and not the placement of the plate.

In type V and type VI fractures, the surgeon should always begin with the less comminuted tibial plateau so that one side can be reduced and provisionally buttressed while the other side is reconstructed. For provisional fixation, the proximal cancellous screws should be directed posteriorly to engage the posterior cortex, which may in some cases be the only cortex left intact. As in fractures of the distal tibia, it is necessary first to reestablish the normal length, and this is clearly best and easiest to accomplish on the side of least comminution. Occasionally, however, the comminution may be so severe that it is impossible to reconstruct either side. Under these circumstances, we have found it best to fix a T plate distally on the medial side and a T buttress plate or a longer plate similarly contoured on the lateral side. These two plates are then used as a lateral scaffolding between which the fragments of the tibia are erected. A bar bolt can then be inserted through the plates proximally to tie them together.

Some surgeons have encountered complications with double plating of these complex fractures and have been recommending minimally invasive techniques, such as blind reduction of the articular depressions (Marsh et al. 1994), indirect reduction of the fractures, percutaneous cannulated screw fixation of the fragments, and external fixateur frames for buttressing (Marsh et al. 1994; Stamer et al. 1994). We feel that blind reduction of the articular surfaces defies fundamental rules of articular fracture surgery. Joints require anatomical reduction of their surfaces, because positive step-off deformities as small as twice the thickness of the articular cartilage can have disastrous consequences for the survival of the articulation (Llinas et al. 1993, 1994). We continue to recommend reduction of the articular components under direct vision.

In our hands, double plating of complex fractures has rarely resulted in any soft tissue complications. We have been very cautious and have always delayed surgery in high-velocity complex injuries to allow the soft tissue injuries to heal. We have also used indirect reduction techniques and percutaneous screws, where possible, to minimize on soft tissue exposure and bone devitalization. In open fractures and in fractures complicated by a compartment syndrome, the surgeon does not have the luxury of time. In these fractures, immediate surgery and immediate stabilization is necessary. Under these circumstances we have either delayed metaphyseal reconstruction or we have used the hybrid frame. Delayed metaphyseal reconstruction means that once the joint was reduced and stabilized with a minimal amount of internal fixation, we bridged the joint with an external fixateur and carried out the metaphyseal reconstruction once the soft tissue envelope was closed, which at times required a rotation or a free flap. The other technique which we have employed successfully is to reduce and fix the joint component of the fracture and use the hybrid ring fixateur consisting of a circular frame and a small crossed wire under tension proximally and then a half-frame and large pins distally as a means of maintaining reduction of the metaphysis and diaphysis. One should not use the large-pin external fixator for buttressing these complex fractures. We have found, as have others, that the large-pin half-frame is associated with an unacceptable incidence of infection of the proximal pins and consequent septic arthritis. We cannot recommend the large pin frame for buttressing of these fractures either alone or in combination with one buttress plate.

We prefer to carry out the articular reconstruction with the limb exsanguinated and a pneumatic tourniquet inflated. This controls bleeding and improves visualization, which leads to a more accurate articular reconstruction. In order to shorten the tourniquet time as well as the time the tibial wound is left open, we prefer to obtain our cancellous bone from the donor site and close that incision before the tibial reconstruction is begun.

19.4.6 Internal Fixation of Different Fracture Types

19.4.6.1 Type I

Type I wedge fractures of the lateral plateau (see Fig. 19.2) can usually be fixed with only cancellous lag screws and washers. In young people with a strong cortex, buttressing is not required, but this fracture type in an older individual requires a buttress plate to prevent redisplacement which might occur on axial loading, the result of muscular contraction alone without actual weight-bearing.

19.4.6.2 Type II

In addition to the lateral wedge, type II fractures have articular depression (see Fig. 19.3). Because this fracture occurs in older, more osteoporotic bone, the surgeon cannot rely on lag screws alone to prevent redisplacement of the fragments. A buttress plate is almost always a must.

19.4.6.3 Type III

In the type III, central depression fracture, the lateral cortex is intact circumferentially (see Fig. 19.5). Thus, theoretically, there is no need for a buttress plate and no need for any lag screws because, first, there is nothing to lag together and, second, the lag screws cannot support the articular fragments, nor can they hold up the bone graft. The hole which has to be made in the lateral cortex weakens the bone. The cortex is also very thin and fragile. Although these factors have to be judged at the time of surgery, we have nevertheless frequently buttressed the lateral cortex to prevent its possible subsequent fracture and displacement. In addition, the lag screw, if passed under the elevated portion of the plateau, will be of some help in keeping it elevated.

19.4.6.4 Type IV

Type IV fractures of the medial plateau (see Fig. 19.6) should be buttressed even in young individuals. The frequently avulsed intercondylar eminence with the attached cruciate ligaments should be either fixed back in place with a lag screw or held reduced with a loop of wire tied under tension over the intact anterior cortex.

The posterior split wedge fragment should not be forgotten; it requires a second buttress plate posteromedially.

19.4.6.5 Type V

If surgery is performed, type V bicondylar fractures require buttressing on both sides (see Fig. 19.7). Lag screws alone are never enough to prevent displacement.

19.4.6.6 Type VI

In type VI fractures, the metaphysis is dissociated from the diaphysis; therefore, at least one of the two buttress plates must be strong and long enough to bridge to the diaphysis and act either as a compression or a neutra-

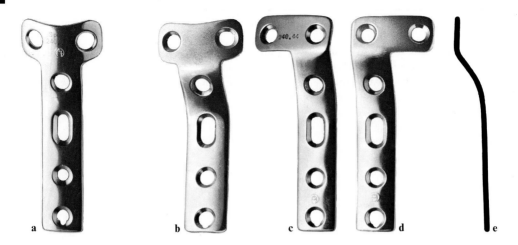

Fig. 19.18 a–e. The different plates available for internal fixation of the proximal tibia. **a** Four-hole T plate. **b** T buttress plate. **c, d** L buttress plates. **e** The double bend of the tibial plateau buttress plate can be seen in profile. (From Müller et al. 1979)

lization plate (see Fig. 19.9). It should be a narrow 4.5 dynamic compression (DC) plate rather than a long T plate. The T plate is too flexible for this purpose (see Fig. 19.18). The tibial condylar buttress plate is ideally suited as a lateral buttress in these situations.

19.4.7 Ligament and Meniscal Repair

Every effort should be made to preserve the menisci. Torn menisci should be repaired if at all technically possible (Wirth 1981; Hohl and Moore 1983; see also Sect. 19.4.2). We have performed open meniscal repair for years, taking the view that even a failed repair which would subsequently lead to a meniscectomy would be better than immediate meniscectomy, because of the protective effect of the meniscus on the underlying articular cartilage. To date we have not had to carry out a secondary meniscectomy. We believe that disrupted collateral ligaments and capsules should also be meticulously repaired. Similarly, if a cruciate ligament is avulsed with a piece of bone, the bone should be reduced and fixed in place. If the cruciate ligament is disrupted in its substance, then we believe that such a disruption should be ignored and repaired at some point in the future if instability makes this necessary. Such a rupture requires a primary ligamentous substitution, which necessitates a period of immobilization to ensure healing. In the presence of a fracture the joint must not be immobilized, because this will lead to permanent stiffness.

19.4.8 Postoperative Care

The postoperative care of fractures of the tibial plateau is governed by the findings at surgery and the degree of stability achieved by the internal fixation. If, at the time of the open reduction and internal fixation, a satisfactory reduction has been achieved of both the joint and metaphysis, and if the internal fixation is stable, then we apply a padded dressing to the knee and elevate the extremity with the knee in 45°–60° flexion on a Böhler-Braun splint. We do not believe in padded compression dressings as an effective means of controlling postoperative swelling; this is far better achieved with the suction drainage which we use routinely for the first 24–48 h. After the first 2–3 days, once we are satisfied that the wound is healing without any complications, we encourage the patient to begin active motion of the knee. The patient has usually regained full extension and at least 90 % flexion by the end of the first week and full flexion by the end of the second or third week. The advent of continuous passive motion machines (CPM) has greatly facilitated the postoperative care of these patients and improved their prognosis. At the end of the surgical procedure, a light, unobstructive dressing is applied to the extremity. The machine is set to permit full extension and flexion to 40°–60°, which is increased to 90° as quickly as the patient will allow. Initially, the patients do not tolerate rapid cycling. We have found that one full flexion and extension every 2 min is a comfortable pace. With time, it is possible to increase the rate as well as the degree of flexion. It is usually possible to cease continuous passive motion at the end of the first week, and the patients are able to carry on with their rehabilitation without reliance on passive aids.

We feel that major intra-articular fractures should be treated immediately after surgery with a CPM because of its influence on articular cartilage healing. Splinting as described should be used only if a CPM is not available.

Regardless of how stable the reduction, we do not allow weight-bearing for 10–12 weeks. We believe in early active motion, since it not only ensures a return of motion to the knee and good function of the soft tissue envelope, but also has a beneficial effect on the healing of the articular cartilage (Mitchell and Shepard 1980; Salter et al. 1980, 1986). Early weight-bearing can lead not only to loss of reduction, joint incongruity, and malalignment, but it can also interfere with the healing of articular cartilage by loading the tissue when it is not sufficiently mature to accept the load.

If, at the time of surgery, the diagnosis of a disrupted collateral ligament is either confirmed or established, then the disruption should be repaired. Because early motion is necessary to prevent stiffness and because the ligamentous repair must be protected from lateral bending forces which could disrupt the repair, we protect such a knee in a cast brace. This protects the ligamentous repair from lateral bending forces and permits full mobilization. In the presence of a fracture, we use polycentric joint hinges, but do not restrict the range of motion. The knee in the brace is then mobilized with a CPM as described.

If, at the end of surgery, we judge the internal fixation to be unstable, then we protect it from overload. If only one plateau is involved, a cast brace with the knee stressed in the direction of the uninvolved plateau provides adequate protection. If both plateaux are involved,

the surgeon must decide whether sufficient longitudinal stability has been achieved to prevent shortening. If doubt exists, then such a knee must be mobilized on a splint with skeletal traction for at least 3–4 weeks before it is transferred to a cast brace for the remainder of healing period.

19.5 Summary and Conclusions

Fractures of the tibial plateau involve a major weight-bearing joint. Thus, to achieve good joint function the surgeon must strive to achieve joint congruity, axial alignment, stability, and a satisfactory range of motion. If the fracture is stable, the joint congruous, and the alignment acceptable, then closed treatment is the method of choice (Fig. 19.19). Early motion must be instituted, however, because if immobilized, even with closed treatment, the knee will stiffen permanently. Joint instability and significant incongruity are clear indications for surgical treatment. The majority of these fractures occur in the fifth and sixth decades, and at least 50 % of the patients who underwent surgical treatment had some degree of osteoporosis (Schatzker et al. 1979). Thus, age and osteoporosis cannot be employed as an argument against open treatment. The patients who underwent surgical treatment had, on average, at least three times the degree of depression of their articular surface, and

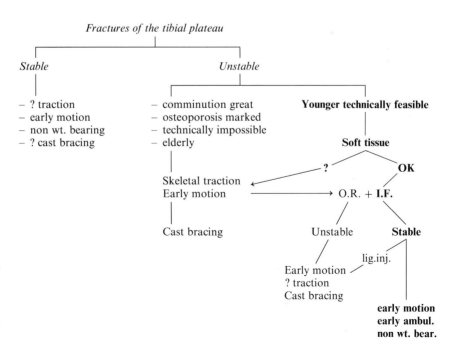

Fig. 19.19. An algorithm for the treatment of tibial plateau fractures. *O.R. + I.F.*, open reduction and internal fixation; *wt*, weight; *lig.inj.*, ligament injury; *ambul.*, ambulation

yet the overall results of surgical treatment were better than those of closed treatment (Schatzker et al. 1979). Therefore, the degree of joint depression should not prevent surgery being performed. We have stressed the following:

1. *Atraumatic anatomical reduction.* This ensures the reconstruction of joint congruity and axial alignment which, in the presence of intact ligaments, will also ensure joint stability.
2. *Elevation of the plateau en masse.* Depressed, comminuted impacted articular fragments must be handled as a continuum and elevated by pushing from below on the whole area of depression until it reexpands. This ensures the proper reduction of the fragments, enhances their stability, and, where possible, preserves their blood supply.
3. *Bonegrafting of the defect in the metaphysis.* The elevation of the depressed articulation leaves a defect in the metaphysis which must be bonegrafted to prevent redisplacement.
4. *Stable internal fixation.* The vertical fracture lines in the articular surface and metaphysis must be stabilized with the aid of compression by means of lag screws. This greatly enhances articular cartilage healing and regeneration (Mitchell and Shepard 1980). The metaphysis must be buttressed to prevent redisplacement due to axial load. Stable fixation eliminates pain and makes early motion possible.
5. *Early motion.* Early motion is necessary for the preservation of joint motion and soft tissue function. Furthermore, it has a profoundly beneficial effect on cartilage regeneration (Salter et al. 1980, 1986).

Based on these principles, we have achieved an acceptable result in 89% of patients treated, which is better than the results achieved with other methods of treatment (Schatzker et al. 1979).

These excellent results can be obtained in patients in whom the tibial plateau fracture is an isolated injury. Patients with head injury and unconsciousness, and particulary those with spasticity and rigidity, cannot mobilize their knees nor cooperate subsequently with a rehabilitation regimen. Their results are compromised. This is also true of polytrauma patients with other serious injuries and patients with severe open fractures. It is the severity of the open wound which ultimately determines the outcome. Early stable fixation of the articular surfaces and a delayed and staged metaphyseal reconstruction have minimized the complications and greatly improved the outcome in these very difficult injuries.

•••

References

Apley AG (1979) Fractures of the tibial plateau. Orthop Clin North Am 10:61–74

Hohl M, Hopp E (1976) Ligament injuries in tibial condylar fractures. J Bone Joint Surg 58A:279 (abstr)

Hohl M, Moore TM (1983) Articular fractures of the proximal tibia. In: McCollister Evarts C (ed) Surgery of the musculoskeletal system, vol 7. Churchill Livingstone, New York, pp 11–135

Kennedy JC, Bailey WH (1968) Experimental tibial plateau fractures. J Bone Joint Surg 50A:1522–1534

Llinas A, McKellop HA, Marshall GJ, Sharpe F, Bin Lu MS, Kirchen M, Sarmiento A (1993) Healing and remodelling of articular incongruities in a rabbit fracture model. J Bone Joint Surg 75A:1508–1523

Llinas A, Lovasz G, Park SH (1994) Effect of joint incongruity on the opposing articular cartilage. Annual AAOS meeting, Los Angeles, CA

Manley P, Schatzker J (1982) Replacement of epiphyseal bone with methylmethacrylate: its effects on articular cartilage. Arch Orthop Traumatol Surg 100:3–10

Marsh JL, Smith ST, Do (1994) Outcome of severe tibial fractures. Annual OTA meeting, Los Angeles

Mitchell N, Shepard N (1980) Healing of articular cartilage in intra-articular fractures in rabbits. J Bone Joint Surg 62A:628–634

Moore TM, Harvey JP Jr (1974) Roentgenographic measurement of tibial plateau depression due to fracture. J Bone Joint Surg 56A:155–160

Müller ME, Allgöwer M, Schneider R, Willenegger H (1979) Manual of internal fixation, 2nd edn. Springer, Berlin Heidelberg New York, p 257

Müller ME, Nazarian S, Koch P, Schatzker J (1990) The comprehensive classification of fractures of long bones. Springer, Berlin Heidelberg New York

Rasmussen PS (1973) Tibial condylar fractures. J Bone Joint Surg 55A:1331–1350

Roberts JM (1968) Fractures of the condyles of the tibia. J Bone Joint Surg 50A:1505–1521

Salter RB, Simmonds DF, Malcolm BW, Rumble EJ, MacMichael D (1980) The biological effects of continuous passive motion on the healing of full-thickness defects in articular cartilage: an experimental investigation in the rabbit. J Bone Joint Surg 62A:1232–1251

Salter RB, Hamilton HW, Wedge JH, Tile M, Torode IP, O'Driscoll SW, Murnaghan J, Saringer JH (1986) Clinical application of basic research on continuous passive motion for disorders and injuries of synovial joints: preliminary report of a feasibility study. Techniques Orthop 1(1):74–91

Schatzker J, McBroom R, Bruce D (1979) The tibial plateau fracture. The Toronto experience. Clin Orthop 138:94–104

Shrive N (1974) The weight-bearing role of the menisci of the knee. J Bone Joint Surg 56B:381 (abstr)

Stamer DT, Schenk R, Staggers B, Aurori K, Aurori B, Behrens F (1994) Bicondylar tibial plateau fractures treated with a hybrid ring external fixator: a preliminary study. Annual AAOS meeting, Los Angeles, CA

Walker S, Erkman MJ (1975) The role of the menisci in force transmission across the knee. Clin Orthop 109:184–192

Wirth CR (1981) Meniscus repair. Clin Orthop 157:153–160

20 Fractures of the Tibia

M. Tile

20.1 Introduction

The management of the tibial fracture remains controversial despite advances in both nonoperative and operative care. Orthopedic opinion is often cyclic, and in no area of orthopedic endeavor is this better seen than in the management of the fractured tibia. Orthopedic surgeons with an interest in orthopedic history would be well advised to study this particular fracture, which reflects the cyclic changes in opinion so clearly.

During our orthopedic residency and careers as clinicians, we have been subjected to this full cycle. During our residency, we were taught that most tibial fractures were best treated by open reduction and internal fixation; unfortunately, the surgery was often inadequately performed and indifferent results were achieved, with many serious complications. This, in turn, led to an extreme nonoperative approach, championed on the North American continent by Dehne et al. (1961) and Sarmiento (1967). In the preceding era, this nonoperative approach had been popularized by Böhler (1936) of the Viennese School.

The introduction of the AO/ASIF method of fracture care led to a renewed interest in internal fixation based on sound biomechanical and biological principles. In the hands of the AO/ASIF surgeons, marked improvement was reported in the results of operative fracture care (Allgöwer 1967). However, many problems remained, reflected in yet another cycle in operative care, i.e., which is the best method. At present, the intramedullary nail, previously in some disrepute, has become the implant of choice, which in turn reveals further difficult problems.

It is obvious that there is no perfect method of treating all tibial fractures. Different circumstances demand differing approaches to the same problem. At the present time, improved methods of both nonoperative care of the fractured tibia, using functional casts, cast braces, or splints and operative care, using the principles and implants of the AO group (Müller et al. 1979), where indicated, should allow decision making to be based on logical principles, which in turn should resolve the so-called controversy of the fractured tibia. We should reject the theories of dogmatists which state that "all tibia fractures must be treated nonoperatively" or, conversely, that "all tibia fractures should be treated operatively." It is time to remove this type of dogma from our thinking and to individualize the treatment for each patient.

Logical management of any tibial fracture can only flow from a precise knowledge of its natural history. For the individual case, the natural history is dependent upon the personality of the particular fracture to be treated. Once the personality has been determined by a careful clinical and radiographic assessment, and compared to the natural history of similar fracture types, a treatment protocol for that particular patient will become relatively clear. This knowledge will also allow the surgeon to carefully weigh and balance the alternative methods of management and clearly outline them to the patient. Where clear-cut alternative treatment methods exist, the surgeon should not play God, but should allow the patient to share in the decision-making process.

20.2 Natural History

Most fractures of the tibia will heal if treated by nonoperative means – this fact is undeniable. Watson-Jones and Coltart (1943) stated that "if immobilized long enough, all fractures will eventually heal."

Charnley (1961) stressed the importance of the soft tissue hinge on the healing process of the tibial fracture. He recognized that fractures with an intact periosteal hinge did well, whereas those with gross displacement, indicating complete periosteal rupture, did less well. He recommended primary surgery for the tibial fracture with an intact fibula and for any tibia with a gap at the fracture following reduction. Astutely, he recommended early bone grafting procedures for fractures with predictably poor results.

Nicoll (1964), in a definitive study of 705 tibial fractures treated prior to the widespread use of the early weight-bearing method, was able to clearly describe the natural history of the tibial shaft fracture treated nonoperatively. It was he who coined the term "personality of the fracture," by which the eventual outcome of each case could be predicted. The major factors affecting the outcome were:

440 ·

Chapter 20   **Fractures of the Tibia**

1. The amount of initial displacement
2. The degree of comminution
3. The amount of soft tissue damage in the open fracture
4. The presence or absence of sepsis

The incidence of favorable outcome for fractures managed by nonoperative means ranged from 91% in the "good personality" types to 61% in the "poor personality" types and to only 40% if sepsis was involved. These figures indicate a significant complication rate with many poor functional results in all categories. In order to improve upon these results, two major schools of thought evolved, one stressing the importance of early weight bearing to the ultimate function of the limb, the other, the importance of stable internal fixation.

· ·

20.2.1 Nonoperative School

Bohler (1936) had recommended that all major tibial fractures be treated with skeletal traction for 3 weeks followed by a weight-bearing plaster cast until healing was complete. However, Watson-Jones and Coltart (1943) clearly showed that traction for tibial shaft fractures had a deleterious effect on the rate of union.

Dehne eliminated the preliminary period of skeletal traction and instituted immediate weight bearing for the patient in a long-leg cast with the knee extended. In 1961, he and his colleagues reported good functional results with no nonunions.

In 1967, using the combination of early weight-bearing casts and functional braces, Sarmiento reported no nonunions in 100 consecutive fractures of the tibial shaft. His biomechanical and clinical studies indicated few complications with early weight bearing, and many benefits. Excessive shortening was not the problem it was expected to be – the fracture rarely shortened beyond its initial displacement, the average being 1.9 cm (Fig. 20.1). Weight bearing on the injured extremity allowed early functional rehabilitation, thus preventing joint stiffness, swelling, and other complications, while also having a beneficial effect on fracture healing. Other reports by

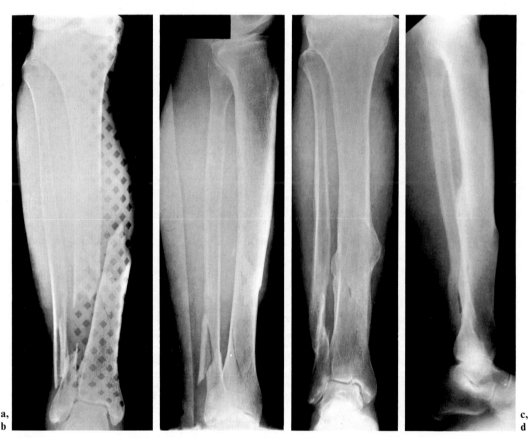

a,
b

c,
d

Fig. 20.1 a–d. Nonoperative management of a spiral tibial fracture. **a,b** Anteroposterior and lateral radiographs of a 59-year-old woman showing a markedly displaced fracture of the tibia and fibula. Note also the undisplaced butterfly fragment.

c,d Closed manipulation under general anesthesia and plaster immobilization for 12 weeks resulted in firm bony union and an excellent functional result with shortening of only 1.1 cm

Sarmiento and Latta (1981) and Sarmiento et al. (1989) corroborated the above results. In this latter study, 780 tibial shaft fractures were treated by a cast followed by a prefabricated functional brace. The average time to application of the brace was 3.8 weeks for closed and 5.2 weeks for open fractures. Factors influencing healing were the soft tissue injury, the initial displacement, the degree of comminution, and the condition of the fibula. There were 20 nonunions, average healing occurring in 17.4 weeks for the closed and 21.7 weeks for the open fractures. A total of 90% of the fractures healed with less than 10 mm of shortening and acceptable angulation.

Brown (1974) soon confirmed these improved results. Thus, the simple addition of early weight bearing positively altered the natural history of the tibial fracture without affecting the safety factor inherent in closed treatment.

Oni et al. (1988) prospectively studied 100 consecutive tibial shaft fractures treated by closed means. Only four cases had failed to unite at 30 weeks, and the majority united by 20 weeks. Closed treatment was a long-leg cast for 4–6 weeks followed by a patellar-bearing cast. Residual shortening and angulation were acceptable, but 43% of patients had restriction of ankle and/or subtalar motion.

Thus, all of these studies indicate that the vast majority of tibial fractures will heal with nonoperative treatment and will result in good functional limbs, if the patients follow the prescribed programs.

20.2.2 Operative School

In 1957 the AO group, studying the poor functional results then being obtained by nonoperative treatment, placed open reduction and stable internal fixation on a firm scientific basis. They believed that the failure of surgical treatment, leading to its widespread condemnation at the time, was mainly the result of poor surgery. Stable internal fixation would, they believed, eliminate the complications resulting from plaster immobilization, i.e.,, "plaster disease."

Careful documentation by devotees of that method have indicated excellent functional results with no sacrifice of fracture healing, as a study of the excellent papers of Rüedi et al. (1976), Allgöwer and Perren (1980), Karlstrom and Olerud (1974), and others will indicate. Complications in their hands were minimal (Tables 20.1–20.4).

Thus, it would appear that both schools have achieved the same end by markedly different means, i.e., excellent functional results with few complications.

From the above reports, it is self-evident that nonoperative management will achieve satisfactory results in the majority of tibial fractures, without the need for surgery. Are the arguments of the proponents of the operative school cogent enough to sway us into adopting their approach, i.e., almost universal operative management of displaced tibial fractures? We doubt it; therefore, we recommend that most tibial fractures can be managed nonoperatively unless a clear indication for surgery exists, as will be noted later in this chapter. Even the argument about plaster disease needs careful scrutiny.

Table 20.1. Results of 617 cases of fracture tibias, treated by stable internal fixation (from Allgöwer and Perren 1980)

Fracture site	Type	Total (n)	Late disability (<20%)	
			(n)	(%)
Shaft of	Closed	535	6	1.1
the tibia	Compound	45	8	17.7
Distal tibia	Intra-articular	37	3	8.1
Total		617	17	2.7

Total of four fully controlled series: 1958/1959, 1959/1960, 1961/1962, and 1962/1963. None of the patients received insurance compensation for permanent partial damage of more than 20% (total invalidity being taken as 100%).

Table 20.2. Follow-up of 435 consecutive tibial shaft fracture with dynamic compression (DC) plate fixation (from Allgöwer and Perren 1980)

	Fracture (n)		Total
	Closed	Open	(n)
DC plate fixation	334	101	435
Follow-up	323	95	418
Personal	300	88	388
X-ray and questionnaire	23	7	30
No follow-up	2	–	2
Died	9	6	15

Table 20.3. Functional results 1-2 years after dynamic compression (DC) plate fixation of 323 closed fractures of the tibial shaft (from Allgöwer and Perren 1980)

	Patients	
	(n)	(%)
Good[a]	317	98
Acceptable[b]	6	2
Poor[c]	–	–
Total	323	100

[a] Functional recovery compatible with normal professional and extraprofessional activities.
[b] Occasional complaints (pain, fatigue), normal professional, reduced extraprofessional (sports) activities.
[c] Any of the following: significant pain in tibiotarsal or knee joints, reduced professional activities, nonunion, amputation.

Table 20.4. Functional results 1-2 years after dynamic compression (DC) plate fixation of 95 open fracutres of the tibial shafts (from Allgöwer and Perren 1980)

	Patients	
	(n)	*(%)*
Good[a]	84	88.3
Acceptable[b]	8	8.0
Poor[c]	3	3.5
Total	95	100

[a] Functional recovery compatible with normal professional and extraprofessional activities.

[b] Occasional complaints (pain, fatigue), normal professional, reduced extraprofessional (sports) activities.

[c] Any of the following: significant pain in tibiotarsal or knee joints, reduced professional activities, nonunion, amputation.

20.2.3 Plaster Disease

As previously indicated, if patients comply with their exercise program of early weight bearing, plaster disease in nonoperative care is rarely significant. Is it, then, alone enough of a reason to recommend universal open reduction for the fractured tibia? Is it, in fact, a real entity and can it be eliminated by an aggressive operative approach?

Plaster disease is, in our opinion, not a disease but a syndrome. This syndrome, characterized by swelling under the cast followed by permanent stiffness in the immobilized joints, has many causes, including the following:

1. An unrecognized compartment syndrome
2. Reflex sympathetic dystrophy
3. Thromboembolic disease
4. Severe soft tissue injury

While it may be true that eliminating the plaster of Paris will improve early function in many cases, it is not true that any of the above will necessarily be eliminated by surgery. Failure to recognize that fact may obscure an impending compartment syndrome and lead to a delay in its diagnosis.

What of the other causes of this syndrome? To answer this question, each of them will now be discussed in turn.

20.2.3.1 Compartment Syndromes

Plaster disease is often mistakenly diagnosed in patients suffering from an unrecognized deep compartment syndrome, which is far more common in fractures of the tibia than we have been led to believe. A perusal of the recent literature will indicate the growing importance of the compartment syndrome in determining the end result of a tibial fracture. The advent of modern monitoring techniques, either intermittent or continuous, as advocated by Rorabeck (1977), Mubarek et al. (1978), and others, makes it possible to prevent this disastrous complication by early diagnosis and aggressive management.

Patients with a tibial fracture who are placed in a well-padded, above-knee plaster rarely have undue or excruciating pain. If they do, a compartment syndrome must be suspected. For example, the patient shown in Fig. 20.2, a 17-year-old girl, sustained a high-energy tibial fracture after being thrown from a horse. She complained of severe pain in the extremity, but never developed any other symptoms or signs of vascular insufficiency. The first 2 months of her treatment were agonizing for her when she attempted to bear weight. As treatment progressed, it became obvious that she had developed an equinovarus foot deformity with clawing of the toes (Fig. 20.2 c,d). Union of the fracture was also delayed for 7 months. This patient represents a typical case of a posterior compartment syndrome leading to Volkmann's ischemic contracture of the deep posterior muscle groups. This syndrome is often misread as plaster disease. The residual equinovarus foot with a cock-up deformity of the great toe is pathognomonic of this condition. Unfortunately, these patients may also have painful hyperesthesia of the foot, a condition most difficult to eradicate.

20.2.3.2 Reflex Sympathetic Dystrophy

This complication, which may occur in any fracture, is occasionally seen in patients with a tibial fracture. The patients often develop massive swelling under the cast and will not bear weight, and a painful, stiff, hyperesthetic foot is often the result. Since this complication is not specific to the form of treatment, operative or nonoperative, it should not be taken to be plaster disease.

20.2.3.3 Thromboembolic Disease

The functional result is also affected by the presence of deep vein thrombosis in the injured extremity. This, in turn, may lead to chronic edema in the extremity with all the sequelae of that condition. We believe the incidence is higher in patients who have been kept in plaster for long periods and that this is a true indication of plaster disease. However, precise data on this matter is unavailable at present, and it must be remembered that deep thromboembolism may also occur following surgery.

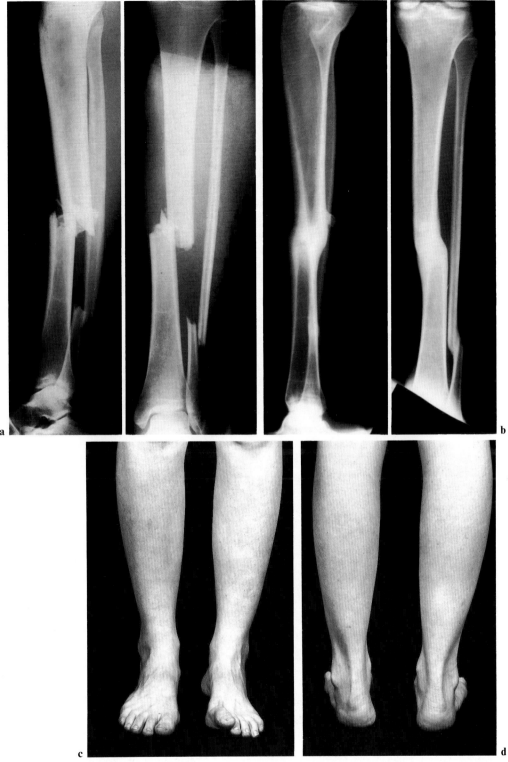

Fig. 20.2 a–d. Deep posterior compartment syndrome. **a** Lateral and anteroposterior radiographs of a 17-year-old girl injured when thrown from a horse. The patient complained of severe pain in the extremity following reduction of this fracture but never developed any other signs or symptoms of vascular insufficiency. **b** The fracture eventually united after 7 months in plaster. **c,d** The photographs show the classic appearance of a deep posterior compartment syndrome. Note the equinovarus foot and the cock-up deformity of the left great toe, as well as the varus position of the heel on the posterior view. The patient also complained of painful paresthesia. Secondary reconstructive surgery (a triple arthrodesis) was required but success was only partial. (From Tile 1980)

444 •••

Chapter 20   **Fractures of the Tibia**

20.2.3.4 Severe Soft Tissue Injury

The functional result is often compromised by significant soft tissue damage. In some instances, when the soft tissue damage is so major that it includes loss of muscle, the damage will be permanent no matter which mode of treatment is chosen. However, stabilization of the fracture in patients with major soft tissue damage will allow early motion of the soft tissues, ensuring more rapid rehabilitation and a better final result. Recent studies by Salter et al. (1980) have stressed the importance of the postoperative use of continuous passive motion. We believe that this technique, when combined with stable fracture fixation, will in the future allow much quicker and better rehabilitation of the patient with a major soft tissue injury associated with fracture.

Thus, if plaster disease is not truly a disease, and open operative treatment aids only cases with major soft tissue injury and perhaps lowers the incidence of thromboembolic disease, without altering the problem of the compartment syndrome or reflex sympathetic dystrophy, what factors, if any, favor operative treatment of the tibial diaphyseal fracture? The answer will be made clearer by a study of the factors influencing the natural history of the tibial fracture.

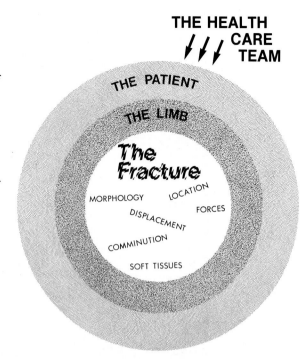

Fig. 20.3. The personality of an injury is determined by a careful appraisal of the patient, the limb, the fracture, and the expertise of the health care team. (From Tile 1984)

20.2.4 Factors Influencing the Natural History

In order to justify any open operation on the tibia, we must clearly define those characteristics of the fracture which adversely affect its ability to heal satisfactorily with normal function, i.e., affect the natural history of the fracture. Such factors do exist and may be present in the fracture itself, the limb, or the patient, and they are modified by the experience and expertise of the health care team (Fig. 20.3). By carefully weighing and balancing all of these factors for each particular patient, i.e., by assessing the personality of the injury, the most logical method of treatment should become apparent.

20.2.4.1 Pathoanatomy of the Fracture

The tibia, like the ulna, is an unique anatomical structure. Its anteromedial surface is entirely subcutaneous and its location in the body makes it prone to injury, often associated with high energy. The pathoanatomy of the fracture (i.e., the location, morphology, and degree of displacement) has a marked influence on the outcome of the fracture. As important as the pathoanatomy of the fracture itself is the state of the soft tissues. A careful analysis of the pathoanatomy of the fracture and the

state of the soft tissues will allow the surgeon to identify the personality type to which it most closely relates and thereby predict the expected outcome.

a) Anatomical Site

The natural history of the tibia fracture is influenced by the location of the fracture, whether it is in the diaphysis, the transition zone extending into the metaphysis, or the epiphysis, with or without joint involvement. The response of diaphyseal cortical bone is quite different from that of metaphyseal cancellous bone.

Articular (Epiphysis)
If the fracture extends into either the knee (see Fig. 20.8) or the ankle joint (see Fig. 20.9) and is displaced, then dealing with that aspect of the fracture assumes overriding importance, since the end result will depend upon obtaining a stable anatomical reduction and early motion of the joint.

Metaphysis and Transition Zone
Fractures in the metaphysis or in the transition zone between the metaphysis and the diaphysis may be caused by compressive or tensile forces. If caused by *compressive forces,* the fractures are often crushed and

axially malaligned. Healing of this cancellous bone may be rapid, but in an unacceptable position. Closed reduction of this type of fracture may often leave a gap at the site of crush, with a tendency for the fracture to redisplace into it. Also, disimpaction of the fracture changes it from a stable to an unstable one.

Transition zone fractures caused by *shear forces* may be due to direct or indirect trauma. Those caused by direct trauma, especially in young people, are usually markedly unstable. The same may be true of those caused by indirect trauma, with torsional forces. The force required to fracture the metaphysis of a young patient with normal bone is extreme. A shearing injury through the metaphysis or the transition zone between the metaphysis and diaphysis is therefore a high-energy one and may be associated with considerable instability and displacement. If this displacement results in poor bone apposition, despite adequate non-operative management, difficulties may arise. Since cancellous metaphyseal bone heals quickly if compressed and slowly if displaced, open reduction and compression of some fractures in the metaphysis or the transition zone may be desirable.

Diaphysis

Unstable, displaced diaphyseal fractures of the tibia may be slow to heal. In these cases, the soft tissue enve-lope, which includes both muscle and periosteum, may be grossly disrupted. As a result, maintenance of an acceptable reduction may be difficult and union may be delayed.

b) Morphology

The morphology of the fracture will suggest the type of violence that caused it, whether transverse, short oblique, or spiral, displaced or undisplaced, comminut-ed or not.

Transverse and short oblique fractures, unless associated with a pathological lesion in the bone, are indicative of a more violent force than are spiral fractures. Marked comminution and gross displacement, suggesting complete disruption of the soft tissue, further emphasize the violent nature of the injury.

Therefore, it is possible for a pattern of injury to emerge from a study of these factors. A high-energy injury caused by shearing forces is usually transverse, comminuted, and markedly displaced, while spiral fractures with minimal displacement and minimal comminution represent examples of low-energy injury (Fig. 20.4). Definite personality traits of the injury will become more apparent if the state of the soft tissues is considered.

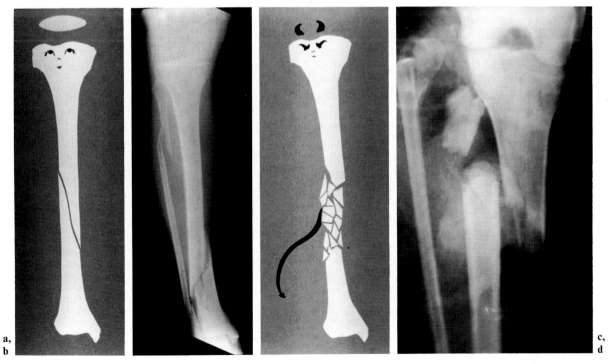

a,
b

c,
d

Fig. 20.4 a–d. Personality traits of tibia fractures. **a,b** A "happy" tibia fracture, a low-energy spiral fracture caused by rotation. **c,d** An "unhappy" tibial fracture, transverse, severely comminuted, and usually open

20.2.4.2 Soft Tissue Injury

The state of the soft tissues is at least as important as the morphological appearance of the fracture. Open fractures of the tibia will be considered in more detail later in this chapter. Suffice it to say here that the more violent the trauma, the more likely the presence of major soft tissue damage.

This soft tissue damage may be overt, with an open wound, or presumed, with massive swelling, ecchymoses, and instability of the fracture. These closed fractures may be accompanied by complete disruption of the soft tissue envelope, leading to hematoma and massive edema and thereby causing increased compartment pressure and tension on the skin. Fracture blisters may appear early and will greatly influence the management decisions. If the fracture is open, the site and size of the laceration and the degree of muscle damage and possible contamination are all important factors. Tscherne and Gotzen (1984) have classified soft tissue injury associated with closed fractures. This classification is discussed fully in Chap. 21 and later on in this chapter (Sect. 20.3.1.2).

20.2.4.3 Other Injuries to the Limb

The presence or absence of other injuries in the same limb will greatly affect the natural history of a tibial fracture. Fractures of the pelvis and acetabulum may require long-term bed rest, and the beneficial effect of early weight bearing is thus out of reach. Fractures of the femur associated with fractures of the tibia usually have a major injury to the knee associated with them. This injury, known as the "floating knee," has a poor prognosis with nonoperative treatment.

The presence or absence of an arterial or nerve injury or an early compartment syndrome will greatly influence the decision making in the management of a tibial fracture. An arterial injury in particular has a gravely deleterious effect on the prognosis of a tibial fracture.

Dickson et al. (1994) have studied the effect of an arterial lesion in the limb on the healing of a tibial fracture in the same limb. They found a direct correlation; those patients with an arterial injury had a significantly greater incidence of delayed or nonunion.

20.2.4.4 Patient Factors

a) General Considerations

It is important to carefully assess the general state of the patient. His or her age is important at the two extremes. In skeletally immature patients, open reduction of the

tibia is almost never indicated. In older individuals, on the other hand, having decided that open reduction and internal fixation are strongly indicated and important, the surgeon may find him- or herself faced with extremely osteoporotic bone in which it is impossible to achieve stable internal fixation. Therefore, the physiological age of the patient, especially with reference to the presence of osteoporosis, is important.

The patient's occupation and recreational habits should be known so that there can be no major disparity between the expectation of the patient and the expectation of the surgeon with respect to the quality of the end result. This is especially true in the case of the professional athlete.

Finally, the pretrauma general medical state of the patient must be considered prior to the patient's subjection to a general anesthetic.

b) Polytraumatized Patients

Patients with injuries to many body systems have a high risk of developing respiratory complications. If these patients are rapidly mobilized, especially in the upright position, many of these complications may be prevented or reversed (Border et al. 1975). Therefore, current surgical practice would indicate that early stabilization of fractures and rapid mobilization of the polytraumatized patient are beneficial to both the fracture and the patient (McMurtry et al. 1984).

In the tibia, however, this is not a prime indication for surgery, since patients can be mobilized with a plaster cast. However, when associated with other fractures in the same limb, some type of stabilization of the tibia, whether internal or external, is often desirable.

20.2.4.5 The Health Care Team

A realistic assessment of the health care team is often difficult, but in deciding upon the management of a tibial fracture this assessment becomes vital. Where clear alternatives to treatment exist, a route must be chosen that will not only give superior results, but will also be safest for the patient. Good nonoperative management is far preferable to poor operative management, the results of which can be disastrous. The patient may be left with the worst of both worlds – the trauma of inadequate surgery superimposed upon the trauma of the injury, which often compromises the results and exposes the patient to needless risk, especially of sepsis. Therefore, surgeons must appraise their own ability and that of their team in order to achieve the type of stable fixation that we have been stressing before embarking on operative care of a tibial fracture. The surgeon must have available a complete armamentarium of modern internal and external fixation devices. For open reduction and internal fixation, the infection rate in any institution should not exceed 2 % and should preferably be well below 1 % for elective orthopedic surgery. If the team is not experienced in modern biomechanical principles and methods of fixation, the surgeon should decide whether the surgical indications in a particular patient are definite or relative. If definite, the patient should be referred to another center, and if relative, nonoperative means should be employed.

20.2.5 Summary

At the worst end of the personality scale is the grossly displaced, highly comminuted, open fracture with skin loss and vascular compromise; at the best end, the spiral, minimally displaced, closed fracture (Fig. 20.4). Fractures, however, do not come in neat packages with specific labels, nor with absolute – i.e., good or bad – personalities. Each patient is unique, his or her injury falling somewhere in the spectrum. By determining the specific characteristics of the fracture and by predicting how those characteristics will affect its natural outcome, the surgeon will have taken the first and most logical step in the management of that fracture. That initial management decision will have far greater influence on the final outcome of the fracture than any amount of attempted late rehabilitation.

20.3 Assessment

A careful clinical and radiographic assessment, looking for those factors which will affect the natural history, is the first important step in management.

20.3.1 Clinical Assessment

20.3.1.1 History

Precise details of the injury are important, as obtained either from the patient or from reliable witnesses. From the history alone, the surgeon may be able to suspect the nature of the injury.

The *general patient profile* is of great importance and will affect the medical treatment. Of importance are the age, both chronological and physiological, the general medical state, and especially the expectations. The expectations of a professional athlete will be considerably different from those of a sedentary, physically inactive individual, and this will affect the treatment decision considerably.

20.3.1.2 Physical Assessment

A careful general physical examination is mandatory as it is in any injured patient corresponding to the primary survey of the American College of Surgeons (1981). The limb must also be inspected *locally* for the degree of soft tissue damage, the presence of an open wound, the degree of deformity and instability, the neurovascular state, and the presence of a compartment syndrome. If a compartment syndrome is suspected, pressure measurements using a monitoring device are mandatory. Continuous monitoring is being successfully used in some centers to ensure early detection of a deep compartment syndrome (Fig. 20.5).

a) Soft Tissue Assessment

The evaluation of the skin and the soft tissues is of prime importance, as it will lead the surgeon to an appreciation of the degree of violence of the injury. Attempts have been made to grade the degree of injury for both closed (Tscherne and Gotzen 1984) and open (Gustilo 1982) fractures.

Closed Fractures
The medial border of the tibia is subcutaneous, and the skin and subcutaneous tissues are therefore immediately adjacent to the periosteum. The ends of the tibial fracture frequently puncture this skin, creating an open fracture. If a puncture of the skin does not occur, the soft tissue envelope may be stretched by the hematoma and fracture displacement. However, this skin is unable to stretch very much, which causes excessive pressure on the soft tissues, leading to diminished vascularity and pressure necrosis, as exhibited by fracture blisters and dead skin. Furthermore, the muscles in the leg are encased in firm fibrous compartments which are very sensitive to increases in intracompartmental pressure. Compartment syndromes involving all compartments of the leg, the anterior, the lateral, and the posterior, are not infrequent. Therefore, the degree of soft tissue damage in closed fractures is as important as in open fractures and has major prognostic significance.

Any grading system will be handicapped by individual variations in the patients and observer bias. In managing the individual case, therefore, a careful description of the injury is more valuable than assignment of a number (Fig. 20.3). However, for the purpose of comparing results between centers and different treatment regimens, a numerical grading system is helpful, but none has been universally accepted. The following is a suggested grading system (Tscherne and Gotzen 1984; see also Fig. 20.4):

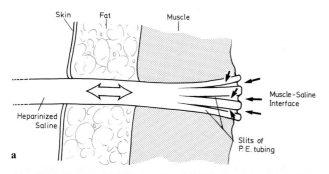

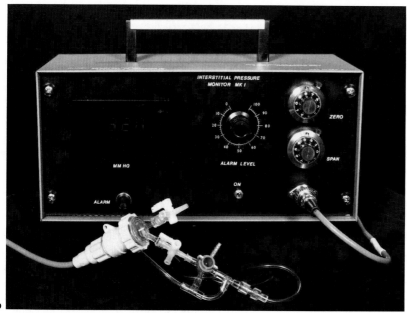

Fig. 20.5 a,b. Continuous compartment monitoring. **a** Position of a slit catheter for measuring compartment pressure. **b** Measuring device for continuous compartment pressure monitoring. (Courtesy of Dr. Cecil Rorabeck)

– Grade 0: little or no soft tissue injury
– Grade 1: superficial abrasion with moderate swelling and bruising of the skin and subcutaneous tissue
– Grade 2: deep contaminated abrasion with tense swelling, excessive bruising, and fracture blisters
– Grade 3: extensive contusion, tense swelling, fracture blisters, with the addition of a compartment syndrome or injury to major vessels

Open Fractures

Many observers have attempted to grade open fractures, but again, in the individual patient, a clear description of the injury is more important than a numerical grade. For example, a grade 1 injury is defined as a small puncture wound (less than 1 cm). However, the location of that small puncture wound is more important than its size. If the puncture wound is on the medial subcutaneous border of the tibia, it might have been caused by relatively low energy, since the skin lies immediately adjacent to the fractured bone. Muscle damage in such a case may be relatively minor (Fig. 20.6 a). However, if the puncture wound is located posteriorly, the bone ends must have penetrated a large mass of muscle to reach the skin. The puncture wound would have been the same size, but the amount of muscle damage is far greater than in the previous case (Fig. 20.6 b). Failure to recognize this fact might have grave consequences for the patient, as inadequate management might lead to gas gangrene.

Therefore, any grading system of open fractures must consider the site of the lesion, the size of the lesion, the degree of muscle damage, the involvement of nerves, tendons, and blood vessels, and, finally, whether a traumatic amputation is present.

The following grading system is relatively widely accepted (Gustilo 1982):

– Grade 1: small puncture wound (<1 cm) with little visible contusion or swelling
– Grade 2: larger wound from without with visible contusion to skin
– Grade 3: severe injury with skin contusion, skin loss, muscle crush or less severe periosteal stripping

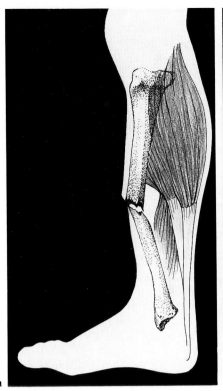 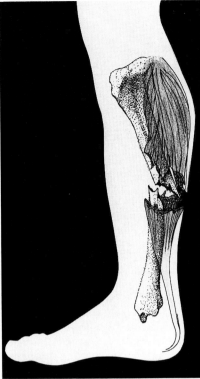

a   b

Fig. 20.6 a,b. Open fracture of the tibia. **a** A high-energy open fracture of the tibia with an anterior subcutaneous puncture wound. Note that the skin may be easily punctured without great damage to muscle. **b** However, the fracture has displaced posteriorly through a massive amount of muscle. Major muscle necrosis may be expected here under a seemingly small skin wound. In this particular situation, inadequate management might lead to grave consequences including gas gangrene. (From Tile 1980)

a) With major muscle loss or nerve or tendon damage
b) With arterial injury
c) With traumatic amputation

b) Bony Assessment

The physical examination of the limb will allow the examiner to assess the stability of the fracture. A careful assessment of the bony injury is essential. All the factors noted in Sect. 20.2.4 must be considered, including the location (articular, metaphyseal, diaphyseal), the morphology (transverse, oblique, spiral), the degree of displacement (high- or low-energy force), and the amount of comminution. Recommendations of radiological techniques are given in the next section.

20.3.2 Radiological Assessment

In the standard examination an anteroposterior, a lateral, and an oblique radiograph will usually allow the surgeon to determine the morphology of the fracture. The radiographs must include views of both the knee and the ankle. If the fracture lines extend into a joint, tomograms are often helpful.

If vascular impairment is suspected, a special examination using arteriography may be indicated.

20.4 Management

20.4.1 Decision Making

The natural outcome of a tibial shaft injury should be a functionally excellent limb and a healed fracture. A decision favoring surgery cannot be taken lightly and must be justified by a careful assessment of the individual fracture. Only if the fracture possesses significant unfavorable personality traits and no major contraindications should surgery be contemplated, and then only by a surgeon and a team well versed in modern operative fracture care. In other words, logical decision making by the astute surgeon depends upon the natural history of the injury, altered by the specific personality traits of the individual case.

Therefore, if no clear indication for surgery exists, the surgeon should proceed with nonoperative treatment.

20.4.2 Nonoperative Treatment

The fracture should be aligned and an above-knee padded plaster applied (Fig. 20.7 a). A general anesthetic is rarely necessary if reduction is carried out shortly after the injury. Gravity reduction with the patient in the sitting position is often all that is required to align the frac-

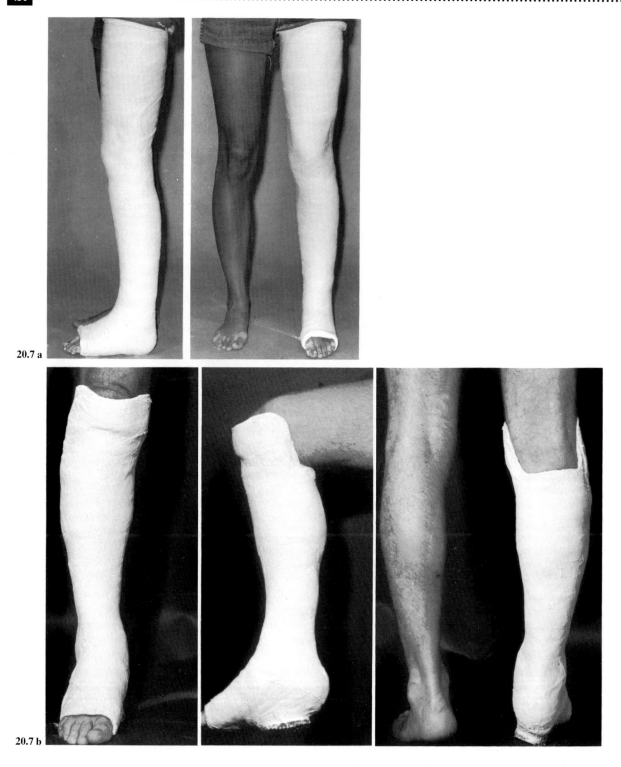

20.7 a

20.7 b

ture. If a padded plaster is not applied, the cast should be split immediately after drying to allow for soft tissue swelling. The patient should be admitted to hospital, the leg well elevated, and the patient closely monitored for any impending compartment syndrome. The use of a continuous monitoring device should rule out the potential catastrophe of a compartment syndrome, as changes in the monitored parameters occur more quickly than the clinical signs and symptoms of pain, pallor, paresthesia, paralysis, and pulselessness and will allow

Fig. 20.7 a–c. Casts and splints in the treatment of tibial fractures. **a** Above-knee walking cast for early weight-bearing treatment in tibial fractures. **b** A functional patellar-bearing below-knee cast. **c** Functional brace allowing ankle and knee motion. (From Sarmiento and Latta 1981)

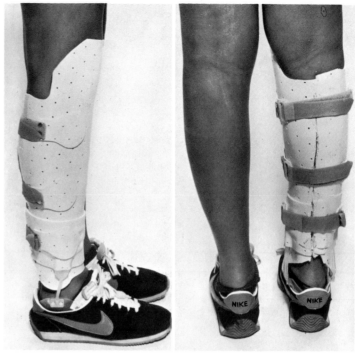

20.7 c

the surgeon to react much quicker to a developing symptom complex.

Once the initial phase of the injury is over, usually in 2 or 3 days, the patient is encouraged to stand upright and begin weight bearing. Many patients have misconceptions about walking on their fractured limb, so a careful educational program should accompany this phase of the treatment. Patients may bear weight on the cast as much as they can tolerate. Usually between the seventh and 14th day, full weight bearing with the use of crutches may be achieved.

When fully weight bearing, the patient may switch to canes as tolerated. Depending on the type of fracture present, the above-knee cast may be converted to a below-knee patellar-bearing plaster (Fig. 20.7 b) or to a functional cast brace between the fourth and eighth week (Fig. 20.7 c). However, there are some fractures that are best left in an above-knee plaster, namely, those occurring close to the knee joint, and those associated with an intact fibula.

With progressive healing, a mobile foot and ankle device is added to the functional splint (see Fig. 20.7 c).

The patient must be carefully monitored throughout the treatment phase: in the early phase to detect the presence of a compartment syndrome, and in the intermediate and later phases to prevent redisplacement of the fracture, leading to malunion, and to detect thromboembolic disease. It must be remembered that many patients with slow fracture healing require protection

for 4–6 months. Failure to recognize this may lead to permanent late displacement of the fracture.

Our motto should be "maximum function in minimum time." With this method, early function is restored to the limb, and most nonindustrial workers can return to their jobs quickly.

20.4.3 Indications for Surgery

If most tibial fractures can be managed successfully by nonoperative means, what, if any, are the indications for surgery?

We have already discussed those factors in the natural history of this injury which may compromise the final result, such as the degree of displacement or instability, the amount of comminution, the presence of an open wound with or without soft tissue or bone loss, and others. Careful assessment of the patient may lead the surgeon to choose an operative approach in order to fulfill the prime aim of fracture care, i.e., a return of the injured limb to full function in the shortest possible time and with relative safety.

A tibial fracture should be fixed for the reasons given below and summarized in Table 20.5.

Table 20.5. Operative indications for tibial fractures

Primary
    Definite
        Associated intra-articular and shaft fracture
        Open fracture
        Major bone loss
        Neurovascular injury
        Limb reimplantation
        Compartment syndrome
        Ipsilateral femoral and tibial fractures ("floating knee")
    Relative
        Unstable fractures – inability to maintain reduction
        Relative shortening
        Segmental fractures
        Tibial fractures with intact fibula
        Transition zone fractures
        Polytrauma
        Enforced bed rest
        High expectations (professional athletes)
Delayed primary
    Failure to maintain reduction
Secondary
    Unacceptable position
    Management of complications

20.4.3.1 Primary Indications

a) Definite Indications

Early assessment of the patient may reveal that operative management of the fracture would be the preferable choice. Under ideal conditions, the situations described below form the more definite indications for surgical intervention, as listed in Table 20.5. The word "definite," as used here, must be preceded by the word "more," indicating that considerable surgical judgment must be exercised in each case.

Associated Intra-articular and Shaft Fractures

Displaced intra-articular fractures in the lower extremity are prime indications for open reduction and internal fixation. If a tibial shaft fracture is associated with a displaced fracture into either the knee or ankle joint, the difficulties of nonoperative management are almost insurmountable. Optimal function can rarely be achieved in these joint injuries without adhering to the basic principles in the management of joint fractures; i.e., anatomical reduction, stable internal fixation, and early motion. In a tibial plateau fracture, the only method by which the surgeon can achieve early motion without operative stabilization is with traction, but if a diaphyseal fracture is also present, this option becomes extraordinarily difficult, if not impossible. Therefore, stabilization of the fracture becomes not only desirable but almost imperative if an excellent functional result is to be obtained.

Diaphyseal fractures of the tibia may be associated with either a tibial plateau fracture into the knee joint or with a fracture into the ankle joint. This combination of a tibial shaft fracture with an intra-articular extension into the knee or the ankle is not uncommon, forming 4.7% of all tibial diaphyseal fractures (Keating et al. 1994). These diaphyseal fractures with extensions into the joint must be anatomically reduced and stabilized using atraumatic techniques. Techniques describing fixation of displaced tibial condyle fractures are described in Chap. 19. Bone grafts are often required to maintain the depressed fragments in their reduced position. Following reduction of the intra-articular fracture, the diaphyseal portion of the injury should be dealt with by plating with a suitable implant. If the metaphysis is greatly comminuted, two buttress plates may be required to restore stability (Fig. 20.8) or occasionally an external fixation frame. This technique of double plating is rarely indicated at this time because of the possible damage to the bone vascularity; therefore, a simple external frame will often suffice as the medial buttress.

Fractures of the tibial diaphysis, especially those in the lower third, associated with a posterolateral butterfly fragment and a displaced lateral malleolar fracture are difficult to manage nonoperatively. Attempts at reducing the ankle often displace the tibial shaft component. Since the posterolateral butterfly is usually connected to the lateral malleolar fragment, only open reduction will allow accurate anatomical restoration and return good, early function to the ankle (Fig. 20.9). Discussion of the distal tibial metaphyseal injury will be found in Chap. 21.

Open Fractures

Treatment of the open fracture of the tibia remains controversial and will be discussed later. However, a consensus of current surgical opinion favors primary stabilization of the open tibia fracture associated with major soft tissue damage. Movement due to imperfect stabilization in plaster may compromise soft tissue healing and may impair the functional result. In our opinion, an improved final result will be achieved by proper stabilization of the fracture, whether by internal or external means, and by sound surgical management of the soft tissue injury.

Major Bone Loss

If a major degree of bone loss is present, the length of the extremity can only be maintained by surgical stabilization of the fracture. Bone loss at the time of injury is always associated with a major open fracture, another definite indication for surgical intervention (Fig. 20.10). Currently, bone transplant techniques would probably be used in this situation.

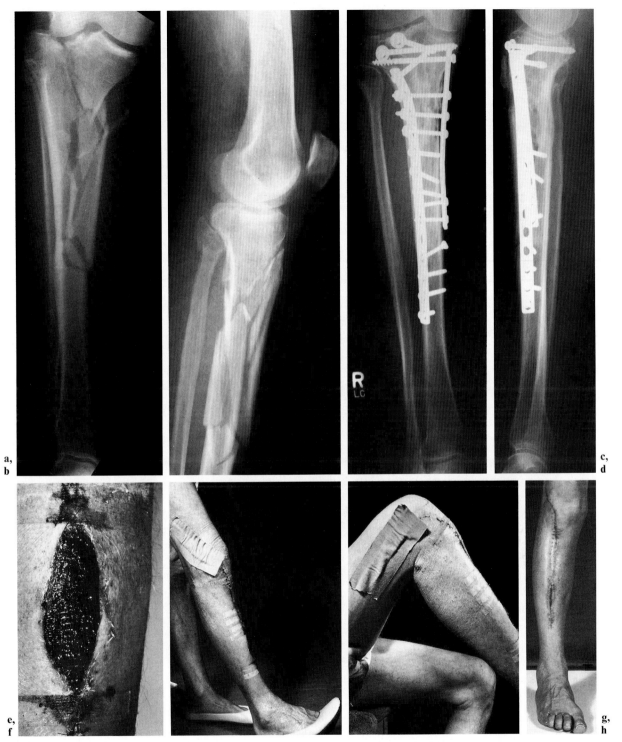

Fig. 20.8 a–h. Associated intra-articular fracture of the knee with tibial shaft fracture. **a,b** Anteroposterior and lateral radiographs of a 60-year-old man who fell 12 feet from a ladder. Note the severe depression of the lateral tibial plateau and severe comminution of both the metaphysis and disphysis of this tibia. **c,d** Anteroposterior and lateral postoperative radiographs showing reconstruction of the joint surface with cancellous lag screws and neutralization of the tibial fracture by a double plate. The medial buttress plate was necessary because of the extreme comminution area and porosity of the bone. A cancellous iliac bone graft was used to fill the gap. Immediate surgery was necessary because of a developing compartment syndrome which in this case was caused by an expanding hematoma rather than increasing edema in the muscle. **e** Postoperatively the lower portion of the wound was left open to avoid tension. **f,g** The state of the limb 10 days postoperatively. Note the excellent knee movement, from full extension to 95° flexion. **h** The lower portion of the incision was allowed to heal by secondary intention and fully epithelialized. The final functional result was excellent. (From Tile 1980)

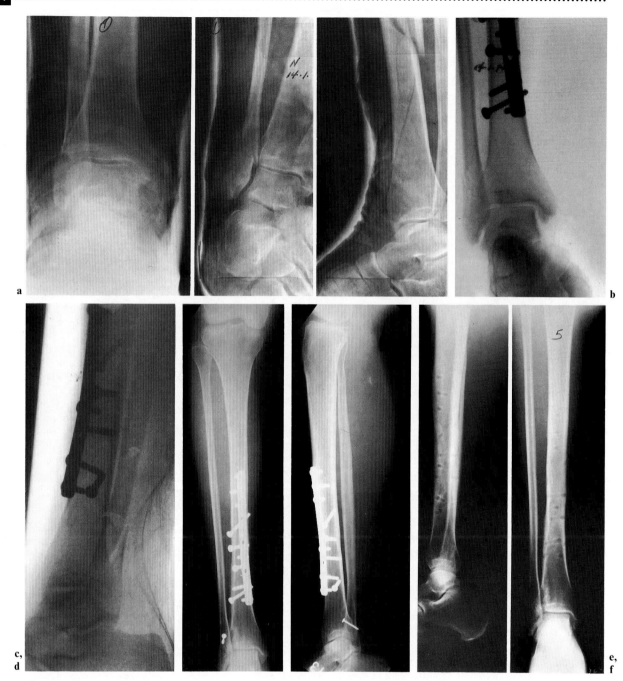

Fig. 20.9 a–f. Fractured ankle associated with tibial diaphyseal fracture. This 29-year-old woman sustained a fracture of the tibia associated with an ankle fracture while skiing. **a** The tibial fracture has a posterolateral butterfly and the lateral malleolus is fractured at the level of the ankle mortise. All attempts to reduce the ankle fracture resulted in displacement at the tibial site, while all attempts to reduce the tibia fracture allowed the ankle to remain in valgus. **b** The anteroposterior intraoperative Polaroid radiograph shows the stable internal fixation by means of three lag screws and a neutralization plate. Note that when the tibia was anatomically reduced the lateral malleolar fracture also reduced with no valgus deformity at the ankle. **c** This is clearly seen on the lateral intraoperative Polaroid radiograph. **d,e** Anteroposterior and lateral radiographs 3 months after surgery show sound primary bone union. A single cancellous lag screw was used to immobilize the fibula. **f** The final appearance at 2 years. The anatomical appearance of the ankle is confirmed by an excellent functional result. (From Tile 1980)

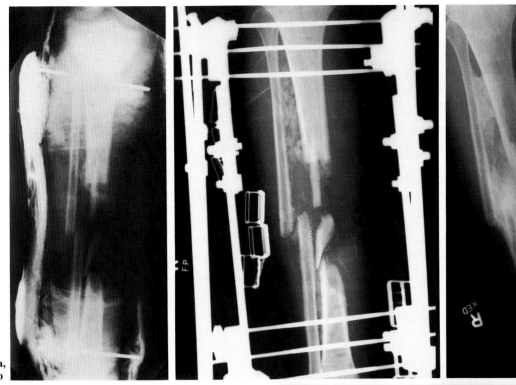

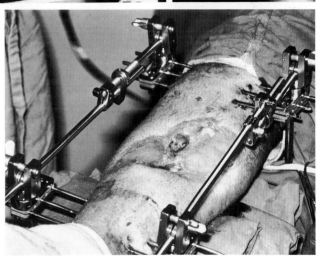

Fig. 20.10 a–d. Open tibial fracture with bone loss.
a Anteroposterior radiograph of a 22-year-old man
injured in a mine accident. This was an open fracture
and much of the tibial shaft was débrided and discarded. The patient was immobilized with a pin above and
below the fracture incorporated in plaster, as seen in
this radiograph. When seen at 5 weeks he had purulent
drainage anteriorly. **b** Treatment consisted of a bilateral
external skeletal fixator and débridement of the anteri-
or wound, followed 2 weeks later by a massive posterolateral bone graft from the tibia to the fibula. **c** The
appearance of the extremity in the bilateral external
fixator. At 8 weeks, a second posterior bone graft was
carried out to span the proximal to distal tibia after
partial consolidation fo the first bone graft had taken
place. **d** The final result at 1 year is of good function in
the foot and ankle and sound union of the fracture.
(From Tile 1980)

Arterial or Nerve Injury

In the past, repair of arterial injuries at the tibial level
has been infrequent, but with refinements in microvascular techniques, it is becoming more common.
Although not essential, stabilization of the fracture
enhances the possibility of successful microvascular
repair, and we recommend it highly in such cases.
Stabilization of the fracture is also desirable following
primary repair of an injured lower extremity nerve.
However, it must be understood that the combination of
an open tibial fracture with a vascular injury gives a
poor prognosis for the limb. In such cases, especially in
a crushing injury, early amputation may be the best form
of treatment in select cases.

Limb Reimplantation

The ultimate open arterial injury is the severed limb. The
advent and advance of microvascular techniques have
made the salvage of severed limbs both possible and
desirable. The first step in such a procedure is to stabilize
the fracture; therefore, limb reimplantation is an absolute indication. However, as stated above, in lesions

through the tibia, especially with crushing, amputation is the treatment of choice.

Compartment Syndrome

We have already stated that compartment syndromes are not uncommon following closed treatment of tibial fractures. The advent of continuous monitoring devices should prevent the disastrous complication of Volkmann's ischemic contracture from occurring. Early recognition, followed by immediate decompression of the involved compartment or compartments, will achieve this end. Following decompression, open reduction through the same incision and stable internal fixation of the unstable fracture are highly desirable and will simplify the further management of the patient (Fig. 20.8). Stability of the fracture will prevent further damage to the soft tissues and will allow early motion of the extremity, which should reduce edema. Also, it will permit the limb to be handled during the many necessary dressing changes and secondary skin procedures without fear of losing the reduction. These advantages so outweigh any theoretical disadvantages that we regard the association of a tibial fracture with a compartment syndrome as a definite indication for stabilization.

Ipsilateral Fractured Femur and Tibia: "Floating Knee" Syndrome

The combination of a fracture of the tibia with a fracture of the ipsilateral femur has given rise to notoriously poor results when both fractures have been treated nonoperatively (Fraser et al. 1978). These fractures are often associated with a severe injury to the knee joint, frequently called the "floating knee." Nonoperative care usually results in impaired knee function and difficulty with one or other fracture. Optimal management consists of stabilization of both fractures, followed by careful evaluation of the knee injury. This, in turn, may be managed by primary ligamentous repair, if necessary, and early active or continuous passive motion.

b) Relative Indications

If any or some of the factors listed below are present in the particular fracture to be treated, they should be taken as more relative indications that operative stabilization is the preferred method of management; again, this should only be undertaken under ideal conditions, as previously outlined.

Relative Shortening

Sarmiento and Latta (1981) stated that most longitudinally unstable tibial fractures of the short oblique or spiral variety do not excessively shorten when placed in a proper cast. They based this assertion on both clinical and experimental observations, and we agree fully with them. However, there are instances, albeit rare, when unacceptable shortening is present at the initial examination (Fig. 20.11). The desirability of carrying out an open reduction, therefore, will depend entirely on the total personality of the injury, as discussed previously. The treatment will obviously differ for a young patient with 3 cm of shortening and high expectation of a cosmetically and functionally perfect result than for an elderly patient with a similar injury. In our opinion, when excessive shortening is present, the surgeon should discuss the treatment options with the patient, who in turn should share in the management decision, based on informed consent.

Segmental Fractures

In our view, proper open reduction will give more satisfactory results in select cases of segmental fracture than nonoperative means. Nonoperative treatment of a segmental fracture is difficult, and, frequently, the final result is compromised by delayed union at one or other site, by malalignment, and by shortening (Fig. 20.12).

Fractures of the Tibia with Intact Fibula

This particular fracture remains controversial. Many surgeons feel that the management of this injury may be nonoperative with no increase in complications (Sarmiento et al. 1989), but others regard the complications to be excessive (O'Dwyer et al. 1993) found that healing of associated fractures with poor personality traits such as open fractures or high-energy displaced fractures was delayed. It is clear that the displaced fractured tibia associated with an intact fibula is difficult, though not impossible, to maintain in plaster. Drift of the tibia into varus is common and difficult to overcome; delayed union and nonunion are also common. Teitz et al. (1980) reviewed 23 patients of more than 20 years of age and found complications in 61%, including six with varus malunion and six with delayed union or nonunion. Therefore, early surgery should be considered for these cases. The key word is *displaced*; a relatively undisplaced fracture may be managed nonoperatively, but grossly displaced fractures, often with disruption of the interosseous membrane up to and including the proximal tibiofibular joint, are best treated operatively. We favor this approach in most cases, allowing the patient to share in the decision. If closed treatment is used, it must be remembered that the plaster must extend above the knee in almost full extension until the fracture is healed, because this fracture may angulate *late* in the treatment cycle.

Transition Zone Fractures

Fractures through the transitional area between the metaphysis and diaphysis are mainly through cancellous

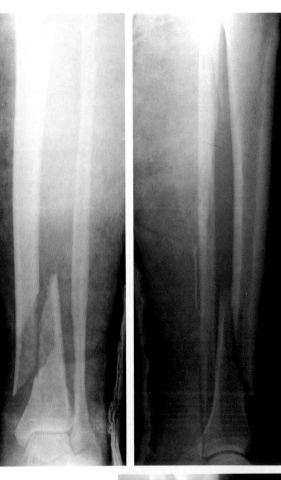

Fig. 20.11 a–f. Transition zone fracture of the tibia into the metaphysis with wide displacement and shortening. **a,b** The anteroposterior and lateral radiographs of this 53-year-old man show a long spiral fracture extending from the lower third into the metaphysis. This fracture occurred during skiing. Two centimeters of shortening are noted. Because of the wide displacement of this fracture, associated with significant shortening, and in consultation with the patient, open reduction and internal fixation were felt to be the preferred treatment. **c** The clinical photograph shows the wide gap present at the time of surgery. **d** Reduction was easily obtained with the use of the AO distractor. Note the two interfragmental screws in position. **e,f** The final result, showing a medially placed neutralization plate and an anatomical reduction. Function returned quickly to the extremity, and the fracture was healed within 10 weeks

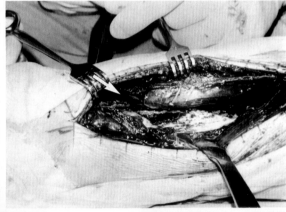

a, b

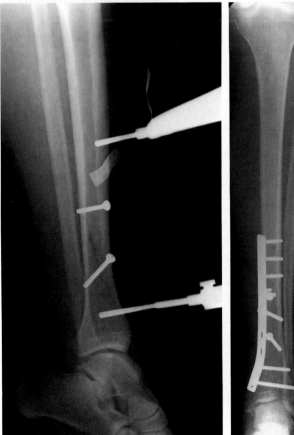

c

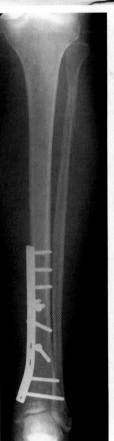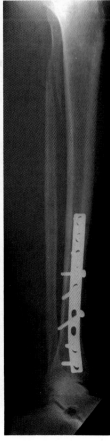

d

e, f

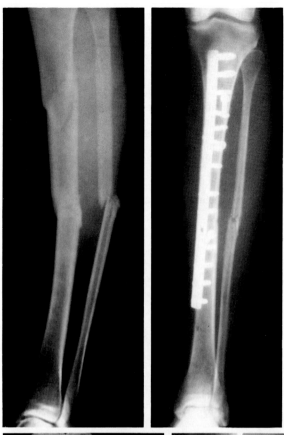

bone, which contains large numbers of osteoblastic cells, and therefore, normally, few problems in healing should be encountered. However, we find that union in these particular fractures in any long bone, especially the tibia, may be delayed (Fig. 20.13).

In the young, the metaphysis and the transition zone between the diaphysis and metaphysis is strong; fractures of this area in young people therefore often mean an injury caused by high violence.

On initial inspection of the radiographs, some degree of comminution and gap may be present, which may persist even after reduction (Fig. 20.13 b). Since cancellous bone heals well if compressed, and often poorly if not, and since compression may be achieved quite simply by interfragmental compression, the entire outlook for the patient and his or her fracture may be changed dramatically by an early decision favoring surgery (see Fig. 20.11).

Fig. 20.12 a–f. Segmental fracture of the tibia. **a,b** Anteroposterior radiograph of a segmental fracture treated by open reduction and internal fixation. **c–f** A patient treated by a closed intramedullary nail distally locked, a preferred technique where technically possible

a,
b

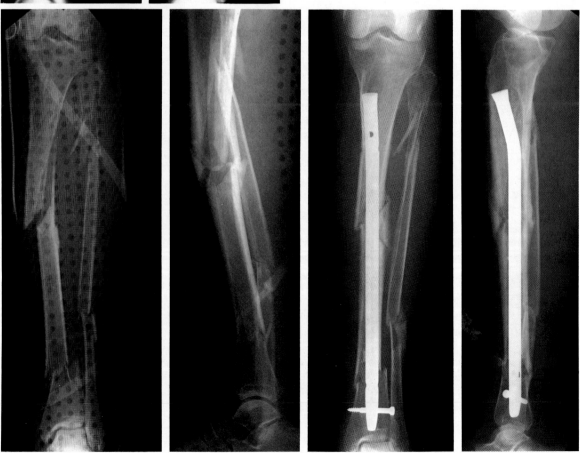

c,
d

e,
f

Fractures through this area may be of two distinct types, the shear type and the compression type, each with their own specific problems. The *shear* injury is characterized by gross instability indicated by a large gap between the fragments and marked comminution. If closed reduction fails to close the large gap often present in these fractures, we favor early stabilization by the appropriate means, usually internal fixation with inter-fragmental compression and a neutralization plate (Fig. 20.9) or a locked intramedullary nail, if technically possible (see Fig. 20.12 c-f). In the elderly population, fractures through this region may almost be considered pathological, since the osteoporotic process has its greatest effect in the metaphysis. Although more commonly associated with delayed union and nonunion in humeral and femoral fractures, osteoporosis can play the same role in fractures of the tibia.

Compression injuries to the metaphysis caused by direct trauma may cause so great a crush that, when reduction has been performed, a large gap will be present at the site of bone compression. Such fractures are notoriously difficult to maintain in the reduced position and consideration should be given to early operative intervention with bone graft. Since this applies more to the so-called pilon fracture than to tibial fractures, it will be discussed more fully in Chap. 21.

Polytrauma

Current surgical practice strongly favors stabilization of lower-extremity diaphyseal fractures in polytraumatized patients. This is especially true in patients in whom the upright position is necessary for treatment of the many chest complications often seen in these individuals. Several studies have shown that the morbidity rate in these patients is diminished if early stabilization of the fractures is performed and the patient is mobilized quickly (Border et al. 1975). Furthermore, these patients had better final functional results of the fracture itself. For the tibia, however, this is only a relative indication because patients with tibial fractures can be maintained in light plaster casts and mobilized early without resorting to surgery.

Conditions Requiring Prolonged Bed Rest

If the patient has a major pelvic ring disruption or injury about the hip joint that will prevent early weight bearing on that extremity, consideration should be given to stabilization of the tibial fracture. However, this is only indicated if careful assessment of the fracture indicates an increased risk of delayed union.

High-Expectation Patients (Professional Athletes)

In some patients, the desire for a perfect result is so high that operative fixation of the fracture becomes preferable to nonoperative treatment. This would be especially true

in professional athletes requiring full knee and ankle motion, especially in sports such as skiing, basketball, or track and field sports. Socioeconomic factors rarely play a part in the decision making for the tibia because most individuals can function very well with the functional weight bearing casts and splints now available.

20.4.3.2 Delayed Primary Indications

Grossly unstable fractures of the tibia may be difficult to maintain in an acceptably reduced position. This is especially true if comminution is extreme. In those cases, shortening and/or angulation may occur in plaster. If this situation arises, we prefer early fracture stabilization when it becomes apparent that closed methods are failing.

20.4.3.3 Secondary Indications

a) Delayed Reduction

Patients referred late with an unacceptable reduction of their fracture will require open reduction if, as often occurs, closed reduction fails. Open reduction may be hazardous, since soft tissue contracture is the rule. The AO/ASIF distractor is an invaluable instrument in such cases, minimizing the need for excessive soft tissue stripping and achieving normal length at the fracture site (see Fig. 20.11).

b) Complications of Fractures

Open methods are required for the management of such complications as delayed union or nonunion, malunion or sepsis. We stress again that surgery should only be carried out according to the strict biological and biomechanical principles outlined in the next few pages and by an experienced surgical team with a full armamentarium.

Having completed the decision-making process and having decided upon operative intervention, we must now decide when to intervene and how to fix the fracture.

20.4.4 Role of Amputation in Severe Tibial Fractures

In the past decade, much has been written about "salvage or amputation" for severe tibial trauma. It is clear that some patients would be better served by an immediate amputation than by futile attempts at limb salvage, which would lead to amputation secondarily. Bondurant et al.

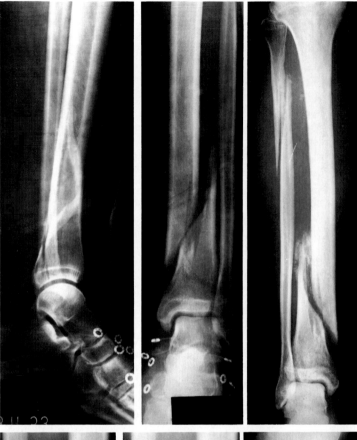

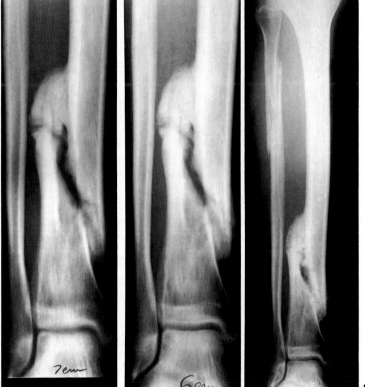

Table 20.6. MESS (*Mangled Extremity Severity Score*) variables

		Points
A.	Skeletal/soft-tissue injury	
	Low energy (stab; simple fracture; „civilian" GSW)	1
	Medium energy (open or multiple Fxs, dislocation)	2
	High energy (close-range shotgun or „military" GSW, crush injury)	3
	Very high energy (above + gross contamination, soft-tissue avulsion)	4
B.	Limb ischemia	
	Pulse reduced or absent but perfusion normal	1*
	Pulseless; paresthesias, diminished capillary refill	2*
	Cool, paralyzed, insensate, numb	3*
C.	Shock	
	Systolic BP always > 90 mm Hg	0
	Hypotensive transiently	1
	Persistent hypotension	2
D.	Age (yrs)	
	< 30	0
	30–50	1
	> 50	2

* Score doubled for ischemia > 6 hours

Fig. 20.13 a–d. Transition zone fracture. **a** This 53-year-old man sustained a long spiral fracture of his tibia and fibula while skiing. He was treated in an above-knee plaster and began weight bearing immediately. **b** In spite of early weight bearing union was delayed (shown here at 5 months). **c** The tomograms taken at 7 months show union to be complete at the periphery but not at the center of the lesion. **d** Bony union was complete at 1 year. The patient's ankle movement was good, but he continued to have tenderness and some pain on weight bearing at that stage; 1 cm of shortening was present. This type of long spiral fracture in the metaphysis, when associated with comminution, a large gap at the fracture site, and shortening, may be considerably delayed in union and therefore represents a relative indication for surgery. (From Tile 1980)

(1988) found that patient outcome was significantly better at lower cost for amputation done primarily. This subject will always depend on many factors in the patient and the surgeon. There is general unanimity that in patients with Gustilo type III fractures with a vascular injury the limb should be amputated primarily (Claude and Stern 1987; Hansen 1987; Lange et al. 1985). Johansen et al. (1983) proposed a mangled extremity score (MESS) to bring an objective measure to a subjective problem (Table 20.6). Gregory et al. (1985) found the use of the MESS score (>20) to be predictive of amputation. The surgeon must assess the general state of the patient, as well as the degree of local injury (vascular, neurological, soft tissue) in making this difficult decision.

20.4.5 Timing of Surgery

The exact timing of operative treatment is extremely important and will have a major bearing on the eventual outcome of the fracture. Ideally, we prefer early to late surgery in tibial fractures, but not if this means operating through excessively traumatized skin or soft tissue. Moreover, in this subcutaneous bone, closed intramedullary techniques are, where possible, preferred to open techniques. The surgeon must carefully weigh and balance the various factors influencing the decision, such as the following:

1. General factors
   - The severity of other injuries in polytraumatized patients
   - The general medical state of the patient
2. Local factors
   - The time elapsed since injury
   - The state of the skin and soft tissues
   - The importance of the surgical indication
   - The type of surgical intervention planned

If the patient is seen shortly after injury and there is a strong indication for surgical treatment, then that surgery should proceed immediately. Swelling is usually minimal at this stage, so already traumatized skin will not be subjected to further damage by pressure, as would happen if treatment were delayed. For open methods, an atraumatic operative technique, evacuation of the fracture hematoma, stable fixation of the bone to prevent further soft tissue damage, and adequate postoperative suction drainage should lead to good wound healing with little trouble.

Closed intramedullary techniques are favored for closed fractures, since no incisions will be made at the fracture site. However, timing is important, since adding a reamed intramedullary nail to an already maximally swollen leg may give rise to a compartment syndrome.

One added advantage of early surgery is the ease of fracture reduction, since no fixed shortening of the soft tissues has occurred. Early restoration of the normal muscle length without contracture allows early painless motion of the extremity.

If, however, the patient arrives late, or for other reasons surgery is delayed beyond 8–24 h after injury, the situation may change dramatically. The extremity may become very swollen and the skin ecchymotic, with areas of fracture blisters. Operative intervention through this type of skin is fraught with obvious danger and may lead to disaster. Therefore, unless a major absolute indication exists, such as an open fracture or a compartment syndrome, it is best to delay surgery until the skin has become revascularized or areas of skin loss have become apparent. The patient should remain in bed, with the limb elevated and inspected frequently. If the fracture is displaced and pressing on the skin, it must be reduced closed to reduce the compression effect on the soft tissues. It is often necessary to delay the surgical intervention for 7–14 days until it is safe to proceed. In this situation, the operative reduction of the fracture becomes difficult and may require the use of a distractor, as described below. If possible, where traumatized skin precludes a surgical incision, the surgeon should turn to closed nailing as the technique of choice, if practicable. Recent advances in nailing techniques, namely, the locking type of nail, have extended the indications for nailing in tibial fractures, making it a more viable option in this particular type of case (see Fig. 20.12 c–f).

In summary, a careful analysis of the individual patient will lead the astute surgeon to the correct decision. Early operative intervention is ideal for patients with a major indication, but it should never be carried out through doubtful skin. In such cases, it is far safer to delay surgery and deal with the late technical difficulties by established techniques.

20.4.6 Surgical Methods

We have now decided which tibial fractures should be fixed and when to fix them. We now turn our attention to the surgical methods. Any operative intervention must be carried out according to strict biological and biomechanical principles with careful attention to detail. The skin incision must be carefully planned and executed and all biological tissue handled with atraumatic techniques. The internal fixation should be stable enough to allow the surgeon to do without most external appliances such as casts or splints. In this decade, fixations such as those shown in Fig. 20.14 are inexcusable. The surgeon must always remember that the weak link in the system is the bone and, therefore, many of the tech-

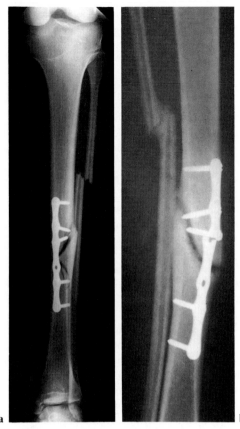

a   b

Fig. 20.14 a,b. How not to do internal fixation. This fracture could have been treated nonoperatively, but the surgeon elected to perform operative intervention. **a** Note that the postero-lateral fragment has not been fixed with lag screws. The screws holding this inadequate plate also enter the fracture, thereby holding it apart. **b** In spite of 16 weeks in plaster, the fracture failed to unite and the plate eventually broke. (From Tile 1980)

niques are not appropriate for patients with extremely osteoporotic bone. If the bone is porotic, but a strong indication for surgery exists, then special techniques must be used, such as cement augmentation followed by external protection of the fixation. Several conflicting factors often coexist, as, for instance, in the case of a displaced fracture in the knee in an elderly individual with osteoporotic bone, so that time and again, the surgeon is required to exercise sound judgment and choose the best treatment for his or her patient.

20.4.6.1 Approaches

The choice of incision is dependent upon many factors, including the degree of skin trauma, the presence of an open wound, the type and location of the fracture, and the type of surgical intervention.

As a general principle, no incision should ever be made directly over a subcutaneous bone. Even a relatively minor stitch abscess or small area of wound necrosis will assume much greater significance if the incision has been made directly over the subcutaneous surface rather than over soft tissue. Also, an incision over bone would limit the location of the implant, since the implant should not be placed directly under the incision, for obvious reasons. This is especially true in the tibia, since the skin over the subcutaneous border of the tibia is often poorly vascularized and skin breakdown not uncommon, but is also true for the ulna, the clavicle, and any other subcutaneous bone.

The periosteum and surrounding anterior muscle mass must be handled with extreme care. The fracture should always be exposed through its torn soft tissue envelope. Only as much intact periosteum should be stripped back as is necessary to expose the fracture. All soft tissue attachments to bone must be preserved and only atraumatic reduction techniques used.

a) Standard Anterolateral Approach

Our standard incision is made 1 cm lateral to the subcutaneous anterior border of the tibia, lying over the anterior compartment muscle mass (Fig. 20.15). This incision offers many advantages including:

1. *Extensile exposure.* The entire tibia from knee to ankle may be exposed through this incision. At the upper end, it may be carried laterally to expose the lateral tibial plateau, and at the ankle it may be carried either laterally or medially to expose the tibial articular surface. Therefore, it is truly an extensile approach and any tibial fracture can be fixed through this incision. Since the incision is over soft tissue only and not over bone, minor problems in the incision assume less importance. The major potential problem is at the distal end, in the region of the anterior tibial tendon. In this area, the incision should curve just medial to the tendon. Great care is necessary to ensure that the tendon sheath remain closed if possible; if it is opened, it should be resutured so that the tendon itself is not directly under the incision.
2. *Open wound treatment.* In open fractures, the wound should be left open. If under excessive tension, the wound in a primary open reduction and internal fixation for a closed fracture must also be left open (see Fig. 20.8). With careful planning of the incision, the bone and implants will remain covered.
3. *Medially based flap.* Since the incision is lateral to the subcutaneous surface, the skin flap will be based medially, in an area of higher vascularity, and skin sloughs will not normally occur. It is important, how-

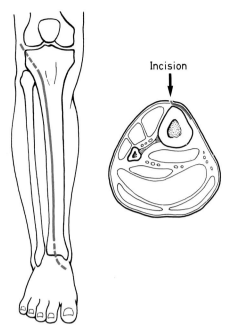

Fig. 20.15. Anterolateral approach to the tibia. The incision is made 1 cm lateral to the anterior crest of the tibia on the anterior tibial muscle mass. This incision allows the surgeon to raise a medially based flap which can then cover any internal fixation on either the lateral or medial surface of the tibia. If a wound breakdown occurs, this incision has the added advantage of not being directly over the fixation or the bone

ever, that the subcutaneous tissues be handled with great delicacy. Since the skin is vascularized from its deep surface, it is essential that the entire subcutaneous layer be taken with the skin when the medially based flap is raised and the anterior surface of the tibia exposed, otherwise skin necrosis will ensue.

Note: If the patient has had a recent incision along the posteromedial border of the tibia, an anterolateral incision should not be made, as the area between the two incisions is poorly vascularized and major necrosis of the flap may ensue. Under these circumstances, the previous incision should always be used.

Presently, there is a tendency to carry out biological plating without exposing the fracture site. This may be performed using this incision, but tunneling under the central part of the tibia, using only the ends of this incision for fixation.

b) Posteromedial Approach

The posteromedial incision, made 1 cm posterior to the medial border of the tibia, is useful for decompression of the deep posterior compartment of the leg. Open reduc-

tion may be performed using the subcutaneous surface or the posterior surface of the tibia if necessary (Fig. 20.16).

c) Posterolateral Approach

The posterolateral approach with the patient in the prone or lateral position is excellent for secondary bone grafting procedures, especially if the anterior skin is badly traumatized (Fig. 20.17 a, b). It may also be used in open fractures with skin loss and ensuing sepsis. Care should be taken not to violate the anterior compartment in those cases. An added advantage is the possibility of incorporating the fibula in the grafting procedures if there is a gap in the tibia due to bone loss (Fig. 20.17 c–i).

d) Incision for Closed Nailing

In suitable cases, closed nailing techniques with or without locking devices, will be ideal, with the added advantage of not further traumatizing the skin at the fracture site. We prefer a longitudinal incision just medial to the tibial tubercle, with the point of bone perforation dependent on a central siting on the preoperative radiograph. Thus, the entry may be central, by splitting the patellar tendon (Fig. 20.18), or medial, beside the tibial tubercle.

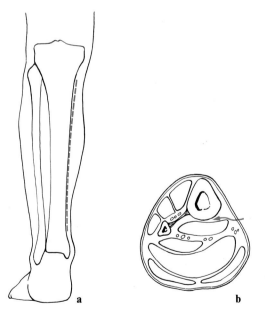

Fig. 20.16 a,b. Posteromedial approach to the tibia. This approach should rarely be used in acute trauma. **a** The incision is made 1 cm posterior to the medial border of the tibia over the muscle mass. **b** The posterior surface of the tibia may be approached by raising a small skin flap, as shown in the cross-section

20.4.6.2 Reduction Techniques

The 1990s is the era of biological reduction and fixation techniques. Atraumatic handling of the soft tissues has always been a hallmark of the AO method, but was over-shadowed by biomechanical stability. In the tibial shaft, both are essential, i.e., atraumatic reduction and fixation techniques as well as retention of biomechanical stability.

The resurgence of intrameduallary nailing led to the concept of indirect reduction technqiues. Fractures managed by intrameduallary nailing, even if not anatomically reduced, often healed quickly, because all soft tissue to bone was retained. In the tibia, intrameduallary techniques are now preferred, which may be yet another pendulum swing. In the era prior to locking nails, Lottes (1974) showed excellent results with an unreamed nail and a cast.

If tibia fractures are to be treated openly with plates, all soft tissues to bone must be retained. Reduction may be gently obtained with traction or with the use of a distraction device (Fig. 20.19)

Reduction should restore length, restore alignment, and restore stability, but it may do so without necessarily being absolutely anatomical in the tibial diaphysis.

20.4.6.3 Fixation

We have stressed the importance of atraumatic techniques for the skin and soft tissues; careful handling of the skeletal tissue is equally vital. As the soft tissue cover on the tibia is sparse, indiscriminate handling of the bone may destroy all vestiges of soft tissue attachment, which in turn may lead to death of the skeletal tissue, delayed union, and, possibly, implant failure.

Rationale for Implant Selection

Careful planning is required to achieve stable fracture fixation. The preoperative radiographs must be of excellent quality, capable of showing all possible lines of comminution, as this will affect the type and position of the implants. Preoperative drawings should be made from these radiographs. With them the surgeon can carefully plan the internal fixation and instruct the operating room personnel about the necessary implants. The method of internal fixation chosen will, in turn, direct the type of incision used. For the tibia, many methods are available for achieving stable fixation, including:

1. Splintage with intramedullary devices
   – Rigid – reamed
   – Stable – unreamed ± locking

   – Flexible
2. Internal fixation – biological plating
   – Compression – interfragmental lag screws
   – Axial compression with tension band plates
   – Neutralization plates
   – Buttress plates
3. External fixation – may compress, neutralize, or buttress
4. Combined methods of internal and external fixation

The selection of any particular method of stabilization depends upon a knowledge of the natural history of the fracture, namely, those factors which make up the personality of the injury. This includes a careful assessment first of the soft tissue injury and then of the fracture pattern. Both must be considered in any management plan. Of equal importance in the decision-making process is the state of the bone, i.e., whether it is normal or osteoporotic and therefore unable to hold screws.

The first step in decision-making regarding the method of fixation is a careful assessment of the soft tissue injury, whether the fracture is a closed fracture or an open fracture.

Closed Fractures

As indicated previously closed injuries themselves may be further classified (Tscherne and Gotzen 1984). Since

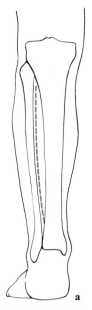
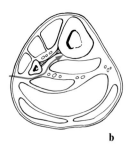

Fig. 20.17 a, b. The posterolateral approach to the tibia. **a** The skin incision, with the patient in the prone position. **b** The dissection proceeds posterior to the peroneal muscles, along the interosseous membrane, to the posterior aspect of the tibia. Exposure of the posterior of the middle third of the tibia is excellent. This approach is excellent for tibial nonunions, especially with poor anterior skin

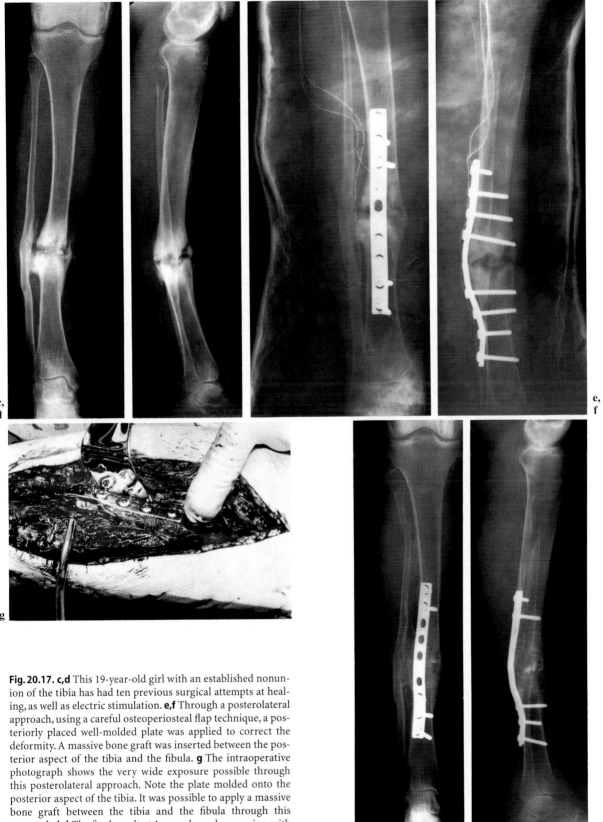

Fig. 20.17. c,d This 19-year-old girl with an established nonunion of the tibia has had ten previous surgical attempts at healing, as well as electric stimulation. **e,f** Through a posterolateral approach, using a careful osteoperiosteal flap technique, a posteriorly placed well-molded plate was applied to correct the deformity. A massive bone graft was inserted between the posterior aspect of the tibia and the fibula. **g** The intraoperative photograph shows the very wide exposure possible through this posterolateral approach. Note the plate molded onto the posterior aspect of the tibia. It was possible to apply a massive bone graft between the tibia and the fibula through this approach. **h,i** The final result at 1 year shows bony union with cross-union to the fibula

466 •••

Chapter 20   Fractures of the Tibia

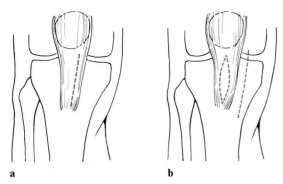

Fig. 20.18 a,b. Incision for closed nailing. **a** This incision should be longitudinal, just medial to the tibial tubercle and extending proximally to the patella, along the medial third of the patellar tendon. **b** The deep portion of the incision is developed either along the medial subcutaneous border of the tibia or through the split patellar tendon. The preoperative radiographic assessment will determine the entry point of the nail

Fig. 20.19 a,b. Biologic reduction techniques. **a** If open reduction and plate fixation are to be used for tibial fractures, reduction techniques must be atraumatic and where possible indirect. Two examples include the articulating tension device used to distract the fracture, in this place with a butterfly fragment against the plate attached distally. Virtually no dissection is required of the main fragments, thereby ensuring blood supply. **b** The same effect can be obtained with the use of the AO distractor, allowing indirect reduction through traction while maintaining blood supply

the tibia is subcutaneous, high-energy injury without laceration of the skin may produce an even worse soft tissue injury than a puncture wound which is open. Therefore, the skin and subcutaneous tissues need to be examined for contusion, edema, fracture blisters (traumatic bullae), skin avulsions from the underlying tissues, and finally vascular and neurological injury. Closed soft tissue injury which is of low grades, i.e., very little damage, may be amenable to any technique in our armamentarium, but high-grade soft tissue injuries must be carefully managed, usually by closed means to avoid the complications of skin necrosis and sepsis. After careful examination of the soft tissue injury the surgeon must then determine the location and morphology of the fracture itself: firstly, whether it is articular, metaphyseal, or diaphyseal, and secondly, the degree of comminution of the fracture itself.

Associated Articular Fractures with Shaft Fractures. Displaced articular fractures of the ankle or knee require anatomical reduction of the joint surface whether associated with other fractures in the tibia or not.

In *closed* fractures with a low grade soft tissue injury, open reduction and internal fixation with interfragmental lag screws is the method of choice. Buttress plates are usually required for the metaphyseal component but great care must be taken to preserve the blood supply to the bony fragments (see Fig. 20.8). If the diaphysis is involved, the plate fixation may be extended to that frac-

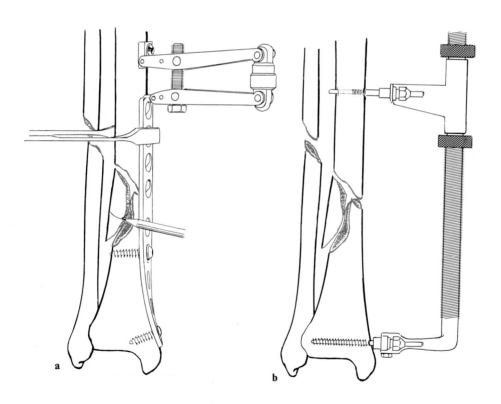

ture from the metaphysis or other combinations may be used, such as screws and plates at the joint and intramedullary devices in the shaft. Careful preoperative planning is essential if such combinations are to be used.

In patients that have a high-grade soft tissue injury and a metaphyseal fracture, different techniques may be required. The current trend is to use minimal internal fixation of the joint surface by percutaneous techniques under image intensification. Limited small incisions may be used to elevate joint fractures; alternatively, the joint may be examined under arthroscopy and the articular surface reduced under arthroscopic vision. Kirschner wires and/or cannulated screws are used to fix the articular portion of the fracture. If the skin and soft tissues have returned to a normal state, open surgery can be done safely. In many of these high-energy polytrauma patients, the metaphyseal portion of the fracture is better managed by external means. External frames, either standard varieties or a ring fixator, associated with a standard proximal or distal fixation depending on whether the knee or ankle is involved, are highly recommended. This will allow stability of the fracture and adequate soft tissue healing without endangering the underlying bone or subjecting patients to an increased risk of skin necrosis and/or sepsis.

Therefore, the principles of articular anatomical reduction and stabilization of the metaphysis or shaft fractures are adhered to, but the technology involved varies with the soft tissue injury. Under ideal circumstances open reduction and internal fixation with careful atraumatic techniques will afford excellent results, but under less than ideal circumstances a standard ring fixator with a limited percutaneous approach under arthroscopic or image intensification will be safer for the patient.

Metaphyseal (Nonarticular) Fractures. In nonarticular closed fractures of the metaphysis, the method of internal fixation of metaphyseal fractures most favorable will depend on the exact location of the fracture (proximal or distal), the degree of comminution, the state of the bone, and the state of the soft tissues.

In ideal circumstances, with a low-grade soft tissue injury and normal bone, fractures close to the joint are best managed by plate fixation, depending on the degree of comminution. For unicortical comminution, one plate will suffice; for bicortical comminution, two plates are occasionally used. Under ideal circumstances, if the surgeon is well versed in biological fixation techniques. The area of comminution should be bridged without disturbing the blood supply to viable bone fragments. Alternatively, the medial cortex may be buttressed with a simple external frame (Fig. 20.20). Fractures within the metaphysis but more removed from the joint may be managed by plating or by a locked intramedullary nail, if careful preoperative planning indicates that this is technically possible (Fig. 20.21).

In *osteoporotic* bone, screws may not hold. Therefore, postoperative immobilization may be necessary if plates are used. Flexible intramedullary pins may be desirable in such cases.

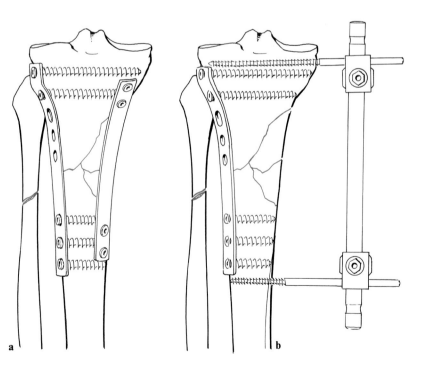

Fig. 20.20 a,b. In metaphyseal fractures of the proximal tibia with bicortical comminution various forms of fixation may be required. **a** A laterally placed plate bridging the area of comminution is supplemented by a medial buttress which, as noted, also bridges the comminuted area, leaving all blood supply to bone intact. **b** A simple external fixator may also be used as a medial buttress and has the advantage of buttressing the comminuted area without disturbing the blood supply to the fragments

468 •••

Chapter 20   **Fractures of the Tibia**

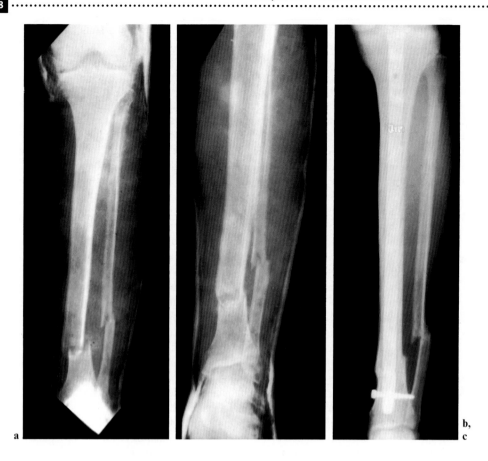

Fig. 20.21 a–c. Closed nailing for metaphyseal fracture. **a** Anteroposterior radiograph of the tibia of a 22-year-old poly-traumatized man. **b** Excessive valgus deformation is visible. **c** The closed nailing of this distal fracture was achieved with a single distal locking screw following careful preoperative planning

Early open surgery should not be attempted through severely traumatized skin, which is often present in fractures of the distal tibia. In these cases, the limb should be elevated and immobilized in traction or external fixation, and surgery performed after the blisters have disappeared and the skin has revascularized.

In the distal tibia with severely traumatized skin and soft tissues in a closed injury, it is more prudent to use external fixation, with a standard anterior or Delta external frame or a distal ring fixator attached to a standard two-pin configuration in the upper tibia (see Chap. 21). This will allow excellent healing of the soft tissues without a traumatic event of incising them.

Fixation of the Fibula. In the distal tibia, especially under conditions of a severe soft tissue injury where open surgery is not contemplated, a lateral incision and open reduction and internal fixation of the fibular frac-

ture may be extremely helpful in restoring length and in achieving some lateral stability in conjunction with the external fixator. The tendency for valgus deformation will be resisted by this technique.)

Intramedullary Nails. The tendency to extend the indications for locked intramedullary nails to fractures in the proximal and distal metaphysis needs to be reexamined. In the distal tibia, if two distal locking screws can be inserted, this is the method of choice where skin and soft tissue lesions preclude an open operation. However, in the proximal tibia, it has been extremely difficult to achieve stability with the very proximal fractures. This has allowed early drifting of the fracture into valgus deformation, and many series now show unacceptable positions following this technique. It is preferable to use an alternative technique, such as external fixation, where open surgery is contraindicated. Should the surgeon find that the locked nail is not stable and is drifting into valgus, the additional use of a temporary fixator may rescue the unpleasant situation. The recently introduced pinless fixator may be indicated for a 6-week period during the initial healing phase to prevent valgus deformation. Other techniques for this particular situation include a biological plating through two small incisions by tunneling the plate under the lateral muscles. The plate must be prebent anatomically from the radiographs.

Diaphyseal Fractures. In closed fractures of the diaphysis, the methods available include open reduction and internal fixation with interfragmental screws combined with neutralization plates, tension band plates, or intramedullary devices, both rigid and flexible.

Since the circulation of the pretibial skin is so precarious, even in the best of circumstances, e.g., a low-grade soft tissue injury, closed methods of internal fixation of closed fractures are preferable to open methods. A standard or locked intramedullary nail inserted by closed techniques offers good stability for all fracture types. Even fractures with extreme comminution may be statically locked at both ends to prevent shortening (see Fig. 20.27 c).

Reaming is required to achieve stability with the standard nail. Therefore, the surgeon must be alert to the possibility of a postoperative compartment syndrome. The rigid intramedullary nail is technically demanding, but is relatively safe, can be inserted by closed techniques, and gives good stability, thereby allowing early motion and inspection of the soft tissues. It is the method of choice for closed shaft fractures requiring stabilization, especially if the skin or soft tissues are compromised.

Because of the incidence of compartment syndrome, many surgeons prefer the use of an unreamed tibial nail in all circumstances. The advent of locking for diaphyseal fractures has allowed good stability to be obtained with two locking screws at either end of the nail. The solid nature of the nail makes it biomechanically stronger; therefore, smaller sizes can be used unreamed. There is some evidence that would support a reduced infection rate in this solid nail. At this time, the debate with respect to reaming versus unreaming in closed diaphyseal fractures of the tibia is unresolved. Haas et al. (1993) have reported the use of the new solid, unreamed tibial nail for shaft fractures with severe soft tissue injury, both open and closed. They had considerable complications, but concluded that the unreammed tibial nail with locking could be an alternative to the external fixator in the treatment of tibial shaft fractures with severe soft tissue injury. There was a low rate of sepsis and a reduction in the healing period. Riemer and Butterfield (1993) compared reamed and nonreamed solid core nailing of the tibial diaphysis after external fixation and felt that nonreamed solid core nails were efficacious and were preferable to reamed nails to reduce the incidence of sepsis in that situation.

Flexible rods have gained popularity, but do not offer full stability except in relatively stable fracture types such as the transverse fracture. They are easy to insert and do not require reaming, but they require some postoperative external splintage.

Open Fractures

Open fractures in the tibia, a subcutaneous bone, are relatively common. The most widely used classification is that of Gustilo and Anderson (1976), but other classifications including the AO (Tscherne and Gotzen 1984) are valid. A new comprehensive classification is attempting to grade the soft tissue injuries, either open or closed, in association with the bony injuries, which will be helpful in decision making. If the skin laceration is along the anteromedial subcutaneous border, the overall soft tissue injury is minimal and the surgeon may procede as if he or she were dealing with a closed fracture, as noted above. The methods of fixation will, therefore, depend upon location and morphology of the fracture as well as the preference of the surgeon. However, should the open fracture be of a high grade with severe soft tissue damage to muscle, then alternate methods are required to prevent long-term complications.

Where the vascularity to the distal limb is interrupted at the level of the tibia fracture, attempts at restoration of the circulation and salvage of the limb are often fruitless and an early decision to limb ablation must be made. This is especially true in severe crush injuries.

However, if sensation is present on the plantar aspect of the foot, preservation of the limb may be more useful to the patient than even the best prosthesis (Fig. 20.22 a–d).

Associated Articular with Shaft Fractures. Following a careful assessment of the open soft tissue injury, the location and morphology of the underlying fracture must now be examined.

In *open* as in closed injuries, the principle of anatomical reduction of joint fractures must be adhered to. The above methods are valid, i.e.,, interfragmental screw fixation and buttress plating. The major concern is timing. In general, for grade I or II open fractures, the joint should be fixed at the time of the initial surgery following cleansing and débridement. In severe grade III injuries, the surgeon must be guided by the circumstances of the case. Again, we favor immediate fixation of these injuries to allow early motion, but factors may militate against this and cause delay. These factors may be local, such as extreme contamination or vascular compromise, or they may be general factors precluding a complex, lengthy joint reconstruction. In general, as in closed fractures, the tendency in grade 3 open fractures is for anatomical reduction of the joint by minimal dissection and fixation devices with stabilization, either a standard or ring fixator or combination.

Every effort should be made to close the joint with soft tissue and to stabilize the metaphyseal and diaphy-

470 ·

Chapter 20   **Fractures of the Tibia**

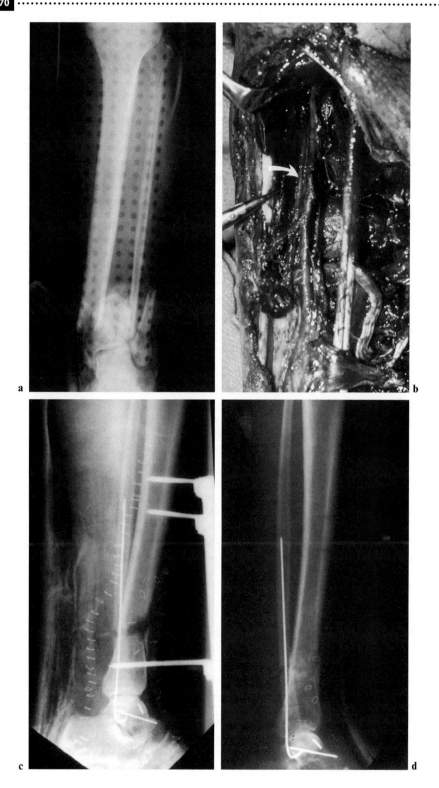

Fig. 20.22 a–d. Open fracture to the distal tibia with vascular injury. **a** This 19-year-old man was injured in a motorcycle accident. He had an open fracture of his distal tibia as noted in the anteroposterior radiograph. The posterior tibial nerve was intact, giving him sensation to the sole of this foot, but all arteries to the foot were severed. **b** The posterior tibial artery was resutured *(white arrow)* The foot viability was maintained. **c** The skeletal injury was treated with an anterior external fixator as well as internal fixation of the talar fracture. **d** The result at 2 years was good. Viability of the talus was maintained; the fracture healed with sensation on the sole of his foot. His result is certainly much better than a prosthesis

seal components, allowing the joint to be managed with continuous passive motion.

Open Metaphyseal Fractures. Under ideal circumstances in grade I and grade II open metaphyseal fractures, plating techniques may be used primarily. Careful planning should permit coverage of the implant. If a locked nail device is to be used, it should be delayed until soft tissue healing has taken place. As indicated in our discussion previously, a locked intramedullary nail may not afford good stability to proximal metaphyseal fractures, and biological plating, ring fixators, other forms of external fixation, or a combination of a locked nail with a pinless fixator may be better methods of choice (see Fig. 20.33). In grade III open fractures of the metaphysis, external fixation devices, especially with severe comminution of the bone, are the methods of choice. The specific type of external fixator will depend on the experience of the surgeon, but again, for this area ring fixators are becoming more popular at this time.

In grade III open fractures, external skeletal fixation is the method of choice.

Open Diaphyseal Fractures. The management of the open diaphyseal fracture of the tibia requires careful surgical judgment; the consequences of the wrong initial decision may be very grave, in some instances leading to amputation. An open tibial fracture with a distal vascular injury leads to an amputation in 60 % of cases (Lange et al. 1985). Therefore, the initial decision must be the desirability or otherwise of *limb salvage*. This decision will depend on general factors in polytraumatized patients as well as on local factors, including the type of vascular trauma, the degree of bone and muscle loss, and the severity of nerve involvement. In polytraumatized patients with severe open tibial fractures associated with distal vascular injury and skin, muscle, and bone loss, amputation may be the most prudent choice. However, if the posterior tibial nerve is intact, affording good sensation to the plantar aspect of the foot, preservation of the limb may be worthwhile (see Fig. 20.22).

Immediate Management. Since the first edition of this book was published there has been a considerable pendulum swing towards intramedullary nailing devices for open diaphyseal fractures of the tibia shaft. In the grade I and some grade II injuries with adequate soft tissue cover, all methods available in our armamentarium may be used to achieve stability. These include intramedullary devices, rigid or flexible, reamed or unreamed, internal plating devices inserted by biological techniques, external fixators, or a combination of the above. In the past, intramedullary devices were felt to be contraindicated in open fractures because of damage to the intramedullary blood supply after the bone has had

damage to the periosteal blood supply. This theoretical disadvantage in the grade I and grade II fractures has been tested by several prospective studies. These studies have shown no increase in infection rate and have had good healing times, and while complications such as broken screws have been frequent the overall results have been satisfactory. Open reduction and internal fixation using intrafragmental screws and plates inserted by strict biological techniques, without interference of the blood supply and discarding of all dead bone, will give acceptable results (Tile et al. 1985; Clifford et al. 1988) in the grade I and grade II fractures. In grade III open fractures, a controversy still exists in spite of many excellent prospective studies comparing external fixators to intramedullary nails.

Therefore, for most grade I and grade II open diaphyseal fractures, any of the above methods is suitable. We favor immediate cleansing and débridement of the wound (discarding any devitalized bone not attached to soft tissue), intravenous antibiotics, and primary open wound care with secondary closure. The type of fixation used will depend on the morphology and exact location of the fracture. If the wound is in such a location to fully expose the fracture, I favor plating on the lateral aspect, bridging the area of comminution and burying the plate under the anterior muscle mass (Fig. 20.23). The low-contact dynamic compression (LCDC) plate offers advantages to the vascularity of the cortex and the results have been good (Clifford et al. 1988). Where the wound is small, I favour adequate débridement and management with a solid intramedullary locked nail unreamed. Alternatively, the patient may be managed nonoperatively as previously described above.

For higher-grade open fractures (grade II), I use the same decision-making process, but in cases where there is severe muscle damage may revert to an external fixator.

For severe open fractures (grade III), we recommend an external skeletal frame, usually a half-frame configuration with cross-linkages. Primary internal fixation with plates or intramedullary nails has lead to an unacceptably high sepsis rate. Prior to application of the frame, a culture is taken from the wound, which is then cleansed and débrided. Intravenous antibiotics, usually cephalosporins, and adequate tetanus prophylaxis are given immediately. Following débridement, the wounds are left open and covered with a wetting agent such as acriflavine with glycerin.

The use of unreamed locked intramedullary devices for grade III open fractures has gained prominence in the last few years. Several comparison studies conclude that it is at least as effective, if not more so, than using an external fixator and has acceptable complication rates. With proper wound management and meticulous débridement of all dead bone, intramedullary infection, which was so prevalent in the early decades of nailing,

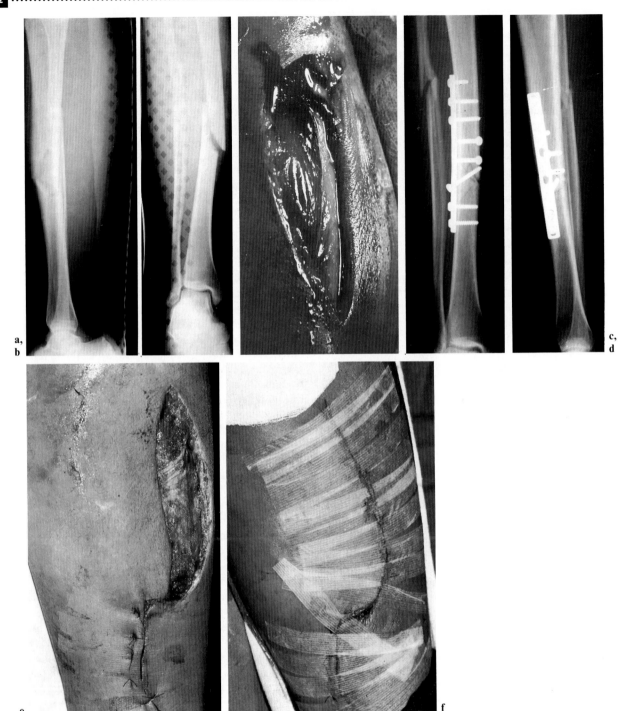

a,
b

c,
d

e

f

Fig. 20.23 a–f. Open fracture treated by internal fixation. **a** This 19-year-old sky diver was injured when her parachute opened only 200 feet from the ground. The radiographs show a high-energy, short, oblique tibial fracture with a butterfly fragment. **b** There was massive skin avulsion. **c,d** Very little muscle damage was found, and it was therefore elected to treat this fracture with cleansing, débridement, and primary internal fixation, using lag screws and a plate placed on the lateral surface of the tibia under the anterior tibial muscle mass. Note the interfrag-mental screws fixing the butterfly fragment and the lag screw across the fracture site through the plate, increasing the stability of the system. **e** The laceration was left open postoperatively, but the surgical incision was closed. **f** The avulsion flap 5 days after injury. The flap was viable and exhibited no swelling, with a good layer of granulation tissue covering the remainder of the wound. At that time skin tapes were used to close the wound.

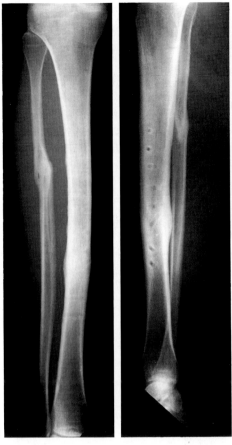

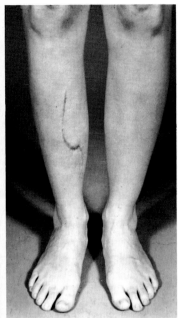

Fig. 20.23 g,h The bone after metal removal. **i** The patient had an excellent functional result and returned to competitive sky diving. (From Tile 1980)

g

h

has not been a major problem. Therefore, in the grade III tibia fracture the decision making is based on the wound and the amount of muscle damage, and these are not black and white determinations of grade III fractures, but shades of grey or a continuum. Unless the surgeon is involved in a clinical trial, the choice of fixation method will need to be individualized and will depend very much on the experience of the surgeon and the institution in which he or she works.

Subsequent Management. Patients with a diaphyseal fracture of the tibia must be told that the initial treatment of the fracture is only the first step in the management and that many other procedures may be required. Subsequent treatment is dependent upon many factors, such as the degree of soft tissue injury and the degree of bone injury. All are influenced by the general state of the patient and the presence or absence of sepsis in the wound.

Specific considerations relating to soft tissue injury include whether the injury involved no skin loss, skin loss only, or skin, muscle, and other soft tissue damage. Similarly, assessment of the bony injury will take into account whether the injury has been anatomically

reduced and stabilized, whether it is one with marked comminution precluding anatomical reduction, or whether it is one with both comminution and bone loss. In addition to the above, the presence or absence of sepsis must be taken into consideration.

Although we will describe the subsequent management of the soft tissue and bone elements separately, it is obvious that they require concurrent treatment.

Management of the Soft Tissues. Since the wounds will have been left open in virtually all cases, we recommend that the first dressing change be carried out in the operating room 2 days postoperatively. The treatment of the soft tissue depends upon the degree of soft tissue injury:

- *No skin loss.* If the wound has been left open and there is no definite skin loss, the wound may be left to granulate and heal by secondary intent, or, if clean and not tense, it may be closed secondarily with suture or tapes by the fifth postoperative day (see Fig. 20.21). Good healing may be anticipated.
- *Skin loss.* If the patient has sustained loss of skin, this loss may be either over muscle or over bone. If over muscle and small, it may be left to granulate by secon-

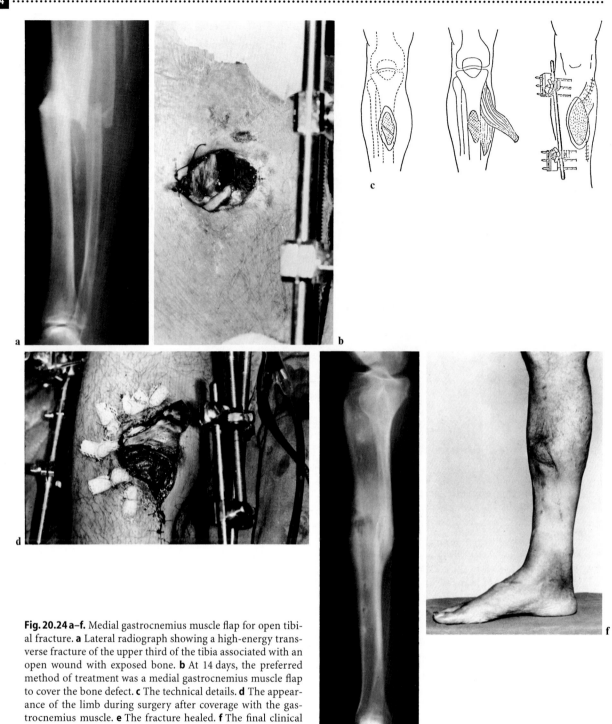

Fig. 20.24 a–f. Medial gastrocnemius muscle flap for open tibial fracture. **a** Lateral radiograph showing a high-energy transverse fracture of the upper third of the tibia associated with an open wound with exposed bone. **b** At 14 days, the preferred method of treatment was a medial gastrocnemius muscle flap to cover the bone defect. **c** The technical details. **d** The appearance of the limb during surgery after coverage with the gastrocnemius muscle. **e** The fracture healed. **f** The final clinical result at 1 year is excellent

dary intent; if larger, it should be managed with a split-thickness skin graft applied when the wound is granulating, usually 5–7 days after trauma. If it is over the subcutaneous border of the tibia and the bone is exposed, the same treatment may be implemented,

i.e., it should be allowed to granulate by secondary intent if the wound is small, or a split-thickness skin graft should be applied directly onto the bone if granulation tissue has covered the bone. However, large split-thickness skin grafts applied directly to bone have a tendency to break down, and we have found the long-term outlook to be much better if a gastrocnemius muscle flap is rotated to cover the defect on the subcutaneous border of the tibia. Therefore, with bone exposed, the preferred treatment is to cover the exposed bone with muscle. We believe that this increases the vascularity to the bone and almost ensures bony union. This procedure should also be carried out in a granulating wound 5–14 days after trauma (Fig. 20.24).

– *Composite soft tissue loss.* We have already indicated that in polytraumatized patients with a vascular injury and a massive soft tissue wound involving skin and muscle, with or without neurovascular damage, there may be a case for primary amputation. In the isolated fracture, however, primary amputation is rare unless the soft tissue injury is unsalvageable. In patients who have skin and muscle loss and whose limb has been revascularized, secondary treatment also depends upon whether or not the bone is exposed. If the bone is not exposed, split-thickness skin grafts should be applied to the granulating wound. For cases in which it is exposed, many sophisticated forms of management are now available. For smaller wounds in the diaphysis, a myofascial flap using the gastrocnemius muscle is the treatment of choice (Fig. 20.24). If the wound is too massive, precluding the above procedure, a free muscle flap using the latissimus dorsi muscle is indicated (Fig. 20.25). Finally, if the muscle and skin loss is associated with bone loss, a composite free flap from the iliac crest may be indicated.

None of these procedures can be carried out unless the wound is clean and granulating, for if carried out in the face of sepsis they will undoubtedly fail.

Management of the Bony Injury. Subsequent management of the bony injury will also depend on many factors, not the least of which is the soft tissue component previously discussed. For the bony injury, several possibilities also exist:

– *Anatomical reduction.* If an anatomical reduction has been achieved and the fracture stabilized by either internal or external fixation, it is unlikely that further surgical intervention will be required. In the vast majority of patients in this situation, the tibial fractures will heal within an appropriate period, namely 16–20 weeks.

– *Comminuted fractures with no bone loss.* If the patient has had a comminuted fracture with no bone loss, the need for subsequent bone-grafting procedures will be dependent on the particular local circumstances. Factors influencing the decision include the degree of comminution, the original method of management, and the degree of soft tissue injury. Therefore, the decision regarding bone grafting must be individualized for each case.

If the wound is small (grade I) and the fracture has been fixed secondarily with a stable intramedullary nail, bone grafting will usually be unnecessary. For the comminuted fracture treated with open reduction and internal fixation but where the degree of comminution does not allow anatomical reduction, bone grafting is highly desirable. This is also true for patients treated with an external skeletal frame.

– *Bone loss.* If fragments of bone have been lost due to the original trauma or subsequently due to débridement, bone-grafting is essential, no matter whether treatment is open reduction and internal fixation or external skeletal fixation (see Fig. 20.10). Bone et al. (1993 have recently reported favorable results of open tibial fractures with early bone-grafting when healing has been delayed.

– *Method of bone grafting.* Bone grafting may be performed anteriorly, posteriorly, or may be part of a composite free flap. If there has been no major skin or soft tissue loss anteriorly, a cancellous bone graft inserted through the original wound at the time of wound closure is acceptable (anterior approach). However, if the anterior soft tissues are poor, then the posterolateral approach is far more desirable. Because of the subcutaneous position of the tibia and the severe damage often inflicted upon the anterior subcutaneous soft tissues, the *posterolateral route* of bone grafting is usually far more desirable and physiological than the anterior approach (see Fig. 20.17). The incision is made just posterior to the fibula. The cutaneous branch of the peroneal nerve must be protected. Access to the posterior compartment is between the peroneal and posterior compartment muscle masses; the interosseous membrane should not be violated. Osteoperiosteal flaps should be raised from the fibula to the posterior aspect of the tibia proximal and distal to the fracture. If major bone loss is present, the bone graft should be carried to the fibula. A large amount of cancellous bone graft may be obtained from the posterosuperior iliac spine. If bone loss is minimal, the cancellous bone graft should be placed only along the posterior aspect of the tibia. This procedure should be preplanned and carried out approximately 3 weeks after injury, when much of the swelling has disappeared and the soft tissues have healed.

– *Massive bone loss.* Cases with a major degree of bone loss in the tibia require careful individual decision making. If bone loss is partial, i.e., unicortical, then the posterolateral cancellous bone graft is the procedure of choice (see Fig. 20.17). Most of these fractures will heal and good functional results should ensue. If

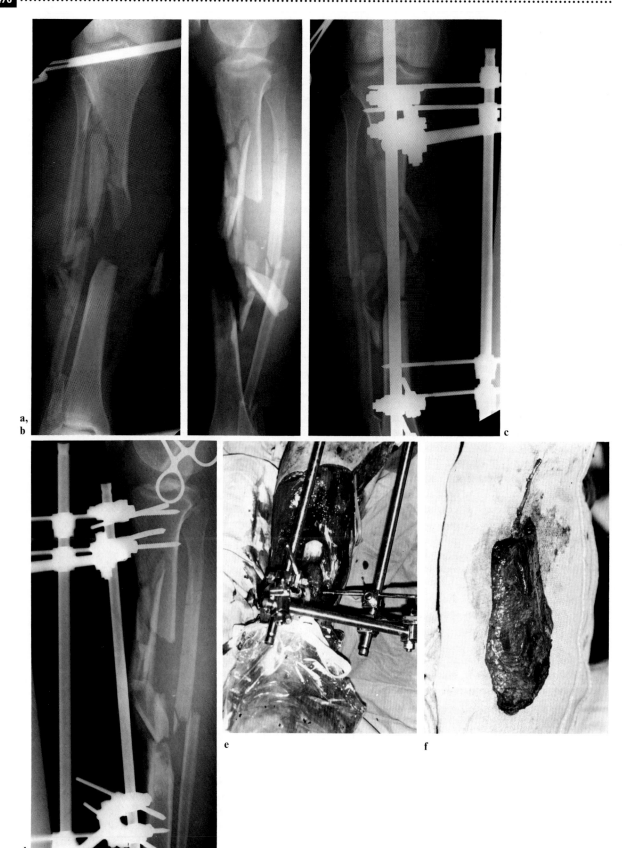

a,
b

c

d

e

f

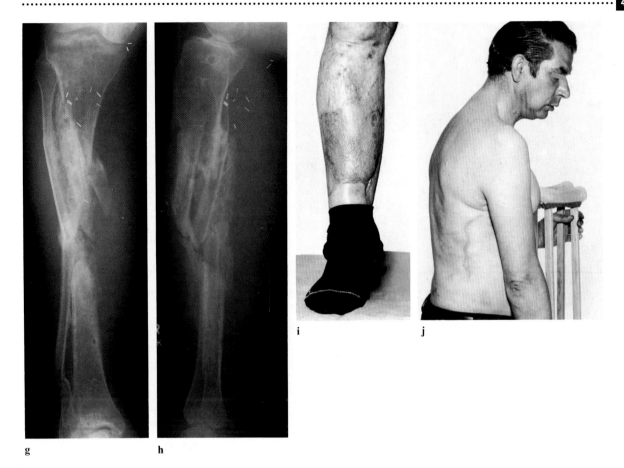

g   h   i   j

Fig. 20.25 a–j. Open fracture of the tibia with bone loss treated with a latissimus dorsi free muscle flap. **a,b** This 39-year-old man sustained an open fracture of the tibia and fibula with skin, muscle, and bone loss. Initial treatment consisted of wound cleansing, débridement, and removal of dead bone. **c,d** The fracture was stabilized by external skeletal fixation using an anterior and medial half-frame joined in a triangular fashion. Definitive management included a massive cancellous bone graft through a posterolateral approach as well as a free latissimus dorsi flap for anterior soft tissue coverage. **e** Intraoperative photograph showing the extent of soft tissue coverage by the free latissimus dorsi muscle flap. **f** Muscle flap postoperatively. **g,h** Bone union was complete at 6 months. **i** The appearance of the limb. **j** The donor site of the latissimus dorsi free muscle graft. The patient's overall shoulder function was good

the bone loss is massive and bicortical, the posterolateral cancellous graft still may be the procedure of choice. In such cases, we have often placed a massive posterolateral bone graft and, secondarily, after anterior wound healing, placed a cancellous bone graft anteriorly as well (see Fig. 20.10). The more massive cases of bone loss may be managed in several ways after adequate soft tissue coverage. These methods include a vascularized fibular graft augmented with cancellous bone, a composite flap of bone muscle and skin from the anterior iliac crest (see Fig. 20.25), a free

muscle flap, or as is most common at this time traction osteogenesis using bone transport (Ilizarov). It should be stressed that most cases can be adequately managed using the simpler posterolateral bone graft techniques.

c) Techniques

Having examined the rationale for implant selection, we will now examine fracture fixation techniques, including stable intramedullary nails inserted either open or closed, locked or unlocked, flexible intramedullary nails, open reduction and internal fixation using lag screws and plates, external skeletal frames, and, finally, combinations of the above.

Intramedullary Nailing

Stable Nailing. The intramedullary nail is the ideal method of fixation for the transverse or short oblique fracture of the midtibial diaphysis.

With newer locking techniques, these indications have been extended to include more comminuted and more proximally or distally placed fractures. Locking the nail

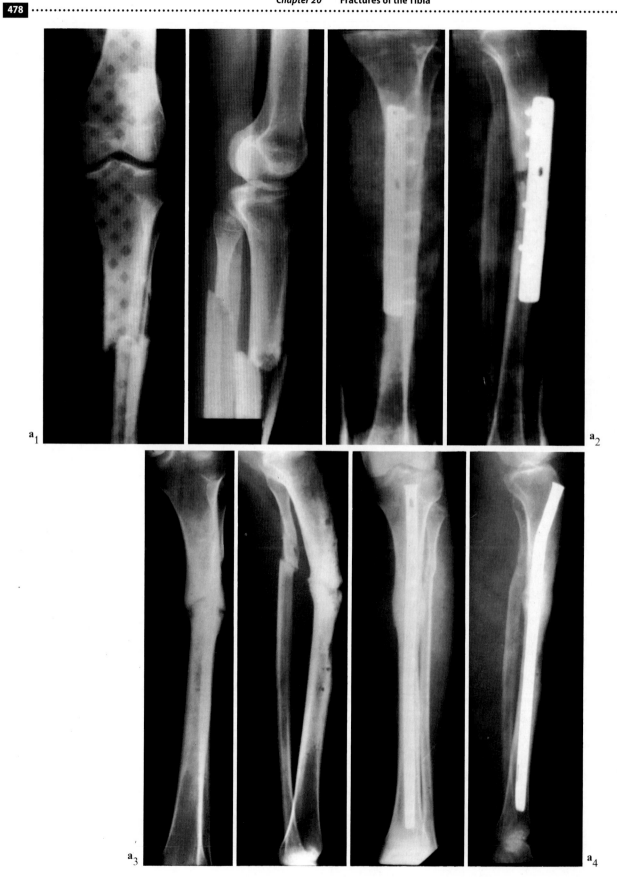

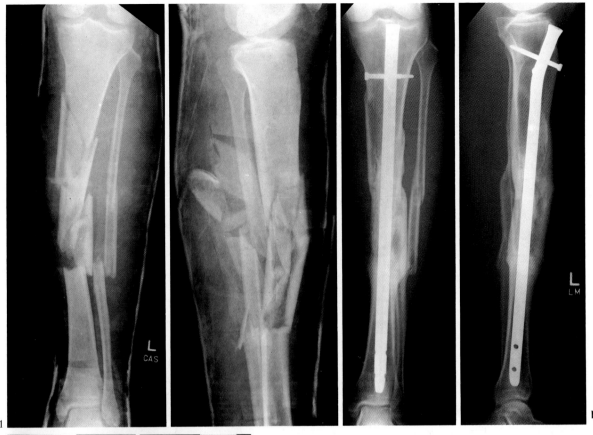

b₁   b₂

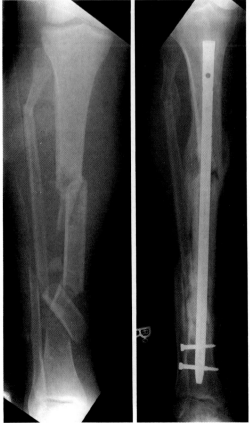

Fig. 20.26 a–c. Examples of closed intramedullary nailing.
a Intramedullary nail with no locking. *1*, Tranverse fracture of
the upper third of the tibia with significant displacement. *2*,
Open reduction and internal fixation using a plate. *3*, Nonunion
9 months after fracture. No sepsis was present in this case. *4*,
Treatment with a stable reamed intramedullary nail. No locking was necessary in this nail because of the extreme sclerosis
at the fracture site allowing firm fixation of the nail. Solid union
occurred and excellent function returned. **b** Fractured tibia
with proximal lock. *1*, Anteroposterior and lateral radiographs
showing a severely comminuted fracture of the middle third of
the tibia. *2*, Treatment consisted of a closed intramedullary nail
with a proximal lock. In this particular fracture configuraion,
preoperative planning indicated sufficient fixation by the nail
in the distal fragment for a distal lock not to be necessary. The
proximal fragment required locking because of the proximal
location of the fracture. Union was complete in 4 months.
c Closed intramedullary nailing with distal lock. *1*, A severely
comminuted segmental fracture of the middle to distal third of
the tibia. *2*, Preoperative planning indicated reasonable stability in the proximal fragment, so only a distal lock was used. At
10 weeks healing had progressed. Fig **26 d** see p. 480

c₁   c₂

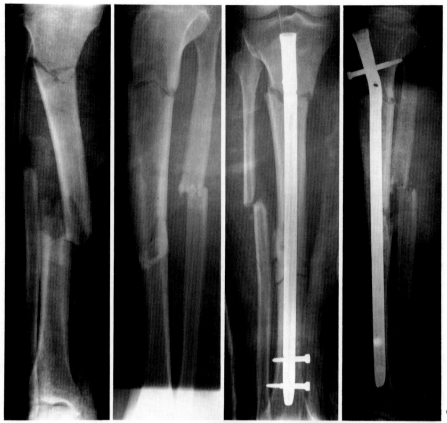

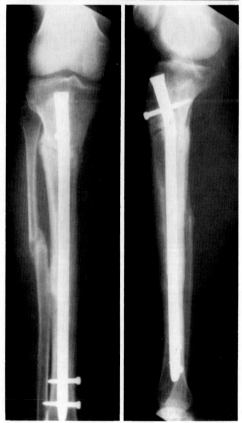

Fig. 20.26 d. Fracture of the tibia with proximal and distal lock. *1*, Anteroposterior and lateral radiographs of segmented tibial fracture. *2*, In this case it was felt that both a proximal and distal lock were necessary. The distal lock may not have been essential since the distal third of the bone is intact. *3*, The radiographs show sound healing at 6 months

at one end prevents rotation, thus permitting its use in more proximal or distal fractures; locking it at both ends allows a severely comminuted fracture to be fixed with little chance of excessive shortening. Since this technique has shown some problems, especially with proximal fractures, considerable expertise and judgement must be exercised before it is applied to difficult cases.

If preoperative planning indicates that the intramedullary nail is the ideal treatment, then a choice must be made between closed and open methods.

Closed nailing has several advantages and is the preferred method where possible. It allows the surgeon to operate at a site proximal to the fracture and not interfere with the already traumatized and poorly vascularized skin on the anterior tibial border; therefore, skin necrosis leading to infection is rare. Theoretically, the infection rate should be lower than with open nailing, although this is controversial.

As we have mentioned, any remaining soft tissue is left attached to the bony fragments, so as to enhance healing. Intramedullary reaming will allow bone-forming cells in the reamed debris to be deposited at the fracture site, further enhancing healing. Since the tibia is a subcutaneous bone, the technique of closed nailing is relatively easy, although the addition of locking techniques is more difficult. Reduction may be aided by direct finger palpation and a traction table is not essential; indeed, most surgeons now prefer to operate on a standard radiolucent table with image intensification.

For closed nailing the patient is placed on the fracture table with the knee in the flexed position or on a radiolucent table with the knee flexed. A longitudinal incision is made, as previously described. After bone perforation, a guide wire is placed into the medullary cavity and extended across the fracture site, which should be reduced. Visualization is afforded by the image intensifier. The entry point is extremely important, especially with the long, sloping nail configurations.

Reamed Nailing. Reaming is still the preferred method of many centers and with surgeons who feel that reaming is essential to achieve stability, but the amount of reaming will be dependent on the fracture configuration, the amount of comminution, and the presence or absence of a segmental component. The size of the nail and therefore the amount of reaming can be determined by measurements with the ossimeter on the preoperative radiograph. In stable fracture configurations, the medullary canal should be reamed to a size necessary to achieve 2 cm of stable bone proximal and distal to the fracture. If this can be achieved, no locking techniques are necessary.

If reaming cannot achieve this stability because of unicondylar or bicondylar comminution, then the use of a proximal or distal locking screw is essential. If the fracture is proximal, the nail must be locked proximally to prevent rotation. Likewise, if distal, it must be locked distally to avoid rotation. However, if bicortical comminution is present, the nail must be locked both proximally and distally to prevent both rotation and shortening (Fig. 20.26).

Following reaming, the appropriate nail is assembled and driven across the fracture. The locking screws are inserted using the appropriate jigs and siting devices as necessary and the wound closed. Stability should be tested under the image intensifier so that proper postoperative planning can ensue.

Few surgeons still use open reaming techniques. The advantages of *open* intramedullary nailing of a tibial fracture are more theoretical than practical. Open reduction allows the surgeon to anatomically reduce the fracture, to add cerclage wires or antirotation plates as necessary, and to instantly check the stability he or she has achieved. In addition, bone grafts may be added if anatomical reduction has not been achieved. The major

disadvantages are possible problems with the soft tissues, such as skin necrosis and sepsis, and possible devitalization of attached bone fragments; in our opinion, these outweigh the advantages. Also, the addition of the locked nail to our armamentarium has almost eliminated the need for open techniques.

Unreamed Nails. As previously noted, unreamed tibial nails have now been almost elevated to the rank of "conventional wisdom," especially for open fractures. The closed solid nail has the theoretical advantage of less infection. The strength of the nail allows a small size and obviates the necessity for reaming, and locking will allow stability to be obtained. The theoretical advantage is less damage to the intramedullary blood supply. The disadvantage is less stability to the fracture construct. Early studies have shown it to be effective but with many complications, including loss of position when the indications are extended to the metaphysis and a 10 %–14 % incidence of broken screws. Delayed healing is prevalent, leading to early bone-grafting being suggested in these circumstances.

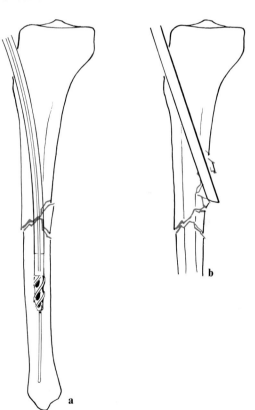

Fig. 20.27 a,b. Posterior insertion of the intramedullary nail. **a** The guide wire and the reamer, being flexible, may enter the distal fragment easily. **b** However, when the relatively rigid nail is inserted, it may be driven posteriorly, shattering the cortex. This complication can be prevented by changing the entry point and by not using undue force in driving in the nail

Complications of Nailing. Intramedullary nailing of the tibia is fraught with the same *complications* as it is in other long bones; there are, however, problems specific to the tibia, and these are outlined below.

1. *Posterior insertion.* Because the point of insertion of the nail is anterior, the nail will naturally tend to be driven against the posterior cortex (Fig. 20.27). The surgeon may be lulled into a false sense of security by the ease with which the flexible reamers navigate the shaft. The more rigid nail, however, may be driven posteriorly, shattering the cortex, and forcing the surgeon to abandon the procedure and change the management to an external frame, internal fixation with a plate, or a cast. Changing the method of fixation to a plate, after the intramedullary blood supply has been destroyed by reaming, obviously has sinister implications and must be avoided. Usually, a cast will not confer enough stability to be used in this situation. This leaves an external frame as the treatment of choice.

   The best choice of all, however, is prevention: no undue force should be used to drive in the tibial nail. The fracture must be continually visualized during nailing, either directly in open nailing or radiographically in closed nailing. If resistance is met, the nail should be removed and a smaller nail used or further reaming performed. Moving the entry point proximally and fully flexing the knee may further aid the surgeon who meets this difficulty.

2. *Rotational and vertical instability.* These potential problems have been eliminated by careful planning and the use of the locked nail.

3. *Compartment syndrome.* Reaming into a closed compartment may cause a compartment syndrome, which must be dealt with by immediate decompression. This complication is relatively frequent, leading many centers to monitor the compartment pressures of all patients undergoing closed tibial nailing.

Flexible Nails. The major advantage of flexible nails is ease of insertion, and the major disadvantage poor stability. No reaming is necessary, so the risk of precipitating a compartment syndrome is diminished. We have generally not used this technique because of its main problem, i.e., lack of sufficient stability to allow external splints and casts to be discarded.

Open Reduction and Internal Fixation. The use of open reduction and internal fixation using screws and plates has sharply decreased in the past decade with the advent of the locking nail. However, there are still many situations where this technique must be used, and in many centers it remains the operative treatment of choice.

The incision is made as described above, 1 cm lateral to the anterior border of the tibia over the anterior tibial muscle mass (see Fig. 20.15). The most frequently used implants are the 4.5-mm LCDC plates and 4.5-mm cortical screws, used either as lag screws or to fix the plate to bone. In the metaphyseal area, the 6.5-mm cancellous screws are also used, either the lag screw type (for interfragmental compression) or the fully threaded type (for fixation of the plate to the metaphyseal bone).

We favor placement of the plate on the lateral surface of the tibia, especially when used in open fractures. The plate will thus be buried under the anterior tibial muscle mass even when there is significant skin loss (Fig. 20.28).

In this era of biological plating, areas of comminution in the bone are bypassed. If they are connected to viable tissue and are easily reduced without destroying the tissue, intrafragmental screws may be placed through these fragments using the previous technique (Fig. 20.28 a,b). However, often dissection of these fragments will devitalize them, leading to delayed union and possible sepsis. Therefore, this area of comminution should be bypassed or bridge-plated . The technique has come to be known as biological plating (Fig. 20.28 c).

The major unresolved question is how to achieve stability with the use of biological plating. This technique requires longer plates and possibly fewer screws. I believe we need the same guidelines as previously stated with the longer plate. If an area of comminution is to bridged and the plate lengthened, the same number of cortices should be used as would have previously been used with intrafragmental compression, i.e., seven cortices on each side of a tibia fracture. Biomechanically, the most important screws are the ones at the ends of the plate and the ones closest to the fracture. These screw holes must be filled or the fracture will lose stability and displace if early rehabilitation is attempted (Fig. 20.28 d–f). In some instances, with biological plating, the fracture line is not opened at all. The plates are inserted through small incisions proximal and distal to the fracture. The disadvantage here is that screws through the central portion of the plate, so important for stability, are often left out. They could be inserted through stab wounds under image intensification.

Therefore, the use of the implant depends on the fracture type. For the pure transverse and short oblique fracture, a properly molded LCDC plate may achieve axial compression and is placed on the lateral surface of the tibia under the soft tissues. Biological plating is indicated for severely comminuted fractures. For pure spiral fractures, a cerclage wire well placed atraumatically may help with reduction and a biological plating may be carried out.

A word about titanium: many of the implants are now being made of titanium, a metal which is less rigid and more biologically compatible. The screws, however, are

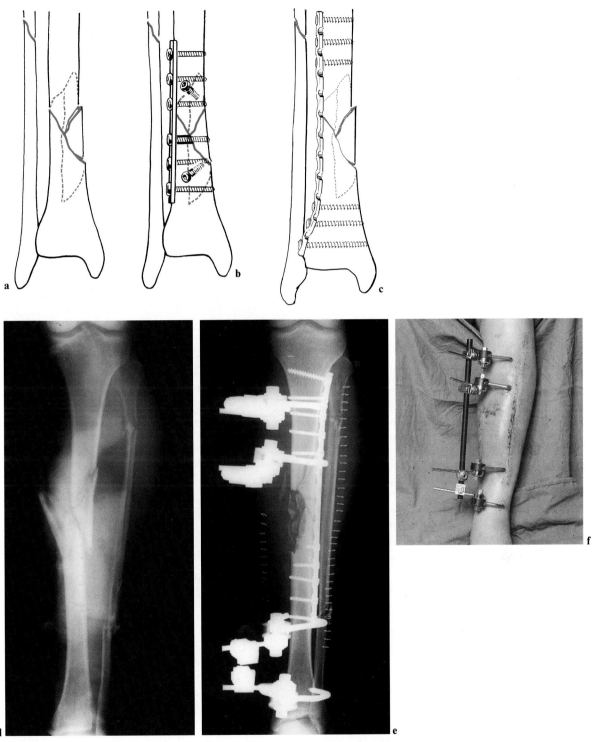

Fig. 20.28a–f. Fixation of tibial fracture with lateral plate. **a** Tibial fracture with posteromedial butterfly. **b** The butterfly fragment is fixed with two interfragmental screws. We favor placement of the plate – in this case a 4.5-mm dynamic compression (DC) plate – on the lateral surface of the tibia under the anterior tibial muscle mass. Any screws crossing the major fracture line should be lag screws, as shown. **c** If reduction of the comminuted fragments requires devitalization this area should be left completely alone (biologic plating) and the area by-passed. Note the use of the LCDC plate, the increased length of the plate to achieve biomechanical stability and no screws crossing any of the fracture lines. The surgeon should take care to leave all viable tissue undissected and the plate is used to by-pass this area. **d** Open comminuted fracture of the mid shaft of the tibia. Three large fragments of cortical bone were discarded because they were completely stripped of soft tissue and were avascular. **e** A long bridge plate was applied to the lateral surface of the tibia without any stripping of periosteum or interference with blood supply. Note the long plate at 5 days. Cancellous bone grafting was used to fill the gap and a pinless fixator inserted medially because of the massive bone loss

more brittle and great care must be taken when tightening a titanium screw, as the head may break if it impinges the plate. Also, surgeons should refrain from using lag screws since they will be extremely difficult to remove with ingrowth into the titanium surface. The preferred technique, therefore, is overdrilling and the use of a cortical screw even at the ends of the plate in the metaphysis. Otherwise, caution is required during removal, as the screws may break.

Because of the subcutaneous position of the tibia with its relatively poor blood supply, it is essential that atraumatic techniques be used during open reduction and internal fixation of this bone.

Preoperative planning should guide the surgeon's choice of incision and implants. Several types of comminution are recognized, such as the posterolateral, posteromedial, and anterior torsional butterfly. However, the principles of management remain the same for all.

External Skeletal Fixation. The recommended method of frame configuration has changed considerably over the past decade. The double frame with pins crossing the anterior compartment of the tibia resulted in significant complications: anterior compartment syndromes, permanent impairment of dorsiflexion, and injury to neurovascular structures were not uncommon. In addition, the rigidity of the double frame significantly impaired bone healing. For that reason, a simple anterior half-frame is now recommended, as shown in Fig. 20.29. In cases of bicortical comminution or major bone loss, a medial half-frame may be added to the fixation and further stability achieved by triangulation, as shown in Fig. 20.30.

As in the past edition of the book, the double frame disappeared in favor of the anterior half-frame or Delta frame. In this decade, the use of ring fixation in the tibia, especially at the metaphyseal ends, has gained popularity. The ring fixator can be used as two rings or a single ring adapted to a standard fixator and may be an excellent method of stabilization in certain fracture patterns, as has been previously discussed.

Also, for more temporary fixation, the pinless fixator may have advantages (see Fig. 20.28 d,e).

Combined Minimal Internal with External Skeletal Fixation. In some open fractures a combination of minimal internal fixation with interfragmental screws followed by the use of external skeletal fixation as a neutralization frame may be the most desirable. This combination should be employed when major fragments in the open fracture can be simply fixed with interfragmental screws without further soft tissue damage. In these instances, the use of the external skeletal frame as a neutralization frame may be preferable to the further soft tissue stripping necessary for application of a neutralization plate internally.

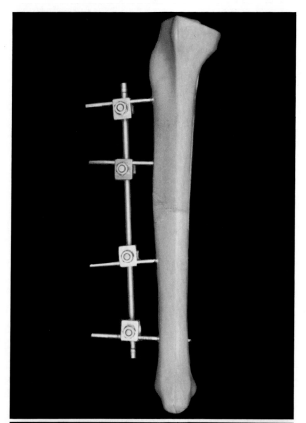

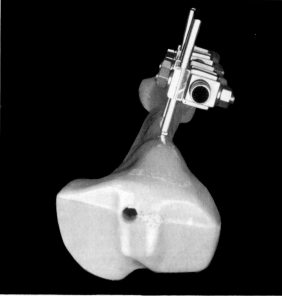

Fig. 20.29. Unilateral anterior half-frame in the anteroposterior direction on the tibia. (From Hierholzer et al. 1985)

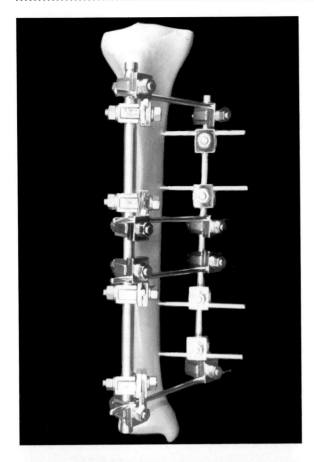

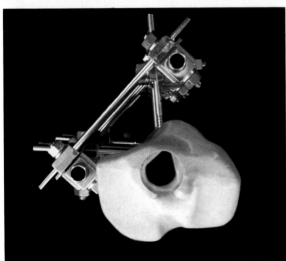

Fig. 20.30. Anteroposterior and medial half-frames joined in a triangular fashion to increase stability. (From Hierholzer et al. 1985)

Bone Grafts. Cancellous bone grafts should be considered in all cases in which an anatomical reduction has not been achieved. They should always be performed where bone loss is present or where the area of comminution is so great that healing is likely to be retarded beyond the limits of the implant. In such circumstances, the stability of the system is provided only by the implant. Since anatomical reduction of all the fragments is technically impossible, they can provide no direct stability to the fracture. Devitalization of the fragments makes delayed union likely; therefore, the addition of a bone graft is necessary to prevent this delay and the implant failure which usually follows. As we have previously indicated, in open fractures treated with an external fixator, delayed union is so common that we prefer early elective bone grafting in almost all cases, usually to be performed 2–3 weeks after injury (see Fig. 20.28 d–f).

Since the posterior skin and soft tissues are usually the better preserved, we prefer the posterolateral approach in most cases (see Fig. 20.17). Using this approach the grafts are under a muscle layer, which will hasten their vascularization. If large gaps are present, the grafts may be used to bypass the tibia; this is done by applying them to the fibula proximal and distal to the fracture, creating a tibiofibular diastasis. The results of such posterior bone grafting are excellent, and the technique is therefore highly recommended.

20.4.6.4 Wound Closure

a) Primary Wound Closure

The next major decision to be made concerns skin closure. In closed fractures, if the skin can be closed with meticulous, tension-free, atraumatic techniques, then this is the preferable course. Suction drainage should always be used to prevent hematoma formation. Not infrequently, however, it is extremely difficult to close the skin without tension. In this situation, it is far safer to leave a portion of the wound open than to close it under tension and risk the possibility of skin necrosis and sepsis. Therefore, the dictum to be followed is: "Close if possible, but not at all cost."

If the incisions have been well planned and are away from the subcutaneous border, and if the implant has been carefully placed so that it is buried under soft tissue, then little harm will come from leaving the skin open. On the fifth day, when granulation tissue has appeared, it is usually a simple matter to either secondarily suture or tape the wound, if the swelling has subsided.

When two incisions have been used, one over the fibula and one over the tibia, the more important incision

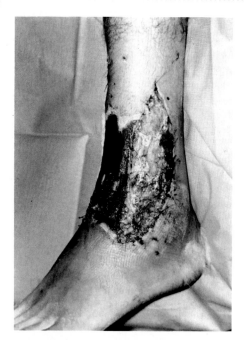

Fig. 20.31. A relaxing incision on the lateral aspect of the lower leg resulted in complete loss of the anterior flap. This necrotic flap was excised. Subsequently, the anterior tibial tendon also became necrotic and required excision

should be closed and the other one left open, to be closed secondarily when possible.

There are, however, exceptions to the above rule. Sensitive structures such as tendon, nerve, artery, and joint should not be left open (we do not consider bone to be a sensitive structure). Other techniques may be required to close the tissues over these sensitive structures. This is especially true at the distal end of the tibial incision, where the anterior tibial tendon may become exposed and, if it does, may die, with serious consequences.

Rotating a skin flap along the anterior border of the distal tibia in an acute injury is a dangerous procedure and cannot be recommended. Too often, we have seen loss of this flap and exposure of the underlying tendon, resulting in its death (Fig. 20.31).

b) Delayed Primary and Secondary Wound Closure

Wounds not associated with skin loss may be sutured on the fifth day after trauma if they are clean, granulating, and free of tension; if small, they may be left to heal by secondary intent.

Wounds associated with significant skin or muscle loss require careful consideration. In most cases, a simple split-thickness skin graft will be sufficient cover for

the clean, granulating wound and may be applied at the first or second dressing change.

If devitalized bone is exposed and granulation delayed, we favor an early muscle pedicle graft for coverage (see Fig. 20.22). Care must be taken to remove the area of devitalized bone. Cancellous bone grafting is almost always required to aid union.

Finally, the occasional open tibial fracture with major bone and soft tissue loss will be best treated by a free microvascular composite graft, but only in a well-vascularized, noncontaminated bed (see Fig. 20.23).

20.4.6.5 Postoperative Course

a) Immediate Postoperative Course

At the end of the operative procedure, the surgeon must realistically appraise the situation at hand. The skin must be carefully assessed, whether the wound is closed or open; if closed, the degree of tension, if any, must be gauged. The surgeon must be completely honest regarding the degree of stability achieved for the particular fracture.

If the surgeon feels that excellent stability of the fracture has been achieved and the bone is of normal strength, then motion of the extremity may be started early. The leg should be elevated with the ankle splinted at 95° dorsiflexion. Under ideal conditions, the splint may be removed on the second postoperative day and the patient encouraged to move the ankle. The splint should be reapplied after exercise and at night until the patient has regained normal dorsiflexion function; otherwise a disastrous plantar flexion deformity will develop. Patients should sleep with their splints on for at least 2–3 weeks following injury.

Early motion of the ankle should be delayed (a) if there is concern about the stability of the fracture or (b) if soft tissue healing would be jeopardized. In both of these situations, the leg should remain splinted until the surgeon is satisfied that the dangerous period is over. In some instances of severe porosis or comminution, a cast or cast brace must be retained until union is complete. This is preferable to an otherwise inevitable implant failure with its related problems.

b) Follow-Up

Careful follow-up is required in order to monitor the race between implant failure and bone union. If the patient exhibits good soft tissue healing and sound stability of the internal fixation system, feather weight-bearing can be started forthwith and gradually

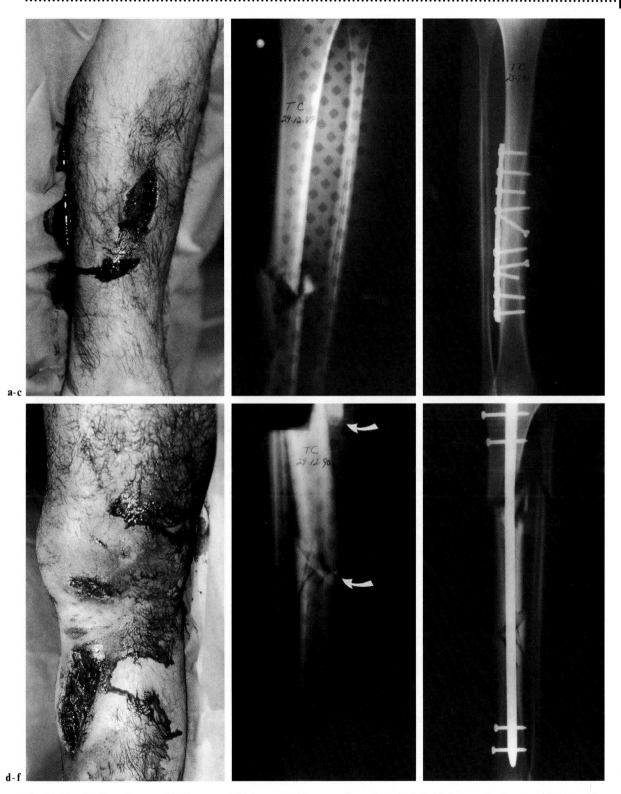

a-c

d-f

Fig. 20.32 a–f. Bilateral open tibia fractures. This 55-year-old man was a pedestrian hit by a car. He sustained bilateral open tibial fractures. **a** On the right the clinical photograph shows the extent of the wound of this wedge type tibia fracture with a butterfly. **b** This was treated with an LCDC plate. In this case the fragment could be restored without destroying the blood supply. **c** Uneventful healing by primary bone union is noted in the radiograph. The patient's functional outcome with this limb is excellent. **d** On the left side he sustained an open fracture. The wound was in the metaphysis in close proximity to the knee as shown in the photograph. **e** This was a segmental fracture seen at the *two white arrows*. This was treated with an unreamed tibial locked nail. **f** Note at 1 year the proximal fracture is ununited and the fracture has drifted into varus, a not unusual complication when nails are used in fractures that are this proximal

increased, depending on the radiographs, which should be taken at 3-weekly intervals. The average tibial fracture will be healed at 16–20 weeks, when more normal activities may be initiated.

Careful decision making according to these guidelines should make good functional results possible for the majority of patients with this difficult fracture (Allgöwer and Perren 1980; Karlstrom and Olerud 1974). However, the final chapter in this difficult fracture has yet to be written, as the case in Fig. 20.32 illustrates.

20.5 Conclusions

In spite of all the efforts of the past decade to improve the outcomes of patients with fractures of the tibia, especially open fractures of the tibia, disability from this particular diaphyseal fracture is greater than any other, mainly due to the high-energy nature of the injuries affecting this subcutaneous bone. Many prospective studies have been performed, examining the intraobserver error in determining the grade of closed and open soft tissue injuries. Clearly, fractures at the ends of the tibia involving the metaphysis, with or without articular involvement, are more difficult to manage than those of the diaphysis. In this past decade, studies have shown that intramedullary nails, previously thought to be dangerous for this open fracture, have in fact given satisfactory results where meticulous attention to débridement has been performed. In fact, the published results are better in open fractures than those with external fixation. There have been no recent studies on comparing biological plating to other forms of fixation, but in our own experience, again with meticulous attention to detail and with the new implants, this technique for grade I and grade II open fractures has been excellent.

When faced with an open or severely damaged closed tibia fracture, the surgeon is faced with many choices. Decison making is based on the fracture factors and the patient factors. With vascular injury associated with severe nerve injury in polytrauma, limb ablation is the method of choice. If protective sensation is present, attempts to restore limb function may be fruitful. With minimal soft tissue injury standard techniques for fixation of either the joint, the metaphysis, or the diaphysis may be chosen. With open reduction and internal fixation, the methods of choice in the articular and metaphyseal area is closed intramedullary nailing, either reamed or unreamed, and locked as necessary for the diaphysis.

Where the soft tissue injury is major, closed techniques at both the joint and the diaphysis which include minimal internal fixation through percutaneous techniques, arthroscopic visualization for articular fractures, and closed intramedullary nails unreamed and locked for diaphyseal fractures become the preferred methods.

For grade I or II open wounds, the surgeon may procede as for the ideal circumstances noted previously in both the articular and nonarticular fractures.

The grade III open fractures, no matter what method is chosen, have a significant complication rate. The use of unreamed solid intramedullary locked nails has been found to be safe as long as all dead and devitalized tissue has been removed. Alternatively, types of external fixators have remained the method of choice.

Acute treatment is only the first stage of management, and patients must share in the decisions made for follow-up surgical care to both skin , soft tissues, and bone, which include secondary closure, bone-grafting, and various forms of skin-grafting and flaps.

Certainly, the results of open tibial fractures have improved significantly with these techniques over the past two decades as compared to original descriptions with nonoperative care and casts, as described by Nicoll (1964). Hopefully, by continued adherence to strict biological and biomechanical principles, results will continue to improve.

References

Allgower M (1967) A healing of clinical fractures of the tibia and rigid internal fixation. The healing of osseous tissue (reprint). National Academy of Science/National Research Council, pp 81–89

Allgower M, Perren SM (1980) Operating on tibial shaft fractures. Unfallheilk/Traumatology 83(5):214–218

American College of Surgeons (1981) Advanced trauma life support system. American College of Surgeons, Committee on Trauma, Park Ridge, IL

Bohler J (1936) Treatment of fractures. Wright, Bristol, p 421

Bondurant F., Cotler H. Buckle R et al (1988) The medical and economic impact of severely injured lower extremities. J Trauma 28:1270

Bone L, Stegemann P, McNamara K (1993) External fixation of severely comminuted and open tibial pilon fractures. Clin Orthop Rel Res 292:101–107

Border JR, LaDuca J, Seibel R (1975) Priorities in the management of the patient with polytrauma. Prog Surg 14:84–120

Brown PW (1974) Early weight bearing treatment of tibial shaft fractures. Clin Orthop 105:165–178

Chapman MW, Mahoney M (1979) The role of early internal fixation in the management of open fractures. Clin Orthop 138:120–131

Charnley J (1961) The closed treatment of common fractures, 3 rd edn. Livingstone, Edinburgh

Claude RJ, Stern PJ (1987) Severe open fracture of the tibia. J Bone Joint Surg 69A(6):801–807

Clifford RP, Beauchamp CG, Kellam JF, Webb JK, Tile M (1988) Plate fixation of open fractures of the tibia. J Bone Joint Surg [Br] 70B 644–648

Dehne E, Metz CW, Deffer P, Hall R (1961) Nonoperative treatment of the fractured tibia by immediate weight bearing. J Trauma 1:514–535

Dickson K, Katzman S, Delgado et al (1994) Delayed unions and nonunions of open tibial fraactures. correlation with arteriography results. Clin Orthop 302:189–193

Fraser RD, Hunter GA, Waddell JP (1978) Ipsilateral fractures of the femur and tibia. J Bone Joint Surg [Br] 60B:510–515

Gregory RT, Gould RJ, Peclet M et al (1985) The mangled extremity syndrome (M.E.S.): a severity grading system for multisystem injury of the extremity. J Trauma 25:1147

Gustilo RB (1982) Management of open fractures and their complications. Saunders, Philadelphia (Monographs in clinical orthopaedics, vol 4)

Gustilo RB, Anderson JP (1976) Prevention of infection in the treatment of one thousand and twenty-five open fractures of long bones. J Bone Joint Surg 58A:453

Haas N, Krettek C, Schandelmaier P (1993) A new solid unreamed tibial nail for shaft fractures with severe soft tissue injury. Butterworth/Heinemann, London–

Hansen ST (1987) The type 111C tibial fracture. Salvage or amputation. J Bone Joint Surg [Am] 69(6):799–800

Hierholzer G, Ruedi T, Allgower M, Schatzker J (1985) Manual of the AO/ASIF tubular external fixator. Springer, Berlin Heidelberg New York

Johansen K, Daines M, Howey T et al (1990) Objective criteria accurately predict amputation following lower extremity trauma. J Trauma 30 (5):568–573

Karlstrom G, Olerud S (1974) Fractures of the tibial shaft: a critical evaluation of treatment alternatives. Clin Orthop 105:82–115

Keating JF, Kuo RS, Court-Brown C (1994) Bifocal fractures of the tibia and fibula. J Bone Joint Surg 76B

Lange RH, Bach AW, Hansen ST Jr, Hansen KH (1985) Open tibial fractures with associated vascular injuries: Prognosis for limb salvage. J Trauma 25(3):203–208

Lottes JO (1974) Medullary nailing of the tibia with the triflange nail. Clin Orthop 105: 253–266

McMurtry RY, Saibil E, Tile M (1984) General assessment and management of the polytraumatized patient. Williams and Wilkins, Baltimore, pp 41–56

Mubarek SJ, Owen GA, Hargens AR et al (1978) Acute compartmental syndromes: diagnosis and treatment with the aid of the Wick catheter. J Bone Joint Surg [Am] 60A:1091–1095

Müller ME, Allgower M, Schneider R, Willenegger H (1979) Manual of internal fixation, 2nd edn. Springer, Berlin Heidelberg New York

Nicoll EA (1964) Fractures of the tibial shaft. A survey of 705 cases. J Bone Joint Surg [Br] 46B:373–387

O'Dwyer KJ, DeVriese L, Feys H et al (1993) Tibial shaft fractures with an intact fibula. Injury 24(9):591–594

Oni OO, Hui A, Gregg PJ (1988) The healing of closed tibial fractures. The natural history of union with closed treatment, J Bone Joint Surg (Br) 5: 784–786

Oni OO, Hui A, Gregg, PJ (1988) The healing of closed tibial fractures. The natural history of union with closed treatment. J Bone Joint Surg (Br) 70(5):784–786

Reimer BL, Butterfield S (1993) Comparison of reamed and non reamed solid core nailing of the tibial diaphysis after extrenal fixation: a preliminary report. J Orthop Trauma 7(3):279–285

Rorabeck C (1977) Pathophysiology of the anterior compartment syndrome. Surg Forum 28:495–497

Ruedi TH, Webb JK, Allgower M (1976) Experience with a dynamic compression plate (DCP) in 418 recent fractures of the tibial shaft. Injury 7(4):252–257

Salter RB, Simmonds DF, Malcolm BW et al (1980) The biological effect of continuous passive motion on the healing of full thickness defects in articular cartilage – an experimental investigation in the rabbit. J Bone Joint Surg [Am] 62A(8):1232–1251

Sarmiento A (1967) A functional below-knee cast for tibial fractures. J Bone Joint Surg [Am] 49A:855–875

Sarmiento A, Latta LL (1981) Closed functional treatment of fractures. Springer, Berlin Heidelberg New York

Sarmiento A, Gersten LM, Sobol PA et al (1989) Tibial shaft fractures treated with functional braces. Experience 780 fractures. J Bone Joint Surg [Br] 71(4):602–609

Teitz CC, Carter DR, Frankel VH (1980) Problems associated with tibial fractures with intact fibulae. J Bone Joint Surg [Am] 62A:770

Tile M (1980) Fractures of the tibia: indications for open reduction of tibial fractures. In: Leach (eds) Controversies in orthopaedic surgery. Saunders, Philadelphia

Tile M (1984) Fractures of the pelvis and acetabulum. Williams and Wilkins, Baltimore

Tile M, Beauchamp CB, Kellam JF (1985) Open fractures: is primary stabilization desirable? In: Uhthoff HK (ed) Current concepts of infections in orthopaedic surgery. Springer, Berlin Heidelberg New York

Tscherne H, Gotzen L (1984) Fractures with soft tissue injuries. Springer, Berlin Heidelberg New York, p 24

Tscherne H, Lobenhoffer P (1993) Tibial plateau fractures. Management and expected results. Clin Orthop 292:87–100

Watson-Jones R, Coltart WD (1943) Slow union of fractures: with a study of 804 fractures of the shafts of the tibia and femur. Br J Surg 130:260–276

Worlock P, Slack R, Harvey L, Mawhinney R (1994) The prevention of infectionin open fractures: an experimental study of the effect of fracture stability. Injury 25(1):31-38

21 Fractures of the Distal Tibial Metaphysis Involving the Ankle Joint: The Pilon Fracture

M. TILE

21.1 Introduction

The pilon fracture, a metaphyseal injury extending into the ankle joint, is difficult to treat successfully by any method. If the fracture into the ankle joint is displaced, the basic principles of open anatomical reduction and stable internal fixation, followed by early motion *if technically possible*, are valid. It is in this particular area, to an extent equaled perhaps only by fractures of the acetabulum, that the words "if technically possible" loom large, for this fracture is often so comminuted that technical difficulties cannot be overcome.

In the past decade, the soft tissue injury has received much attention, which has resulted in a considerable change in the bony treatment, from an emphasis on rigid internal fixation to more limited techniques of internal fixation, even percutaneous techniques in association with external fixation (Bone et al. 1993; Teeny and Wiss 1993; Leone et al. 1993).

The major problems affecting the natural history of this injury may be summarized as follows:

1. The nature of the injury
2. The state of the bone
3. The state of the soft tissues
4. Technical difficulties

21.2 Natural History

21.2.1 Nature of the Injury

Fractures in cancellous bone are subject to either compressive or shearing forces, each inflicting its own particular type of lesion on the bone (see Figs. 21.1, 21.2). Compressive forces cause severe impaction, while shearing or tensile forces cause marked disruption of the bone and soft tissues without impaction, resulting in gross instability. A fracture caused by a combined shear, and compressive load may present a lesion with both impaction of the articular surface and instability of the metaphysis as well as damage to the soft tissues due to the lack of muscle cover to the medial border of the tibia.

In the distal tibia and ankle, an area predisposed to high-energy trauma, either force may be operative. Severe compression injuries are seen in patients falling from a height; whereas shearing injuries are often seen in skiing injuries, the so-called boot-top fracture, or major motor vehicle trauma. It is with the complex force patterns of high-energy motor vehicle trauma that both types of injuries may be seen.

The prognosis of the injury depends on the amount of articular damage compared to the metaphyseal damage, as is clearly evident in Fig. 21.1 and is reflected in the revised classification.

21.2.1.1 Axial Compression

a) Tibia

Articular Cartilage. Severe compression (Fig. 21.1a) usually causes impaction of the articular surface, often with marked comminution (Fig. 21.1b,c). On some occasions, the comminution is so great that anatomical repair of the articular surface is virtually impossible. If surgical repair is attempted, small avascular pieces of articular cartilage and subchondral bone may have to be discarded, leaving gaps on the joint surface. Osteoarthritis will inevitably follow no matter what form of treatment is used.

Metaphysis. Fractures of the distal metaphysis caused by compression associated with a rotation force often severely impact the metaphyseal bone, causing unacceptable axial malalignment (Fig. 21.1d). The result of uncorrected axial malalignment in the lower extremity is abnormal stress on the distal joint, which in time will destroy it. Since the upper extremity is not subjected to the major weight-bearing stresses of the lower extremity, some leeway is permissible, especially about the shoulder. However, in the lower extremity, anatomical alignment is necessary to prevent these major forces of weight-bearing from destroying the joint.

Therefore, when these impacted fractures are reduced by closed manipulation, an extremely large periarticular gap is formed (Fig. 21.1d–m). Nature abhors a vacuum – if treated nonoperatively, the distal fragment may tend to

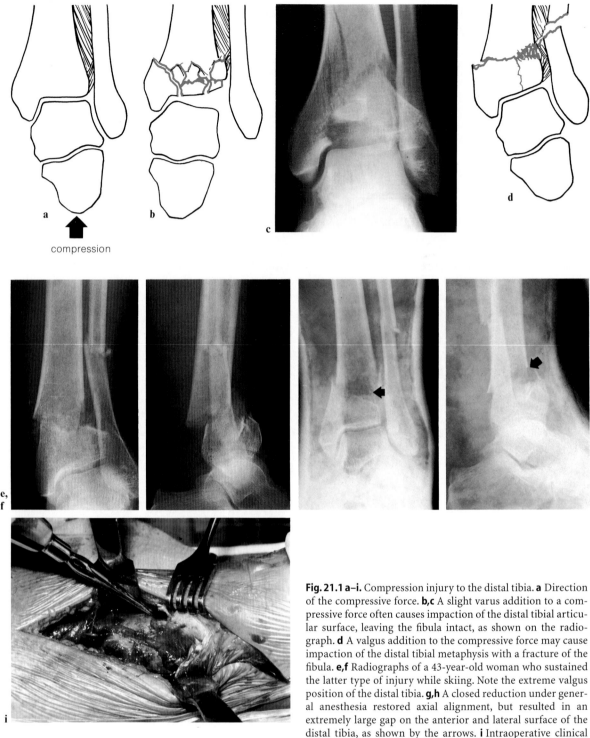

compression

Fig. 21.1 a–i. Compression injury to the distal tibia. **a** Direction of the compressive force. **b,c** A slight varus addition to a compressive force often causes impaction of the distal tibial articular surface, leaving the fibula intact, as shown on the radiograph. **d** A valgus addition to the compressive force may cause impaction of the distal tibial metaphysis with a fracture of the fibula. **e,f** Radiographs of a 43-year-old woman who sustained the latter type of injury while skiing. Note the extreme valgus position of the distal tibia. **g,h** A closed reduction under general anesthesia restored axial alignment, but resulted in an extremely large gap on the anterior and lateral surface of the distal tibia, as shown by the arrows. **i** Intraoperative clinical photograph showing the large gap through which a curette has been passed. **j,k** Operative treatment was undertaken to prevent loss of reduction and consisted of intramedulary fixation of the fibula, restoration of the articular surface, and bonegrafting of the distal metaphysis of the tibia and stabilization with a cloverleaf plate. **l,m** The final result after plate removal 3 years following injury is excellent

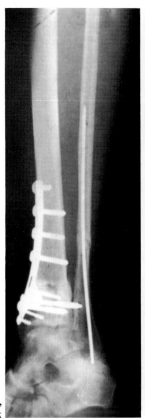 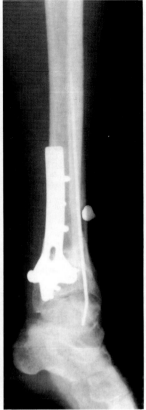 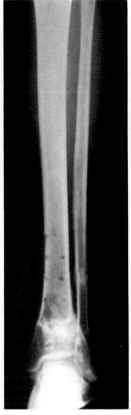 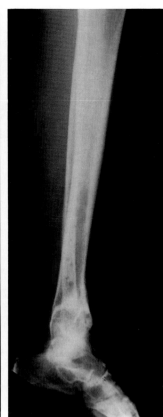

j,
k

l,
m

displace into that gap in the postreduction period, necessitating multiple reductions. Also, since the compression fracture has been disimpacted, and since cancellous bone heals poorly under such conditions, union may be delayed. This, in turn, will require prolonged immobilization of the limb with resultant poor ankle function.

b) Fibula

In many compression injuries the fibula may remain intact, which it never does in the shearing-type injury. With an intact fibula, the ankle is often driven into varus with severe impaction of the medial part of the tibial plafond (Fig. 21.1 b, c).

21.2.1.2 Shear (Tension)

a) Tibia

Articular Cartilage. Pure shearing or tensile forces, free of axial loading and usually rotatory in nature, may spare the articular surface (Fig. 21.2 a,b). Minor cracks may appear at the joint surface, but severe impaction is rare. The long-term prognosis, therefore, is more favorable than for injuries with major articular compression.

Metaphysis. The shear injury to the distal tibia produces an unstable injury with a disrupted soft tissue envelope. Although the articular surface may be relatively intact, the unstable nature of the bony injury, if treated nonoperatively, often requires immobilization, with resultant stiffness of the ankle.

b) Fibula

The fibula is always fractured, usually as a result of a valgus external rotation force (Fig. 21.2b). The fibula fracture is usually transverse or short and oblique in nature, with a butterfly fragment. However, on occasion, the fib-

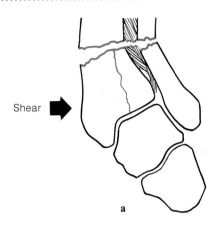

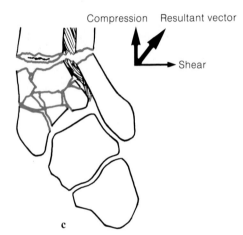

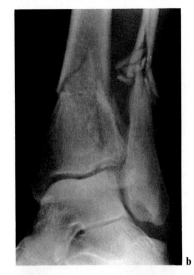

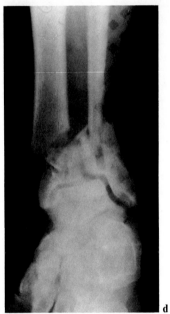

Fig. 21.2 a–d. Shearing injury to the distal tibia. **a** The shearing force in valgus which fractures the fibula as well as the distal tibial metaphysis. **b** Anteroposterior radiograph showing a fracture of this type with comminution of the fibula. **c** Shearing injury of the distal tibial metaphysis combined with a compression force, resulting in severe comminution of the articular cartilage. **d** Radiographic appearance of such a case

ula is markedly comminuted, making any reconstruction difficult.

21.2.1.3 Combined

Severe high-energy trauma may produce a combined injury, with both shearing and axial compressive forces (Fig. 21.2 c,d). It is obvious that the lesion found in a particular patient, i.e., the personality of the individual fracture, is the result of a resolution of these forces. Therefore, a spectrum of possible injury exists, depending on the involvement of the articular surface, the metaphysis, and the fibula (Fig. 21.3). The natural history

will in a large measure depend on these factors and will significantly affect one's management decisions.

21.2.2 State of the Bone

In younger patients with good-quality bone, the surgeon may expect that the holding power of the screws will be satisfactory. However, like fractures in many other areas of the body, metaphyseal fractures of the distal tibia often occur in elderly patients with osteoporotic bone, which makes stable internal fixation difficult to obtain.

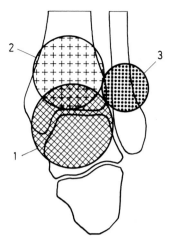

Fig. 21.3. The three important anatomical zones to be considered in the decision making and prognosis of the pilon fracture. *1*, articular surface; *2*, metaphysis; *3*, fibula

21.2.3 State of the Soft Tissues

The importance of the soft tissues in open fractures has been stressed in the medical literature for decades. Tscherne and Gotzen (1984) stressed the equal importance of the state of the soft tissues in closed fractures. Their grading system is particularly appropriate to the distal tibial fracture, where major soft tissue damage is so common and the consequences of soft tissue loss so disastrous. Tscherne and Gotzen's grading of soft tissue injuries for closed fractures is as follows:

– Grade 0: little or no soft tissue injury (Fig. 21.4 a)
– Grade I: significant abrasion or contusion (Fig. 21.4 b)

Fig. 21.4 a–d. Grading system of soft tissue injury in closed fractures. **a** Grade 0: little or no soft tissue injury. **b** Grade 1: superficial abrasion *(shaded area)* with local contusional damage to skin or muscle. **c** Grade 2: deep contaminated abrasion with local contusional damage *(shaded area)* to skin and muscle. **d** Grade 3: extensive contusion or crushing of skin or destruction of muscle *(shaded area)*. (From Tscherne and Gotzen 1984)

– Grade II: deep contaminated abrasion with local contusional damage to skin or muscle (Fig. 21.4 c)
– Grade III: extensive contusion or crushing of skin or destruction of muscle; also subcutaneous avulsions, decompensated compartment syndrome, or rupture of a major blood vessel (Fig. 21.4 d)

In this particular injury, the state of the skin and subcutaneous tissue is of overriding importance. Notoriously poor soft tissue healing, often measured in months, is common about the distal tibia. Venous drainage is often inadequate, leading to chronic edema and stasis ulceration. A high-energy injury may severely traumatize this poorly vascularized tissue, either by direct or indirect forces. Since much of the tibia at the ankle is subcutaneous, the skin and subcutaneous tissues, lacking the protection of muscle, may be traumatized by the fracture fragments from within, without an open wound being present. The resultant massive swelling may lead to the early formation of post-traumatic bullae. Skin necrosis may ensue, especially if the surgeon has chosen to further traumatize the skin with an ill-advised surgical procedure. Therefore, the timing of the surgery and delicate, atraumatic handling of the soft tissues are of vital importance in the management of this fracture.

21.2.4 Technical Difficulties

We have already discussed some of the important technical difficulties, such as severe comminution of the articular surface, impaction of cancellous bone, weak osteoporotic bone, and the precarious state of the soft tissues. In addition to these factors, exposure of the distal tibia to fully visualize the articular surface of the ankle is difficult, which further compounds the problem.

21.2.5 The Dilemma

A classic "catch 22" situation is obvious: i.e., nonoperative care may result in persistent joint displacement and a poor outcome, but surgical treatment, in turn, is

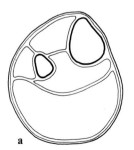

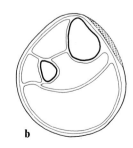

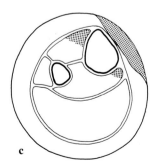

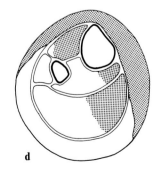

a   b   c   d

fraught with many difficulties. Good results may therefore be difficult to achieve by any method for some of these fractures.

The literature on this subject, sparse as it is, reflects this dilemma. Most reports indicate the need for anatomical restoration of the distal tibia but feel the difficulties and the risks involved are too great. Williams et al. (1967) and Ruoff and Snider (1971) therefore recommend traction methods as an alternative to open reduction, with the occasional use of percutaneous pinning in internal fixation of the fibula. However, their number of cases was too small to be significant.

Conrad (1970) described the lateral tibial plafond fracture associated with trimalleolar ankle fractures and made a plea for their anatomical open reduction. However, that injury is different from the so-called *explosion* or pilon fracture of the distal tibia, and the conclusions are therefore inapplicable.

The European literature is more extensive, but reaches similar conclusions. Bonnier (1961), DeCoulx et al. (1961), and Fourquet (1959) all reported large series treated by both open and closed methods, with 43%, 45%, and 50% functional results, respectively. No definite trends were noted.

The reports of Rüedi and Allgöwer (1969) began to shed light on this dilemma. They adhered to the principles of the AO/ASIF group, i.e.:

1. Reconstruction of the fibula (if fractured)
2. Reconstruction of the articular surface of the tibia
3. Cancellous bone-grafting of the gap in the distal tibial metaphysis
4. A medial or anterior tibial buttress plate to restore stability

At a 4-year review they were able to show good functional results in 74% of their 84 patients with pilon fractures.

The same group of patients were reviewed again 9 years after surgery: few had regressed and many had improved their previous rating (Rüedi 1973). For the first time in the literature, these reports indicated that this fracture was amenable to meticulous anatomical open reduction, stable internal fixation, and early motion.

Further reports by Heim and Naser (1977), Rüedi and Allgöwer (1979), and Szyszkowitz et al. (1979) confirmed these findings. The further publications by Rüedi and Allgöwer came from Basel, where 50% of the injuries were caused by high-energy motor vehicle trauma, unlike their original report, in which most were caused by skiing injuries. They were able to achieve excellent results in 69.4% of their cases, in spite of the shift of the injuries to a higher energy type.

However, Kellam and Waddell (1979) indicated in a study of 26 distal tibial pilon fractures that results were more often linked to the type of fracture than to their management. With open reduction of the shearing type

Table 21.1. Treatment results of different types of fracture (from Kellam and Waddell 1979)

Results	Compression type (%)	Shearing type (%)
Excellent	37	70
Adequate	16	14
Poor	47	16

injury without major joint impaction, they achieved good results in 84% of the patients, a figure comparable to the Swiss group. However, in the severely impacted, comminuted compression type, they achieved only 53% good results (Table 21.1). However, the results obtained by operative treatment were superior to those obtained by nonoperative treatment.

21.2.6 Summary

Have we, at this time, solved our dilemma? The answer, to a certain extent, is yes – but only to a certain extent. The final result of any lower-extremity joint injury is dependent upon the ability of the surgeon to achieve an anatomical reduction of the joint surface. If this cannot be achieved by closed means, then open reduction is indicated. If we are to embark upon that course for the distal tibial fracture, it behooves us to pay particular attention to the timing of the operation, to the handling of the soft tissues, and to the precise details of the internal fixation. This, in turn, will avoid many of the complications and should improve the functional results.

However, there will be some fractures in this area that by virtue of their articular cartilage destruction will defy even the most expert surgeon. Also, the soft tissue injury in some patients may be so severe that open reduction is hazardous and therefore other techniques must be performed. In those cases, the prognosis resides more in the injury itself than in the treatment, and poor functional results, often ending in ankle arthrodesis, may be expected (see Fig. 21.11).

21.3 Classification

The Rüedi-Allgöwer (1969) classification of distal tibial fractures is based on the degree of displacement of the articular fragments. Fractures are graded as follows:

- Grade I: articular fracture without significant displacement
- Grade II: articular fracture with significant articular incongruity
- Grade III: severely comminuted and impacted articular fracture

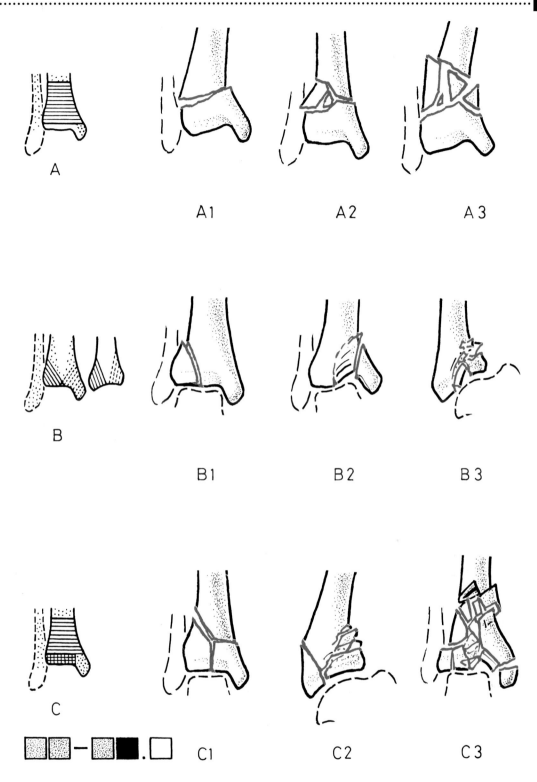

Fig. 21.5. Comprehensive classification of distal tibial fractures. *A1* Extra-articular fracture, metaphyseal simple; *A2* Extra-articular fracture, metaphyseal wedge; *A3* Extra-articular fracture, metaphyseal complex; *B1* Partial articular fracture, pure split; *B2* Partial articular fracture, split-depression; *B3* Partial articular fracture, multifragmentary depression; *C1* Complete articular simple, metaphyseal simple; *C2* Complete articular fracture, articular simple, metaphyseal multifragmentary; *C3* Complete articular fracture, multifragmentary

21.3.1 Comprehensive Classification

Since the previous edition of this book, the AO group have proposed the comprehensive classification of all fractures (Müller et al. 1990) using the alpha-numeric code: type A, B, and C in order of severity (Fig. 21.5). This classification in the distal tibia is based on the Ruedi-Allgower classification and may be very useful in prognosis, since it clearly defines the following:

– Type A: extra-articular fractures (Fig. 21.5 a)
– Type B: partial articular fractures which involve only a part of the articular surface, leaving the other part intact and connected to the tibial shaft (Fig. 21.5 b)
– Type C: complete articular fractures in which the articular surface is comminuted and separated from the tibial shaft (Fig. 21.5 c)

This classification does not include the fibular lesion, but it does have value in predicting the prognosis of the injury.

21.3.2 Use of Classification in Decision Making

This classification is excellent for documentation purposes and we recommend it. However, to help us with the management of the individual patient the classification

must, as with other fractures, be expanded. Each case is different and must be individually assessed. We have learned that by answering a series of questions rather than by adhering to a precise, unbending classification, logical decision making will follow. The important questions to ask are related to the state of the fibula, the articular surface of the tibia or talus, and the metaphyseal region of the tibia, as given in the following sections.

21.3.2.1 Fibula

Is the fibula fractured? In cases where it is intact, the injury has usually been caused by a severe varus compression force, often crushing the medial portion of the tibial articular surface (see Fig. 21.1 b,c). Also, the intact fibula acts as a post, stabilizing the important

Fig. 21.6 a–d. Pilon fracture with good prognosis. **a,b** Anteroposterior and lateral radiographs of a 32-year-old man injured while skiing. Note the comminution to the distal tibial metaphysis, the fracture of the fibula, and the valgus and anterior displacement. The distal tibial articular surface is relatively intact, with only one small undisplaced fracture through it. **c,d** The intraoperative radiographs show the fixation of the fibula with a Rush rod, the stabilization of the lower-third tibial fracture with two interfragmental screws, and the provisional stabilization of the articular surface with four Kirschner wires. No bone graft was required in this case

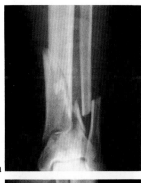
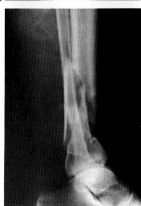
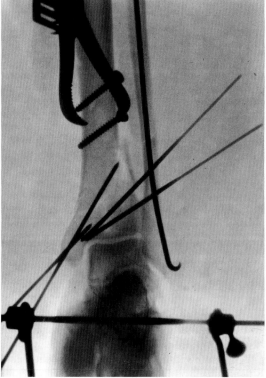
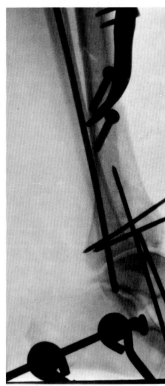

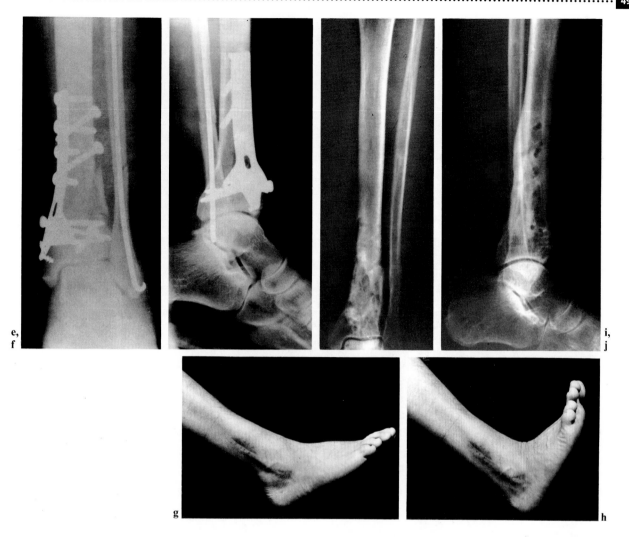

e,
f

i,
j

g

h

Fig. 21.6. e,f The postoperative radiographs at 6 weeks show early union. **g,h** The patient's function at that time showed almost normal ankle motion. Note the use of indirect reduction and no attempt to fix all fragments, thereby maintaining bone vascularity. **i,j** The final result after plate removal shows normal articular cartilage and normal axial alignment. The patient had an excellent end result

lateral aspect of the joint, the surgical implications of which are obvious. If the fibula is fractured, then the force involved is usually a valgus shear with resultant severe injury to the lateral aspect of the joint (see Fig. 21.1 d,e).

21.3.2.2 Articular Surface of the Tibia

Is the articular fracture displaced and, if so, is it a relatively uncomminuted fissure (type B1, C1) or a grossly comminuted shattered lower end of the (tibia type B3,

C3) (Fig. 21.2)? Severe impaction and comminution of the articular surface may be irreparable; the final outcome of the case will therefore be more dependent on the answers to these questions than to any others.

21.3.2.3 Distal Tibial Metaphysis

Is the bone in the lower tibial metaphysis normal or osteoporotic? Is the fracture severely comminuted? Is there axial malalignment? Is there impaction of the cancellous bone which will cause a large gap following reduction?

21.3.3 Personality of the Fracture

The above are the important questions to ask before embarking upon the treatment of a pilon fracture. The answers to these questions as well as all others will pre-

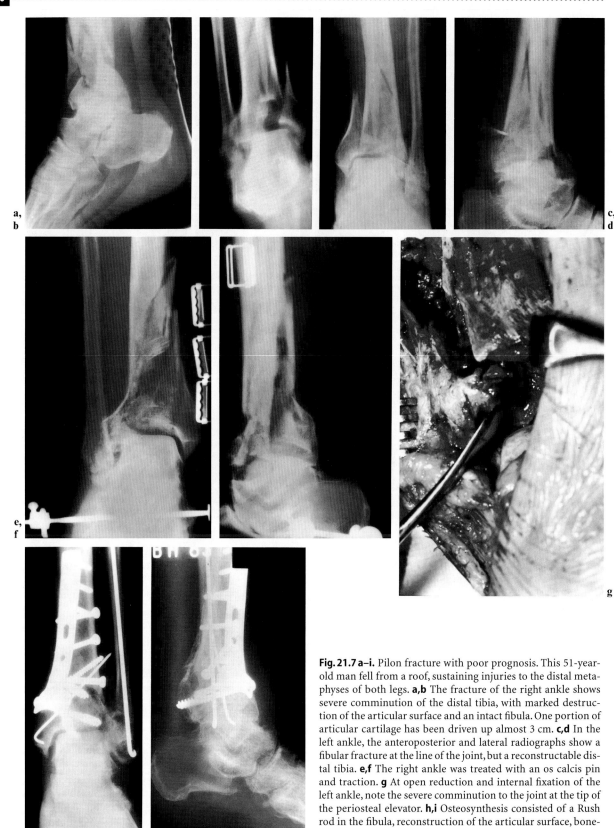

Fig. 21.7 a–i. Pilon fracture with poor prognosis. This 51-year-old man fell from a roof, sustaining injuries to the distal metaphyses of both legs. **a,b** The fracture of the right ankle shows severe comminution of the distal tibia, with marked destruction of the articular surface and an intact fibula. One portion of articular cartilage has been driven up almost 3 cm. **c,d** In the left ankle, the anteroposterior and lateral radiographs show a fibular fracture at the line of the joint, but a reconstructable distal tibia. **e,f** The right ankle was treated with an os calcis pin and traction. **g** At open reduction and internal fixation of the left ankle, note the severe comminution to the joint at the tip of the periosteal elevator. **h,i** Osteosynthesis consisted of a Rush rod in the fibula, reconstruction of the articular surface, bone-grafting, and stabilization with a T plate

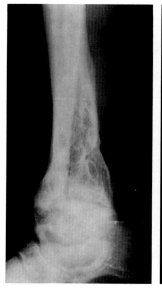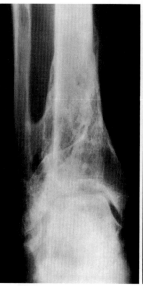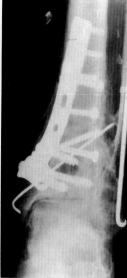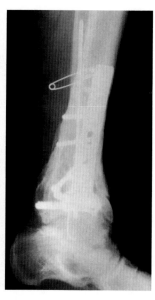

j

k,
l

Fig. 21.7 j–l. The final result 8 years later shows good bony union bilaterally. Both ankles show osteophytes and joint narrowing and both are painful, the right being slightly worse than the left. The result in traction was almost equal to that afforded by internal fixation. The prognosis was determined more by the original injury to the articular cartilage than by the method of treatment

cisely define the personality of the fracture. The personality of the fracture is dependent not only on the *fracture factors* discussed in the previous section, but also on the degree of the soft tissue injury. In addition, and equally as important, there are *patient factors* such as the age of the patient, the state of the bone, the associated injuries, and the general medical state. A consideration of all these factors will lead the surgeon to a logical management decision for each patient. Many permutations and combinations are possible. For example, an undisplaced fracture into the ankle joint with marked comminution and displacement of the metaphysis is suitable for careful reconstruction. Because the articular surface is not beyond repair, with ideal treatment an excellent result should be expected (Fig. 21.6).

By contrast, in the case of a severely comminuted impacted fracture of the articular surface of the ankle joint, with or without axial malalignment in the metaphysis, even the most careful open reduction may fail to restore joint congruity, which will inevitably lead to a poor result. In such a case, so much articular comminution is present that surgery cannot possibly restore it. Open reduction should therefore be avoided and traction methods employed (Fig. 21.7).

Also important is the soft tissue injury. Using the Tscherne and Gotsen classification, the type 0 and 1 soft

tissue injury may be suitable for standard open reduction and internal fixation techniques, using atraumatic techniques, but type 2 and 3 soft tissue injuries will usually require alternative methods, such as minimal internal fixation combined wtih external methods (Fig. 21.8).

All of these factors must be considered when comparing the results of different modalities, so as not to compare apples with oranges, as we have said before.

21.4 Assessment

Theoretically, the decision-making process should be relatively easy in this major weight-bearing joint fracture (Fig. 21.9). Since we believe that any *displaced* fracture of a major weight-bearing joint requires anatomical reduction, stable internal fixation, and early joint motion for optimal end results, then any such fracture in the distal tibia should be treated in that manner. However, because of the problems previously stated of severe bone comminution, osteoporosis, and poor soft tissues, exceptions have to be made.

As with all fractures, a careful assessment of the patient, the limb, and the injury, taking into account the expertise and experience of the surgeon, will aid in the decision-making process.

21.4.1 Clinical

General details of the medical history will reveal the chronological and physiological age of the patient and his or her general medical state and ambitions. The future expectations of the patient must be respected,

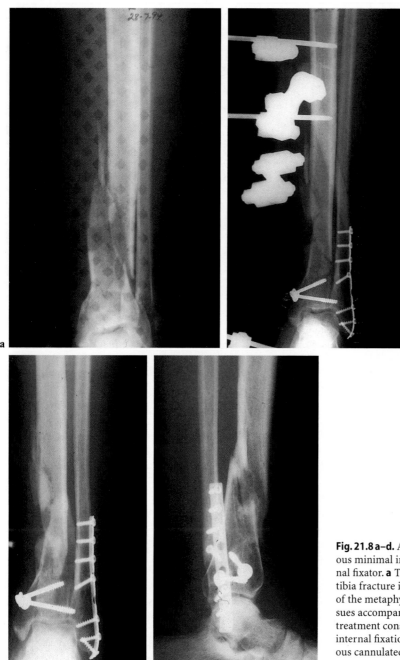

Fig. 21.8 a–d. A pilon fracture treated with percutaneous minimal internal fixation of the joint and an external fixator. **a** The anteroposterior X-ray reveals a distal tibia fracture into the joint with marked comminution of the metaphysis. A major injury to skin and soft tissues accompanied this fracture. **b** Because of that, treatment consisted of fixation of the fibula, minimal internal fixation fo the joint surface using percutaneous cannulated screws, and application of an external fixator as seen in the anteroposterior radiograph. **c,d** Good healing occurred as noted on the anteroposterior radiograph and the lateral radiograph

especially in the case of the professional or amateur athlete.

The specific details of the mechanism of injury are important, as they will suggest to the surgeon the type of force involved. The violence exerted upon both the soft and skeletal tissues will vary considerably depending upon the mechanism of injury, whether a motor vehicle

or motorbike accident, a fall from a height, or, in an older individual, a simple fall at home.

As always, a general physical examination is essential to assess the medical state of the patient.

Examination of the limb will reveal evidence of neurovascular damage and other skeletal injuries. A careful examination of the local area will reveal any lacerations

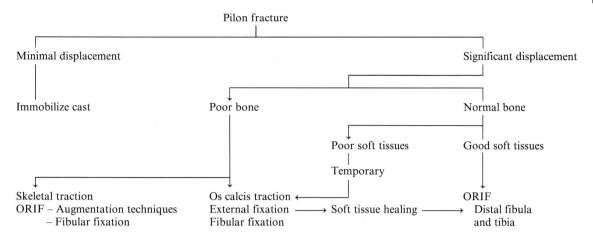

Fig. 21.9. Decision-making algorithm for pilon fractures. *ORIF,* open reduction with internal fixation

at the fracture site. The degree of swelling and ecchymosis or the presence of fracture blisters will have considerable bearing on the management decision, for an incision made through damaged skin may lead to a surgical disaster.

21.4.2 Radiological

In any articular fracture, it is imperative that a careful radiological assessment be carried out. All too often, major operative decisions are made on the basis of poor radiographs. The surgeon is then surprised during the operation by the number of fracture fragments present, and the injury may prove inoperable. The number of *surgical surprises* must be reduced by surgeons demanding good anteroposterior, lateral, and oblique radiographs of the ankle as well as both anteroposterior and lateral tomograms. Computed tomograms (CT) are invaluable in determining comminution of the articular surface, and the newer three-dimensional CT can be very helpful in the overall planning of the surgical procedure (Fig. 21.10).

A careful radiographic assessment will clearly reveal the number of articular fragments and will greatly aid in the treatment decision; then, if surgery is indicated, careful preoperative planning is possible.

After this careful assessment, the surgeon must fully discuss the injury with the patient and allow him or her to participate in the treatment decision. If the prognosis for that particular injury is poor, the patient should be so informed. If there is any chance that the surgeon may wish to do a primary ankle arthrodesis, the patient must be told of this prior to surgery; otherwise, misunderstandings (and possibly litigation) may follow.

21.5 Indications for Surgery

21.5.1 Minimal Displacement

If the preoperative assessment has indicated an *undisplaced* fracture, immobilization in a cast followed by a cast brace will lead to an acceptable result (Fig. 21.9). Patients with this kind of fracture usually have a partially intact soft tissue envelope, which favors rapid union and allows early motion.

21.5.2 Significant Displacement

If significant displacement is noted – that is, if large fragments of the articular surface of the joint are displaced, or the metaphysis is grossly malaligned – surgery is indicated.

21.5.2.1 Operable

The determination of the operability of the fracture, employing logical surgical judgment, will be the next step in the decision-making process. If surgery is chosen, failure to achieve the stated goals of anatomical reduction and stable internal fixation will lead to the *worst of both worlds,* i.e., the added trauma of the surgery inflicted upon an already severely injured extremity. It will also destroy all of the soft tissue hinges, so that nonoperative traction methods cannot be used successfully. Therefore, this initial decision is extremely important and must be based on a careful assessment of the radiographs, including the tomograms, as well as the soft tissues.

If the bone is deemed to be normal, the degree of joint comminution not excessive, and the metaphysis reconstructible, then early operation is indicated, but only through satisfactory soft tissue (see Fig. 21.6).

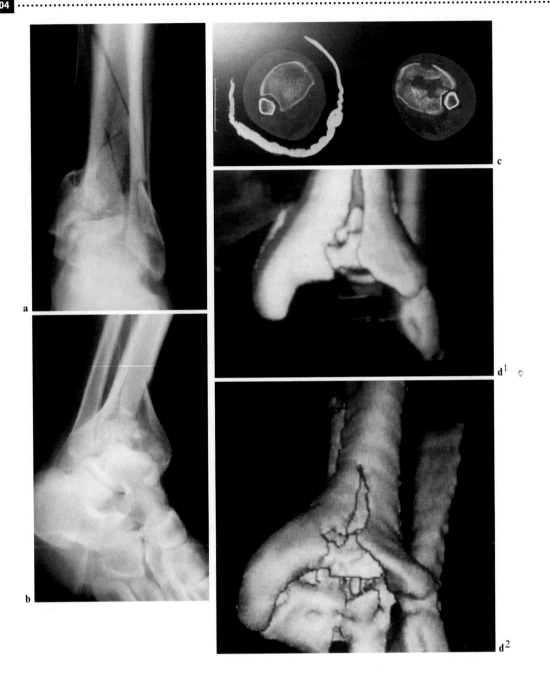

Fig. 21.10 a–d. Computed tomographic (CT) examination of pilon fracture. **a,b** This 33-year-old man was injured in a cycling accident. He sustained a severely comminuted left pilon fracture (C type) as noted on the anteroposterior (**a**) and lateral (**b**) radiograph. **c,d** The plain CT (**c**) shows the lesion with crush of articular cartilage but this is better seen on the three-dimensional (3D) CT (**d**) with the talus subtracted. In that view the overall pattern of the fracture is noted, as well as the extreme comminution of the joint surface. CT and 3D CT examinations are extremely helpful for operative decision making in pilon fractures

a) Immediate Surgery

If the soft tissue is adequate for a major surgical procedure, then an open reduction and internal fixation should be carried out immediately. However, many patients are seen late and the skin and soft tissues are not suitable for surgery because of the presence of marked swelling or fracture blisters (see Fig. 21.7), and for these patients surgery must be delayed.

b) Delayed Surgery

Patients in whom surgery has to be delayed should be taken to the operating room, where under general anesthesia a *closed reduction* should be performed, correcting any angular displacement which may be impinging on the soft tissues. If the joint is subluxated, it must be reduced. If this reduction can be maintained in a plaster slab with a bulky dressing, the patient should be immobilized in this way. The limb should be elevated on several pillows and the patient encouraged to exercise limb and toes. If the instability is so marked that adequate alignment cannot be maintained, then an *os calcis traction pin* should be inserted and the patient kept on a Böhler-Braun frame to elevate the extremity: alternatively, an external frame may be used to allow the soft tissues to heal (see Fig. 21.7 e,f). Many types of frames have been advanced, and most incorporate the os calcis to the tibia. The ring fixator has also been successfully used in these situations.

In association with the frame in patients whose anterior skin is too poor for an early operative procedure but whose lateral skin is satisfactory, immediate open anatomical reduction of the fibula with delayed tibial fixation can be performed. This restores limb length, affords partial stability to allow the soft tissues to heal, and prevents the common drift to valgus of the tibia. (Fig. 21.11)

Also, if the articular surface is amenable, percutaneous fixation of the articular fragments in reduced position using X-ray control may be definitive (see Fig. 21.8). Cannulated screws are helpful. Occasionally, a small incision may be made to allow the insertion of a periosteal elevator, which will help with reduction of the articular fragments.

If a tradional open reduction is contemplated, the surgeon should wait until the skin and soft tissue have returned to a reasonable state before performing the surgical procedure on the tibia. This may require 7–10 days of elevation of the limb. During this period, revascularization of the traumatized soft tissues will occur. If the skin and soft tissues never return to an acceptable state, then traction or external fixation must become the definitive treatment. In that particular situation, prior fibular fixation will prove markedly advantageous.

21.5.2.2 Inoperable

If the preoperative assessment indicates that the bone is so osteoporotic or the degree of comminution is so great that surgery, even by the most expert hands, cannot restore and stabilize the joint, then other methods of treatment must be sought.

a) Skeletal Traction

With the patient under general anesthetic, a closed reduction should be carried out, the fracture being viewed under the image intensifier. If the fragments become reasonably aligned, a Kirschner wire should be inserted into the os calcis and the patient treated in traction for 6–8 weeks until the fracture has shown some consolidation. During this period, early motion of the ankle is encouraged.

Alignment must be maintained during this period, so frequent radiographs are necessary. If the alignment cannot be maintained because of a tendency to valgus deformation, fixation of the fibula, if fractured, should be considered as outlined above. This will prevent displacement and may greatly simplify the management in traction.

The surgeon must be certain that the ankle joint is not immobilized in the dislocated position. We have seen a number of patients treated nonoperatively with the ankle in the dislocated position – needless to say, with disastrous results.

Therefore, if a closed reduction is attempted but fails, the surgeon must discover the cause of this persistent dislocation. Usually, the medial soft tissues, such as the posterior tibial tendon, the neurovascular bundle, or the flexor digitorum longus, are caught in the fracture. In one such case, the surgeon even fixed the fibula but left the ankle joint dislocated in traction (Fig. 21.12). Further surgery at 4 weeks revealed the posterior tibial tendon to be interposed between the main tibial fragments.

b) External Skeletal Fixation

An external frame, os calcis to tibia, may be used in place of skeletal traction. This will allow the patient to be out of bed, but will prevent motion of the ankle, unless one of the newer frame designs is used which allows motion.

c) Primary Arthrodesis

If the patient has good bone but the degree of comminution is so excessive that an anatomical reduction cannot be carried out, then the surgeon could consider primary arthrodesis (Fig. 21.13). In our opinion, this is rarely indicated and, as stated previously, must be thoroughly discussed with the patient preoperatively to avoid misunderstanding and possible litigation. The advantage of primary arthrodesis is that it not only stabilizes the ankle, but allows early mobilization of the remainder of the foot, which is so important with ankle arthrodesis. However, with an os calcis traction pin and elevation,

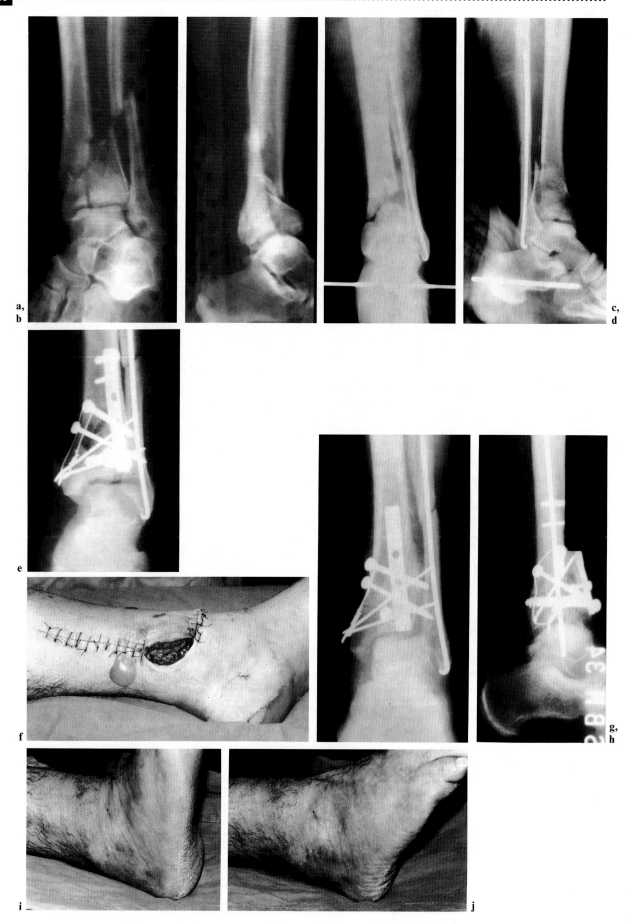

a,
b

c,
d

e

f

g,
h

i

j

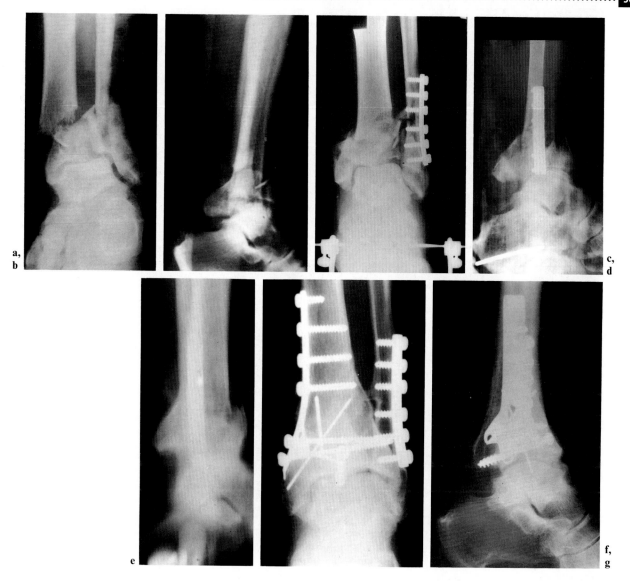

a, b

c, d

e

f, g

Fig. 21.12 a–g. Posterior tibial tendon entrapment. **a,b** This 29-year-old workman fell from a roof, sustaining a severely comminuted intra-articular open pilon fracture of the left ankle. Initial treatment consisted of débridement of the wound, stabilization of the lateral malleolus, insertion of an os calcis pin, and subsequent os calcis traction. The original medial wound was left open. **c,d** The immediate postoperative radiographs show the position of the fracture postoperatively. On the lateral radiograph (**d**), the ankle joint is clearly dislocated along with the anterior fragment of the distal tibia. **e** This is better illustrated in the lateral tomogram. The posterior tibial tendon was interposed between the two bone fragments of the distal tibia and was not seen at the initial débridement. The dislocation was subsequently recognized at 3 weeks and open reduction, position, and internal fixation of the distal tibia were performed. **f,g** Two years following injury, some joint narrowing and sclerosis is noted, indicative of an early osteoarthritis. The patient's function at that time was fair

◀ **Fig. 21.11 a–j.** Immediate fibular fixation, delayed tibial fixation. **a,b** This 42-year-old workman fell from a scaffold and sustained an open pilon fracture. On the night of admission, the wound was cleansed and débrided. **c,d** The fibula was fixed with a Rush rod and an os calcis pin was inserted for skeletal traction on a Böhler-Braun frame. On the seventh day after injury, open reduction and internal fixation of the tibial fracture were performed. **e** The postoperative radiograph shows the excellent reconstruction of the joint surface with interfragmental screws, Kirschner wires, and a dynamic compression (DC) plate. A bone graft was used in this case. **f** The original open portion of the wound was left open, and the remainder sutured. **g,h** Three years following injury, the bone has healed and the ankle joint has remained congruous and stable. **i,j** The patient has 5° dorsiflexion to 20° plantar flexion

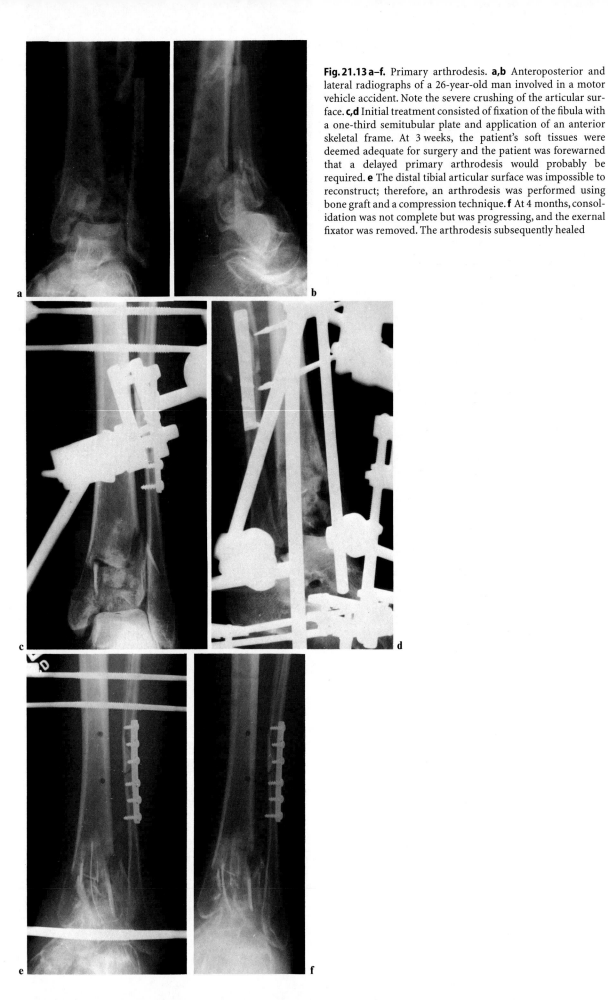

Fig. 21.13 a–f. Primary arthrodesis. **a,b** Anteroposterior and lateral radiographs of a 26-year-old man involved in a motor vehicle accident. Note the severe crushing of the articular surface. **c,d** Initial treatment consisted of fixation of the fibula with a one-third semitubular plate and application of an anterior skeletal frame. At 3 weeks, the patient's soft tissues were deemed adequate for surgery and the patient was forewarned that a delayed primary arthrodesis would probably be required. **e** The distal tibial articular surface was impossible to reconstruct; therefore, an arthrodesis was performed using bone graft and a compression technique. **f** At 4 months, consolidation was not complete but was progressing, and the exernal fixator was removed. The arthrodesis subsequently healed

mobilization of the ankle and foot are also possible; therefore, unless the situation is completely hopeless, we prefer this approach to primary arthrodesis.

21.6 Surgical Technique

21.6.1 Timing

The timing of any surgical procedure around the distal tibia must be carefully determined, depending on the particular circumstances of the case. Many questions remain unanswered.

Should the surgery be performed soon after the injury, before the development of severe soft tissue swelling and fracture blisters, or is it best to delay to allow the skin and soft tissues to recover? Also of clinical significance is whether fragments of bone are impinging on the skin and soft tissues; if so, they must be reduced or soft tissue healing may be delayed; ulceration may even occur. If the closed soft tissue injury is assessed according to Tscherne and Gotzen (1984; see Fig. 21.4), the open reduction and internal fixation may be performed early in grade 0 or 1 injuries, but in higher grades, delay is more prevalent. While waiting, fibular fixation is beneficial, as is traction or external fixation. Open fractures should also be dealt with immediately. The wounds should be cleansed and débrided. Precise preoperative planning is required to safely incorporate the wounds into the surgical incisions and to optimally place the implants.

In grade 2 and 3 soft tissue injuries where massive swelling and traumatic bullae are already present, surgery is hazardous and must be avoided. As previously mentioned, any dislocation must be reduced, and the limb should be elevated in a bulky dressing if stable or, if unstable, with a traction pin in the os calcis.

An external fixator will serve the same purpose, i.e., immobilization to allow soft tissue healing and traction to maintain length (Fig. 21.14). One or two pins in the tibia joined to one pin in the os calcis will be sufficient to maintain traction on a temporary basis. Usually 7–10 days are required for the soft tissues to recover sufficiently to allow safe reconstruction of the fracture.

In these circumstances, alternative treatment should be used, including limited internal fixation of the joint fracture with external fixation. This may be a wiser choice rather than risking a wound breakdown in the ankle area, which may lead to sepsis and a disastrous result.

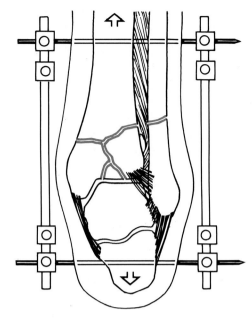

Fig. 21.14. External fixator to maintain temporary traction in a pilon fracture

21.6.2 Approach

21.6.2.1 Soft Tissue

Careful planning of the skin incision is essential. Given the choice, the favored incision runs just lateral to the anterior surface of the tibia and just medial to the tibialis anterior tendon, extending distally over the anterior portion of the medial malleolus (Fig. 21.15). However, the incisions might have to be modified depending upon the presence of lacerations or traumatized skin. The lateral incision for the fibular fracture should be posteriorly placed to increase the bridge between the two incisions (Fig. 21.15 b).

Delicate handling of the skin in this area is imperative. It is relatively avascular, and improperly raised flaps and traumatic handling of the skin will result in necrosis with its ensuing problems. The surgeon must take great pains to be certain that the flap raised over the lower tibia is of full thickness, i.e., contains both skin and subcutaneous tissue right up to the periosteum. If the subcutaneous layer is entered, the blood supply will be compromised and necrosis of the skin may ensue. This in turn often leads to sepsis and a disastrous result.

For more limited approaches to the distal tibia, only the distal end of the anterior incision is used. Placement of the limited incision will also depend on the size and location of the fragments.

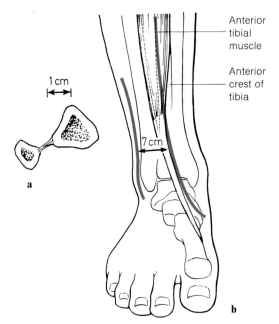

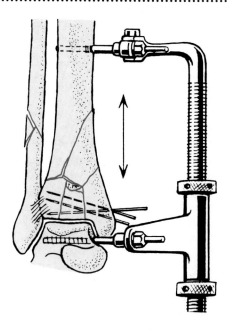

Fig. 21.15 a,b. Surgical approach to fractures of the distal tibia (pilon fractures). The incision for the distal tibia should be medial to the tibialis anterior tendon, crossing the ankle joint and then curving slightly medially. This incision should be well lateral to the anterior subcutaneous surface of the tibia (**a**). The lateral incision should be posterior to the most prominent portion of the lateral malleolus and fibula, the surgeon being certain to keep as wide a bridge of skin as possible between it and the medial incision (**b**). (Adapted from Müller et al. 1979)

Fig. 21.16. Indirect reduction using the distractor and temporary fixation of the joint fragments with Kirschner wires. Internal fixation then can be applied to the fibula. (From Müller et al. 1991)

21.6.2.2 Skeletal Tissue

As in all metaphyseal fractures, especially those involving a joint surface, exposure of the joint should be through major tears in the soft tissue envelope (see Fig. 21.17 a,b). This will preserve the remaining soft tissue attachments to the fracture fragments and facilitate stabilization of the comminuted metaphyseal fragments. Also, in order to maintain bone viability, these soft tissue attachments must be preserved by using indirect reduction techniques, such as the AO distractor (Fig. 21.16).

Because the area in the distal tibia is such a difficult area for healing due to limited blood supply, atraumatic techniques including indirect reduction are essential to achieve satisfactory results. In this area, clearly *biology* is more important than *biomechanics*.

21.6.3 Technique of Internal Fixation

21.6.3.1 Without Fibular Fracture

If the fibula is intact, lateral stability of the ankle mortise is maintained. Usually, however, the tibial fracture exhib-

its comminution and impaction of the joint surface (see Fig. 21.2 c).

A large intact fragment usually remains with the fibula and is used as a guide to the articular reconstruction. The large medial vertical fragment may be carefully retracted with a rake retractor, thus exposing the articular surface (Fig. 21.17 a,b). All soft tissue attachments to this fragment must be retained. If a central depressed articular fragment is found, it must be restored to its anatomical position and provisionally fixed with Kirschner wires (1.6–2.0 mm) (Fig. 21.17 b). A cancellous bone graft will hold the articular fragments in place, and then the medial vertical fracture is reduced, thus "closing the book" (Fig. 21.17 c). This type of fracture is akin to the usual type of depressed proximal lateral plateau fracture. The large medial fragment is stabilized with interfragmental lag screws and a medial buttress plate, usually the T or cloverleaf type (Fig. 21.17 d–h).

21.6.3.2 With Fibular Fracture

If the fibula is fractured (Fig. 21.18 a), the four steps in the reconstruction are as follows:

1. Reconstruction of the fibula (Fig. 21.18 b)
2. Open reduction of the tibial articular surface and metaphysis (Fig. 21.18 c)

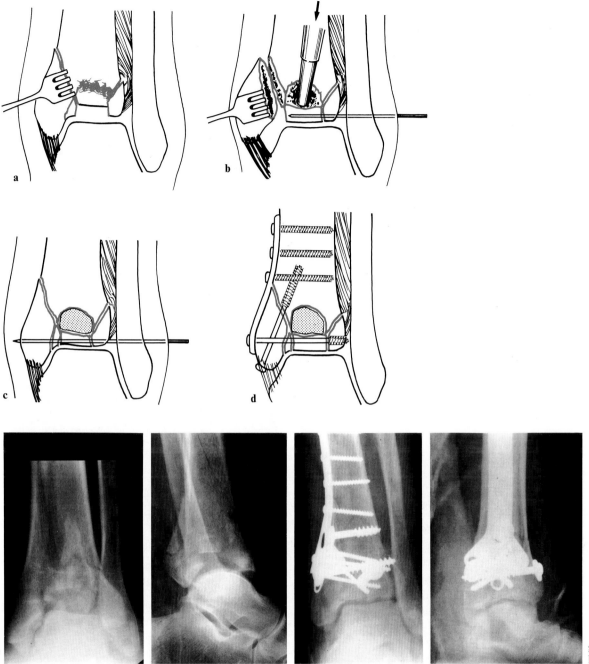

Fig. 21.17 a–h. Technique of open reduction and internal fixation in a pilon fracture with an intact fibula. Since the fibula is intact, lateral stability of the ankle mortise is maintained. A large tibial fragment usually remains with the fibula and is used as a guide to articular reconstruction. **a** The large medial vertical fragment is retracted with a rake retractor. Working through the fracture in order not to destroy soft tissue, the articular fragments are restored to the anatomical position and provisionally fixed with 2-mm Kirschner wires. **b** Atraumatic indirect reduction techniques must be used. **c** Any gap is filled with cancellous bone to hold the articular fragments in place. **d** The tibia is then buttressed with a medial buttress plate and lag screws as indicated. **e,f** Anteroposterior and lateral radiograph of a 23-year-old man involved in a motor vehicle accident. Note the intact fibula and the articular crush. **g,h** Reconstruction by the above method using a cloverleaf plate, with excellent articular reconstruction

512 ·

Chapter 21   **Fractures of the Distal Tibial Metaphysis Involving the Ankle Joint**

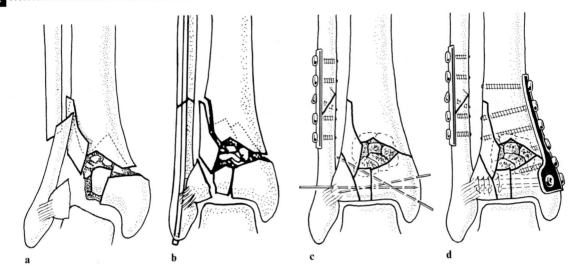

a   b   c   d

Fig. 21.18 a–d. Pilon fracture reconstruction with fibular fracture. **a** Pilon fracture with intra-articular comminution and fibular fracture. **b** Step 1: reconstruction of the fibula by either an intramedullary rod or a one-third semitubular plate. **c** Steps 2 and 3: reconstruction of the articular surface of the distal tibia and provisional fixation with Kirschner wires. The metaphysis is reduced with the atraumatic, indirect techniques. The resultant gap is filled with cancellous bone graft. **d** Step 4: application of a medial buttress plate (T plate). (Adapted from Müller et al. 1979)

3. Cancellous bone-grafting of the metaphyseal defect (Fig. 21.18 c)
4. Application of a buttress plate to the anterior or medial cortex of the tibia (Fig. 21.18 d)

a) Fibular Reconstruction

The fibular reconstruction should be performed using standard AO/ASIF techniques (Fig. 21.18 b).

If the fracture is transverse, an intramedullary Steinmann pin or Rush rod may be used. This has the added advantage of a short incision and minimal dissection on the lateral side, which makes the medial approach and closure much simpler. Restoration of fibular length is essential, but less than perfect rotational stability of the fibula is acceptable in the pilon fracture since stability of the tibia is restored. In the usual bi- or trimalleolar ankle fracture, it is imperative to achieve rotational stability of the fibula, and therefore intramedullary devices in the fibula are contraindicated. However, in the particular type of fracture with which we are dealing here, i.e., the pilon fracture, intramedullary devices in the fibula are ideal if the fibular fracture is transverse and not comminuted.

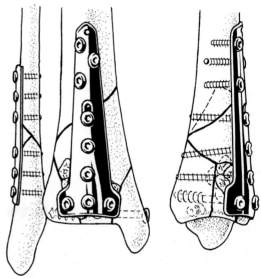

Fig. 21.19. Spoon plate as an anterior buttress plate. As the situation dictates, an anterior buttress may be more desirable than a medial buttress, and for this situation the spoon plate is an excellent implant. (From Müller et al. 1979)

If the fibula is comminuted, the fracture should be fixed with interfragmental compression screws and a one-third semitubular plate as a neutralization plate. If the fibula is grossly comminuted, it is extremely important to be certain that full length is restored to the fibula. The fibula is connected to the lateral articular fragment of the tibia; therefore, its proper length is the key to the reduction of this tibial articular surface. Shortening of the fibula will cause malreduction of the major tibial fracture.

In rare instances, there may be so much comminution of the fibula that primary fixation of this bone is impos-

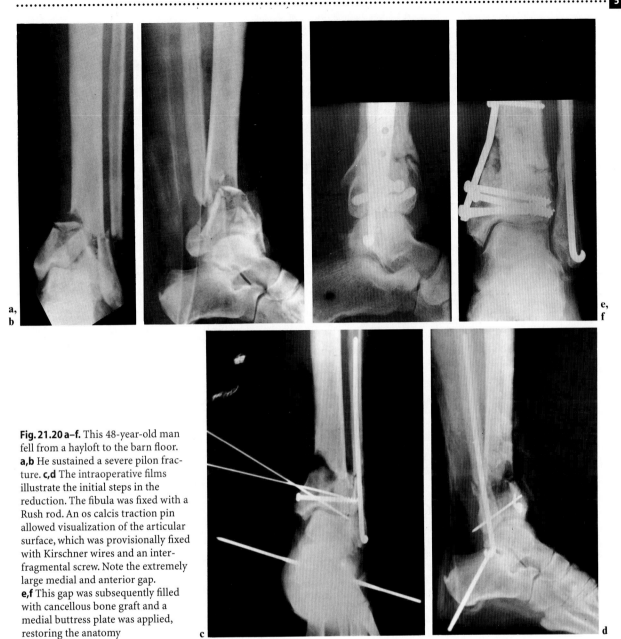

Fig. 21.20 a–f. This 48-year-old man fell from a hayloft to the barn floor. **a,b** He sustained a severe pilon fracture. **c,d** The intraoperative films illustrate the initial steps in the reduction. The fibula was fixed with a Rush rod. An os calcis traction pin allowed visualization of the articular surface, which was provisionally fixed with Kirschner wires and an interfragmental screw. Note the extremely large medial and anterior gap. **e,f** This gap was subsequently filled with cancellous bone graft and a medial buttress plate was applied, restoring the anatomy

sible. In those circumstances, articular reconstruction of the tibia should proceed first, and fixation of the fibula be undertaken afterwards if technically possible. However, failure to reconstruct the fibula at all is a major error in judgement and may jeopardize the tibial reconstruction, as the tendency of the ankle to drift into valgus will be difficult to overcome. Stabilization of the fibula is therefore an essential part of the treatment (see Fig. 21.23).

b) Articular Reconstruction of the Tibia

After fixation of the fibula, articular reconstruction should proceed in a logical fashion. The articular surface should usually be reduced first. The key to the articular reconstruction is the lateral fragment, which should be in the anatomically correct position if connected by the inferior tibiofibular ligament to the already anatomically fixed fibula. Each of the major fragments should be reduced and carefully fixed with Kirschner wires. If only major fragments are involved, the reduction is relatively easy and should be anatomical (Fig. 21.18 c).

Chapter 21   **Fractures of the Distal Tibial Metaphysis Involving the Ankle Joint**

514 ....

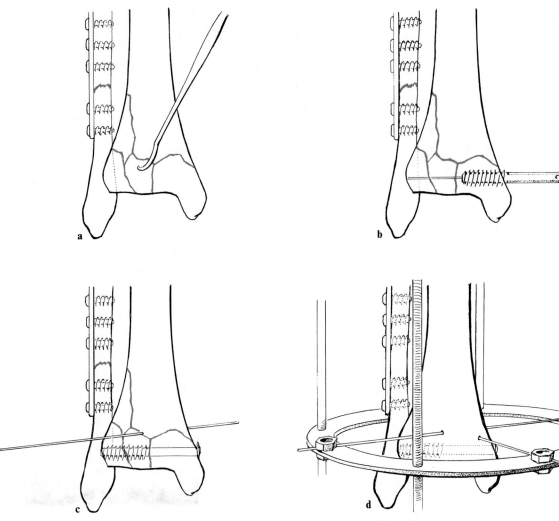

Fig. 21.21 a–d. Reduction and fixation techniques with poor soft tissues. **a** If the distal fibular tissues allow and the fibula is fractured, anatomic open reduction and external fixation of the fibula should proceed first. **b** Using traction techniques to reduce the fracture (see Fig. 21.26), or through a limited anterior approach using a periosteal elevator to reduce the articular fragment, Kirschner wires are inserted. If the articular fragments are reduced, cannulated screws are inserted over the Kirschner wires for fixation. Also a bone graft may be inserted through this approach. **c** Other fragments may be held using the above wires or other fine wires, attached to a ring fixator for axial stability (**d**)

If gross comminution of the metaphysis is present, the surgeon should first focus his or her attention on an accurate reconstruction of the articular surface. The articular fragments should be provisionally fixed with 1.6-mm Kirschner wires and then held with large cancellous screws if possible.

Following temporary fixation of the articular surface, the axial alignment of the metaphysis must be obtained.

It is essential that the fragments retain their soft tissue and vascularity; therefore, indirect techniques must be used. Several techniques are possible, including a skeletal distractor, external fixation, or the use of a plate connected to the articular fragment and a distraction device (Fig. 21.16).

c) Cancellous Grafting

A cancellous bone graft, which may be taken prior to surgery or simultaneously by a second operative team, is then impacted into the large metaphyseal gap (Fig. 21.18 c). Small fragments of articular cartilage which have not been fixed with Kirschner wires and are not small enough to discard may be held in place between the cancellous bone graft and the dome of the talus. Their stability, however, must be ensured, so that they do not fall out into the joint and act as a loose body. The cancellous bone graft should be fully impacted to restore stability to the distal fragment.

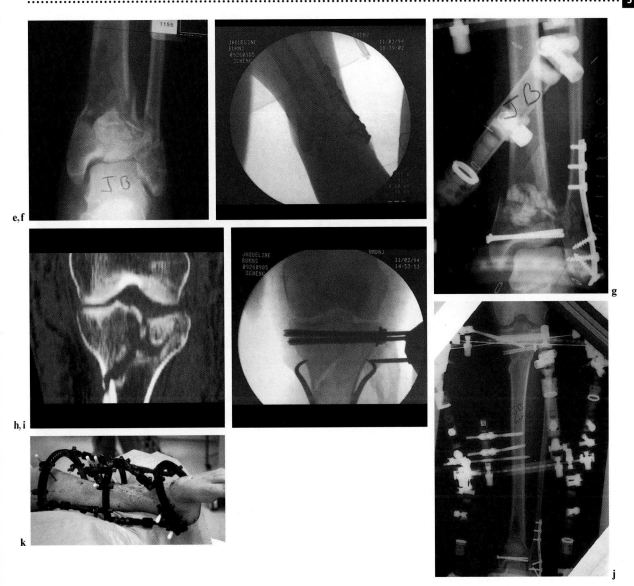

Fig. 21.21 e–k. Minimal internal fixation and ring fixator in polytrauma with poor soft tissues. This 40-year-old woman was involved in a motor vehicle accident. She sustained a pelvic ring injury, a segmental femur fracture, a fracture of her right tibia, as well as the illustrated fracture of her left tibial plateau, and an open pilon fracture. Because of her polytrauma and poor soft tissues it was elected to treat the left tibial fractures with minimal internal fixation and a ring fixator. The severe comminution of the ankle joint is noted in the radiograph (**e**), and after fibular fixation in the intraoperative radiograph (**f**). **g** The joint surface was anatomically reduced and fixed with two cannulated screws. **h,i** Note the severe comminution of the tibial plateau on the intraoperative radiograph (**h**) and the intraoperative film showing the two cannulated screws in place on the image intensifier (**i**). **j** The final position, including the ring fixator, is noted on the radiograph. **k** The position of the ring fixator and the soft tissues is seen in the photograph. The fracture healed in good position and the patient has excellent function. (Courtesy of R. Schenk, Newark, NJ, USA)

d) Medial Tibial Cortex Buttress Plate

To ensure the anatomical reduction of this provisionally fixed tibia, a buttress plate must be applied either anteriorly or medially, depending upon the area of comminution (see Fig. 21.6). The medial buttress plate may be either of the T plate or cloverleaf variety (see Fig. 21.6). The cloverleaf plate is weak and should only be used in those situations where the comminution is so great that multiple screw holes are required for the fixation of the articular surface. In most cases, the T plate is a better implant. If the comminution is anterior, the anterior or spoon plate will give far better fixation and is recommended (Fig. 21.19). These general principles are well illustrated in Fig. 21.20.

516 ....

Chapter 21   **Fractures of the Distal Tibial Metaphysis Involving the Ankle Joint**

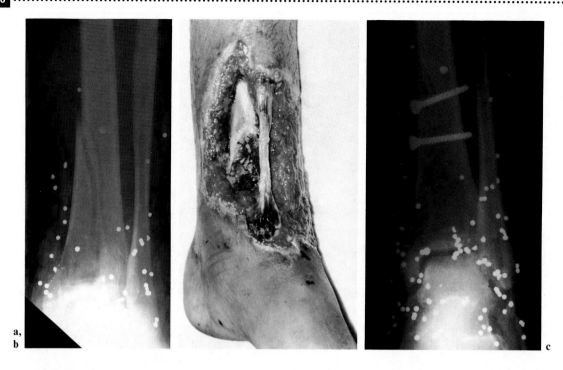

a,
b

c

Fig. 21.22. a Radiograph of a 29-year-old man with an open fracture of the right ankle due to a gunshot. **b** After débridement, the surgeon attempted a relaxing incision, resulting in complete necrosis of the skin and anterior tibial tendon. **c** The fracture was secondarily fixed with two interfragmental screws and the wound débrided and skin grafted

With compromised soft tissue, external fixation as a medial buttress is a better choice than a plate.

If it becomes obvious to the surgeon after the start of the surgical procedure that the bone is too weak to hold a screw, the situation may be improved by using low-viscosity polymethyl methacrylate bone cement in the screw hole or at the fracture site. However, we would recommend this procedure only in older individuals. In these cases, the Kirschner wires should be retained as definitive forms of internal stabilization and should not be removed until union is complete. Early motion will not be possible, so the final result may be compromised.

21.6.4 Fixation Techniques with Poor Skin and Soft Tissue (Grade 3)

If the soft tissues are compromised, as in grade 2 or 3 injury (Tscherne), then the surgeon should use alternative, safer techniques, which may not give as much biomechanical stability, but will respect the relative avascular environment of the distal tibia and the ankle.

Fibular Fixation. If the fibula is fractured, it should be fixed first as described in the previous section, if the lateral skin allows (Fig. 21.21 a).

Articular Reconstruction. Articular reconstruction will depend on the fracture type; in type B lesions, reconstruction through a limited approach or even percutaneously using cannulated screws may be indicated (Fig. 21.21 b). However, in type C grossly comminuted fractures, reduction may be difficult, or even impossible. In all cases, the key to reduction of the joint fragments is the lateral fragment attached to the fibula.

Metaphyseal Reduction. With poor skin, the metaphyseal lesion should be stabilized by an external fixator, either a ring fixator, a standard type, or the presently popular combination type (Fig. 21.21 c,d).

Bone Graft. If a limited approach has been used, a bone graft may be used, as previously indicated.

21.6.5 Wound Closure

If both incisions can be closed without tension, this should be done, primarily over suction drains. Very commonly, however, suturing both incisions will cause undue tension on one or the other wound. When this is the case, it is far better to leave a portion of one wound open than to close it under tension, since this will undoubtedly result in skin necrosis. It is best to close the tibial wound

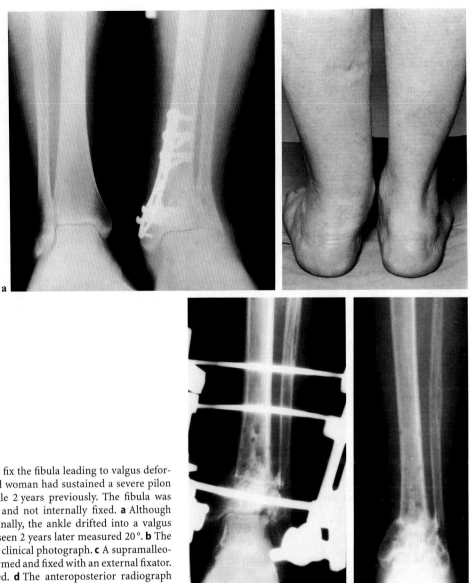

Fig. 21.23 a–d. Failure to fix the fibula leading to valgus deformation. This 41-year-old woman had sustained a severe pilon fracture to her left ankle 2 years previously. The fibula was extremely comminuted and not internally fixed. **a** Although anatomically fixed originally, the ankle drifted into a valgus deformity, which when seen 2 years later measured 20°. **b** The deformity is seen on the clinical photograph. **c** A supramalleolar osteotomy was performed and fixed with an external fixator. Correction was obtained. **d** The anteroposterior radiograph shows the osteotomy healed and the good position of the ankle joint

because of its proximity to the anterior tibial tendon, the subcutaneous border of the tibia, and the major metal implant. The lateral wound may be left open along all or a part of its length. If the lateral skin incision has been correctly made, posterior to the fibula, then the fibular plate will be covered by the skin flap and few problems will ensue. This lateral wound may then be closed on the fifth to tenth postoperative day with fine sutures or skin tapes.

Note: in this area, the surgeon should not attempt to rotate skin flaps to ensure skin closure. The skin in this area may be so traumatized that the entire flap may be rendered avascular and become necrotic, causing a major surgical disaster (Fig. 21.22). It is far better to leave one wound open and close it secondarily than to undertake ill-advised primary plastic procedures.

21.6.6 Postoperative Care

21.6.6.1 Early

In the immediate postoperative period a bulky dressing and posterior slab are applied to the ankle in the neutral position and the extremity is elevated to reduce swelling.

The course of the patient's postoperative care will depend upon the surgeon's honest appraisal of the

518 ....

Chapter 21   **Fractures of the Distal Tibial Metaphysis Involving the Ankle Joint**

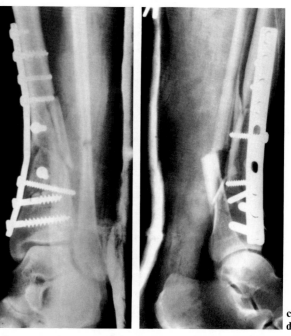

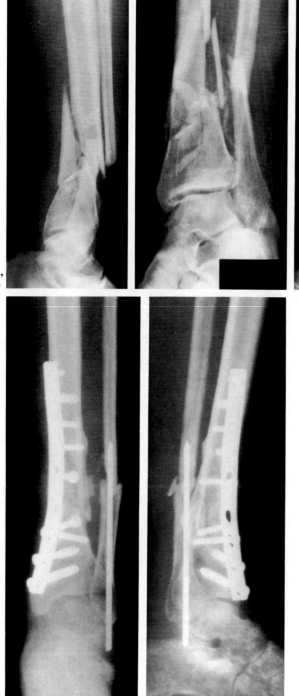

Fig. 21.24 a–f. Failure to fix the fibula with varus deformation. **a,b** Lateral and anteroposterior radiographs of a 27-year-old woman with a pilon fracture involving both the tibia and the fibula. **c,d** Immediate postoperative radiographs showing the varus position of the distal tibia. The fibula was not fixed. **d** Note the recurvatum deformity. **e,f** An attempt to secondarily fix the fibula failed to anatomically reduce the tibial fracture. The final result was fair

stability achieved by surgery. If the bone quality is good and the surgeon has been able to achieve stable internal fixation, then the dressing and splint are removed on the second postoperative day and motion is encouraged. The stabilized fracture is relatively painless, many patients being able to move their ankle comfortably as early as the second postoperative day. To prevent a troublesome equinus deformity from developing, the ankle must be maintained in a right-angled splint when the patient is not exercising; once an equinus deformity has developed, attempts at correction by rehabilitation may be tedious and prolonged, and they are often unsuccessful.

If the surgeon is in doubt about the stability of the fracture at the conclusion of the operation, he or she should insert an os calcis pin for skeletal traction to protect the osteosynthesis or use an external fixator. Preservation of the anatomical reduction is essential to the long-term result and should not be compromised by early motion.

The use of the traction pin will allow early motion of the ankle while affording protection to the internal fixation. The pin is generally required for 4–6 weeks, when healing of the cancellous bone has usually progressed

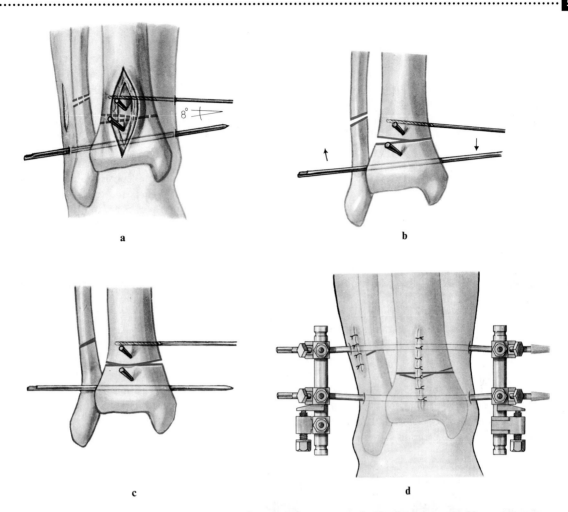

Fig. 21.25 a–d. Stable fixation with two Steinmann pins and external fixators. **a** A small segment of the fibula is resected and a Steinmann pin inserted parallel to the distal articular surface of the tibia. From the medial side and proximal to the planned osteotomy a 3.2-mm drill bit is inserted into the tibia. This drill bit should subtend the desired angle of correction with the Steinmann pin. Two Kirschner wires are inserted into the ante-rior crest, one on each side of the osteotomy. They serve to control the rotational alignment as well as the angulation of the osteotomy. **b** The osteotomy is carried out between the Kirschner wires. **c** The deformity is corrected. **d** The drill bit is removed and replaced with a Steinmann pin. The osteotomy is reduced and compressed with two external fixators. (From Müller et al. 1979)

sufficiently to remove it. A cast brace with a moving ankle piece may then be applied until bone union is complete.

21.6.6.2 Late

The patient must be carefully monitored clinically and radiologically. A patellar-bearing weight-relieving caliper may be used after 6 weeks if healing is progressing well. This allows the patient to bear partial weight with the aid of crutches. The splint should be regularly removed for ankle exercises. If the patient has no pain and the radiograph indicates no problems with the implant, bone union is usually complete at 10–16 weeks and full weight bearing may be resumed. This will, of course, depend upon other factors, such as the degree of comminution, the size and incorporation of the bone graft, and the state of the soft tissues.

21.7 Common Pitfalls of Treatment

Since the pilon or distal tibial metaphyseal fracture is fraught with major problems in management, it seems relevant to mention here many of the common pitfalls we have encountered in our practice when the principles stated above have been compromised.

21.7.1 Poor Decision Making

Poor decision making is probably the commonest cause of grief with this fracture. In some cases, operable fractures are treated nonoperatively, with poor results, while in others shattered fractures, obviously nonoperable, are treated operatively, with a similar outcome.

21.7.2 Operating Through Poor Skin

Operating through severely traumatized skin with fracture blisters constitutes a great error of judgement and often leads to a major disaster, occasionally even an amputation.

Alternative methods of management have been described and will lead to fewer complications.

21.7.3 Technical Difficulties with the Fibula

If the fibula length is not restored, the ankle will tend to drift into valgus (Fig. 21.23), while if the normal valgus curve of the fibula is not restored, the ankle will assume to varus position (Fig. 21.24). The resulting axial malalignment will cause difficulty with the gait and eventual degenerative arthritis in the ankle.

21.7.4 Technical Difficulties with the Tibial Fracture

Previously there was a tendency among surgeons to fix the articular position of the joint and ignore the metaphyseal crush, i.e., to do only one half of the job. This is a common error, usually leading to axial malalignment and a poor final result.

Furthermore, failure to fill the large metaphyseal gap with bone graft may allow the articular fracture to displace, with adverse late consequences.

At this time, attempts are usually made to fix the metaphysis, but unfortunately the methods used often do not reflect the newer techniques of biologic fixation which are extremely important in this anatomic area.

21.7.5 Poor Postoperative Care

Over-optimistic assessment of the operative stabilization and the state of the bone often leads the surgeon to institute early motion of the ankle. If the assessment was wrong, the inevitable result will be collapse of the fixation and loss of the anatomical reduction.

A major cause of grief is failure to splint the ankle at postoperatively. The resulting equinus deformity may be difficult to deal with. There is no excuse for this preventable complication.

21.8 Late Reconstruction: Supramalleolar Osteotomy

If the patient has continuing pain following union of a pilon fracture, careful clinical and radiographic assessment will determine whether the articular cartilage of the ankle joint has been so damaged that arthrodesis of the ankle is the only alternative or whether the articular surface is satisfactory and axial malalignment is the major cause of the problem. In instances of the latter, a supramalleolar osteotomy will restore axial alignment, usually restore normal foot mechanics, and be very helpful to the patient. Careful preoperative planning is essential to the correct performance of this operative procedure. The osteotomy may be fixed with an external fixation device under compression or with internal fixation, which, if possible, is preferable (Figs. 21.25, 21.26). Even in instances where there is damage to articular cartilage, supramalleolar osteotomy may prove to be of major help to the patient without resorting to arthrodesis. The patient in Fig. 21.27, a 29-year-old school teacher, had a marked varus deformation with a medial indentation of the distal tibial articular surface. She had great difficulty in walking. A supramalleolar osteotomy was performed, correcting the varus deformity, and in spite of the articular defect her ankle continues to function well 8 years after surgery.

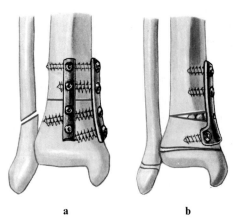

a   b

Fig. 21.26.a Two semitubular plates used for the fixation of a supramalleolar osteotomy in an adult. **b** In children, where the deformity results from a premature partial closure of the epiphyseal plate, we prefer an open wedge osteotomy, which restores some length and corrects the deformity. The defect is bone-grafted and the osteotomy fixed with a small T plate. (From Müller et al 1979)

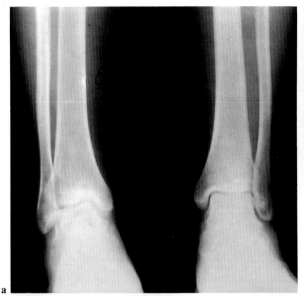

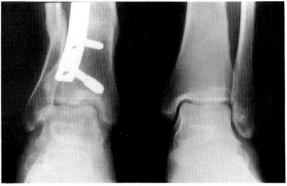

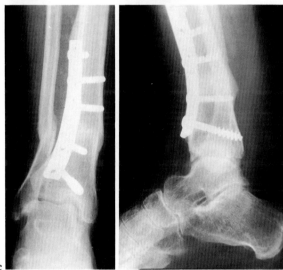

Fig. 21.27 a–c. Varus deformation requiring supramalleolar osteotomy. **a** Comparative standing anteroposterior radiographs of both ankles showing the severe varus deformation of the right ankle, due to an impacted fracture of the distal tibial articular surface. The patient had severe pain and difficulty walking with the right foot. A supramalleolar osteotomy was performed with fibular osteotomy, and the tibial osteotomy was internally fixed. **b** The comparative radiograph now shows correction of the varus deformity. **c** Anteroposterior and lateral radiographs taken at 1 year showing the healed osteotomy and the excellent anatomical position. Eight years following osteotomy, the patient's ankle is still functioning well with only minimal discomfort

References

Bone L, Stegemann P, McNamara K, Seibel R (1993) External fixation of severely comminuted and open tibial pilon fractures. Clin Orth Rel Res 92:101–107

Bonnier P (1961) Les fractures du pilon tibial. Thesis, Lyons

Conrad RW (1970) Fracture dislocations of the ankle joint in the impaction injury of the lateral weight bearing surface of the tibia. J Bone Joint Surg 52A:1337

DeCoulx P, Razemon JP, Rouselle Y (1961) Fractures du tibial pilon. Rev Chir Orthop 47:563

Fourquet D (1959) Contribution a l'étude des fractures récentes du pilon tibial. Thesis, Paris

Heim U, Naser K (1977) Fractures du pilon tibial: resultats de 128 osteosynthèses. Rev Chir Orthop 63(1):5–12

Kellam JF, Waddell JP (1979) Fractures of the distal tibia. J Trauma 8:593–601

Müller ME, Allgöwer M, Schneider R, Willenegger H (eds) (1979) Manual of internal fixation, 2nd edn. Springer, Berlin Heidelberg New York

Müller ME, Nazarian S, Koch P, Schatzker J (1990) The comprehensive classification of fractures of long bones. Springer, Berlin Heidelberg New York

Müller ME, Allgöwer M, Schneider R, Willenegger H (eds) (1991) Manual of internal fixation, 3rd edn. Springer, Berlin Heidelberg New York

Rüedi T (1973) Fractures of the lower end of the tibia into the ankle joint: results 9 years after open reduction and internal fixation. Injury 5:130

Rüedi TP, Allgöwer M (1969) Fractures of the lower end of the tibia into the ankle joint. Injury 1:92

Rüedi TP, Allgöwer M (1979) The operative treatment of intra-articular fractures of the lower end of the tibia. Clin Orthop 138:105–110

Ruoff AC, Snider RK (1971) Explosion fractures of the distal tibia with major articular involvement. J Trauma 11:866

Szyszkowitz R, Marti R, Wilde CD, Reschauer R, Schloffmann W (1979) Die offene Reposition und Verschraubung der Talusfrakturen. Hefte Unfallheilkd 133:41–48

Teeny SM, Wiss DA (1993) Open reduction and internal fixation of tibial plafond fractures: variables contributing to poor results and complications. Clin Orth Rel Res 292:108–117

Tscherne H, Gotzen L (1984) Fractures with soft tissue injuries. Springer, Berlin Heidelberg New York

Williams CW, Langston J, Sander A (1967) Comminuted fractures of the distal tibia into the ankle joint. J Bone Joint Surg 49A:192

22 Fractures of the Ankle

M. Tile

22.1 Introduction

22.1.1 Basic Principles

As in all fractures through the articular surface of a major weight-bearing joint, optimal treatment for fractures of the ankle follows the basic tenet: restoration of the normal anatomy is required to prevent development of secondary arthritis. The anatomical reduction may be obtained by closed means, but often, in unstable fractures, it cannot be maintained. The most precise method of restoring and maintaining the anatomy of the unstable ankle injury is open reduction and internal fixation. As an added advantage, modern stable internal fixation may allow early motion and will usually ensure a satisfactory outcome.

22.1.2 Anatomical Considerations

22.1.2.1 Stability

Stability is imparted to the ankle by its bony configuration and its complex ligamentous system. The dome of the talus is held snugly in the ankle mortise by a cup-like structure consisting of the adjacent articular surfaces of the tibia and fibula. At the ankle, these two bones are held together by the interosseous membrane and the strong syndesmotic ligaments, the anterior tibiofibular ligaments, and the strong posterior tibiofibular ligaments (Fig. 22.1 a). Only minor degrees of motion are possible at the intact distal tibiofibular joint. Further stability is imparted by the medial and lateral collateral ligaments and the intervening joint capsule.

The medial or deltoid ligament is a fan-shaped structure consisting of two portions, a superficial and a deep (Pankovich and Shivaran 1979; Fig. 22.1 b). The deep portion, in turn, consists of two parts: the deep anterior talotibial ligament, originating from the anterior aspect of the medial malleolus and distally inserting on the medial side of the talus, and the deep posterior talotibial ligament, running from the posterior aspect of the medial malleolus posteriorly to the medial aspect of the talus. The superficial portion, the tibiocalcaneal band, consists of a continuous fan-like structure connecting the anterior colliculus of the medial malleolus to the navicular bone, calcaneus, and talus. The tendon sheaths of the posterior tibial and flexor digitorum communis muscles are contiguous with the deltoid ligament.

On the lateral aspect, stability is maintained by the complex lateral collateral ligament, consisting of three portions (Fig. 22.1 c). Functioning as the anterior cruciate ligament of the ankle, the anterior talofibular ligament connects the anterior portion of the fibula to the talar tubercle, thereby preventing anterior displacement of the talus in the ankle mortise. The importance of this ligament in ankle pathology has been greatly underestimated. The calcaneofibular ligament limits inversion by its attachments from fibula to calcaneus. The posterior talofibular ligament runs horizontally and medially, completing the lateral stabilizing mechanism and limiting posterior and rotatory subluxation of the talus.

22.1.2.2 Congruity

The ankle joint is fully congruous in all positions of the talus, from full plantar flexion to full dorsiflexion (Inman 1976). Previous teaching held that the talus, narrower posteriorly than anteriorly, would be unstable in the ankle mortise when plantar flexed. However, Inman postulated that both the talar and tibial articular surfaces are segments of a cone or frustum, with the apex located medially (Fig. 22.2 a); therefore, during the normal ankle motion of dorsiflexion to plantar flexion, the dome of the talus rotates around its laterally placed base (Fig. 22.2 b). The smooth and congruous motion of the normal ankle depends upon an anatomical and stable lateral malleolar complex to accommodate the longer excursion of the larger lateral border of the talus. As each segment of the cone rotates, full congruity is maintained in all positions. Further work in our laboratory using latex injection into the joint confirmed the congruous nature of the joint.

Using standard radiographic techniques in normal subjects, Gollish et al. (1977) also ascertained that the normal ankle has no talar tilt either in valgus or varus in the stance phase of gait and is fully congruous in that position (see Fig. 22.8 a, b).

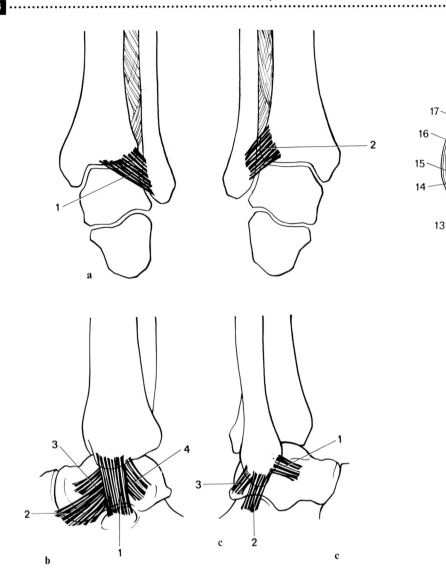

Fig. 22.1. a *Left,* the anterior *(1)* and posterior *(2)* tibiofibular ligaments (syndesmotic ligaments): *Right,* cross-section of the ankle showing the syndesmotic ligaments. *1,* anterior tibial tendon; *2,* neurovascular bundle: anterior tibial nerves and vessels; *3,* extensor hallucis longus; *4,* extensor digitorum longus; *5,* saphenous vein; *6,* tibia; *7,* posterior tibial tendon; *8,* flexor digitorum longus tendon; *9,* neurovascular bundle: posterior tibial nerves and vessels; *10,* flexor hallucis longus tendon; *11,* Achilles tendon; *12,* sural nerves; *13,* posterior syndesmotic ligament; *14,* peroneous longus tendon; *15,* peroneous brevis tendon; *16,* fibula; *17,* anterior syndesmotic ligament. **b** The medial (deltoid) ligament. Note the fan-shaped insertion of this ligament, which contains two portions, a superficial *(1)* (the tibiocalcaneal band) and a deep one, a part of which becomes the spring ligament (**2**). The deep portion has two parts, a deep anterior talotibial ligament *(3)* and a deep posterior, talotibial ligament *(4)*. **c** The lateral ligament. This ligament has three parts, the anterior talofibular ligament *(1),* the calcaneolfibular ligament *(2)* and the posterior talofibular ligament *(3)*

22.1.2.3 Physiology

Although the ankle joint remains congruous, some motion does occur at the distal tibiofibular joint during normal gait. In the stance phase, a lateral thrust occurs from the talus to the lateral malleolus. This force is then transferred back to the tibia through the interosseous membrane (Fig. 22.3). The lateral malleolus, therefore, is a weight-bearing structure, maintaining approximately one sixth of the body weight (Elmendorff and Petes 1971).

22.1.2.4 Pathoanatomy

Several important clinical considerations arise from the preceding comments. First, since the ankle liga-

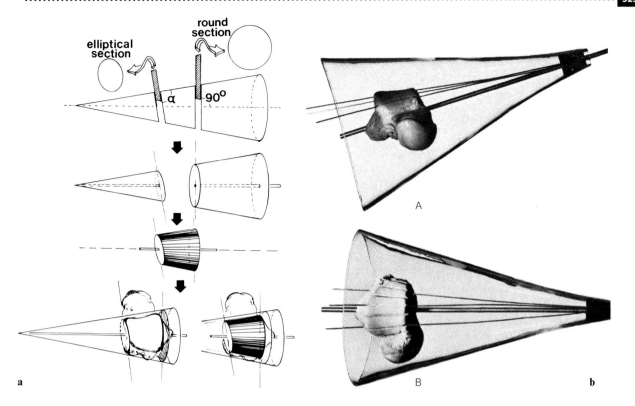

Fig. 22.2. a Pictorial representation of present concept of construction of the trochlea of the talus. A frustrum is cut from a cone. The section cut at 90° to the axis of the cone is circular when projected onto a transverse plane of the cone; this corresponds to the fibular (lateral) facet. The section cut obliquely is elliptical; this corresponds to the tibial (medial) facet. Note that the fibular facet, being farther from the apex of the cone, possesses greater dimensions. With minor modifications, a section of the frustrum is converted into the trochlea of the talus. The anteroposterior curve of the fibular facet is an ellipse because of the oblique orientation of the conical surface of the trochlea when viewed from above. **b** *A* Talus mounted inside transparent glass cone and oriented so it is viewed from the front. Note that while the superior surface of the trochlea is horizontal, the axis is oblique, causing both the glass cone and the conical surface of the trochlea, as outlined by the Kirschner wires, to be slanted. *B* View from above the glass cone with enclosed talus, which has not been moved. Note that because of the obliquity of the axis and the slant of the glass cone *(A)*, the open base of the glass cone is now viewed as an ellipse. Attention is called to the resultant parallelism between the edge of the glass cone and the curvature of the lateral edge of the trochlea. (From Inman 1976)

ments are vital for the stability of the joint, they must be considered as important as the bone in the assessment of the injury. On clinical examination, the presence of local tenderness, ecchymoses, and swelling at the site of a ligamentous attachment, in the absence of a radiologically proven fracture, should alert the sur-

geon to a major ligamentous disruption. Demonstration of a subluxation of the talus in the ankle mortise, occasionally under general anesthesia, will confirm the resultant instability. Second, since the joint is fully congruous in all positions of ankle motion, it follows that even minor abnormalities in the ankle mortise will alter the biomechanics of the joint and may result in major long-term problems. Therefore, restoration of ankle congruity is imperative if secondary osteoarthritis is to be avoided.

Finally, contrary to previous belief, the lateral side of the joint is of vital clinical importance for both stability and congruity and must therefore be anatomically restored. Shortening or rotatory displacement of the fibula will markedly affect the articular contact area between the talus and the tibia.

Willenegger (1979) showed that a 2°–4° tilt in the vertical axis of the lateral malleolus displaced the talus 2 mm laterally, while a 2–3 mm posterior displacement of the lateral malleolus moved the vertical axis of the talus by 10°, both reducing the contact area on the talar dome significantly (Fig. 22.4). Using latex in combination with dye techniques, Gollish et al. (1977) found similar results.

Ramsay and Hamilton (1976), using a black carbon transference technique, determined the contact area in 23 dissected tibiotalar articulations, with varying displacements of the talus laterally. The greatest reduction

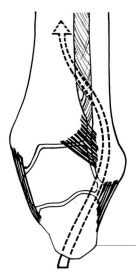

Fig. 22.3. Approximately one sixth of the body weight is transferred through the fibular malleolus to the tibia

in contact area occurred during the initial 1 mm of lateral shift, the average reduction being 42%.

Therefore, the incongruity resulting from a malunited lateral malleolus places the joint in a subluxated position (Fig. 22.5). This will in turn decrease the joint surface contact area, with a concomitant rise in the surface pressure, and lead inevitably to degenerative changes.

Fig. 22.4 a,b. Reduction in the contact area of the talar dome with the tibial plafond by **a** a tilt in the vertical axis of the lateral malleolus and **b** a posterior displacement of the vertical axis of the talus. (From Müller et al. 1965)

Displacements on the medial side, with an intact lateral malleolus, do not have the same biomechanical significance.

········

22.1.3 Natural History

Are these theoretical facts borne out clinically? The answer is a definite yes. The final result clearly relates more to restoration of joint congruity than to any other single factor. Minor degrees of incongruity usually lead to early symptoms and eventual osteoarthritis, and gross incongruity to early dissolution of the joint (Figs. 22.6, 22.7). Many surgeons have argued that the case for careful restoration of the anatomy has been overstated, since few cases of ankle fracture eventually require an arthrodesis or arthroplasty. Although it is true that patients tend to tolerate symptoms in the ankle better than in the knee or hip joint, a plausible explanation may be that the ankle acts in tandem with the complex hindfoot mechanism and may in part be protected by an intact and functioning subtalar joint. However, patient complaints following ankle fracture are frequent, especially when the anatomy has not been restored (Gollish et al. 1977).

Willenegger and Breitenfelder (1965) reported that all cases of inadequate reduction showed signs of secondary osteoarthritis within 18 months of injury.

Hughes (1980) reported a comparative series of ankle fractures from three major centers. Poor restoration of the anatomy led to poor results, no matter what treat-

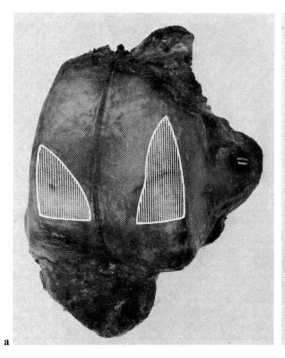

a

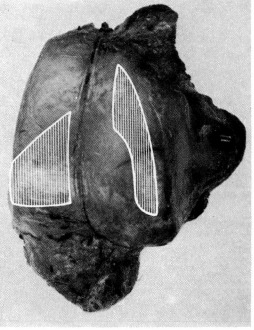

b

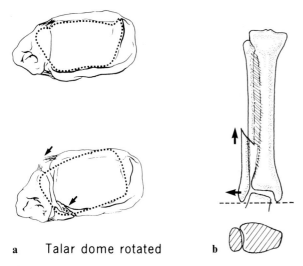

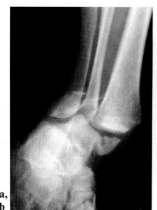

a   Talar dome rotated   b

Fig. 22.5 a,b. A shortened, malrotated lateral malleolus places the joint in a subluxated position, as shown in cross-sectional drawings (**a**) and diagram (**b**). (**b** From Müller et al. 1965)

ment method was employed. As one might expect, fractures treated by closed means had significantly poorer results than those treated by open means, because of the difficulty in maintaining the reduction. However, some fractures treated by open reduction also had a poor outcome, due to inadequate anatomical restoration.

Gollish et al. (1977) found similar results. Objective criteria were used to assess the adequacy of reduction achieved and to correlate that with the clinical outcome. The parameters chosen were talar tilt and mortise width. Twenty-five patients with normal ankles had these two

parameters measured on a standard 15° internal oblique view, as illustrated in Fig. 22.8 a.

For the measurement of talar tilt, three lines were used (Fig. 22.8 b). One line was drawn to join the tips of the medial and lateral malleoli, another parallel to the surface of the tibial plafond, and a third parallel to the talar surface. Two angles (T, t) were then measured, with the difference between them constituting the talar tilt. The mean (valgus or varus) talar tilt in the control group was not significantly different from 0.00, the normal range being from –1.5° to +1.5°.

The mortise width was calculated as follows: a line drawn 5.0 mm distal and parallel to the talar dome intersects four cortices at points $a, b, c,$ and d (Fig. 22.8 c). The mortise width was then taken as the length $ab–cd$, measured in millimeters. The normal mortise width was 4.0 mm, with a range of 2.0–6.0 mm.

The results of 77 prospectively documented ankle fractures were as follows. Out of 36 cases in which both talar tilt and mortise width were normal, 35 (97.2 %) had a good clinical result. In 41 cases the measurement of either or both parameters was outside the normal range; of these, 21 (51.2 %) had a result rated fair or poor. The difference between these two groups is statistically highly significant. This demonstrates that the final result of the treatment of an ankle fracture is chiefly dependent upon anatomical joint restoration.

Surgical reconstruction has improved the final results in fractures of the ankle, but precise attention to all details, especially anatomical reduction, is of course mandatory. The result of a lateral malleolus fixed with shortening or malrotation will be poor. Careful study of

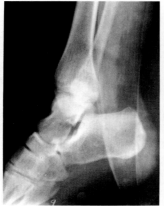

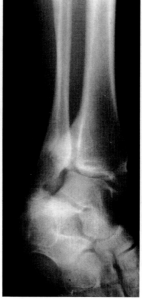

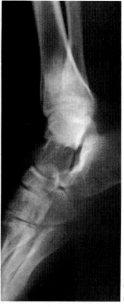

a, b

c, d

Fig. 22.6. a,b Bimalleolar fracture with severe displacement. Closed reduction under general anesthesia and cast immobilization was the definitive treatment. **c,d** Note the severe valgus deformity and early osteoarthritis 1 year after fracture

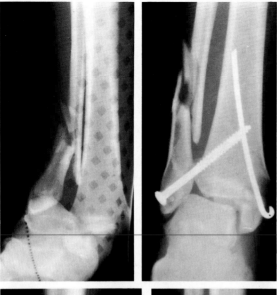

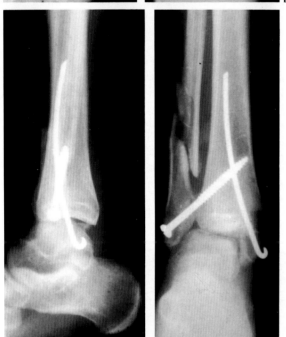

Fig. 22.7 a,b. Severe trimalleolar fracture managed by open reduction and internal fixation. Note the malreduction of both the medial and the lateral malleolus. The medial malleolus is fixed in a nonanatomical position by the Rush rod; the fibula is shortened and the talus is in valgus. **c** Further talar tilt is noted at 6 weeks. **d** Radiographs 2 years following surgery indicated severe osteoarthritis of the ankle joint

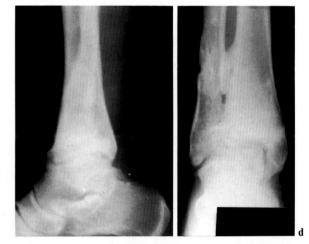

the parameters, talar tilt, and mortise width on the *films* will avoid these errors.

22.1.4 Mechanism of Injury

In a series of experiments using fresh amputation specimens, Lauge-Hansen clearly described the mechanisms of ankle injury and the resultant pathological anatomy (Lauge-Hansen 1942). From his studies, he proposed a classification of ankle injury based on the position of the foot at the moment of trauma and the direction of the injurious force. Essentially, he described two major

directional forces acting upon the ankle, supination and pronation. These are complex forces:

- *Supination* of the foot is a combination of inward rotation at the ankle, adduction of the hindfoot, and inversion of the forefoot. This combined force may be called adduction, internal rotation, or inversion (Fig. 22.9 a).
- *Pronation* of the foot is a combination of outward rotation at the ankle, abduction of the hindfoot, and eversion of the forefoot. This combined force is usually called abduction, external rotation, or eversion (Fig. 22.9 b).

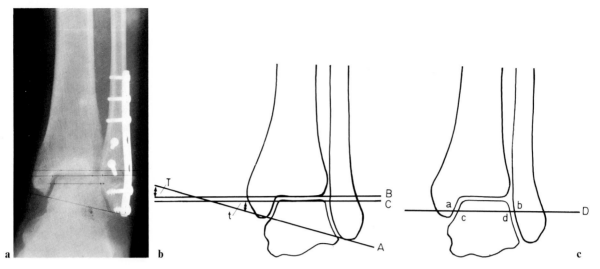

Fig. 22.8 a–c. Measurement of valgus talar tilt and mortise width. **a** Radiograph showing lines of measurement. **b** For the measurement of talar tilt three lines are used: one line is drawn to join the tips of the medial and lateral malleoli *(A)*, another parallel to the surface of the tibial plafond *(B)*, and a third parallel to the talar surface *(C)*. Two angles *(T,t)* are measured, with the difference between them constituting the talar tilt. **c** Calculation of the mortise width. A line *D* is drawn 5 mm distal and parallel to the talar dome. This intersects four cortices, *a–d*. The mortise width is calculated as the length *ab* minus *cd*, measured in millimeters

These forces, which act in opposite directions, produce markedly different injury patterns in the ankle.

Pankovich (1979) has interpreted the above terminology as follows: pronation and supination indicate the position of the foot as it rotates around the subtalar joint axis; internal (inversion) and external (eversion) rotation of the talus are rotational movements around the vertical axis of the tibia. Abduction and adduction are rotational movements of the talus around its long axis. Adduction forces acting upon the ankle produce avulsions of the lateral malleolus below the ankle mortise or its equivalent lateral ligament. The most common injury to the ankle, the "ankle sprain," is due to this force.

The particular injuries produced by abduction or eversion forces acting upon the ankle joint will depend upon the position of the foot at the moment of trauma.

Lauge-Hansen described these patterns as follows:
- In the *supinated* foot, the medial ligament is relaxed during the initial phase of the injury; therefore, the lateral complex is injured first and the medial last.
- In the *pronated* foot, with the medial ligament under tension during injury, the sequence of injury is reversed, i.e., the medial complex is injured first and the lateral last. Biomechanical studies have emphasized the injury sequence, which is helpful in predicting the degree of instability.

The following account of the pattern of ankle injury, based on Lauge-Hansen's description, helps us to understand the bony and soft tissue pathological anatomy and should therefore be studied by all surgeons treating ankle injuries. Of special importance is Lauge-Hansen's emphasis on ligamentous injury and, therefore, hidden instability. In this description the position of the foot is indicated first, and the force involved second.

22.1.4.1 Supination–Adduction

In the first stage of supination–adduction injury (Fig. 22.10), a transverse avulsion fracture of the fibula may occur distal to the syndesmosis or the lateral liga-

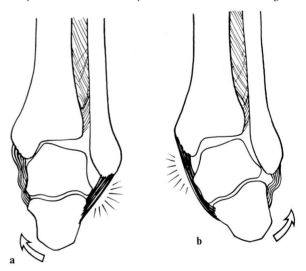

Fig. 22.9 a,b. Effect of foot position. **a** Supination of the foot causes laxity of the medial ligament and tension in the lateral ligament of the ankle. **b** Pronation of the foot causes tension in the medial ligament and laxity in the lateral ligament of the ankle

ment may rupture. Since the lateral injury is distal to the mortise, the syndesmotic ligaments remain intact.

If the adduction force continues, a vertical fracture of the medial malleolus occurs, often with impaction of the joint surface by the subluxating medial talar dome. The posterior structures are usually intact. Occasionally, a fracture may occur in the posteromedial aspect of the tibia, posterior to the medial malleolus. Two types of dome fracture of the talus may occur as the ankle subluxates into varus: on the lateral side, a shear osteochondral fracture, on the medial side, an articular crush (Berndt and Harty 1959).

22.1.4.2 Eversion–Abduction

The combination of eversion and abduction forces produces a shearing rotational injury to the lateral joint complex and avulsion of the medial complex (Fig. 22.11). Three mechanisms are recognized, as described below.

a) Supination–Eversion

This common injury pattern is caused by external rotation of the supinated foot. The following injury sequence occurs:

1. Rupture of the anterior syndesmotic ligament or avulsion of the anterior portion of the fibula (Wagstaffe's fracture) or the anterior tubercle of the tibia.
2. A spiral fracture of the fibula at or above the joint. The fracture begins distally from an anteromedial

position and spirals in a posterolateral superior direction.
3. Rupture of the posterior tibiofibular ligament or avulsion of its posterior tibial insertion.
4. Lastly, as tension is applied to the medial aspect of the joint, avulsion of the medial malleolus or rupture of the deltoid ligament.

b) Pronation–Abduction

With the foot in pronation, the deltoid ligament is under tension and the sequence of injury is therefore reversed. A lateral injury in this pattern always signifies medial instability. In the pronation–abduction pattern, the sequence of injury is as follows:

1. Rupture of the deltoid ligament or avulsion fracture of the medial malleolus.
2. Rupture of the syndesmotic ligaments or bony avulsion of one of their attachments.
3. Oblique fracture of the fibula at or above the syndesmosis. This fracture is more oblique or transverse and is grossly unstable. The interosseous membrane is ruptured up to the level of the fibular fracture. Dome fractures of the talus are common in this shearing fracture.

c) Pronation–Eversion

A pronation–eversion injury is very similar to the previous type, but with subtle differences. The stages are as follows:

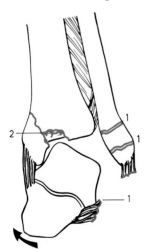

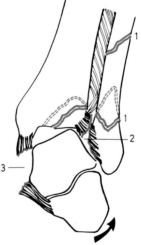

Fig. 22.10. Mechanism of injury: supination–adduction force. In the first stage, a transverse avulsion fracture of the fibula may occur distal to the syndesmosis or the lateral ligament may rupture *(1)*. With a continuing adduction force, a vertical fracture of the medial malleolus occurs, often with impaction of the joint surface *(2)*

Fig. 22.11. Mechanism of injury: eversion–abduction force. A shearing, rotational injury to the lateral joint complex is produced, including a spiral rotational fracture of the fibula *(1)*, a disruption of the syndesmotic ligament *(2)*, and a disruption of the medial ligament or medial malleolus *(3)*

1. Fracture of the medial malleolus or rupture of the deltoid ligament.
2. Rupture of the anterior tibiofibular ligament or avulsion of one of its bony insertions.
3. Fracture of the fibula, at or above the syndesmosis. The fracture is more spiral anterosuperiorly to posteroinferiorly. The interosseous ligament is ruptured up to the level of the fracture.
4. Rupture of the posterior tibiofibular ligament or fracture of the posterior tubercle of the tibia (Volkmann's triangle), leading to instability of the mortise.

A careful perusal of the above descriptions of the injury types will indicate the orderly sequence of the bony and ligamentous injury and will help in the subsequent decision-making process.

22.2 Classification

22.2.1 Introduction

A classification is only useful if it aids in our management of the fracture and if it allows us to compare the results of treatment of similar injuries. For individual patients and their attending surgeons, the former is the more valuable. Unfortunately, none of the existing classifications is wholly satisfactory, and it is far better to precisely define the personality of each individual fracture and use suitable treatment than to memorize an arbitrary classification and attempt to make all injuries fit the common molds.

Although the work of Lauge-Hansen (1942) has allowed us to understand the injury patterns, his classification is cumbersome and difficult to apply clinically. It suggests that the forces acting upon the ankle will always produce a "classic" pattern and will be identifiable from the radiographs, a suggestion difficult to reconcile with the variants seen in clinical practice.

Brunner and Weber (1982), representing the views of the AO/ASIF group, have classified ankle fractures according to the position of the fibular fracture, stating that "the higher the fibular fracture, the more extensive the damage to the tibiofibular ligaments; and the greater the damage, the greater the danger of ankle mortise insufficiency" (Fig. 22.12). A type A fracture is located at or below the syndesmosis, type B at the syndesmosis, and type C above it. However, this classification seems to imply that type C fractures, above the syndesmosis, are more dangerous and, therefore, may have a poorer prognosis than type B and also, by inference, that surgery is always required for such injuries. However, in a review we found no statistical difference between the final results of type B and C fractures (Gollish et al. 1977). Furthermore, the work of Lauge-Hansen (1942),

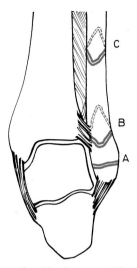

Fig. 22.12. AO/ASIF classification of ankle fractures. The AO/(ASIF classification depends upon the position of the fibular fracture, below (type A), at (type B), or above (type C) the ankle mortise

Pankovich (1979), De Souza Dias and Forester (1974), and Monk (1969) have shown that the supination/external rotation injury may involve the fibula above the syndesmosis without significant medial damage. This common fracture may be stable, may not require surgery, and usually has a good prognosis, in spite of the location of the fibular fracture proximal to the syndesmosis. The key to its stability is the integrity of the posterior tibiofibular ligament or its bony attachments.

Both classifications are useful, the Lauge-Hansen one for outlining the sequence of injury and the importance of ligamentous damage to the stability of the ankle, and the AO/ASIF classification presented by Brunner and Weber for stressing the importance of the lateral joint complex. However, neither can be used in deciding the treatment for any individual fracture. All Lauge-Hansen's types of fracture may be either stable or unstable and, therefore, may require either closed or open treatment; the same may be said for all the AO/ASIF types.

Clearly, there are two distinct types of injury: first, those due to an adduction–inversion force causing a lateral injury below the syndesmosis (see Fig. 22.10), and second, those caused by an external rotation–abduction force, producing an injury to the lateral complex at or above the syndesmosis (Fig. 22.11).

The first type of injury corresponds to the Lauge-Hansen supination–adduction injury and the AO/ASIF type A injury and is characterized by an avulsion fracture of the lateral malleolus and a shear on the medial side. The second type of injury, corresponding to the Lauge-Hansen types supination–eversion, pronation–eversion, and pronation–abduction and to the B and C types of the AO/ASIF classification, is characterized by a torsion or shear fracture of the lateral joint complex and an avulsion of the medial malleolus. With this mechanism, an *isolated* fracture of the medial malleolus or equivalent rupture of the deltoid ligament may also, rarely, occur.

As important as the position of the fibular fracture is the *stability* of the ankle mortise. Injuries caused by inversion (adduction) and those caused by eversion (abduction) may both be stable or unstable; therefore, it is obvious that a clear understanding of the factors causing instability is mandatory.

Stable injuries may be defined as those that cannot be displaced by physiological forces. Simple symptomatic treatment is all that is required for a good result. If physiological forces are applied to an *unstable* fracture, however, it will displace. Anatomical reduction of unstable injuries by closed means may therefore be easy to obtain, but difficult to maintain.

Stability is not a matter of black or white but rather shades of gray, depending on the degree of soft tissue and skeletal damage. Thus, the same fibular fracture above the syndesmosis may be stable or unstable or any grade in between, depending on the amount of ligamentous and capsular damage associated with it. This is the reality of daily medical practice.

In the first edition of this book, we proposed a classification based on two main factors: first, the position and character of the injury on the lateral aspect of the joint, and, second, a clinical and radiological assessment of joint stability.

If stability is defined as the ability of the injured ankle to withstand physiological stress without displacement, what are the factors leading to instability? The stability of the normal ankle (Fig. 22.13) is dependent upon:

1. The lateral malleolus or lateral ligament
2. The medial malleolus or medial ligament
3. The anterior syndesmotic ligaments or their bony equivalents (anterior tibia or fibula)
4. The posterior syndesmotic ligaments or the posterior malleolus

If only one of the above groups is lost, stability of the ankle will be maintained. As each successive group is lost, no matter what the mechanism of the injury, the ankle is pushed further along the stability scale (Fig. 22.13 a). When all four groups are lost, the ankle is completely unstable, held together only by skin. There is

Fig. 22.13 a–d. Ankle stability. **a** The stability scale. **b–d** The stability of the ankle is dependent upon the four bony and ligamentous structures depicted. These structures include the lateral malleolus or lateral ligament *(1)*, the medial malleolus or medial ligament *(2)*, the anterior syndesmotic ligament or its bony attachments *(3)*, and the posterior syndesmotic ligament or posterior malleolus *(4)*. If only one of these groups is lost, stability of the ankle will be maintained. As each successive group is lost, no matter what the mechanism of injury, the ankle is pushed along the stability scale. When all four groups are lost, the ankle is completely unstable, held together only by skin

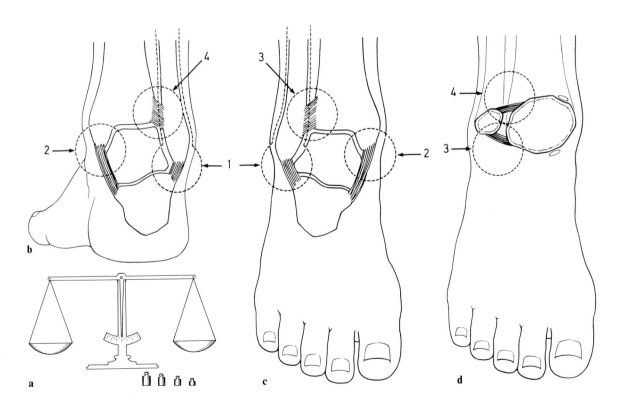

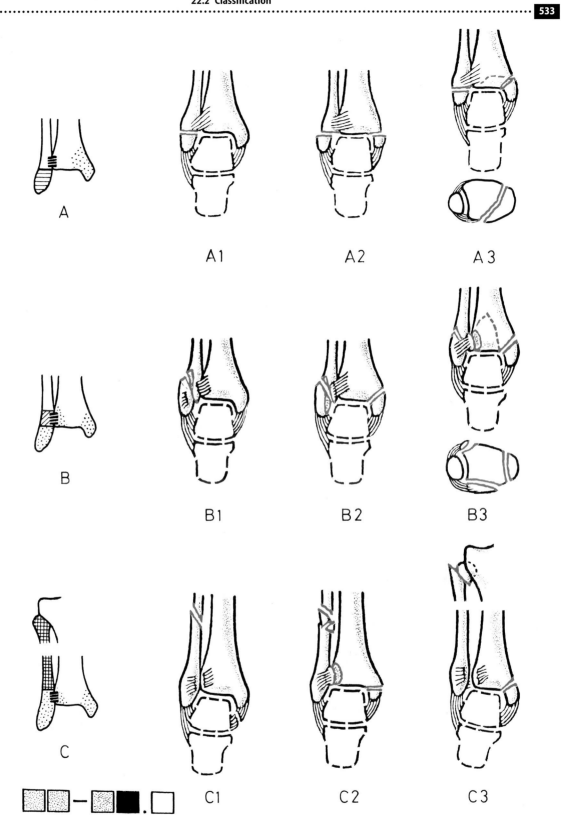

Fig. 22.14. Ankle classification. (From Müller et al. 1991)

534 ....

Chapter 22   **Fractures of the Ankle**

thus a spectrum of instability, and all ankle injuries may be placed anywhere along the stability scale.

Although the classification proposed in the first edition based on stability and the position of the fibular fracture was clinically useful, we have now adopted the comprehensive classifcation of fractures (Müller et al. 1990) using the A,B,C alpha-numeric designation which was developed by the AO group. The fracture pattern is based on the fibular fracture position (Brunner and Weber 1982) and incorporates the concepts previously discussed.

22.2.2 Comprehensive Classification (Fig. 22.14)

The fracture types in this classification, as in the previous AO classification, are based on the position of the fibular fracture; type A fractures are below the syndesmodic ligament, type B are between the anterior and posterior syndesmodic ligaments, and in type C the lateral lesion is above the syndesmotic ligament (see Fig. 22.12).

22.2.2.1 Type A

a) Group A1

Isolated Lateral Lesions. Type A injuries are caused by adduction or inversion forces. The isolated lateral injury may be an avulsion fracture of the fibula (A1.2) or an equivalent rupture of the whole or part of the lateral ligament (A1.1) (Fig. 22.15). The syndesmotic ligament is always intact; therefore, no instability occurs at the syndesmosis.

b) Group A2 Injuries to the Lateral and Medial Side

With continuing inversion, disruption of the anterior capsule occurs, allowing displacement of the fibular avulsion fracture and varus subluxation of the talus in the mortise. At this stage, the varus instability may be recognized on a stress radiograph. With further inversion, the entire talus may be subluxated out of the mortise, rotating only on the intact medial ligament. The entire anterior capsule is torn and the ankle, although congruous, is grossly unstable.

If the ankle is simultaneously subjected to axial loading, a vertical fracture of the medial malleolus may occur together with crushing of the medial talar and tibial articular cartilage. Eventually, the continuing force causes a posteromedial tibial fracture (Fig. 22.16).

Displacement of the talus is indicative of both *incongruity* and *instability* of the ankle. Since both the lateral and medial joint structures are disrupted, the ankle is unstable. Compression of the talus or medial tibial plafond may cause impaction of the articular cartilage, thereby altering the prognosis.

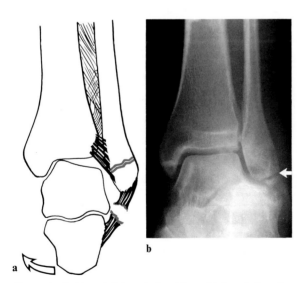

Fig. 22.15 a,b. Type A injury, isolated lateral injury below the syndesmosis. **a** Fracture of the lateral malleolus below the mortise (A1.3) and avulsion of the tip of the malleolus (A1.2) or its equivalent, a rupture of the lateral ligament. **b** Radiographic example of such a fracture (A1.1; *arrow*)

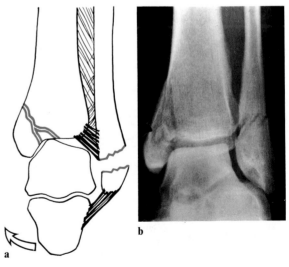

Fig. 22.16 a,b. Type A2 injury, a lateral and medial lesion. **a** Displaced lateral malleolar fracture associated with a vertical fracture of the medial malleolus and impaction of the medial aspect of the tibial plafond. **b** Radiographic example of such a case

22.2.2.2 Type B

The type B lesions are characterized by the fibular fracture at the syndesmosis (Fig. 22.17). Three groups are recognized in order of instability and therefore severity. In these injuries, the anterior syndesmotic ligament ruptures (B1.2), except in completely undisplaced fractures (B1.1).

a) B1 Isolated Lateral Malleolus

These injuries are characterized by an isolated fracture of the lateral malleolus with no clinical or radiographic evidence of a medial injury. The anterior syndesmotic ligament may rupture, but if the medial side is intact, ankle mortise stability is maintained.

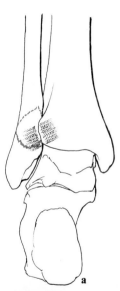

Fig. 22.17 a–c. Type B injury, stable. **a** Fibula fracture at the syndesmosis. In this injury the anterior tibiofibular ligament is torn, but the posterior ligament remains intact. **b,c** This stable pattern is shown in the radiographs

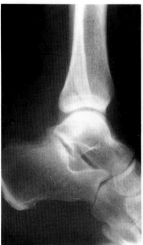
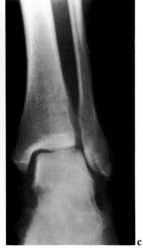

b) B2 Lateral Malleolus and Medial Injury

With an injury to both sides of the ankle joint, the anterior syndesmotic ligament or its equivalent bony insertion to the tibia (Chaput tubercle) or fibula (Le Fort) is always ruptured. These injuries have an unstable ankle mortise and require more vigorous treatment, usually open reduction and internal fixation.

c) B3 Lateral, Medial and Posterior Injury

The key to the stability of the ankle mortise is the posterior syndesmotic ligament complex, i.e., the ligament or its equivalent bony attachment, the posterior tibial tubercle or malleolus (Volkmann triangle fracture; Fig. 22.18). The presence of a posterior lesion always indicates a degree of instability, whether or not the medial structures are disrupted. Complete disruption of the medial structures, associated with a displaced lateral complex, is definite evidence of gross instability.

Remember also that the position of the foot at the moment of injury will determine the sequence of injury, the pronated foot receiving a medial injury first, and the supinated foot a medial injury last. However, no matter what the mechanism, instability must be assumed when an injury to both sides of the joint is accompanied by a posterior syndesmotic ligament injury.

Therefore, the B3 injury is always unstable and is difficult to manage without open surgery.

22.2.2.3 Type C

The type C injuries all have a fibular lesion above the ankle syndesmosis. Usually this is a fracture of the fibula, but occasionally it may be a dislocation of the proximal tibiofibular joint at the knee.

All of the injuries have been described as *unstable* because the lesion above the syndesmosis must rupture the syndesmotic ligaments. This has been disputed by Pankovich (1979), who indicated that, in the Lauge-Hansen supination–eversion mechanism, only the anterior syndesmotic ligament may rupture, with no medial injury, and hence no instability. In the comprehensive classification, this fact is *not* reflected. It is stated that all type C injuries are bifocal, i.e., lateral and medial, and by inference unstable, requiring open reduction and internal fixation. However, many *unnecessary* surgical procedures will be performed if all C lesions are considered bifocal, when in fact many are not, are stable, and can be managed nonoperatively (Fig. 22.19 a,b).

This is another example of the need to treat all patients as individuals and to perform a careful clinical and radiographic assessment of stability and not pre-

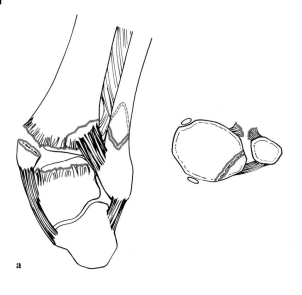

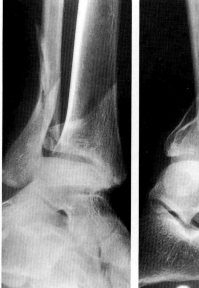

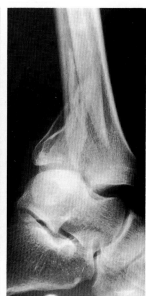

Fig. 22.18 a–c. Type B injury, unstable

judge the cases according to the "cook book" approach, as will be discussed in Sect. 22.3 on assessment of stability of the ankle. Since no classification exists which can cover all contingencies, each case should be treated individually.

In the type C fractures, the presence of a posterior injury designated by subgroup 3 in the classification does always indicate instability, since the key to instability of the ankle is the *posterior disruption* to the posterior syndesmotic ligament or its bony attachments to the tibia (Volkmann fracture) or the fibula.

a) C1 Simple Fracture of the Fibula

In C1 injuries, the fibular fracture is simple, usually oblique and spiral, and as noted above may have an intact medial side (see Fig. 22.19). Fractures of the medial side indicate partial (C1.2) and posterior (C1.3) complete ankle instability.

b) C2 Multifragmentary (Comminuted) Fibular Fractures (see Fig. 22.19)

In C2 fractures, the fibular fracture is multifragmentary and may be associated, as above, with medial (C2.2) or posterior (C2.3) injuries.

c) C3 Proximal Fibular Lesions

The C3 lesions include a proximal fibular fracture or a dislocation of the proximal tibiofibular joint. As in the other type C injuries, the medial side (C3.2) or the posterior side (C3.3) may be disrupted.

22.2.2.4 Isolated Medial Malleolus Fracture

This rare injury (Fig. 22.20) is the first stage of the pronation–eversion injury described by Lauge-Hansen. With that particular mechanism, the medial malleolus or the deltoid ligament is avulsed, but no further injury occurs. Although the ankle is stable, the medial malleolus may be displaced, with resultant incongruity. Since congruity is essential for a satisfactory result, open reduction and internal fixation for the *displaced* medial malleolus fracture is essential. In this classification, this lesion has been considered with the distal tibial area (pilon fracture), but it is really part of the ankle spectrum.

....
22.3 Assessment of Stability

Prior to treatment, a careful clinical and radiological assessment of the ankle is necessary in order to determine the degree of congruity and stability of the joint. These two factors are interrelated but not synonymous: joint congruity is an absolute concept and is essential for a long-term satisfactory result, whereas stability is a relative concept.

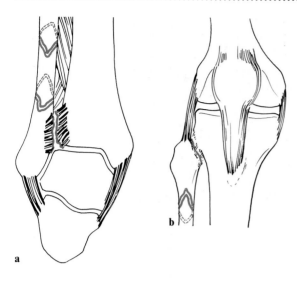

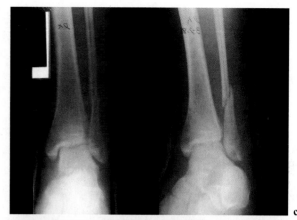

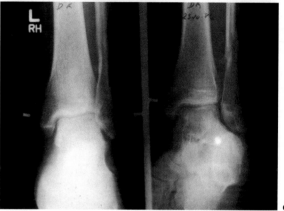

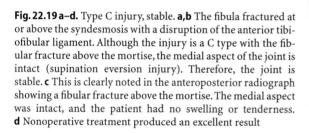

Fig. 22.19 a–d. Type C injury, stable. **a,b** The fibula fractured at or above the syndesmosis with a disruption of the anterior tibiofibular ligament. Although the injury is a C type with the fibular fracture above the mortise, the medial aspect of the joint is intact (supination eversion injury). Therefore, the joint is stable. **c** This is clearly noted in the anteroposterior radiograph showing a fibular fracture above the mortise. The medial aspect was intact, and the patient had no swelling or tenderness. **d** Nonoperative treatment produced an excellent result

These factors may be determined by a precise examination in logical sequence.

22.3.1 Clinical Assessment

22.3.1.1 History

The mechanisms of injury will suggest the degree of violence. Of special importance is the ability of the patient to walk after the injury. A normal patient able to walk reasonably well on the injured ankle is unlikely to have a degree of instability that requires surgery; nevertheless, surgery is occasionally, and perhaps unnecessarily, carried out on such patients. On the other hand, a severe, shearing, high-energy injury due to motor vehicular trauma, for instance, is almost certain to be unstable.

22.3.1.2 Physical Examination

Signs of Injury. Local tenderness, ecchymosis, and swelling, if confined to one side of the ankle, whether lateral or medial, are usually indicative of a stable injury, whereas if these local signs of injury extend to both sides of the joint, instability can be presumed.

Displacement. Obvious clinical displacement always indicates instability.

Instability. Abnormal motion of the talus in the ankle mortise may be felt on clinical examination, either in the conscious patient or during an examination under anesthesia.

22.3.2 Radiological Assessment

Standard radiological assessment must include anteroposterior, lateral, and mortise views (Fig. 22.21). The mortise view, taken at 15° of internal rotation, is *essential* for proper visualization of the inferior tibiofibular syndesmosis.

Tomograms may be of value in assessing the degree of comminution and in outlining talar dome fractures, if present.

For the purpose of this description of the radiographic picture it is necessary for a moment to divide the ankle into its component parts (see Fig. 22.13).

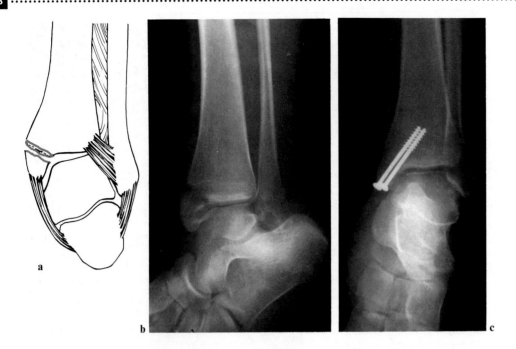

Fig. 22.20. a,b Isolated fracture of the medial malleolus. **c** Because of the unacceptable degree of displacement, this fracture was fixed with two 4.0-mm cancellous screws

Fig. 22.21 a–c. Normal radiographic views of the ankle essential for proper visualization of the ankle joint. **a** Anteroposterior view. **b** Mortise view, taken at 15° internal rotation. **c** Lateral view

22.3.2.1 Lateral Complex: Fibula and Tibiofibular Syndesmosis

Two factors are of importance in the injury to the lateral joint complex: (1) the amount of *shortening* or *displacement* and (2) the *location* and *shape* of the fibular fracture.

The amount of shortening or displacement of the fibular fracture as seen on both the mortise or lateral view

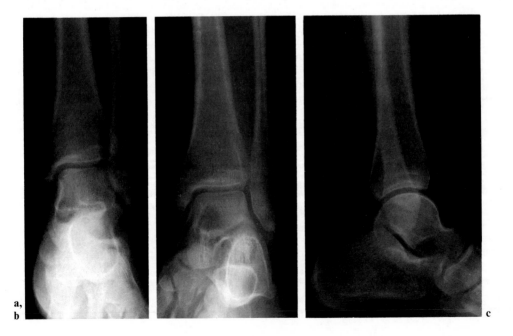

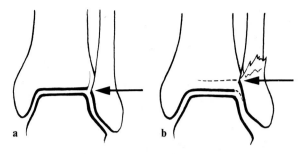

Fig. 22.22 a,b. The tibiofibular line. **a** The subchondral bone plates of the distal tibia and fibula form a continuous line, the tibiofibular line. **b** Any disruption of that line caused by shortening or rotation of the fibula is evidence of displacement of the lateral malleolus

is significant. On the mortise view, any break or gross displacement of the tibiofibular line should be viewed with suspicion (Fig. 22.22). Shortening or lateral displacement of the lateral malleolus is presumptive evidence of a tear in a portion of the syndesmotic ligaments; the presence of an avulsion fracture at one of its attachments is definite evidence of the same (Fig. 22.23). The lateral radiograph will indicate any posterior displacement and shortening of the fibula. Also, posterior subluxation of the talus in the mortise may be associated with a posterior tibial lip fracture or a posterior tibiofibular ligament tear (see Fig. 22.18 b).

The location of the fibular fracture, i.e., below, at, or above the syndesmosis, is also significant, although less so than the degree of shortening or displacement. A

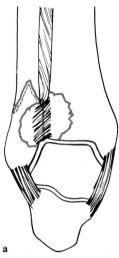

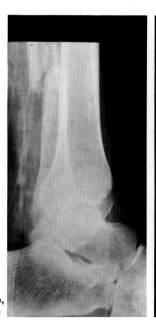
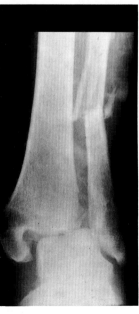
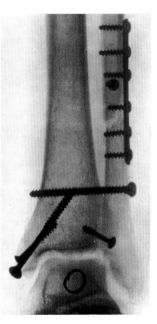
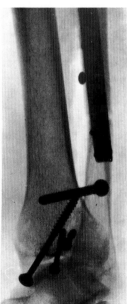

Fig. 22.23 a–e. Displaced lateral malleolus. **a** Avulsion fractures of either the distal tibia or the fibula at either end of the syndesmotic ligament. **b,c** The anteroposterior and lateral radiographs show a fibular fracture 10 cm proximal to the ankle joint. Note also the fractured medial malleolus, increased mortise width, and talar tilt, as well as the avulsion fracture of the tibial end of the anterior syndesmotic ligament. **d,e** Postoperative radiographs show an anatomical reduction of the fibula and medial malleolus as well as a single screw in the avulsion fracture

540 ···

Chapter 22   **Fractures of the Ankle**

transverse fracture below the syndesmosis indicates an avulsion of the lateral complex by inversion forces. External rotational forces disrupt the fibula at or above the syndesmosis. The exact site of the fibular fracture does not indicate the degree of instability present, but the shape of the fracture may: spiral fractures at or above the joint indicate low-energy rotation injuries, whereas short oblique or comminuted fractures at or above the syndesmosis are usually caused by high-energy abduction injuries and are more likely to be unstable (Fig. 22.24).

22.3.2.2 Talus

The talus should be carefully examined for several abnormalities, as follows:

- *Talar tilt.* The normal ankle has *no* valgus talar tilt, and any degree of tilt constitutes the most important sign of tibiotalar incongruity due to instability of the lateral complex (Fig. 22.25). The incongruity may be due to lateral shift of the talus or, more commonly, to external rotation of the talus in the mortise (see Fig. 22.5 a). It should be measured on the mortise view as shown in Fig. 22.21 b.
- *Subluxation of the talus.* The talus may be subluxated either posteriorly or posterolaterally, accompanying the distal fibular fracture, or, rarely, extending into the syndesmosis to lie between the tibia and the displaced fibula (see Fig. 22.2 b).
- *Dome fractures.* Fractures of the dome of the talus are common and can best be seen on the mortise view.

22.3.2.3 Posterior Tibial Process

The surgeon must carefully assess the posterior tibial process for the size and location of the posterior fracture. If associated with a type B fibular fracture, the posterior tibial fragment is always attached to the distal fragment of that fracture by the posterior syndesmotic ligament (see Fig. 22.18 b). The posterior fracture may vary in size from a small posterior tibial avulsion to a large triangular fragment of the posterolateral margin of the tibia (Volkmann's triangle). The latter is probably related to high axial loading as well as rotation at the moment of impact.

If the posterior syndesmotic complex is disrupted, the ankle joint must be unstable. This is clearly seen in Fig. 22.25 a, where *no* fracture of the posterior aspect of the tibia is noted, but the wide displacement of the fibula from the tibia is definite evidence of complex disruption of the posterior syndesmotic complex, hence an unstable ankle mortise.

22.3.2.4 Medial Complex

The following points are of importance:

1. The direction of the fracture
2. The size of the fragment
3. The presence of articular comminution
4. The amount of displacement of the fracture
5. The presence of a posterior fracture

Fig. 22.24 a–c. Abduction injury. **a** An almost transverse fracture just above the mortise, of the kind usually caused by a high-energy abduction force. **b** Anteroposterior radiograph of such a fracture. Note the transverse nature of the fibular fracture just above the syndesmosis. **c** Postoperative radiograph showing an anatomical reduction

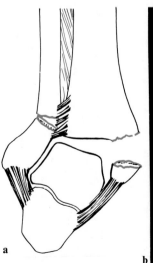
a

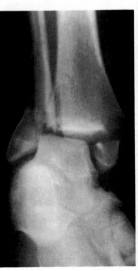
b

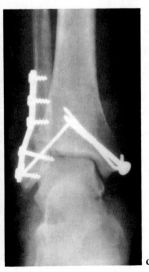
c

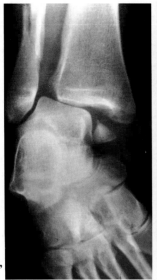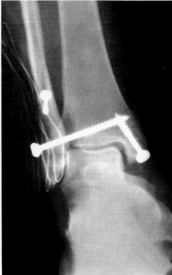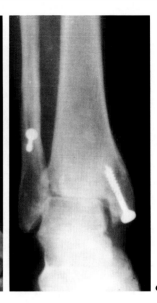

a,
b

c

Fig. 22.25 a–c. Talar tilt. **a** Note the severe lateral displacement of the talus in the anteroposterior radiograph. The fibula is fractured above the mortise and is rotated. Note the space in the syndesmosis, indicating a disruption of both the anterior and posterior syndesmotic ligaments. **b** The immediate postoperative radiograph clearly shows a lack of anatomical reduction. There is increased mortise width and a lateral talar tilt due to shortening and malreduction of the fibula. **c** The end result at 3 years indicated severe osteoarthritis requiring an ankle arthrodesis

Vertical fractures are indicative of inversion injuries and are often associated with comminution of the medial tibial articular surface. If displaced and associated with a lateral injury, rotatory instability and incongruity must be present (see Fig. 22.16).

Transverse fractures at or below the joint level are avulsion types and, if displaced and associated with a lateral and posterior injury, are always definite evidence of an unstable mortise (see Fig. 22.24).

Undisplaced fractures of the medial malleolus without evidence of a lateral injury are stable, although they may be minimally displaced (see Fig. 22.20).

In summary, careful radiological assessment may show definite evidence of instability of the ankle mortise. Of special significance is the degree of talar tilt, either varus or valgus; and the displacement of either the medial or the lateral complex associated with a posterior injury, or both. The degree of instability is always a spectrum, not a black and white concept, so that partial instability to complete instability may be recorded. By combining the radiographic with the clinical assessment, supplemented by examination under anesthesia when necessary, an adequate appraisal of the degree of instability may be made.

22.4 Management

22.4.1 Decision Making

Many ankle fractures can and should be treated nonoperatively; however, physicians are distinguished not by their ability to treat relatively minor injuries, but by their ability to recognize and adequately treat those which, if untreated, will lead to poor results.

The prognosis of the stable types of injury (A1, B1, and some C1) is excellent no matter what treatment is given, but, with improper treatment, that of the unstable types is poor. Very often, in a busy emergency department, the physician is so distracted by mundane problems that the important injuries are not recognized; i.e., he or she cannot see the trees for the forest.

Once the important clinical and radiographic features of the ankle injury, the *personality* of the injury, have been assembled, they must be ordered and considered in logical fashion. It should be remembered that the management decision also depends upon other factors, including the general medical state and expectations of the patient, as well as the condition of the limb and the expertise of the surgical team, i.e., on a careful assessment of the whole personality of the injury and the context of its treatment.

The first step in the decision-making process is to look at the lateral aspect of the joint and determine whether the patient has sustained a type A, type B, or type C injury.

22.4.1.1 Type A

If the fracture in the fibula is at or below the syndesmosis and is transverse, it is a type A fibular fracture of the avulsion kind (see Fig. 22.12 a). Since the syndesmotic ligaments are intact, the ankle mortise must be stable. However, rotatory instability may occasionally occur in injuries of this type if the medial structures are involved. *Warning*: occasionally a shearing, rotational type B injury may appear at the syndesmotic level and lull the surgeon into believing it is a simple transverse avulsion fracture (type A), when in reality it is a dangerous type of type B fracture (see Fig. 22.24).

If the avulsion fracture of the fibula is undisplaced or minimally displaced and *no* lesion is recognized clinically or radiologically on the medial side (A1), then application of a walking cast until the fibula has healed (usually 6–8 weeks) will achieve an excellent result.

If the clinical and radiological examination has revealed an injury to the medial aspect of the joint as well, surgery may be indicated. Surgical indications for the type A injury (see Fig. 22.16) include:

1. A displaced, unstable, lateral malleolar avulsion fracture with major soft tissue disruption, which remains displaced after closed reduction. Failure to close the gap in the lateral malleolar fracture may lead to delayed union or even nonunion, and a compromised clinical result.
2. A displaced fracture of the medial joint complex, including the vertical-type medial malleolus fracture, with or without a fracture of the posteromedial aspect of the tibia.
3. An osteochondral fracture of the medial articular surface of the tibia or the talus.

Although a crush injury to the medial articular surface of the tibia or the talus is listed as an indication for surgery, it must be recognized that precise reconstruction of the joint may be impossible. If the fragments are large enough, they may be supported by cancellous bone graft in the subchondral area; if small, they should be removed. If the articular crush has occurred in isolation, with no medial complex fracture, little can be accomplished by surgery, and early motion, if possible, should be started.

22.4.1.2 Types B and C

The type B and C fractures are considered together, since decision making is similar for both, although the technical details may differ.

These fibular fractures at or above the syndesmosis may be stable or unstable; careful clinical and radiological assessment will reveal which it is in any given case. If

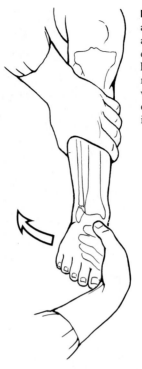

Fig. 22.26. Examination under anesthesia. If uncertainty exists about the stability of the ankle, examination under anesthesia is helpful. In this type B fracture, manipulation of the ankle into valgus may cause a marked opening in the ankle mortise, indicating instability

the surgeon is still uncertain about the stability of the ankle after clinical and radiological assessment, an examination under anesthesia may be found helpful. Under anesthesia, the ankle may be stressed in the presumed direction of injury and checked radiographically with an image intensifier or plain radiographs (Fig. 22.26). If the ankle is stable, very little displacement will occur at the lateral complex with stress abduction and eversion, and nonoperative treatment will be satisfactory.

a) Stable Fractures (B1, some C1)

If little or no displacement is present in the fibula (see Fig. 22.17), and there is no clinical or radiographic evidence of a posterior or a medial injury, nonoperative treatment is indicated, as no further displacement will occur. A good result may be anticipated with merely symptomatic treatment, namely, a below-knee walking cast retained until fibular union is complete. Note that this stable type of ankle injury may occur with a fibular fracture at any level, be it *at or above* the syndesmosis, as previously described. The most common type B or C injury, the supination–eversion variety without medial disruption, may be associated with a fibular fracture at or above the ankle mortise, including an injury to the proximal tibiofibular joint, and may still be classified as stable. Therefore, the proximal position of the fibular fracture alone is not presumptive evidence of mortise

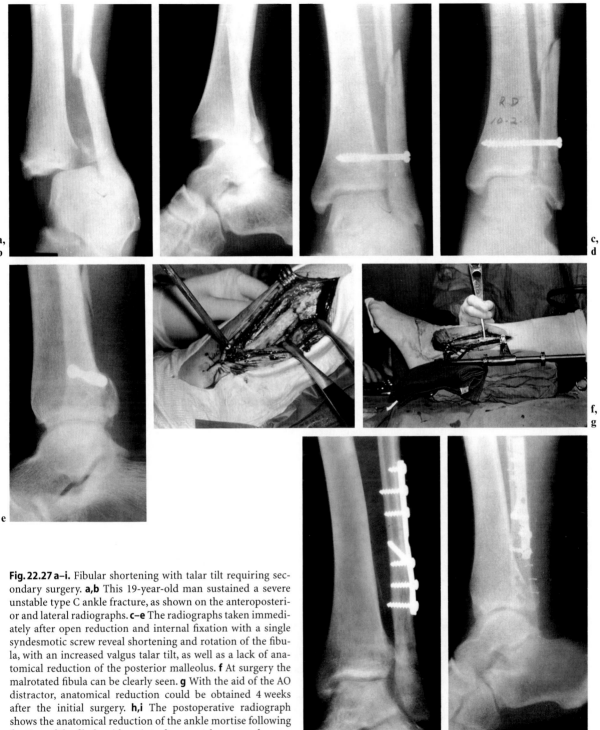

Fig. 22.27 a–i. Fibular shortening with talar tilt requiring secondary surgery. **a,b** This 19-year-old man sustained a severe unstable type C ankle fracture, as shown on the anteroposterior and lateral radiographs. **c–e** The radiographs taken immediately after open reduction and internal fixation with a single syndesmotic screw reveal shortening and rotation of the fibula, with an increased valgus talar tilt, as well as a lack of anatomical reduction of the posterior malleolus. **f** At surgery the malrotated fibula can be clearly seen. **g** With the aid of the AO distractor, anatomical reduction could be obtained 4 weeks after the initial surgery. **h,i** The postoperative radiograph shows the anatomical reduction of the ankle mortise following fixation of the fibula with an interfragmental screw and a one-third tubular plate

544 •

Chapter 22   **Fractures of the Ankle**

instability. The presence of instability must also include an injury to the medial side of the joint and/or the posterior aspect.

b) Unstable Fractures (B2, B3, and most C)

If the original clinical assessment reveals massive swelling, ecchymoses, and tenderness on both the medial and lateral sides of the joint, the surgeon should assume partial or complete instability of the ankle mortise. This will be confirmed by the radiological examination, which may reveal any of the unstable fracture patterns. If instability remains uncertain, especially if the medial injury is to the deltoid ligament, not the medial malleolus, it may be confirmed at examination under anesthesia. The radiographic signs of instability include abnormal valgus talar tilt, increased mortise width associated with shortening and displacement of the fibula, subluxation of the talus, and a fracture of the posterior or medial malleolus or their ligamentous equivalents (see Fig. 22.18). These unstable fractures require *stabilization,* otherwise incongruity will occur, with malunion and poor outcome to be expected. This does not imply that surgery is the only method of stabilization, but in our opinion, it is the best method for most cases.

Having determined that the type B or C injury is unstable, the surgeon should now assess the medial injury, as this injury may influence the management decision as outlined below.

With Medial Malleolar Fracture. Surgical stabilization is the method of choice for the unstable type B or C fracture with an associated medial malleolar fracture. Closed reduction requires a reversal of the mechanism of injury, so the ankle must be immobilized in internal rotation. Not only is this a poor position for the ankle, but the lack of a stable medial post makes redisplacement a common occurrence.

Nonoperative management of this fracture is so fraught with the danger of redisplacement that proper operative treatment is actually the more conservative approach. We believe that an immediate decision favoring open reduction and internal fixation should be made for almost all such fractures; there should be few exceptions.

With Deltoid Ligament Rupture. The presence of a deltoid ligament tear with a type B or C lateral injury also indicates mortise instability, the only difference being a ligament disruption instead of an avulsion fracture of the medial malleolus. Since the implications are the same, the treatment should also be the same. The surgeon should not be lulled into a false sense of security by this injury. Examination under anesthesia will quickly reveal the degree of mortise instability present.

We favor operative stabilization for the fibular fracture, to restore its length and ensure joint congruity. Anatomical reduction of the fibula restores stability to the mortise and greatly simplifies the management of the injury.

We have no quarrel with surgeons who feel that this fracture may be managed by closed means. In this injury, internal rotation of the ankle may anatomically reduce the fibular fracture. The presence of a medial post, namely the intact medial malleolus, *may* ensure that redisplacement will not occur. A word of caution is in order, however: if the postreduction radiograph shows any degree of valgus talar tilt or increased mortise width, a posterior injury with talar subluxation or interposition of the medial ligament or posterior tibial tendon should be suspected, and operative treatment reverted to immediately (Fig. 22.27).

If treated nonoperatively, patients with this injury must be observed closely, at weekly intervals, so that the surgeon may be certain that the reduction is maintained once the soft tissue swelling has subsided. The original

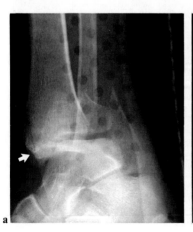 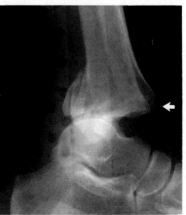

Fig. 22.28 a,b. Subluxation of the ankle. Note the severe ankle subluxation on the anteroposterior (**a**) and lateral (**b**) radiographs. In this situation, the skin may be severely traumatized by pressure from the protruding medial malleolus *(arrows)*. Closed reduction should be performed immediately to eliminate pressure on the skin

a   b

cast must be above the knee so as to maintain the internal rotation of the ankle and must be changed frequently in order to maintain this position. A successful outcome may be expected if careful attention to detail is followed. However, in our opinion the surgical management is simpler, allows early rehabilitation of the ankle, and will in most instances, if done correctly, ensure far better results.

22.4.1.3 Isolated Medial Malleolar Fracture

If displaced, isolated avulsion fractures of the medial malleolus should be treated by surgical stabilization. This will ensure rapid union of the compressed cancellous bone and allow early motion to the joint, with the expectation of an excellent result.

22.4.2 Surgical Technique

22.4.2.1 Tourniquet

We feel that a bloodless field is important for precision surgery, and a tourniquet is therefore recommended.

Fig. 22.29 a–c. Surgical approaches for malleolar fractures. **a** For exposure of the lateral malleolus we prefer an anterolateral (a) to a posterolateral (a') incision. The skin incision follows the anterior border of the fibula and runs parallel to the superficial branch of the peroneal nerve. **b** Incisions for exposure of the medial malleolus: anteromedial (b) or posteromedial (c). The anteromedial incision affords excellent exposure of the ankle joint and is preferred. The posteromedial incision should be used for simultaneous exposure of the medial malleolus and a large posteromedial fragment, which may be fixed by retrograde interfragmental screws. **c** Posterolateral incision (d) for posterior exposure and internal fixation of a fibular fracture associated with a large posterolateral malleolar fracture. The patient is usually in the prone position for maximum exposure. (Adapted from Müller et al. 1979)

22.4.2.2 Timing

Ideally, surgery should be carried out as soon as possible following injury. However, skin problems abound in the vicinity of the ankle, especially over the medial malleolus. If the patient is seen late or if skin viability is questionable, surgery must be delayed to avoid skin necrosis. We have found it prudent on occasion to fix just one injury, if the skin on that aspect of the joint is satisfactory, and delay fixation of the other injury until the condition of the skin improves. If surgery is delayed, any ankle subluxation must be reduced immediately to eliminate pressure on the skin medially (Fig. 22.28).

22.4.2.3 Incisions

a) Lateral Incisions

We prefer an anterolateral to a posterolateral incision (a and a1, respectively, in Fig. 22.29 a). The skin posterior to the fibula is thin and may necrose easier than the thicker anterior skin. Remember also that incisions should never be made over the subcutaneous border of any bone but adjacent to it. This is as true in the distal fibula as it is elsewhere. If skin necrosis does occur, the implant will usually remain covered. In the upper portion of the wound, the superficial peroneal nerve is in jeopardy as it tracks anteriorly across the fibula. It must be protected to prevent injury which would result in a painful neuroma.

b) Medial Incisions

If a longer exposure is required for a vertical fracture, a long anteromedial incision is preferred (Fig. 22.29 b, b). The skin flap, formed with its base posteromedially, usually heals well because of its blood supply from the posterior tibial artery. The saphenous nerve lying adjacent

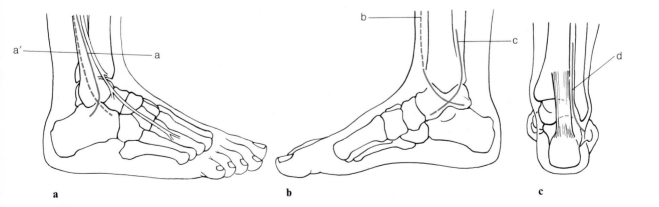

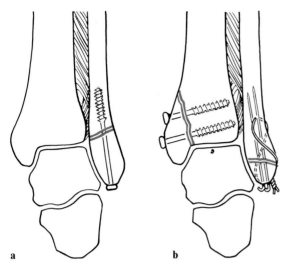

Fig. 22.30 a,b. Fixation of a tranverse avulsion fracture of the lateral malleolus. **a** Fixation with a lag screw. **b** Fixation of the lateral malleolar fragment with a tension band wire and the vertical medial malleolar fracture with two interfragmental lag screws

and immediately lateral to the saphenous vein must be avoided. If a longer anteromedial incision is required, the lateral incision should be made posteriorly to increase the bridge area of skin between them. Usually, in these instances, a small lateral approach will suffice for the avulsion fracture.

For the more typical medial malleolar avulsion fracture, a short anteromedial incision is sufficient to allow fixation of the fracture and inspection of the medial

Fig. 22.31 a–f. Fixation of a type A2 vertical medial malleolar fracture with impaction. **a** Note the marked varus talar tilt with the medial dome of the talus impacting on the articular surface of the distal tibia. **b** The displaced articular fracture must be reduced and held with a bone graft. Provisional fixation with Kirschner wires follows. **c** Definitive fixation with interfragmental screws. **d** Intraoperative anteroposterior polaroid radiograph of such a fracture in an 18-year-old girl. Preoperative planning would have shown the surgeon that a buttress plate was required. **e** Fixation proceeded with an interfragmental lag screw for the fibular fracture and two lag screws for the medial malleolar fracture. No buttress plate was used. **f** The end result was poor because of a varus deformation of the medial fracture and consequently of the dome of the talus

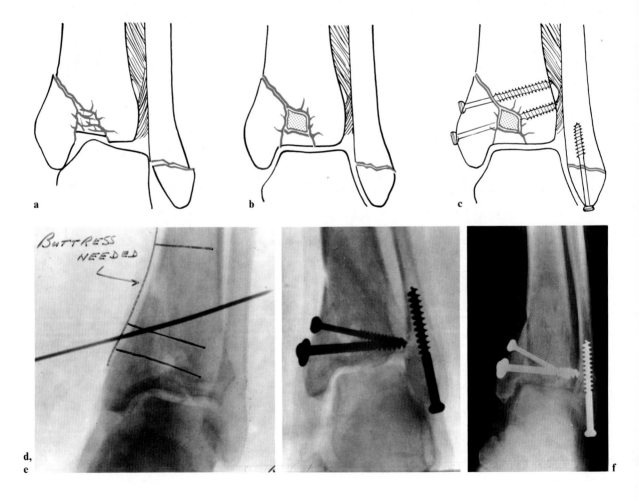

talar dome. If the medial malleolus fracture is associated with a large posteromedial fragment, the posteromedial approach is preferred (Fig. 22.29 b, c).

The skin on both sides of the ankle is very thin and its condition precarious; therefore it must be treated very gently to avoid disastrous complications.

c) Posterolateral Incisions

For patients with a large posterolateral fragment associated with a fibular fracture, the posterolateral approach is preferred, with the patient in the prone position (Fig. 22.29 c, d).

Fig. 22.32 a–d. Failure to restore fibular length. **a** The anterolateral and oblique radiographs of this 19-year-old man show a fibular fracture with shortening and rotation resulting in a valgus talar tile. Open reduction of the fibular fracture was performed immediately. **b** The postoperative radiograph shows the internal fixation of the fibula with a syndesmotic screw. Note the marked mortise widening between the medial malleolus and the medial border of the talus. The obvious reason was a malreduced and poorly fixed fibular fracture. **c** This potentially disastrous complication was recognized and the patient was reoperated upon at 7 days, with accurate fixation of the fibula and restoration of the ankle mortise. **d** The final result at 1 year after removal of the syndesmotic screws was excellent. If such a malreduction is noted on the postoperative radiographs, the surgeon must "bite the bullet", notify the patient, and reoperate to recify the situation as soon as safety permits

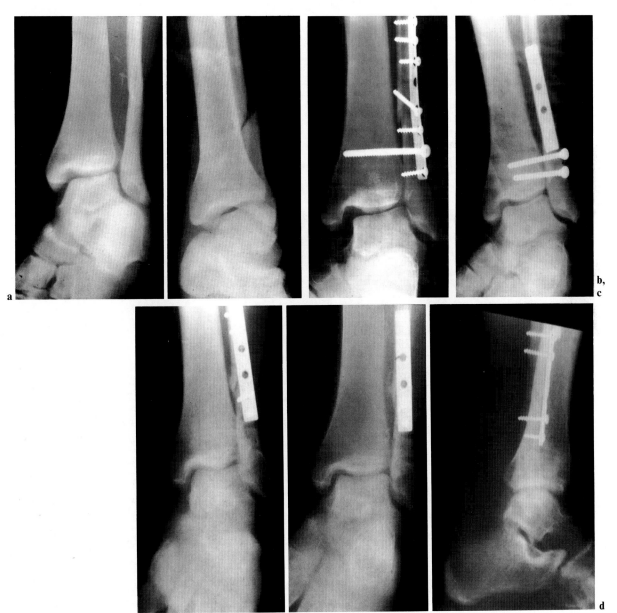

a

b,
c

d

22.4.2.4 Open Reduction and Internal Fixation

Although we have chosen to describe the technique according to the anatomical parts of the ankle, remember that careful preoperative planning of the entire injury is required in order to plan the incisions and the type of internal fixation required.

a) Type A

Lateral Complex. Since the lateral complex (i.e., the lateral malleolus, the syndesmosis, and the posterior tibial tubercle) is the key to the stability of the ankle, it should be inspected first, and if the lateral malleolar fracture is transverse and below the syndesmosis, the

Fig. 22.33 a–c. Fracture dislocation of the ankle with anterior dislocation of the fibula. **a** Anteroposterior radiograph of a 57-year-old man showing a short oblique fracture of the lateral malleolus with diastasis of the distal tibiofibular joint and lateral dislocation of the talus. **b** Lateral radiograph showing the oblique fracture and anterior displacement of the proximal fibular fragment. **c** Full-length lateral radiograph of the tibia showing the distal portion of the fibula displaced anteriorly, the key radiographic finding in this injury. (From Schatzker and Johnson 1983)

following method is recommended. As this injury is truly an avulsion fracture with a ligamentous attachment, dynamic compression cannot be obtained; it may therefore be fixed by a screw or with a tension band wire, which will achieve static compression (Fig. 22.30). We prefer the latter for small fragments and for osteoporotic bone, in which screw fixation is usually unsatisfactory.

The lateral talar dome should always be inspected for osteochondral fragments which, if present and small, should be discarded, and if large, should be replaced and fixed with articular pins or a small screw. As much of the torn anterior capsule and synovium as possible should be resutured.

Medial Complex. If the type A injury has a medial fracture, it is usually of the vertical shear variety A2, A3). This should be carefully inspected for the following important lesions:

1. Articular crush of the medial surface of the tibia or talar dome
2. Comminution of the cortex
3. Posteromedial fracture of the tibia

Careful preoperative planning and intraoperative inspection is required to arrive at the most appropriate

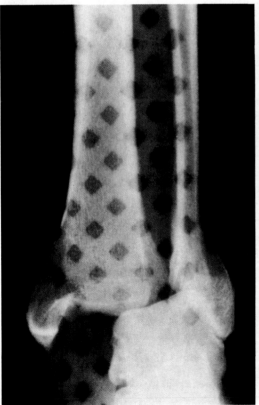
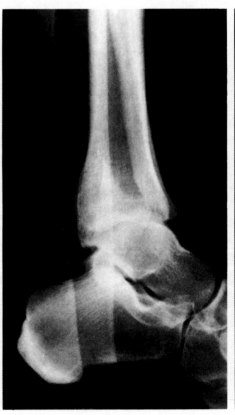
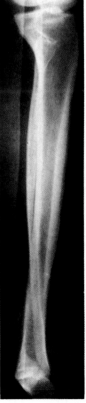

a,
b

c

method of fixation. If the fracture is a single cleavage through good bone, with no comminution, then screw fixation with at least two malleolar or large cancellous lag screws will suffice (Fig. 22.30 b).

If inspection reveals an articular crush to the tibia, considerable surgical judgement is required. If the crushed area is large enough to affect joint congruity, then the articular surface should be restored and a bone graft inserted above it to maintain this position (Fig. 22.31 a, b). Any small, loose fragments should be discarded. If the crushed area is small and does not affect joint congruity or joint biomechanics, it should be left alone in the hope that early motion will allow adequate healing of the area.

If the medial talar dome is crushed, the same principles apply. However, elevation of the crushed talar dome is difficult and the result may be unsatisfactory. A crush to either the tibia or the medial talar dome will adversely affect the prognosis, and the patient should be so informed.

If the proximal portion of the vertical fracture is comminuted, a buttress plate is required. Failure to apply this will result in redisplacement and loss of joint congruity, as shown in Fig. 22.31 d–f. The plate may be a small dynamic compression (DC) plate, a one-third, a T, or a cloverleaf plate.

If the bone is too small for screw fixation, multiple Kirschner wires should be retained as definitive fixation, with, of course, postoperative cast immobilization.

Fig. 22.34 a–e. Soft tissue interposition blocking reduction. **a,b** Lateral and anteroposterior radiographs of an 18-year-old boy injured in a motorbike accident. **c** The tibia is protruding through the skin. An attempt at closed reduction failed because of the interposition of the posterior tibial tendon and the neurovascular bundle *(arrow)*.
d,e Radiographs taken 1 year after anatomical reduction, bone graft, and internal fixation

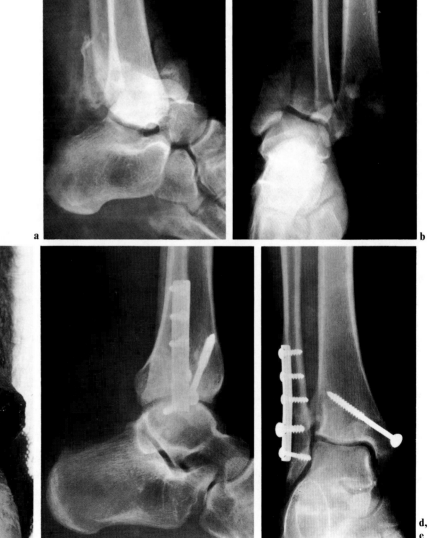

b) Types B and C

With the type B and C pattern (i.e., a fibular fracture at or above the syndesmosis), ankle stability will depend upon anatomical reconstruction and stable fixation of the lateral complex, and, therefore, this area should be fixed first.

Lateral Complex. Anatomical reduction of the lateral joint complex is essential to ensure normal ankle biomechanics. It should therefore be approached first and provisionally fixed. Fibular length must be restored; the most satisfactory method for this is by open reduction and internal fixation of the fibula. When open reduction and internal fixation are accomplished, the lateral malleolus will return to its normal position in the ankle mortise. Failure to restore the normal length and rotation of the fibula is the commonest error made in surgery for ankle trauma, unfortunately leading to many poor results (Fig. 22.32).

Although the first step is reduction of the fibular fracture, the surgeon may find this impossible. If the fibula *cannot* be reduced, the cause may be one of the following:

1. The lateral malleolus may be stuck behind the tibia and only be removable manually at surgery, often with considerable difficulty (Schatzker and Johnson 1983; Fig. 22.33).
2. Soft tissue may be interposed on the medial side, blocking reduction. The entrapped soft tissue is usually an avulsed deltoid ligament which retracts into the joint or, less commonly, the posterior tibial tendon caught in the medial malleolar fracture. Occasionally, all of the medial structures may be driven through the disrupted syndesmosis (Fig. 22.34).

In these situations, it is necessary to correct the medial interposition problem before completing the lateral stabilization; otherwise an anatomical reduction will be impossible to obtain.

Fibula. The fibular fracture must be carefully assessed. If it is in the *diaphysis,* the basic rules for diaphyseal fractures apply. However, in this injury, it is essential that fibular length is restored anatomically and that rotation is correct. Therefore, although gentle handling of soft tissues is important and indirect reduction techniques may be used (see Fig. 22.27), anatomical reduction is mandatory with respect to length and rotation. A transverse fracture is fixed with a tension band plate, a comminuted or spiral fracture by interfragmental screws, and a neutralization plate. The most satisfactory implant is the 3.5-mm DC plate, the low-contact DC (LCDC) plate, and the new 3.5-mm cortical screws, especially in the diaphysis (Fig. 22.35), or the one-third tubular plate for more distal fractures.

If the fibular fracture is in the *metaphysis* (i.e., the lateral malleolus), it is usually spiral and comminuted. Open reduction is performed directly and provisionally held by Kirschner wires. If the bone is *good* and will hold a screw, stabilization can be obtained by interfragmental compression with lag screws and a neutralization plate placed posteriorly or posterolaterally if possible, to prevent the fracture from slipping. The most commonly used implants are the one-third tubular plate, the 3.5-mm and 4.0-mm cancellous screws, and the 3.5-mm cortical screws (Fig. 22.36 a). Where possible, the plate should be applied posterolaterally to achieve the antiglide function (Brunner and Weber 1982; Fig. 22.36 b).

Poor or osteoporotic bone is, however, common in the lateral malleolus, and the screws may not hold

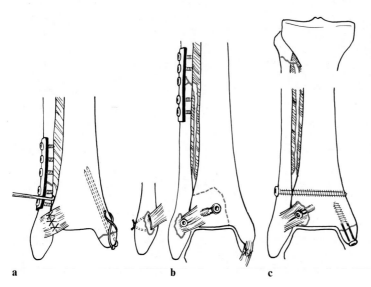

Fig. 22.35 a–c. Fixation of the fibular diaphysis. **a** If the fracture is distal, the one-third tubular plate is the preferred implant. The stability of the syndesmosis should be tested and its anatomical reduction assessed. If anatomical reduction cannot be maintained, a position screw is indicated. The syndesmotic ligament may be resutured. **b** Fracture in the fibular diaphysis may be fixed with a 3.5-mm dynamic compression (DC) plate or a one-third tubular plate, depending on the size of the bone. Avulsion of the bone from either end of the syndesmotic ligaments should be fixed with lag screw. **c** For fracture of the proximal fibula too high for internal fixation or dislocations of the proximal joint, a syndesmotic position screw may be indicated. (From Müller et al. 1979)

a   b   c

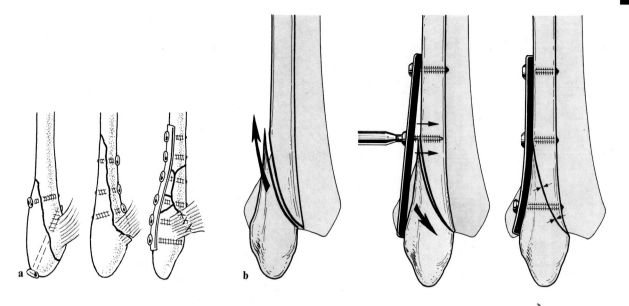

Fig. 22.36 a,b. Fixation of the fibular malleolus. **a** Various methods for fixation of the fibular malleolus using interfragmental lag screws and a one-third tubular plate. A plate is essential in all cases of comminution or osteoporosis. (From Müller et al. 1979). **b** Antiglide plate with supplementary interfragmental compression. A one-third tubular plate applied to the posterior surface of the fibula is attached first proximally and then distally. The plate prevents proximal gliding of the distal fragment. If possible, a lag screw should be inserted through the plate to provide supplementary interfragmental compression. (From Brunner and Weber 1982)

securely. In this case, the Kirschner wires used for provisional fixation should be retained and supplemented with further Kirschner wires across the fracture into the tibia (Fig. 22.37). Fixation will not be entirely stable, but anatomical reduction will be maintained if a supplemental external cast is applied. Since maintenance of anatomical reduction is vital to a satisfactory final result, it must *not* be sacrificed to early motion, which, in our opinion, is of secondary importance in the ankle. Attempted early motion with imperfect lateral fixation, whether by a plate or by Kirschner wires, has ruined many otherwise satisfactory operations and created many difficult problems for both patient and surgeon.

Once the fibula is reduced and fixed, we must turn our attention to the other part of the lateral joint complex. An intraoperative radiograph at this point will confirm the anatomical reduction and is recommended. No talar tilt should remain, the mortise should be anatomical, and the tibiofibular articular line should be restored. If the fibula is not anatomically reduced, the fixation *must* be removed and the cause found and rectified at this stage. Surgeons who fail to do so are deceiving them-

selves and dooming their patient's ankle, for fixation of the fibula in a shortened or rotated position will often cause rapid dissolution of the ankle joint (see Fig. 22.25). The usual reason for persistent valgus talar tilt is a comminuted fibular fracture in which proper length has not been restored.

Posterior Lesion. If the fibular length has been restored and anatomically fixed, any posterior malleolar avulsions which are attached to the distal fibular fracture should be anatomical. If the fragments are small, no treatment is indicated, but if large, they should be dealt with surgically. This will eliminate any gap in the articular surface, reduce postoperative pain, allow early motion, and, most importantly, make certain that posterior displacement of the talus cannot occur. Fragments larger than 20% of the joint surface should be viewed with suspicion and those larger than 33% of the articular surface should definitely be fixed (Harper et al. 1988).

The approach to the posterior fracture will depend upon its size and location. If the fragment is thick and on the medial side, fixation is best done by a retrograde cancellous screw inserted from the anterior tibial surface to the posterior malleolar fragment (Fig. 22.38a). It should be remembered, however, that the posterior fragment may be thin, and the cancellous screw threads inserted in a retrograde manner may cross the fracture, thereby displacing it. If the retrograde technique is used, 3.5-mm cortical screws, with the proximal hole overdrilled, are preferable to cancellous screws, the threads of which may cross the fracture line. Therefore, if the posterior fragment is thin or is lateral, a direct posterolateral approach is preferable (Fig. 22.38b). The patient is placed in the prone position. Both the fibular and poste-

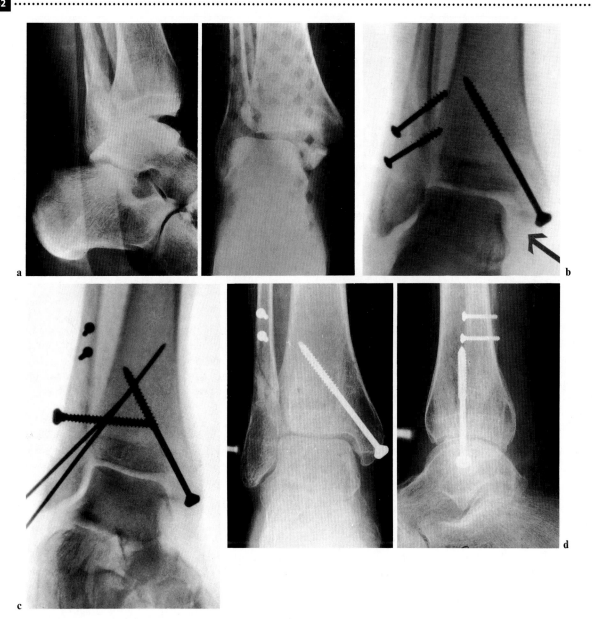

Fig. 22.37 a–d. Fixation of the lateral malleolus in osteoporotic bone. **a** Lateral and anteroposterior radiographs of a 44-year-old man with a type II unstable fracture of his ankle. **b** The immediately postoperative polaroid radiograph shows a malreduced fibula with a marked talar tilt and increased mortise width. The patient was referred for further treatment 5 weeks following the first operation. Reoperation was planned through the fibula, which was osteoporotic by this time. **c** The intraoperative polaroid film shows the use of Kirschner wires to fix the distal fibula as well as a position screw and interfragmental screws on the main fractures. **d** The final result at 5 years is good. The ankle is anatomical, but the patient has some stiffness and discomfort in the joint

rior malleolar fractures may be exposed posterolaterally. Exposure is not difficult, and fixation of the fibular fracture is relatively straightforward. Fixation of the posterior malleolar fracture is much easier in this way than by a retrograde anterior screw, since compression can be obtained directly with cancellous lag screws (Fig. 22.39 a–e).

Syndesmosis. After reduction and stabilization of the fibula and the posterior fragments, the syndesmosis should now be inspected openly or tested for instability (see Fig. 22.33 a). If all the fractures have been anatomically fixed, the distal tibiofibular joint should be anatomical; if it is not, as previously stated, the fibular

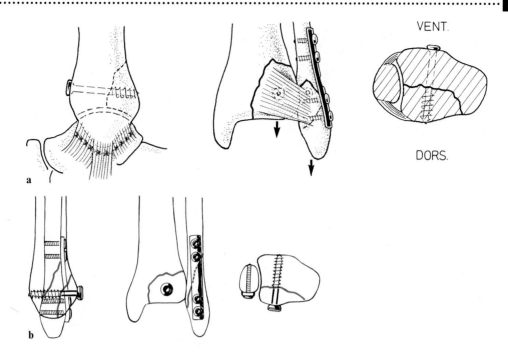

VENT.

DORS.

Fig. 22.38 a,b. Fixation of the posterior malleolar fragment. **a** Large fragments of the posterior malleolus may be fixed with a retrograde screw. (From Müller et al. 1979). **b** If the posterior malleolar fragment is thin and laterally placed, the best approach is posterolateral. With the patient in the prone position, the small fragment can be fixed with an interfragmental cancellous lag screw and the fibular fracture plated from its posterior aspect

reduction must be inspected. The distal tibiofibular joint, if anatomically reduced, should be stable and rarely requires a screw to hold it. Large avulsion fragments from the fibula or tibia should be internally fixed (see Fig. 22.35 b, c). On some occasions, the entire interosseous membrane and both anterior and posterior ligaments are disrupted. In those cases, if the surgeon is concerned about the stability of the joint, a syndesmotic screw may be inserted from the fibula into the tibia just above the distal tibiofibular joint. The screw must not be a lag screw but a position screw, taped on both sides in order not to compress the distal joint, which might limit ankle motion (see Fig. 22.33 c). This screw should be removed prior to unprotected weight-bearing, usually at 6–8 weeks.

High Fibular Fracture. It has been suggested that the high fibular fracture should not be fixed but the mortise restored by a low screw from the fibula to the tibia. Considerable danger exists in this approach. If the fibula was shortened, it is difficult to be certain that length has been restored, and the screw may therefore fix it in a shortened position. We believe that all displaced fibular fractures except those in the upper third should be openly fixed directly, rather than the surgeon relying on a mortise screw to restore fibular length (see Fig. 22.25 a–d). In the upper third of the fibula, direct fixation is impractical and dangerous to the peroneal nerve, so a syndesmotic screw is the only alternative there, but care must be taken to ensure\ normal fibular length (Fig. 22.40 a–g).

Medial Complex. Having fixed the important lateral joint complex, we can now turn our attention to the medial malleolus. Two possibilities are present:

– *Deltoid medial collateral ligament tear.* With an anatomically restored lateral complex, little is gained by resuture of the medial ligament, so we recommend repair only if the ligament is interposed between the medial malleolus and the talus, blocking reduction of the talus.
– *Medial malleolar avulsion.* An avulsed and displaced medial malleolus is ideally treated by open reduction and internal fixation. If the bony fragment is small or osteoporotic, the best technique is tension band wiring using two 2-mm Kirschner wires and no. 18 gauge wire (Fig. 22.41 a). If the bony fragment is large and through good bone, a malleolar screw beginning anteriorly and directed posterolaterally will stabilize the fragment. Rotational stability may be maintained by a second screw, usually a 4.0-mm cancellous screw, or by a Kirschner wire, or by two 4.0-mm cancellous screws (Fig. 22.41 b). Great care should be exercised in handling the medial malleolus, as it is small and may

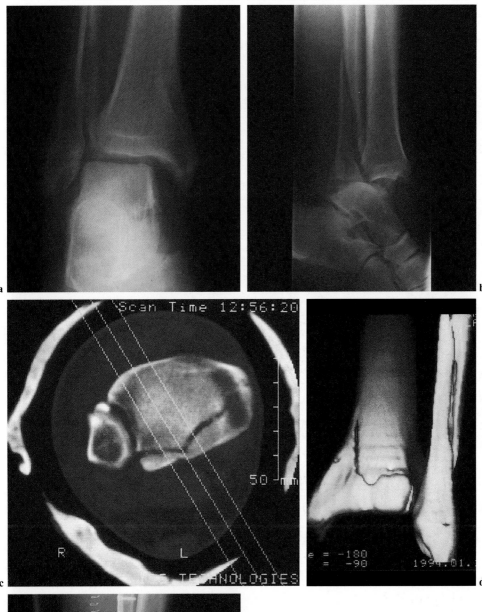

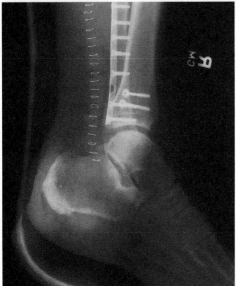

Fig. 22.39 a–e. Fixation of posterior malleolar fracture. This patient, age 19, sustained a fracture-dislocation of the ankle. **a** The anteroposterior radiograph shows the wide medial displacement. **b** The extent of this injury is best seen on the lateral radiograph showing posterior dislocation of the talus, in the ankle mortise with a fracture of the fibula. **c** A computed tomography (CT) scan shows the extent of the posterior malleolar fragment, also clearly seen on the three dimensional CT (**d**). **e** A direct posterior approach was made, the fibula fixed with a one -third semi-tubular plate and two lag screws inserted through the posterior malleolar fracture, as noted on the lateral radiograph. The end result was excellent

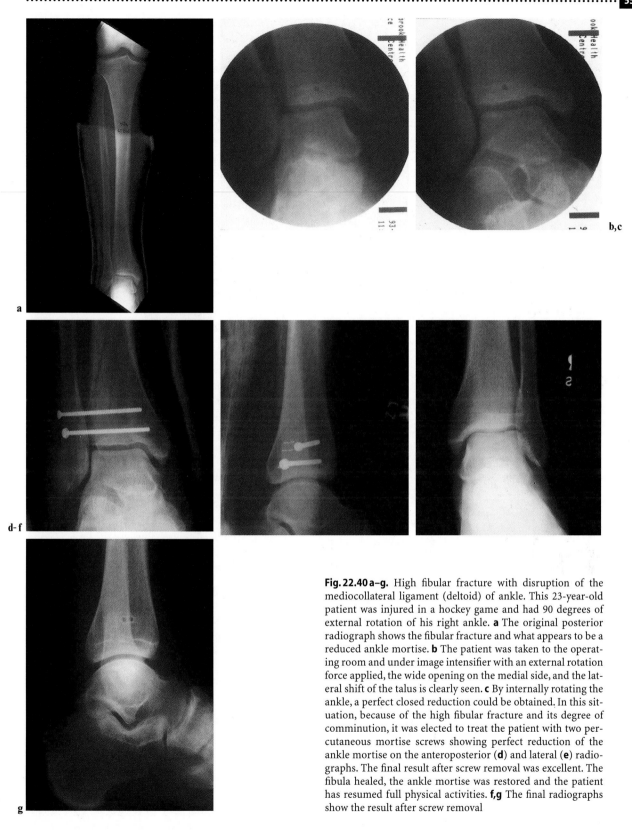

Fig. 22.40 a–g. High fibular fracture with disruption of the mediocollateral ligament (deltoid) of ankle. This 23-year-old patient was injured in a hockey game and had 90 degrees of external rotation of his right ankle. **a** The original posterior radiograph shows the fibular fracture and what appears to be a reduced ankle mortise. **b** The patient was taken to the operating room and under image intensifier with an external rotation force applied, the wide opening on the medial side, and the lateral shift of the talus is clearly seen. **c** By internally rotating the ankle, a perfect closed reduction could be obtained. In this situation, because of the high fibular fracture and its degree of comminution, it was elected to treat the patient with two percutaneous mortise screws showing perfect reduction of the ankle mortise on the anteroposterior (**d**) and lateral (**e**) radiographs. The final result after screw removal was excellent. The fibula healed, the ankle mortise was restored and the patient has resumed full physical activities. **f,g** The final radiographs show the result after screw removal

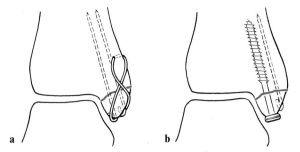

Fig. 22.41 a,b. Fixation of the medial malleolar avulsion. **a** If the fragment is small, a tension band wire technique is preferable. **b** If the fragment is larger, a 4.0-mm cancellous screw or a malleolar screw supplemented with an antirotation Kirschner wire will afford good fixation

shatter. The surgeon usually has only one opportunity to fix this fracture and should plan for it carefully. The medial malleolus will not respond well to multiple attempts at fixation.

22.4.3 Wound Closure

Atraumatic wound closure is required for the thin skin of this area. A small suction drain is helpful in the lateral incision to prevent hematoma formation.

Fig. 22.42 a–d. Ankle fractures in the elderly. **a,b** Anteroposterior and lateral radiographs of a type II unstable fracture of the ankle in a 78-year-old man. The *arrow* in **a** points to the noticeable increase in the mortise width. Because of the marked osteoporosis it was elected to treat this fracture with closed manipulation, anatomical reduction, and fixation of the fibula with a percutaneously inserted Rush rod. **c,d** The final result at 1 year was excellent

22.4.4 Postoperative Program

22.4.4.1 Immediate Management

A well-padded dressing supported by a splint holding the ankle at a right angle is *imperative*. Failure to provide this will result in an equinus deformity because of the disruption of the anterior capsule. In our experience, this is one of the major errors made in the treatment of ankle injuries and may ruin even the most expert internal fixation. During the early postoperative period, the limb should be elevated in order to prevent edema. When the patient has regained active control of the dorsiflexor muscles, usually on the second to fourth postoperative day, the splint may be removed for exercises. However, it must be retained at night or when not exercising to prevent equinus deformity.

22.4.4.2 Early Motion

In the ankle, anatomical reduction should never be compromised for early motion. The final results of treatment depend more on joint congruity than on early motion. If the surgeon is concerned about the stability of the internal fixation or the quality of the bone, especially in the lateral malleolus, the system should be protected until union is well advanced. Failure to do so will court disaster. We have seen expertly fixed lateral malleoli fall apart due to injudicious early motion, while a study in our center showed little difference between the final results of fractures moved early and those moved late (Gollish et al. 1977).

If the internal fixation is stable and the bone is good, then motion may be started as outlined above and continued until rehabilitation is complete.

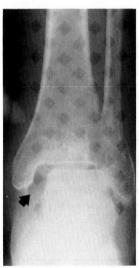
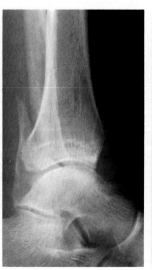
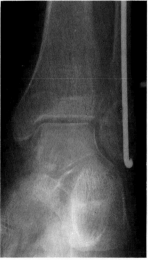
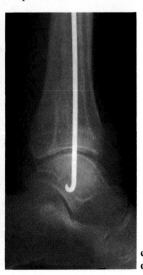

a, b

c, d

The patient is carefully monitored for clinical and radiological signs of implant failure. If none are present, partial weight-bearing may be started by the fourth to sixth week, and full weight-bearing by the 12th week, after which the patient may complete his or her rehabilitation program.

At the first sign of impending implant failure, corrective measures must be applied. As mentioned previously, congruity of the joint is all-important. If therefore, the implant seems to be in danger of failing, but congruity is present, the patient should be put in a non-weight-bearing plaster until union has occurred. If congruity has been lost by implant failure, then further surgery must be performed (see Fig. 22.37). However, this surgery may be extremely difficult because of the high porosity of the bone, and only stabilization with Kirschner wires may be possible. Postoperative immobilization is imperative until bony union has occurred.

22.5 Special Problems in Ankle Fractures

22.5.1 Open Ankle Fractures

The principles of management of open fractures of the ankle have been previously stated and do not differ from the principles of closed ankle trauma. Anatomical reduction is essential. After careful wound débridement and cleansing the ankle fracture should be fixed stably and anatomically with the smallest amount of implant possible. The trauma wounds should be left open, while the incisions may be closed. This treatment protocol will result in good results as reported by Franklin et al. (1984) and Bray et al. (1988).

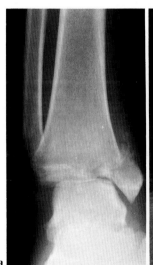
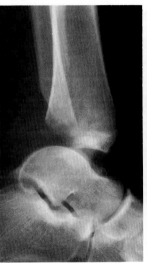
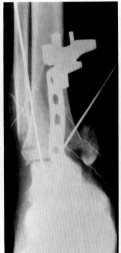
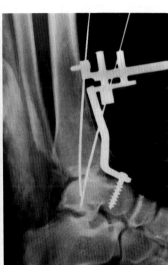
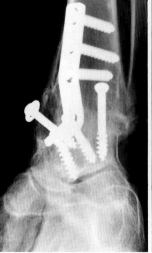
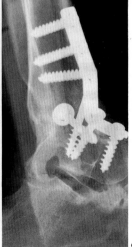

Fig. 22.43 a–c. Primary ankle arthrodesis due to bone loss. **a** Anteroposterior and lateral radiographs of a 21-year-old man injured in a motorcycle accident. The distal fibula and a portion of the distal tibia were extruded through an open wound onto the roadway and were never found. Primary treatment consisted of cleansing and débridement of the wound and cast fixation. At 2 weeks it was elected to perform a primary ankle arthrodesis with the full consent of the patient. **b** The intraoperative radiograph shows the provisional fixation with Kirschner wires and the application of a dynamic compression (DC) plate with tension device. Further bone graft was inserted. **c** The result at 2 years shows sound bony union. The patient has regained excellent movement in this foot and has an excellent functional result. This form of ankle arthrodesis gives a high rate of fusion and allows the surgeon to obtain and maintain an excellent position for the arthrodesis

22.5.2 Ankle Fractures in the Elderly

While the same principles apply to the management of joint injuries in the elderly, the achievement of stable internal fixation by standard techniques in these patients is extremely difficult. This is especially true in articular or periarticular fractures, since the cancellous bone of the metaphysis is often osteoporotic and cannot hold a screw. Also, vascularity in the lower extremity may be compromised, resulting in wound necrosis.

Open reduction and internal fixation in this age-group must therefore be approached with care. If vascularity to the limb is diminished, standard techniques of open reduction and internal fixation should be avoided. Instead, percutaneous techniques through small stab wounds may suffice to restore some stability to the ankle while not compromising the skin or the limb. Since screws do not hold in the osteoporotic bone, techniques of Kirschner wire fixation supplemented by tension band wires are preferable. We have also used Rush rods inserted percutaneously into the lateral malleolus to

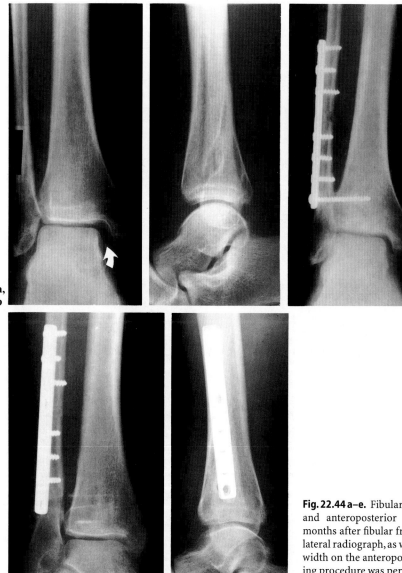

Fig. 22.44 a–e. Fibular lengthening for malunion. **a,b** Lateral and anteroposterior radiographs of a 22-year-old man 8 months after fibular fracture. Note the malunited fibula on the lateral radiograph, as well as the increased talar tilt and mortise width on the anteroposterior view *(arrow)*. A fibular lengthening procedure was performed, using the AO distractor and a 1-cm bone graft inserted between the fibular ends. **c** The postoperative radiograph shows restoration of the ankle mortise. **d,e** The result at 1 year shows restoration of the ankle mortise and union of the osteotomy. The final clinical result is good

restore some stability and length to the lateral joint complex. While perfect rotatory stability cannot be obtained by this method, the addition of a cast will usually be sufficient to prevent displacement of the mortise (Fig. 22.42).

In the ankle, as elsewhere in fracture of the elderly, caution is advised before embarking on standard techniques of open reduction and internal fixation. Beauchamp et al. (1983) reported on the results of ankle fracture management in the elderly. Complications in this group were higher with open than with closed treatment, which resulted in poorer results in those treated by open means. We believe that by careful planning, including assessment of the vascular status of the limb, by using techniques of Kirschner wires or Rush rods inserted percutaneously or through small incisions, and by the addition of plaster casts, complications can be avoided and satisfactory results obtained.

Fig. 22.45 a–d. Supramalleolar osteotomy for malunion. This 56-year-old woman had sustained a fracture of her tibia and medial malleolus while skiing 12 years prior to presentation. **a** Note the varus deformation of the tibial fracture and the severe varus tilt to the talus. **b** The lateral radiograph shows advanced osteoarthritis with a large anterior osteophyte and joint narrowing. The patient had severe pain. **c,d** A supramalleolar osteotomy associated with joint débridement and removal of the anterior osteophyte restored her alignment, increased her motion, and relieved much of her pain

22.5.3 Primary Ankle Arthrodesis

Primary ankle arthrodesis is rarely indicated in the management of ankle trauma. Even in cases of severe comminution in osteoporotic bone, one does better to revert to os calcis traction and early motion than primary fusion. It is only in the rare instance where reconstruction of the joint is impossible, especially in open fractures with bone loss, that early ankle arthrodesis may be desirable (Fig. 22.43). However, this must never be done without prior discussion and consent of the patient, otherwise serious medicolegal problems may arise.

Techniques of primary arthrodesis will depend upon the situation at hand and include external fixation and various types of internal fixation with bone grafts.

22.5.4 Fibular Lengthening for Malunion

While it is beyond the scope of this book to discuss late reconstruction procedures, one such procedure in the ankle is worthy of note, namely, fibular lengthening for malunion. The major cause of a malunited ankle fracture is a shortened, externally rotated fibula, resulting from either operative or nonoperative treatment (Fig. 22.44 a, b). Radiographs will show an increased valgus talar tilt, giving the appearance of a smaller joint space, which implies early cartilage loss. This loss of joint space radiographically does not, however, reflect cartilage loss in the first several months following injury. If lengthening is

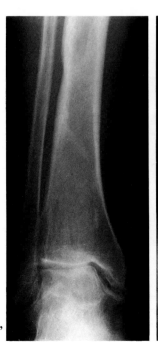
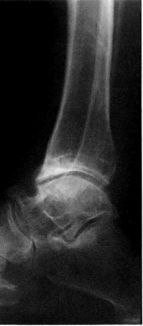
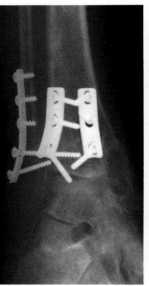
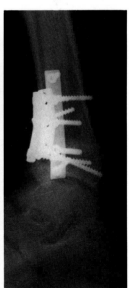

a,
b

c,
d

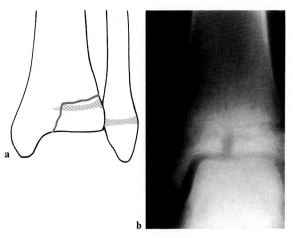

Fig. 22.46 a-b. Lateral epiphyseal separation. **a** The lateral epiphyseal fragment attached to the anterior tibiofibular ligament (juvenile Tillaux fracture) is shown. **b** The radiograph depicts such a fracture

performed in carefully selected cases of fibular malunion, joint congruity can be restored and a good long-term result anticipated. Of course, this depends on the state of the articular cartilage at the time of surgery. If doubt exists about the suitability of a malunited ankle for this procedure, preoperative ankle arthroscopy is indicated.

The technical aspect of the procedure must be carefully planned preoperatively. The exact technique will depend upon the type of malunion. If the fibular fracture

Fig. 22.47 a–c. Triplane fracture of the distal tibia. **a** A three-fragment triplane fracture of the distal tibial epiphysis with an associated fibular fracture. **b** Lateral radiograph of a triplane fracture. **c** Computed tomography (CT) scan showing the coronal split proximal to the physis. (Courtesy of Dr. Philp Spiegel)

is high, the best approach is to osteotomize the lower third of the fibula, distract the osteotomy site to the desired length, insert an iliac crest cortical-cancellous bone graft, and apply a 3.5-mm DC plate (Fig. 22.44 c–e). The restoration of the normal ankle mortise must be verified on intraoperative radiographs. If the fibular fracture is low, osteotomy through the fracture site may be required. In both instances, the use of distractors is essential to achieve the lengthening.

22.5.5 Supramalleolar Osteotomy

Malunion of an ankle fracture may result in a major varus or valgus deformation. If the articular surface is still satisfactory, a supramalleolar osteotomy may restore alignment and preserve ankle function (Fig. 22.45). Careful preoperative planning is essential. The osteotomy is performed through the metaphysis of the tibia and fixation is usually by internal fixation, occasionally by external fixation.

22.5.6 Ankle Fractures in Adolescents

Specific fracture patterns may occur in children at the end of their growth period, usually between the ages of 13 and 15 years. At that particular stage of development, the distal tibial epiphyseal plate may exhibit partial closure, usually on the lateral side. Two types of fracture patterns have been identified, the lateral epiphyseal avulsion (the Juvenile Tillaux fracture; Bonnin 1970) and the triplane fracture (Spiegel et al. 1984).

The lateral epiphyseal avulsion is characterized by a fracture line extending from the articular surface of the

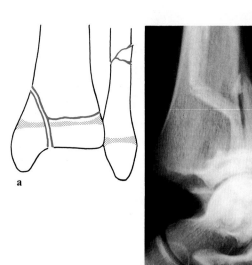
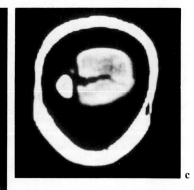

tibia proximally across the epiphyseal plate, then laterally along the physis (Fig. 22.46). This fracture is caused by the anterior tibiofibular ligament in full external rotation.

The triplane fracture (Fig. 22.47) is characterized by two, three, or four fragments in the distal tibial metaphysis. The first fragment is the anterolateral portion of the distal tibial physis (similar to the Tillaux fracture), the second the remainder of the physis extending into the distal tibial metaphysis, and the third the remainder of the distal tibial metaphysis (Fig. 22.47 a). Frequently, the fibula is fractured above the ankle mortise, implicating an external rotation mechanism.

The principle of management for these fractures remains the same as before, i.e., anatomical reduction is essential for good long-term results. Therefore, if the fracture is displaced and closed reduction is not successful, anatomical open reduction and internal fixation, using lag screws and Kirschner wires, are essential.

References

Beauchamp CG, Clay NR, Thexton PW (1983) Displaced ankle fractures over 50 years of age. J Bone Joint Surg 65(3)B: 329–332

Berndt AL, Harty M (1959) Transchondral fractures (osteochondritis dissecans) of the talus. J Bone Joint Surg 41A:988

Bonnin JG (1970) Injuries to the ankle. Darien Community Association, Darien, CT

Brunner CF, Weber BG (1982) Special techniques of internal fixation. Springer, Berlin Heidelberg New York

De Souza Dias L, Forester TP (1974) Traumatic lesions of the ankle joint. Clin Orthop 100:219–224

Elmendorff H, Petes D (1971) Late results of fractures of the ankle. Acta Orthop Unfall Chir 69:220

Franklin JL, Johnson KD, Hansen ST Jr (1984) Immediate internal fixation of open ankle fractures. A report of 38 cases treated with standard protocol. J Bone Joint Surg 66A: 1349–1356

Gollish JD, Tile M, Begg R (1977) Fractures of the ankle. J Bone Joint Surg 59B:510

Hughes J (1980) The medial malleolus in ankle fractures. Orthop Clin North Am 2(3):649–660

Inman VT (1976) The joints or the ankle. Williams and Wilkins, Baltimore

Lauge-Hansen N (1942) Ankelbrud I. Genetisk diagnose og reposition. Dissertation, Munksgaard, Copenhagen

Monk CJ (1969) Injuries of the tibiofibular ligaments. J Bone Joint Surg 51B:330

Müller ME, Allgöwer M, Willenegger H (1965) Technique of internal fixation of fractures. Springer, Berlin Heidelberg New York, p 115

Müller ME, Allgöwer M, Schneider R, Willenegger H (1979) Manual of internal fixation, 2nd edn. Springer, Berlin Heidelberg New York

Müller ME, Nazarian S, Koch P, Schatzker J (1990) The comprehensive classification of fractures of long bones. Springer, Berlin Heidelberg New York

Müller ME, Allgöwer M, Schneider R, Willenegger H (1991) Manual of internal fixation, 3rd edn. Springer, Berlin Heidelberg New York

Pankovich AM (1979) Adult ankle fractures. J Con Ed Orthop 7:17

Pankovich AM, Shivaran MS (1979) Anatomical basis of variability in injuries of the medial malleolus and the deltoid ligament. Acta Orthop Scand 50:217–223

Ramsay PL, Hamilton W (1976) Changes in tibiotalar area of contact caused by lateral tibia shift. J Bone Joint Surg 59A:356

Schatzker J, Johnson R (1983) Fracture-dislocation of the ankle with anterior dislocation of the fibula. J Trauma 23(5): 420–423

Spiegel PG, Mast JW, Cooperman DR, Laros GS (1984) Triplane fractures of the distal tibial epiphysis. In: Spiegel P (ed) Topics in orthopaedic trauma. University Park, Baltimore, pp 153–171 (Techniques in orthopaedic surgery)

Willenegger H (1979) Evaluation of ankle fractures nonoperative and operative treatment. Clin Orthop 138:111

Willenegger H, Breitenfelder (1965) Principles of internal fixation. Springer, Berlin Heidelberg New York

23 Fractures of the Talus

M. TILE

23.1 Introduction

Injuries to the talus occur infrequently, but, when they do, the consequences can be grave. Misconceptions about this injury abound, due mainly to poor comprehension of the blood supply to the talus and to the common practice of comparing dissimilar cases.

Disability arising from talar fractures is due to the major complications of avascular necrosis and of malunion from nonanatomical reduction, which in turn leads to osteoarthritis of the subtalar joint and altered biomechanics of the foot. Also, skin problems are common, often worsened by injudicious surgery. Sepsis may ensue, with severe disability or amputation the likely outcome.

In 1832, Sir Astley Cooper gave in dramatic detail one of the first accounts of the natural history of dislocation of the talus. He describes vividly how "Mr. Downes, on the 24th of July, 1820, had the misfortune to dislocate the astragalus by falling from his horse." In consultation he observed "that I would not operate and that perhaps the skin might give way and the bone become exposed – when we would be justified in removing it." Previous treatment was therefore further pursued: "On the 29th the leeches were repeated and the lotion continued." – "On the 20th of August – . . . there was a great discharge of pus and the astragalus became loose. . . . On Oct. 5, 1820, finding the astragalus very loose, I removed it" (i.e., 10 weeks after the accident). In October, 1821, the patient "had slight motion at the ankle which was gradually increasing."

Syme (1848) recorded 13 patients, of whom only two survived. He recommended primary amputation for open injuries of the talus. Anderson (1919) collected 18 cases of talar injuries occurring in air crashes and named this injury "aviator's astragalus."

Coltart, in 1952, wrote the then definitive work on this subject. He recorded 228 cases, of which 106 were fractures or fracture-dislocations of the talar neck. Most of the subsequent reviews reflect the principles in Coltart's series. He described the natural history of fractures of the talar neck with no displacement, with subtalar dislocation, and with complete dislocation of the body of the talus and indicated the prognosis of each.

As in all fractures, sound management depends upon a return to basic principles. Fractures of the talar neck with displacement demand anatomical reduction and stable internal fixation if closed reduction fails, otherwise the subtalar joint will be adversely affected. However, surgery must not jeopardize the already precarious blood supply to the body of the talus.

Therefore, a precise knowledge of the blood supply to the talus is essential for logical management.

23.2 Anatomical Considerations

The talus is an unique bone, in that 60% of it is covered by articular cartilage and it has no muscular or tendinous attachments (Fig. 23.1).

23.2.1 Vascular Anatomy

The surgical significance of the vascular anatomy cannot be overemphasized. Because of the association of certain fractures and dislocations with avascular necrosis of the body of the talus, the extraosseous and intraosseous vascular anatomy has been the subject of considerable investigation. Lexor et al. (1904), Sneed (1925), Phemister (1940), McKeever (1943), Watson-Jones (1946), Kleiger (1948), and Wildenauer (1950) were pioneers in this field.

Wildenauer (1950) fully described the blood supply of the talus and is credited with being the first to describe the important artery arising from the posterior tibial artery and coursing through the tarsal canal, which is now known to be the most important vessel to the body of the talus. He also pointed out the anatomical distinction between the tarsal sinus and the tarsal canal. The tarsal canal is formed by the sulcus of the talus and the sulcus of the os calcis. It lies obliquely from a posterior medial to an anterior lateral position and opens into the tarsal sinus. In the canal the interosseous talocalcaneal ligament and the artery of the tarsal canal are located. Wildenauer believed that the most important vascular contributions came from the arteries of the tarsal sinus, tarsal canal, and the medial periosteal network.

Further studies by Coltart (1952), Lauro and Purpura (1956), Haliburton et al. (1958), and Montis and Ridola

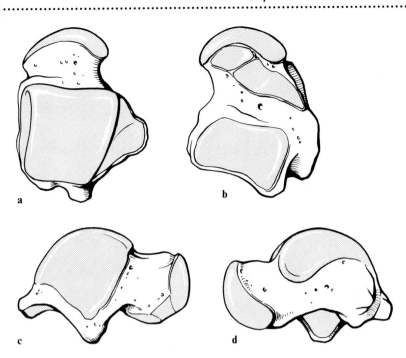

Fig. 23.1 a–d. Anatomical features of the talus. **a** Superior surface. **b** Inferior surface. **c** Lateral aspect. **d** Medial aspect

(1959) added to our knowledge by confirming the studies of Wildenauer, especially the importance of the medial blood supply.

Mulfinger and Trueta (1970) wrote the classic work on this subject, again reaffirming the earlier findings of Wildenauer. Their experimental technique ensured that only the arterial blood supply was injected with contrast medium, offsetting criticism of previous studies.

The important arterial supply to the talus is described in the following sections.

23.2.1.1 Extraosseous Arterial Supply

a) From the Posterior Tibial Artery

Artery of the Tarsal Canal. This important artery usually arises from the posterior tibial artery, 1 cm proximal to the origin of the medial and lateral plantar arteries (Fig. 23.2). From that point, it passes anteriorly between the sheath of the flexor digitorum longus and the flexor hallucis longus muscles to enter the tarsal canal, in which it lies anteriorly close to the talus. Many branches enter the body of the talus from the arterial network in the tarsal canal. Continuing through the tarsal canal into the tarsal sinus, this artery anastomoses with the artery of the tarsal sinus, forming a rich vascular sling beneath the talar neck.

Deltoid Branch. A substantial artery supplying a portion of the medial half of the body of the talus hugs the inner surface of the deltoid ligament of the ankle (Fig. 23.3).

This vessel arises most commonly from the artery of the tarsal canal or directly from the posterior tibial artery, and less frequently from the medial plantar branch of the posterior tibial artery. The surgical significance of this vessel is obvious. First, since most injuries of the talus occur with dorsiflexion and inversion, the medial soft tissues, including this artery, may remain intact and ensure the viability of the body of the talus. Second, medial surgical approaches to the talus may interfere with this vessel, thereby possibly injuring the only remaining blood supply to the talus.

b) From the Anterior Tibial Artery

Superior Neck Branches. The dorsalis pedis artery, a continuation of the anterior tibial artery, sends branches to the superior surface of the neck of the talus.

Artery of the Tarsal Sinus. This artery is always present, large, and always anastomoses with the artery of the tarsal canal. It is formed by an anastomosis of a branch of the dorsalis pedis artery with a branch of the perforating peroneal artery. This lateral blood supply is profuse, with many direct branches into the bone.

c) From the Peroneal Artery

Small branches from the peroneal artery join with branches of the posterior tibial artery to form the posterior plexus around the talus. The perforating peroneal

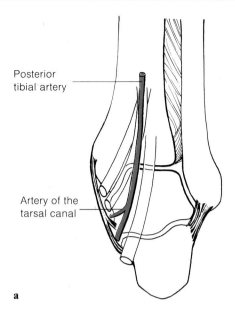

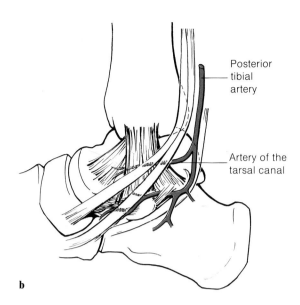

Posterior tibial artery

Artery of the tarsal canal

Posterior tibial artery

Artery of the tarsal canal

a

b

Fig. 23.2 a,b. Extraosseous blood supply to the talus. **a** The artery of the tarsal canal arising from the posterior tibial artery. Note its position along the interior surface of the deltoid ligament. **b** From there, it can be seen entering the tarsal canal

artery contributes to the artery of the tarsal sinus, but in general the peroneal supply to the talus is not considered to be important.

23.2.1.2 Intraosseous

a) Head of Talus

The head of the talus is supplied by two sources, medially by branches of the dorsalis pedis artery and laterally by branches of the arterial anastomosis in the artery of the tarsal sinus (Fig. 23.4).

b) Body of Talus

The *anastomotic artery* in the tarsal canal supplies most of the talar body, through four or five branches on the medial side. This vessel usually supplies almost all of the middle third of the body, except for the extreme superior aspect, and all of the lateral third, except for the posterior aspect.

The *deltoid artery* supplies the medial third of the body (see Fig. 23.4).

Rich anastomoses within the bone were found in almost all cases, especially between the superior neck vessels and the vessels arising from the tarsal canal. In

some people, the artery of the tarsal sinus and the tarsal canal may anastomose within the bone.

23.2.1.3 Summary

From these studies, it may be deduced that:
1. The body of the talus has a rich blood supply through several anastomoses.
2. The major blood supply enters posterior to the talar neck, so that an isolated neck fracture, unless it extended posteriorly into the body, would be unlikely to interfere with the blood supply.
3. An important vessel lies adjacent to the inner surface of the deltoid ligament. Except in cases of total dislocation of the talus and posterior extrusion of the body, this vessel maintains the viability of the talar body, if it is not interfered with surgically.

23.2.2 Mechanism of Injury

23.2.2.1 Common Pattern

Most fractures of the talar neck are caused by a severe dorsiflexion force (see Fig. 23.5). In the Royal Air Force studies (Coltart 1952), forced dorsiflexion of the foot against the rudder bar caused the fracture of the talar neck: hence the term "aviator's astragalus." In our society, most injuries are caused by the complex high-energy forces associated with motor vehicle accidents.

Rotation forces may be added to those of dorsiflexion to complete the injury. Following the talar neck fracture, the body of the talus locks in the ankle mortise. The

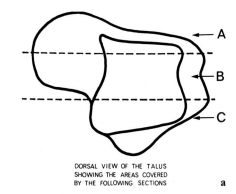

DORSAL VIEW OF THE TALUS
SHOWING THE AREAS COVERED
BY THE FOLLOWING SECTIONS   **a**

DORSALIS PEDIS
ARTERY BRANCHES

DELTOID
BRANCHES

POSTERIOR
TUBERCLE BRANCHES

TARSAL SINUS
BRANCHES

ARTERY OF THE
TARSAL CANAL

POSTERIOR
TIBIAL ARTERY

BLOOD SUPPLY TO THE
MEDIAL ONE - THIRD
OF THE TALUS

DORSALIS PEDIS
ARTERY BRANCHES

POSTERIOR TUBERCLE
BRANCHES

TARSAL SINUS
BRANCHES

ARTERY OF THE
TARSAL CANAL

BLOOD SUPPLY TO THE
MIDDLE ONE - THIRD
OF THE TALUS

LATERAL TARSAL
ARTERY

PERFORATING PERONEAL
ARTERY

ARTERY OF THE
TARSAL SINUS

ARTERY OF THE
TARSAL CANAL
BRANCHES

POSTERIOR
TUBERCLE
BRANCHES

BLOOD SUPPLY TO THE
LATERAL ONE - THIRD
OF THE TALUS

Fig. 23.3 a,b. The deltoid branch. **a** Blood supply to the talus in sagittal sections. The artery of the tarsal canal is shown with the deltoid artery branch arising from it, lying close to the inner surface of the deltoid ligament and entering the body of the talus. **b** Blood supply to the talus in coronal sections. The deltoid branch arising from the artery of the tarsal canal is clearly seen with its relationship to the deltoid ligament and medial malleolus. The other arterial supply, including the perforating peroneal artery, the lateral tarsal artery, the artery of the tarsal sinus, and the dorsalis pedis artery, is also clearly indicated. (From Mulfinger and Trueta 1970)

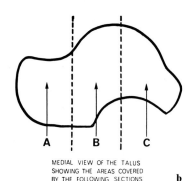

MEDIAL VIEW OF THE TALUS
SHOWING THE AREAS COVERED
BY THE FOLLOWING SECTIONS   **b**

PERFORATING PERONEAL
ARTERY

DORSALIS PEDIS
ARTERY

LATERAL TARSAL
ARTERY

ANASTOMOTIC
ARTERY FROM
DELTOID
BRANCH

ARTERY OF THE
TARSAL SINUS

BLOOD SUPPLY TO THE
HEAD OF THE TALUS

DORSALIS PEDIS
ARTERY BRANCHES

TARSAL SINUS
BRANCHES

ARTERY OF THE
TARSAL CANAL

DELTOID
BRANCH

BLOOD SUPPLY TO THE
MIDDLE ONE - THIRD
OF THE TALUS

TARSAL SINUS
BRANCHES

ARTERY OF THE
TARSAL CANAL

DELTOID
BRANCH

POSTERIOR
TIBIAL ARTERY

BLOOD SUPPLY TO THE
POSTERIOR ONE - THIRD
OF THE TALUS

23.2 Anatomical Considerations

• **567**

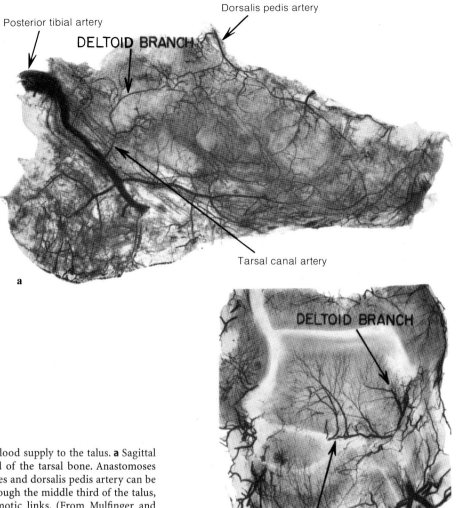

Posterior tibial artery

Dorsalis pedis artery

DELTOID BRANCH

Tarsal canal artery

a

DELTOID BRANCH

Tarsal canal artery

b

Fig. 23.4 a,b. Interosseous blood supply to the talus. **a** Sagittal section of the middle third of the tarsal bone. Anastomoses between the deltoid branches and dorsalis pedis artery can be seen. **b** Coronal section through the middle third of the talus, again showing the anastomotic links. (From Mulfinger and Trueta 1970)

remainder of the foot, including the head of the talus and the os calcis, displaces medially through the subtalar joint (Fig. 23.5).

Continuation of the dorsiflexion force ruptures the intraosseous ligaments between the talus and os calcis as well as the posterior talofibular and talocalcaneal ligaments. The body of the talus is forced posteromedially out of the mortise with the neck fracture, pointing laterally and superiorly. In more than 50 % of such cases the medial malleolus fractures obliquely or vertically (Figs. 23.5 b; see also Fig. 23.12).

Thus, the body of the talus rotates around the intact or partially intact deltoid ligament and eventually rests posterior to the medial malleolus, anterior to the Achilles tendon. The neurovascular structures are rarely injured primarily, but may be secondarily if pressure on them is not rapidly removed.

23.2.2.2 Atypical Patterns

Instead of the usual injury of dorsiflexion, shearing forces may occasionally produce an unusual injury. Shearing forces, acting perpendicular to the cancellous trabeculae, are usually associated with marked instability and displacement, as in the case shown in Fig. 23.6. In this example, the patient's foot was caught in the jaws of a logging machine and his body rotated around the stabilized os calcis and talus, creating an open shear fracture through both bones.

23.2.2.3 Total Dislocation of the Talus

Total dislocation of the talus is a severe injury usually caused by forced, violent, internal rotation and plantar flexion. As the foot displaces, the anterolateral capsule

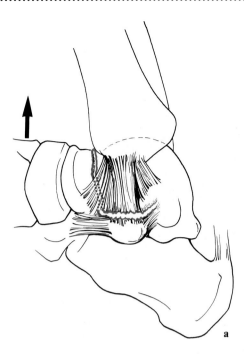

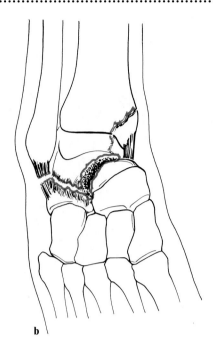

Fig. 23.5 a,b. Talar neck fractures. Most talar neck fractures are caused by a severe dorsiflexion force. **a** The talar neck abuts the anterior portion of the tibia and the continuing force fracture the talar neck. **b** A continuing inversion force ruptures the lateral subtalar ligaments, and often the lateral ligament of the ankle, or causes an avulsion of the lateral malleolus

and the collateral ligaments rupture. Further inversion causes a rupture of the talocalcaneal ligaments allowing the talus to extrude from the ankle mortise, often with rupture of the overlying skin (Fig. 23.7; see also Fig. 23.14).

23.3 Classification and Natural History

Armed with a knowledge both of the rich blood supply of the talus and also of the mechanisms of injury, it is possible to develop a classification of fractures of the talus of considerable prognostic value. The most widely accepted classification of these fractures is a variation on that originated by Coltart (1952), as shown in Table 23.1. Excluded from this classification are the common avulsion fractures of portions of the talus and fractures of the talar dome – so-called osteochondritis dissecans of the talus – since both of these injuries differ in their behavior from the more uncommon fractures of the body and neck.

Clearly, the outcome of these injuries is dependent upon the *type of fracture* and the *degree of violence* causing it. These aspects will also affect the *talar blood supply* and the degree of *subluxation or dislocation of the*

Table 23.1. Classification of fractures of the talus

Fractures of the talar body
Fractures of the talar neck
Type A: Undisplaced fracture of the talar nec
Type B: Displaced fracture of the talar neck with subtalar joint subluxation
Type C: Displaced fracture of the talar neck with dislocation of the body
Subtalar dislocation
Total dislocation of the talus

talar body, the major factors influencing the prognosis of this injury.

23.3.1 Fractures of the Body of the Talus

Simple linear cracks in the body should pose few management problems; the results should be uniformly good with simple treatment.

Major violence may cause severe comminution to the body of the talus, usually defying primary reconstruction. Areas of avascular necrosis and marked incongruity of the subtalar and even the ankle joint combine to make this injury potentially disastrous (Fig. 23.8). Late pain, deformity, and collapse of the talus are common, often requiring secondary reconstruction procedures.

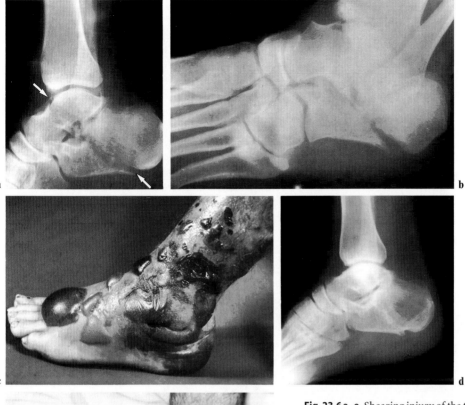

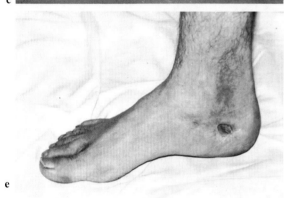

Fig. 23.6 a–e. Shearing injury of the talus. This 21-year-old man had his foot caught in the jaws of a logging machine. **a** His body was then rotated around the stabilized os calcis and talus, creating an open shear fracture through both bones. **b** The oblique radiograph of the foot shows the shearing oblique fracture through the talar neck and calcis. **c** Within 48 h, massive fracture blisters and contusion were evident on the foot and ankle. Nonoperative treatment was the only option because of the soft tissue crush. **d,e** The lateral radiograph and the clinical photograph show the final result 5 years following injury. The fractures have healed, but there was evidence of patchy avascular necrosis of the body of the talus with no collapse. The function of the foot is good. An area on the medial aspect of the os calcis required a split-thickness skin graft

23.3.2 Fractures of the Talar Neck

23.3.2.1 Type A: Undisplaced Fractures of the Talar Neck

Linear fractures of the talar neck with *no* subluxation of the subtalar joint usually have an excellent prognosis with simple management (Fig. 23.9). Ample blood supply is retained in most cases to maintain the viability of the body, and if the hindfoot is truly anatomical, no biomechanical abnormalities will ensue. All major literature reports confirm this, including the reviews of Coltart (1952), Pennal (1963), Hawkins (1970), and Kenwright and Taylor (1970).

23.3.2.2 Type B: Displaced Fractures of the Talar Neck with Subluxation of Subtalar Joint

Any degree of displacement of the fracture through the neck of the talus must be accompanied by a corresponding subluxation of the subtalar joint (Fig. 23.10). Most often, the os calcis and the remainder of the foot subluxate medially, thereby preserving the medial soft tissues even if the medial malleolus is fractured. In this particular type of injury, avascular necrosis leading to collapse of the body is uncommon, but anatomical reduction is required to prevent malunion with resultant foot problems.

570 ·

Chapter 23   **Fractures of the Talus**

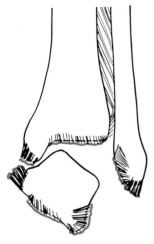

Fig. 23.7. Total dislocation of the talus with disruption of all soft tissue attachments

a) Avascular Necrosis

Although portions of the talar body may become avascular, collapse is rare. The intact medial soft tissue envelope usually retains sufficient vascularity to the body to maintain partial viability. The process of *creeping substitution* is able to strengthen the dead bone at a speed which more than compensates for the tendency of that bone to collapse (see Figs. 23.8, 23.10).

It is wrong to believe that this injury usually results in late problems associated with avascular necrosis. Therefore, aggressive treatment modalities for this injury, such as primary subtalar fusion, should be avoided because the outlook with proper management is favorable. Peterson and Goldie (1975) pointed out in an experimental study that division of the talar neck *with displacement* disrupted the talar blood supply. However, the clinical reviews are clear on this point: i.e., the major-

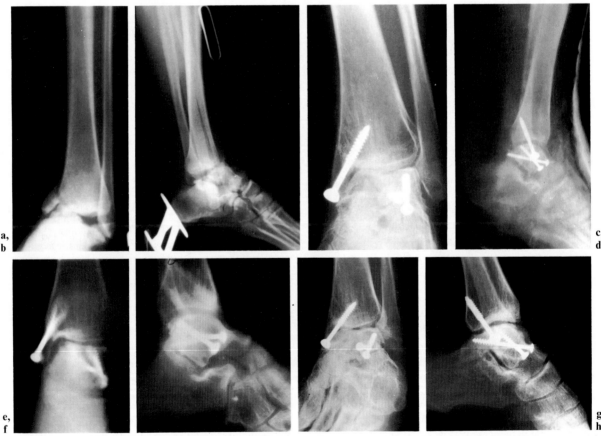

Fig. 23.8 a–h. Fracture through the body of the talus. **a,b** Anteroposterior and lateral radiographs of this 19-year-old woman show a comminuted fracture of the talar neck extending through the body, together with a fracture of the medial malleolus. Treatment consisted of open reduction and internal fixation. **c,d** At 3 months, the anteroposterior and lateral radiographs show union of the medial malleolus. The medial aspect of the talus appears vascularized, whereas the lateral aspect of the talus is sclerotic and avascular. **e,f** Anteroposterior and lateral tomography shows a defect in the distal tibia, allowing varus deformation. **g,h** At 5 years, the talus has not collapsed, but shows a patchy avascular necrosis. The patient has restricted ankle motion and minimal discomfort and functions well in spite of the vascular necrosis

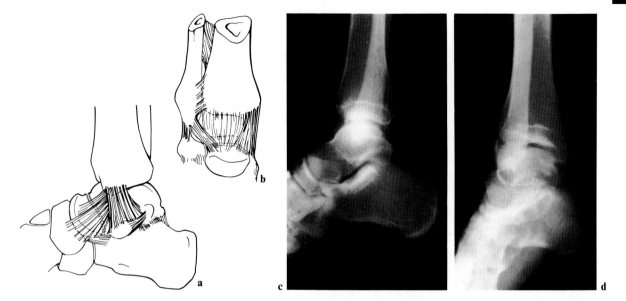

Fig. 23.9 a–d. Type A: undisplaced fracture of the talar neck. **a** Lateral and **b** anteroposterior diagrammatic views. **c** Lateral and **d** anteroposterior radiographs

ity of cases will not develop clinically significant avascular necrosis. Although the reported incidence of avascular necrosis of the talar body in type B injuries is 20%–50%, all authors agree that most cases proceed to bony union with no collapse of the avascular bone. Pennal (1963) reported three cases (33%) of patchy avascular necrosis with no collapse, Kenwright and Taylor (1970) four cases (36%) with no collapse, and Hawkins (1970) 42% with no significant collapse. Recent literature supports the above views (Grob et al. 1985; Comfort et al. 1985; Szyszkowitz et al. 1985).

b) Malunion with Chronic Subtalar Subluxation

In a type B talar neck fracture, malunion is of greater clinical significance than avascular necrosis. If an anatomical reduction is not obtained and maintained, the neck of the talus will heal in an abnormal position (Fig. 23.11). Of necessity, the subtalar joint will remain chronically subluxated. This in turn causes two major problems leading to a poor result: secondary degenerative arthritis and altered foot mechanics.

Secondary Degenerative Arthritis of the Subtalar Joint. This condition may occur early because of the altered joint biomechanics, and is the most frequent cause of unsatisfactory results in type B injuries. Of Pennal's ten cases, the six treated nonoperatively developed these changes, whereas the four treated operatively did not.

Altered Foot Mechanics. If the talar neck heals in the malunited position, the subluxated os calcis at the subtalar joint is usually displaced inwards. Since the remainder of the foot rotates around the subtalar axis through the talar neck and the os calcis, the net effect is a varus heel and foot (Fig. 23.11 b). The normal plantigrade position of the foot is lost, markedly altering the patient's gait pattern.

Therefore, if the talar neck fracture is not anatomically reduced by closed means, open reduction and internal fixation are absolutely imperative.

23.3.2.3 Type C: Displaced Fractures of the Talar Neck with Posterior Dislocation of the Body

Avascular necrosis of the body is inevitable in these injuries (Fig. 23.12) and plays the major role in determining the outcome. The incidence of avascular necrosis approaches 100%, the occasional exception being those cases which retain the deltoid ligament attachment to the talus. I have seen this ligament retained even in an open fracture, as illustrated in Fig. 23.12 c–h. Pennal (1963) reported avascular necrosis in 14 out of 14 cases (100%); however, in one it was patchy in nature. Kenwright and Taylor (1970) reported three out of four (75%) with surprisingly good results. Hawkins reported 18 out of 20 (90%), with three nonunions. Treatment of this injury by all methods resulted in only three satisfactory results. None of the attempts to revascularize the talus early showed any significant effect; therefore, the ultimate prognosis for this injury must be guarded.

Even more sinister is the *open* type C fracture, in Hawkins' series 50% of the total.

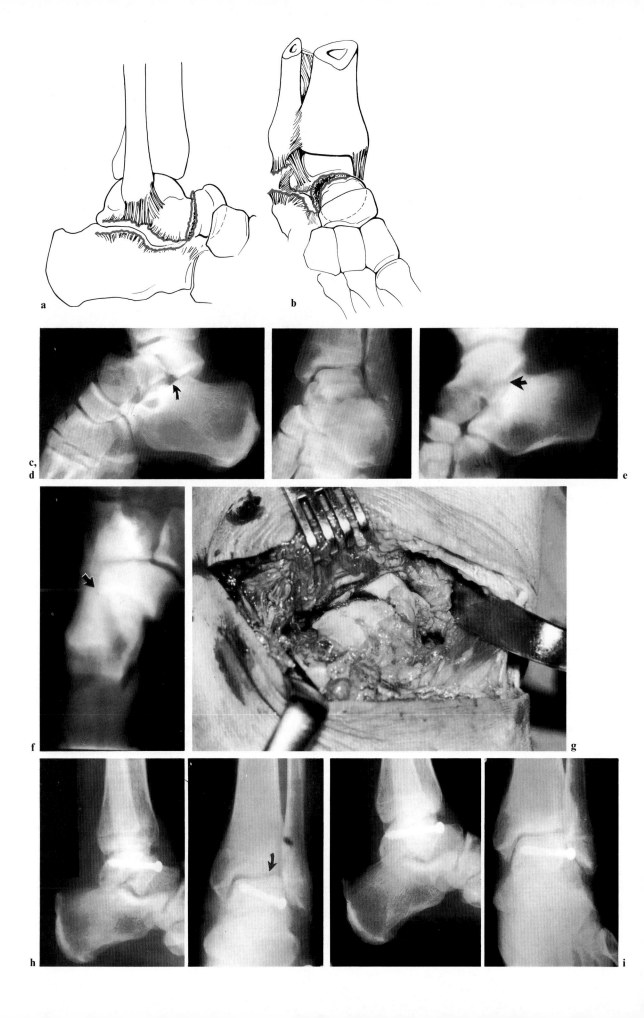

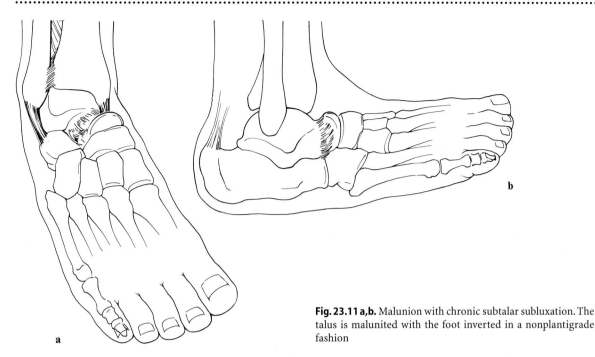

Fig. 23.11 a,b. Malunion with chronic subtalar subluxation. The talus is malunited with the foot inverted in a nonplantigrade fashion

23.3.3 Subtalar Dislocation

This injury (Fig. 23.13), if reduced quickly and anatomically, usually results in good function of the foot and no avascular necrosis of the talus. Late osteoarthritis of the subtalar joint may occur in some cases.

23.3.4 Total Dislocation of the Talus

This injury (Fig. 23.14) is usually caused by violent inversion forces, completely extruding the talus laterally.

◀————————————————

Fig. 23.10 a–i. Type B: displaced fracture of the talar neck with subluxation of the subtalar joint. **a,b** Displaced talar neck fracture. The foot is displaced dorsally and medially with disruption of the lateral subtalar ligament and lateral ligament of the ankle. Note the subtalar subluxation. **c,d** Lateral and anteroposterior radiographs of a 43-year-old man showing a comminuted oblique fracture of the talar neck extending posteriorly into the body. The *arrow* shows the subtalar subluxation. **e** This is clearly seen in the lateral tomograms *(arrows)*. **f** Anteroposterior tomogram showing the oblique nature of the fracture *(arrow)*. **g** This was confirmed at the time of surgery. Through a lateral approach, the fracture was reduced and internally fixed with a single cancellous bone screw. **h** The anatomical appearance is shown in the lateral and anteroposterior radiographs. At 10 weeks, no evidence of radiolucency is noted in the talus, indicating avascular necrosis *(arrow)*. **i** At 62 weeks, increased density is still noted in the talus but there is no evidence of collapse. The patient's talar body never collapsed and he has gone on to an excellent long-term result

Most often, the dislocation is *open*. Usually, all soft tissues are stripped from the bone, and therefore avascular necrosis is certain. Sepsis and skin necrosis are common in the open injury. Of Pennal's ten cases, two required tibiocalcaneal fusion and one an amputation. Detenbeck and Kelly (1969), reporting on nine such cases, of which seven were open, failed to reduce the dislocation closed in all cases. Their dismal results emphasize the seriousness of this injury:

– Eight out of nine patients developed sepsis.
– Seven out of nine patients required talectomy, five with tibiocalcaneal fusion.
– Nine out of nine patients required an amputation for sepsis.

Therefore, this injury has the greatest potential for disaster; often that potential is realized.

23.4 Management

23.4.1 Assessment

Prior to instituting management of the fracture, a careful assessment is mandatory.

23.4.1.1 Clinical Assessment

As always, a complete medical history and physical examination are essential in order to reveal the mecha-

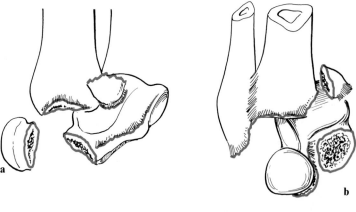

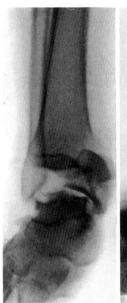
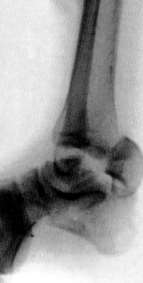
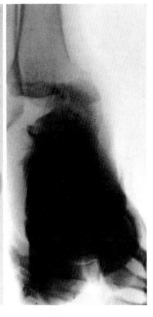

Fig. 23.12 a–c. Type C: displaced fracture of the talar neck with posterior dislocation of the body of the talus. **a,b** Lateral and anteroposterior diagrams showing a talar neck fracture with displacement of the body posteriorly and medially. Note the fracture of the medial malleolus, a common associated injury. **c** Oblique, lateral, and anteroposterior radiographs of an 19-year-old boy with this injury. Note the posteromedial position of the talar body and the fracture of the medial malleolus, as shown in the drawing

nism of injury, the general medical profile of the patient, and the state of the limb. Of great importance is the state of the soft tissues, either the presence of an open wound or, if the wound is closed, the presence of severe skin damage heralding the early onset of fracture blisters and necrosis. Injudicious surgery through such skin may prove disastrous.

23.4.1.2 Radiological Assessment

Standard views of the hindfoot should be supplemented with tomograms and special views, in order to clearly outline the subtalar joint. *Standard views* include an anteroposterior, a lateral, and two oblique views of the foot (see Fig. 23.12). *Tomograms* are in our opinion invaluable (as they are in other fractures) for revealing comminution of the neck and body and incongruity of

the subtalarjoint (see Fig. 23.10 e, f). *Broden's view* (Broden 1949) is excellent for viewing the subtalar joint, especially after a closed reduction (Fig. 23.15 a, b). *Computed tomograms (CT)* of the foot will afford excellent visualization of the fracture pattern, as well as the degree of comminution (Fig. 23.15 c–e).

23.4.2 Decision Making

Careful assessment will reveal the personality of the injury. Following this, the management should become logical.

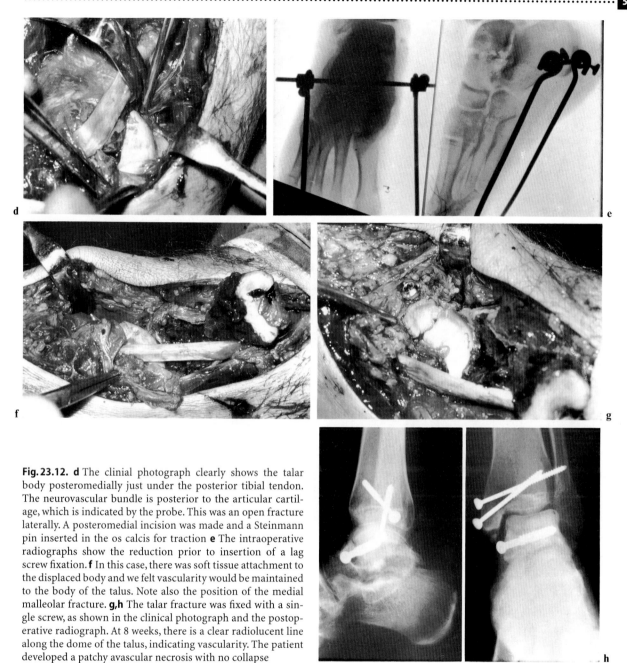

Fig. 23.12. d The clinial photograph clearly shows the talar body posteromedially just under the posterior tibial tendon. The neurovascular bundle is posterior to the articular cartilage, which is indicated by the probe. This was an open fracture laterally. A posteromedial incision was made and a Steinmann pin inserted in the os calcis for traction **e** The intraoperative radiographs show the reduction prior to insertion of a lag screw fixation. **f** In this case, there was soft tissue attachment to the displaced body and we felt vascularity would be maintained to the body of the talus. Note also the position of the medial malleolar fracture. **g,h** The talar fracture was fixed with a single screw, as shown in the clinical photograph and the postoperative radiograph. At 8 weeks, there is a clear radiolucent line along the dome of the talus, indicating vascularity. The patient developed a patchy avascular necrosis with no collapse

23.4.2.1 Fractures of the Body

a) Undisplaced Fractures

For fractures of the body only symptomatic treatment is required, usually a below-knee cast for 6–8 weeks. A good result may be expected.

b) Displaced Fractures

If the fracture is comminuted and displaced, as is all too often the case, the surgeon must assess whether it can be operatively stabilized. If the body is split, it may be possible to perform an open reduction and stable internal fixation using cancellous screws (Fig. 23.16). If the body is completely shattered, the surgeon may immobilize the foot until pain subsides and then begin a rehabilitation program. Most often, the patient will require a secon-

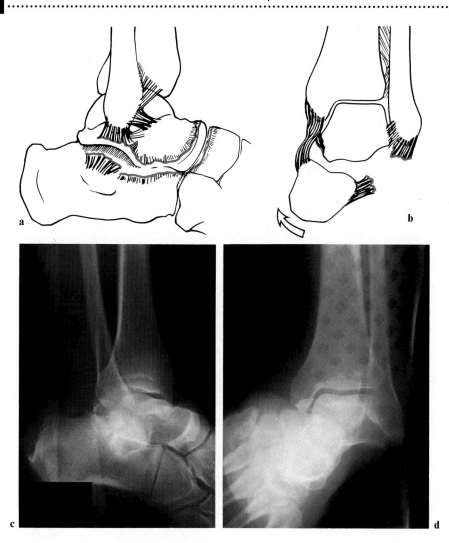

Fig. 23.13 a–d. Subtalar dislocation. **a,b** Lateral and anteroposterior diagrammatic views of a complete subtalar dislocation. Note the disruption of the subtalar and lateral ligaments. **c,d** Lateral and anteroposterior radiographs of subtalar dislocation

dary reconstructive procedure, such as a tibiocalcaneal fusion.

As an alternative for the worst cases, we favor primary excision of the body of the talus and either a Blair-type fusion (Crenshaw 1971, p. 502) or tibiocalcaneal fusion. This procedure should only be performed through skin which has healed sufficiently to avoid necrosis.

23.4.2.2 Fractures of the Talar Neck

a) Type A Fractures

If an assessment of the injury indicates an undisplaced linear type fracture through the talar neck, i.e., a type A injury, simple treatment consisting of immobilization in a plaster cast until the fracture is healed (usually 6–8 weeks) is adequate. The expected result of such

treatment is a healed fracture in perfect position, with no abnormality of the subtalar joint. Avascular necrosis is a rarity and late secondary arthritis of the subtalar joint is also uncommon.

A word of warning however: the assessment of the subtalar joint must be *extensive* and *accurate* and must include all of the radiographic views mentioned above. If there is any question about displacement of the subtalar joint, the injury should be considered a type B injury, which requires anatomical reduction.

b) Type B Fractures

If the fracture of the talar neck is associated with a subluxation of the subtalar joint (type B fracture), anatomical restoration of the neck is essential to restore congruity to the subtalar joint, which, in turn, will restore the normal plantigrade position of the foot. A closed reduc-

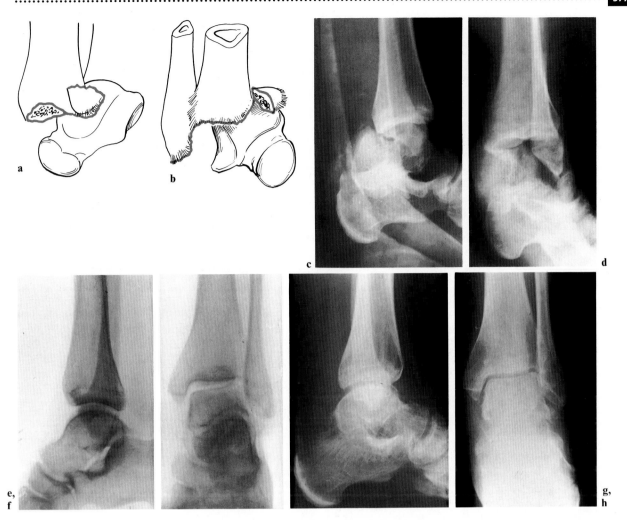

Fig. 23.14 a–h. Total dislocation of the talus. **a,b** Lateral and anteroposterior disagrams showing a complete dislocation of the talus with a fracture of the medial malleolus. **c, d** This injury is cleary seen on the lateral and anteroposterior radiographs of a 29-year-old man involved in a motor vehicle accident. Closed reduction failed to reduce the total dislocation of the talus, and therefore open reduction was necessary. **e,f** The intraoperative Polaroid radiographs indicated the reduction. **g,h** At 6 months, patchy avascular necrosis is evident, but no collapse occurred

tion with general anesthesia may accomplish this task. However, it is again essential that the closed reduction of the talar neck is absolutely anatomical. In our opinion, this is rarely accomplished, so that a common final result with such fractures treated nonoperatively is malunion and chronic subluxation of the subtalar joint (see Fig. 23.10).

In order to avoid this, we recommend *early anatomical open reduction* and *internal fixation* of this injury, if the patient's general state allows. This injury should be considered like any other fracture-dislocation of a weight-bearing joint, of which anatomical open reduction and stable internal fixation are the hallmarks of treatment.

If the surgical approach does not interfere with the remaining medial blood supply, significant avascular necrosis will be rare. Furthermore, since the anatomical reduction of the subtalar joint restores congruity between the dome of the os calcis and the talus, secondary problems in that joint and in the foot will be avoided, resulting in a satisfactory outcome.

In a type B injury there is no indication for primary subtalar fusion in an attempt to restore blood flow to the body of the talus, since the flow is usually ample.

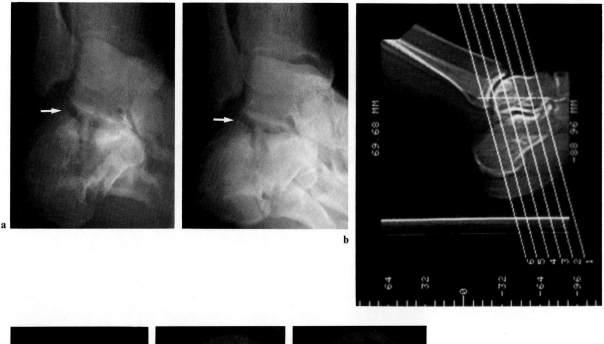

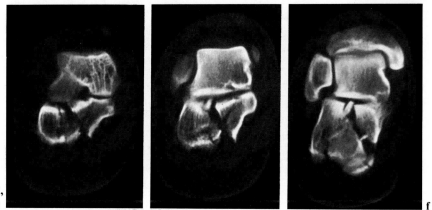

Fig. 23.15 a–f. Broden's view of the subtalar joint. **a,b** The subtalar joint is best seen on Broden's view *(arrows)*. In this case, an os calcis fracture, the precise relationship between the talus and os calcis can be seen. **c–f** Computed tomography (CT) scans of the same patient. Again, note the relationship between the os calcis and the talus

c) Type C Fractures

A fracture of the talar neck with dislocation of the talar body (i.e., type C: see Fig. 23.12), whether open or closed, constitutes a surgical emergency. The extruded body lies posterior to the medial malleolus. Although the neurovascular bundle is rarely injured primarily, pressure on these structures may cause secondary nerve injury or vascular impairment, either arterial or venous. It is therefore urgent that the body of the talus be reduced.

Even under general anesthesia and with a pin inserted in the os calcis, less than 10 % of these injuries can be reduced closed, so little time should be wasted with this maneuver. One or two attempts under image intensification should convince the surgeon that open reduction will be necessary.

Since more than 50 % of patients with this injury have an associated fracture of the medial malleolus, open reduction should be performed medially by turning down the bony fragment (see Fig. 23.12). Care should be taken to preserve any medial soft tissue attachment to the body of the talus, as this may be its only remaining blood supply. Reduction of the body of the talus is then performed manually. This may be a difficult task, requiring full reenactment of the injury in forced dorsiflexion with a Steinmann pin in the os calcis for traction.

Once the body of the talus has been restored to its normal position, the talar neck fracture should then be

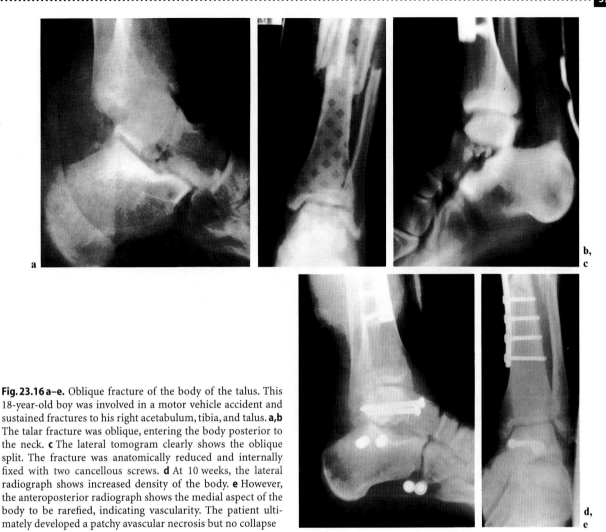

Fig. 23.16 a–e. Oblique fracture of the body of the talus. This 18-year-old boy was involved in a motor vehicle accident and sustained fractures to his right acetabulum, tibia, and talus. **a,b** The talar fracture was oblique, entering the body posterior to the neck. **c** The lateral tomogram clearly shows the oblique split. The fracture was anatomically reduced and internally fixed with two cancellous screws. **d** At 10 weeks, the lateral radiograph shows increased density of the body. **e** However, the anteroposterior radiograph shows the medial aspect of the body to be rarefied, indicating vascularity. The patient ultimately developed a patchy avascular necrosis but no collapse

stably fixed with cancellous lag screws. We favor stable internal fixation, even in cases where the body is free of all soft tissue, unless the body is comminuted or contamination of the wound would make sepsis likely in an open fracture. In those cases, the body of the talus should be discarded and a Blair-type fusion (Crenshaw 1971, p. 502) or a tibiocalcaneal fusion should be performed at the earliest safe opportunity.

Revascularization of the Talus. Is there any method now available to increase the blood supply to an avascular talar body? Phemister (1940) experimentally denuded the articular cartilage from the talus and found that the bone could then be revascularized much more quickly than if the articular cartilage remained. This led some surgeons to perform primary subtalar fusion in an effort to enhance the blood supply to the talar body and prevent collapse of that structure. Sporadic reports in all of the published papers do not support the clinical applica-

tion of this basic principle. The results are very unpredictable, and therefore the method cannot be recommended at this time (Fig. 23.17).

Perhaps in the future direct microvascular techniques to restore the arterial supply of the talus will become possible and will eliminate avascular necrosis. An example of a direct repair of a posterior tibial artery repatir leading to a good result in an open talar dislocation is seen in Fig. 23.18. Until vascular repair is more common, tibiocalcaneal fusion, giving a good stable hindfoot, or fusion from the tibia to the talar head (Blair fusion) are better than talectomy, except in cases of total dislocation of the talus. The condition of the talus in this injury – usually open and completely devoid of all blood supply – is such that it cannot safely be salvaged. Attempts to do so have led to an extremely high rate of sepsis and amputation. "Suitable" treatment would consist of total excision of the talus, either as definitive treatment or combined with a primary or a delayed primary

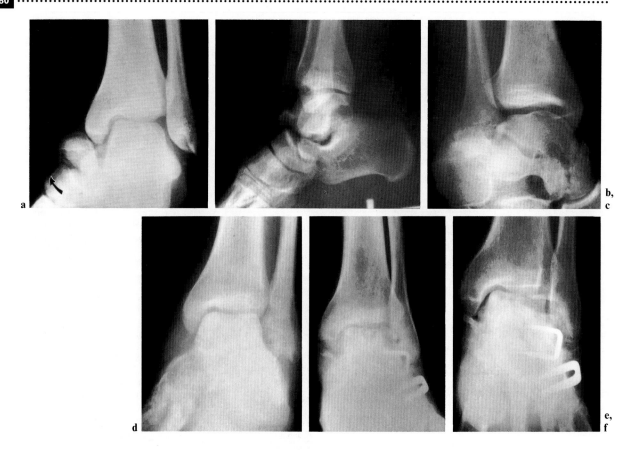

Fig. 23.17 a–f. Avascular necrosis of the talus. **a** Antero-posterior, **b** lateral, and **c** oblique radiographs show a fracture through the talar neck with displacement (*arrow* in **a**). **d** At 24 weeks, the anteroposterior radiograph shows a dense scle-rotic talar body. At this time, a triple arthrodesis was performed in an attempt to bring vascularity to the body of the talus. **e** At 2 years and **f** 3 years, some degree of collapse of the body is noted. The patient has subsequently required further recon-structive surgery and has a poor result

tibiocalcaneal fusion. If sepsis can be avoided by proper soft tissue management, the final result should be satis-factory.

23.4.3 Surgical Technique

23.4.3.1 Timing

The timing of the operative procedure, if operating is indicated, is of vital importance. Obviously, if the frac-ture is open, immediate surgery is indicated. However, if the fracture is closed, careful assessment and planning are required. Dislocation of the body of the talus or the entire talus constitutes a surgical emergency, and if

closed reduction does not succeed, immediate open reduction is called for. The soft tissues must be handled with extreme care. In this situation the wound, if under tension, must be left open.

In a type B fracture-dislocation, the surgeon has more leeway. If the skin is obviously traumatized, sur-gery should be delayed until the swelling has subsided and the skin improves. Incisions should never be made through areas of fracture blister, since the inevitable out-come will be skin necrosis and sepsis (see Fig. 23.6 c). In such cases, the fracture subluxation should be reduced closed, the extremity elevated, and surgery delayed until local conditions are safe.

23.4.3.2 Antibiotics

In this area, we favor the use of prophylactic antibiotics, administration of which should be started prior to the operative procedure. A single intravenous dose of 1 g cefazolin at the time of induction of narcosis, prior to inflation of the tourniquet, will be adequate and should be used for 48 h postoperatively.

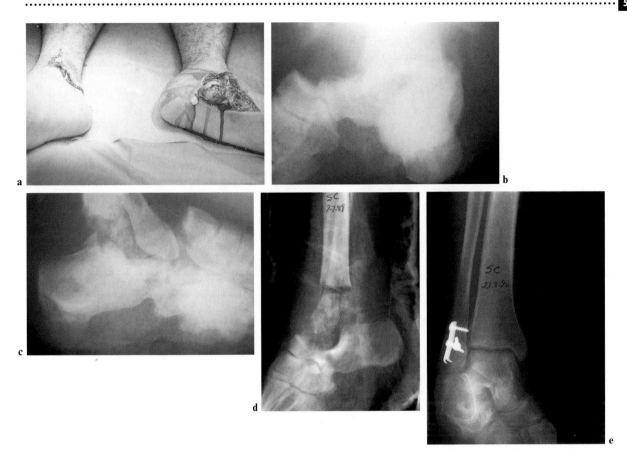

Fig. 23.18 a–e. This 23-year-old man fell five stories when a scaffold collapsed. He sustained bilateral open talar dislocations. **a** The talus has been reduced on the right side back into the ankle mortise. On the left side the entire talus is out through the incision. **b** The dislocated talus on the right. Virtually the entire tibia plafond was missing and was on the roadway. **c** On the left side the dislocation is noted. **d** The missing distal tibia is noted. The patient subsequently had a below knee amputation on that side. On the left side the posterior tibial artery was disrupted. This was repaired directly and the distal fibula fixed. **e** Six months following injury there is radial lucency in the talus indicating vascularity. There was still some soft tissue attachment on the medial side. Re-suture of the posterior tibial artery revascularized the talus through its deltoid branch

23.4.3.3 Tourniquet

In order to achieve an accurate anatomical reduction of the femoral neck, use of a tourniquet, though not mandatory, is desirable.

23.4.3.4 Skin Approaches

The skin on both the medial and lateral aspects of the foot is extremely delicate and must be handled with great care to avoid skin breakdown. The approach to each individual fracture will be dictated by the conditions of the case. Important factors are the type of fracture, the presence or absence of an open wound, and the presence of a medial malleolar fracture.

a) Lateral Approach

If there is no fracture of the medial malleolus, we favor the lateral approach to the talar neck. Two incisions are possible: anterolateral longitudinal (Fig. 23.19 a) and lateral oblique.

The anterior incision is safe and physiological. Unlike the lateral oblique incision, it rarely causes skin breakdown, and for this reason we strongly favor it. In the anterolateral approach, the extensor tendons and neurovascular structures are retracted medially and the ankle joint capsule is divided, allowing exposure of the entire talus (Fig. 23.19 b). Access may also be gained through the interval between the extensor hallucis longus tendon together with the neurovascular bundle medially and the extensor digitorum longus tendons laterally (Fig. 23.19 c), but the advantage of the increased medial exposure through this route is offset by the risk of dam-

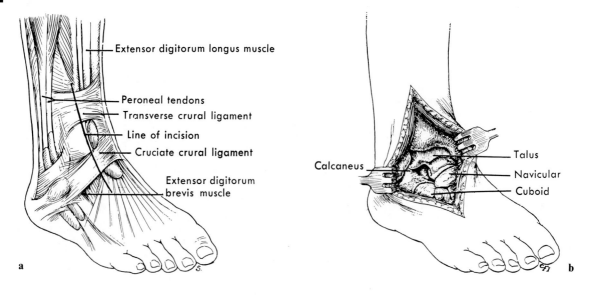

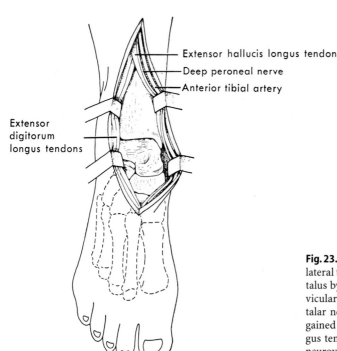

Fig. 23.19 a–c. Anterolateral approach to the talus. **a** Incision lateral to the extensor digitorum longus muscle. **b** Access to the talus by dividing the anterior capsule of the ankle and talonavicular joint. Extension of the incision will allow full view of the talar neck and body. **c** Alternative access to the talus may be gained through a portal between the extensor digitorum longus tendon and the extensor hallucis longus tendon with the neurovascular bundle retracted medially. (Reproduced by permission from Crenshaw 1980)

age to the neurovascular structures, and the lateral portal is therefore preferred.

The oblique lateral incision (Fig. 23.20) affords excellent exposure but is more apt to lead to skin breakdown and should be avoided unless access to the posterior aspect of the talus is required. This approach follows the skin lines obliquely across the talar neck, ending posterior to the fibular malleolus.

The major advantages of these lateral approaches are twofold. First, the lateral is the easiest approach to the

fracture of the talar neck, since simple division of the skin and subcutaneous tissues usually leads one directly into the fracture site, as most of the deep capsular structures are torn. Second, a lateral incision avoids damage to the deltoid artery, which may be present with an intact deltoid ligament. In some cases, this may be the only blood supply to the body of the talus and medial approaches could damage it.

If increased exposure is required on the lateral side, a transverse osteotomy of the fibula may be carried out at

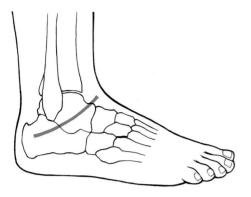

Fig. 23.20. Oblique lateral approach to the talus. (Adapted from Crenshaw 1971)

the level of the mortise. Full access can then be obtained to the body of the talus. At the end of the procedure, the malleolus can be fixed with a malleolar screw through predrilled holes.

b) Medial Approach

If the medial malleolus is fractured, or if the body of the talus is posteriorly dislocated, a medial approach is indicated. A longitudinal incision is made just anterior to the medial malleolus, extending distally across the talar neck, curving slightly posteriorly, long enough to give access to both the talar neck and the ankle joint. The medial malleolus should be retracted posteriorly. Great care must be taken to preserve the attachment, if any, of the deltoid ligament to the malleolus and the talus. If reduction of the dislocated body is difficult, a Steinmann pin should be inserted into the calcaneus so that traction may be applied. At the end of the procedure the medial malleolus should be fixed back with malleolar screws or tension band wires.

23.4.3.5 Stable Internal Fixation

Whether the lateral or medial approach is chosen, stabilization of the fracture is the same. As always, it is extremely important to operate through the fracture site, great care being taken to preserve all soft tissue attachments. This is especially important in comminuted fractures. The talar neck should be reduced anatomically and provisionally fixed with 2.0-mm Kirschner wires. In cases of extreme comminution, the Kirschner wires will serve as definitive fixation, but in all cases it is preferable to fix the fracture with lag screws under compression; this is usually possible from either the medial or the lateral side. The preferable screws are 4.0-mm cancellous lag screws, which may be inserted either ret-

rograde or antegrade depending on the incision used; two or three screws are usually adequate. (Fig. 23.21; see also Figs. 23.10, 23.12, 23.16). Biomechanically, retrograde screws offer better stability but are technically more difficult to insert (Swanson et al. 1992). Cannulated cancellous screws, which may be inserted over the Kirschner wires, are helpful in this situation. In some cases of extreme comminution, a bone graft will be required to fill the gap. In all cases, the subtalar joint should be exposed to ensure perfect congruity.

The cancellous fracture fixed with interfragmental compression should heal rapidly in an anatomical position.

After an osteotomy of the lateral or medial malleolus, or if the medial malleolus is fractured, the bones affected should be stabilized using standard techniques.

23.4.3.6 Postoperative Care

a) Wound Closure

In dealing with open fractures, it is best to leave the lacerated portion of the wound open. Many wounds, even in closed fractures, will be under extreme tension. In these cases, no attempt should be made to close the wound. Areas of sensitive tissue, such as tendon, should ideally be covered, but in some instances it is better even to leave the joint open than to attempt closure under tension. If possible, the patient may return to the operating room on the fifth day for wound closure or skin graft. A bulky dressing with a plaster splint immobilizing the foot in neutral rotation and the ankle at 90° should be applied.

b) Follow-up Care

Recognition and Management of Avascular Necrosis. The specific follow-up care of the patient will depend upon the type of injury and its management. In type A or type B talar neck fractures, the risk of avascular necrosis is minimal, whereas in type C injuries necrosis is virtually certain.

Avascular necrosis of the body of the talus may be suspected as early as 6–8 weeks following injury. Evidence of bone resorption, shown by the presence of subchondral atrophy in the dome of the talus, is de facto evidence of an *intact* blood supply (Fig. 23.22 a,b). In cases in which the blood supply to the talar body is interrupted, bone resorption is impossible; therefore, no subchondral atrophy is seen on the early radiograph and the talar body appears relatively dense (Fig. 23.22 c–e).

Technetium polyphosphate bone scanning, if performed early, may be of some prognostic importance.

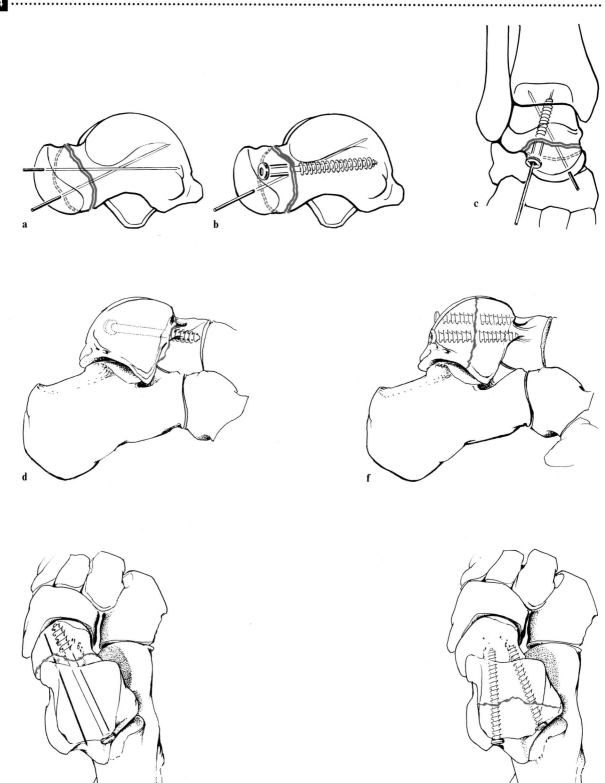

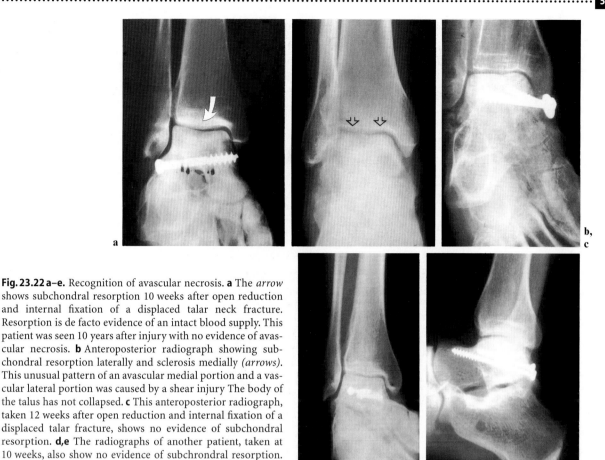

Fig. 23.22 a–e. Recognition of avascular necrosis. **a** The *arrow* shows subchondral resorption 10 weeks after open reduction and internal fixation of a displaced talar neck fracture. Resorption is de facto evidence of an intact blood supply. This patient was seen 10 years after injury with no evidence of avascular necrosis. **b** Anteroposterior radiograph showing subchondral resorption laterally and sclerosis medially *(arrows)*. This unusual pattern of an avascular medial portion and a vascular lateral portion was caused by a shear injury The body of the talus has not collapsed. **c** This anteroposterior radiograph, taken 12 weeks after open reduction and internal fixation of a displaced talar fracture, shows no evidence of subchondral resorption. **d,e** The radiographs of another patient, taken at 10 weeks, also show no evidence of subchrondral resorption. Both of these patients developed complete avascular necrosis of the talar body

Magnetic resonance imaging (MRI) is also a very sensitive indicator of avascular necrosis.

Type A talar neck fractures treated nonoperatively should remain in plaster until bony union has occurred, i.e., usually for 6–12 weeks. Weight-bearing may be started early (after 2–4 weeks) if the fracture is stable.

The postoperative management of *type B* fractures with cancellous screw fixation will depend upon the

---

◄

Fig. 23.21 a–g. Stable internal fixation of talar neck fracture. **a** Provisional fixation is achieved with Kirschner wires. **b** A cancellous lag screw is used to compress the talar neck fracture. **c** A useful technique is insertion of a cannulated screw over the K wire for fixation. The direction of the screw, from medial to lateral or from lateral to medial, will depend on the obliquity of the talar neck fracture as it extends into the body. In general the screw should cross the fracture line perpendicular to the fracture; therefore the obliquity of the fracture will guide the surgeon as to the direction of the screw. **d,e** The screw can also be inserted in a retrograde fashion as noted in the drawings. The screws may be 6.5-mm lag screws (**d,e**) or 3.5-mm cortical screws inserted as a lag screw (**f,g**)

degree of stability of the subtalar joint at the conclusion of surgery. If the joint is stable, motion may be started early, but in cases with an unstable subtalar joint, the foot must be kept in plaster for 8–12 weeks until the capsule has healed. In this group of patients, the final outcome is usually good, even if patchy avascular necrosis of the body of the talus develops. Late collapse of the body is rare, although radiographs and bone scans should nevertheless be carefully monitored. If avascular necrosis is suspected, restricted weight-bearing in a patellar-bearing caliper is advised, although these devices are not completely effective.

In *type C* injury, with the inevitable avascular necrosis (see Fig. 23.17), the follow-up care is controversial. At this time, there is no evidence that attempts at revascularization of the body of the talus will be successful. Bone forage operations and subtalar fusion have been attempted with equivocal results. In our opinion, management should be nonoperative, the patient being fitted with a weight-relieving caliper. If collapse of the body does occur, the treatment options include:

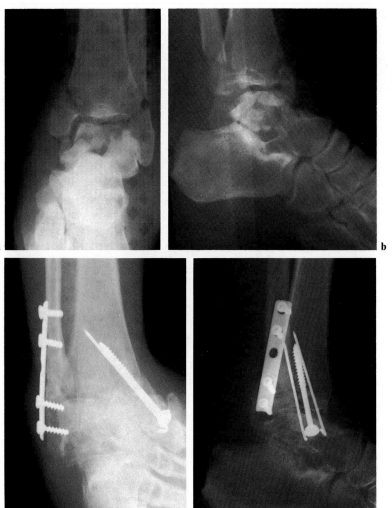

Fig. 23.23 a–d. Comminuted fracture of the body of the talus. **a** Anteroposterior and **b** lateral radiographs showing severe comminution of the body of the talus as well as a fracture of the medial and lateral malleoli of the ankle. This patient also had a severe head injury. The talar fracture was open. Many small fragments of bone had to be discarded, including areas of the articular surface. **c,d** At 9 months, areas of collapse of the talus are seen on the anteroposterior and lateral radiographs. The patient's head injury precluded further reconstructive surgery

1. Excision of the body with fusion of the tibia to the head of the talus (Blair fusion; see Crenshaw 1971, p. 502)
2. Excision of the talus and tibiocalcaneal fusion
3. Tibiotalar-calcaneal fusion through a lateral approach
4. Talectomy (Günal et al. 1993)

It is beyond the scope of this book to describe the surgical techniques of these reconstructive procedures in detail.

23.4.4 Special Problems

23.4.4.1 Open Fractures and Fracture-Dislocations

Open type A and type B talar neck fractures should be managed as previously indicated. Following careful wound cleansing and débridement, the talar neck fracture should be primarily stabilized with cancellous bone screws and Kirschner wires. All soft tissue attachments to the bone must be retained. The wound should be left open and closed secondarily when possible. On occasion, it is safer to let the wound heal by secondary intent than to attempt plastic procedures or wound closure. If the fracture has been stabilized, a careful assessment should be made of the stability of the subtalar and ankle joint. If it is stable, early motion may be initiated, the fracture usually being protected with a below-the-knee splint and hinged ankle device while at rest.

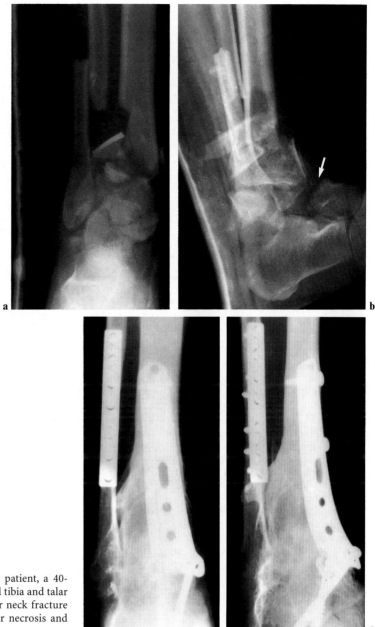

Fig. 23.24 a–d. Tibiocalcaneal fusion. **a,b** This patient, a 40-year-old man, had a severe fracture of the distal tibia and talar neck. Note the severe displacement of the talar neck fracture *(arrow)*. **c,d** He eventually developed avascular necrosis and required a tibiocalcaneal fusion

In type C open fractures with total dislocation of the talus, or in open fractures with a shattered talar body, the situation changes drastically (Fig. 23.23). In these cases, with complete stripping of all soft tissues from the displaced fragments, it is safer to discard the body of the talus and proceed to a tibiocalcaneal fusion. The risk entailed by leaving a large, dead talar body in situ in a potentially contaminated wound is too great, and sepsis is a frequent outcome.

Obviously, each case is different and requires careful assessment, but, in general, the above are the principles favored by us.

23.4.4.2 Comminuted Fractures of the Talar Body

In closed, extremely comminuted fractures of the body of the talus, open reduction and stable internal fixation may be impossible (Fig. 23.24). The late results of this fracture are poor and in some instances, when the skin in the region allows, it is preferable to carry out a delayed primary tibiocalcaneal fusion (Fig. 23.23 a, b). We favor the lateral approach, dividing the fibula 6–8 cm proximal to the ankle joint and rotating it posteriorly. This allows excellent exposure of the entire lateral aspect of the ankle and subtalar joint and the avascular, comminuted talar body can be removed. The fibula can then be used to stabilize the tibia to the os calcis. An iliac crest cancellous graft should supplement the fusion (Fig. 23.24 c, d).

References

Anderson HG (1919) The medical and surgical aspects of aviation. Oxford Medical, London

Broden B (1949) Roentgen examination of the subtaloid joint and fractures of the calcaneus. Acta Radiol 31:85–91

Coltart WD (1952) "Aviator's astragalus." J Bone Joint Surg [Br] 34B:545–566

Comfort TH, Behrens F, Gaither DW, Denis F, Sigmond M (1985). Clin Orthop Res Res 199

Cooper A (1832) Treatise on dislocations and fractures of the joints. London, pp 341–342

Crenshaw AG (ed) (1971) Campbell's operative orthopaedics, vol 1, 5 th edn. Mosby, St. Louis

Crenshaw AG (1980) Surgical approaches. In: Edmunson AS (ed) Campbell's operative orthopaedics, 6 th edn. Mosby, St. Louis

Detenbeck LC, Kelly PJ (1969) Total dislocation of the talus. J Bone Joint Surg [Am] 51A(2):283

Grob D, Simpson LA, Weber BG, Bray T (1985) Operative treatment of displaced talus fractures. Clin Orthop Rel Res 199

Gunal I, Atilla S, Arac S, Gursoy Y, Karagozlu H (1993) A new technique of talectomy for severe fracture-dislocation of the talus. J Bone Joint Surg 75B

Haliburton RA, Sullivan CR, Kelly PJ, Peterson LFA (1958) The extra-osseous and intra-osseous blood supply of the talus. J Bone Joint Surg [Am] 40A:1115–1120

Hawkins LG (1970) Fractures of the neck of the talus. J Bone Joint Surg [Am] 52A(5):991

James S (1848) Contributions to the pathology and practice of surgery, 1 st edn. Sutherland and Knox, Edinburgh, p 26

Kenwright J, Taylor RG (1970) Major injuries of the talus. J Bone Joint Surg [Br] 52B:36–48

Kleiger B (1948) Fractures of the talus. J Bone Joint Surg [Am] 30A:735

Lauro A, Purpura F (1956) La trabecolatura ossea e l'irrorazione sanguina nell'astragalo e nel calcagno. Minerva Chir 11:663–667

Lexor E, Kuliga, Turk W (1904) Untersuchungen über Knochenarterien. Hirschwald, Berlin

McKeever FM (1943) Fracture of the neck of the astragalus. Arch Surg 46:720

Montis S. Ridola C (1959) Vascolarizzazione dell'astragalo. Quad Anatomia Practica 15:574

Mulfinger GL, Trueta J (1970) The blood supply of the talus. J Bone Joint Surg [Br] 52B:160–167

Pennal GF (1963) Fractures of the talus. Clin Orthop 30:53–63

Peterson L, Goldie I (1975) The arterial supply of the talus. Acta Orthop Scand 46:1026–1034

Phemister DB (1940) Changes in bone and joints resulting from interruption of circulation. Arch Surg 41:436

Sneed WL (1925) The astragalus: a case of dislocation excision and replacement; an attempt to demonstrate the circulation in this bone. J Bone Joint Surg 7:384–399

Swanson TV, Bray TJ, Holmes GB (1992) Fractures of the talar neck. J Bone Joint Surg 74A

Syme (1848) Contribution to the pathology and practice of surgery, 1 st edn. Sutherland and Knox, Edinburgh, p 126

Szyszkowitz R, Reschauer R, Seggl W (1985) Eighty-five talus fractures treated by ORIF with five to eight years of follow up study of 69 patients. Clin Orthop Rel Res 199

Watson-Jones R (1946) Fractures and joint injuries, vol 2, 3 rd edn. Livingstone, Edinburgh, pp 821–843

Wildenauer E (1950) Die Blutversorgung des Talus. Z Anat Entwicklungsgesch 115:32

24 Fractures of the Calcaneus

M. Tile

24.1 Introduction

The management of fractures of the os calcis remains highly controversial. This irregularly shaped tarsal bone, commonly injured in falls and motor vehicle accidents, has been the subject of a great number of publications (Bohler 1931; Palmer 1941; Essex-Lopresti 1993; Lindsay and Dewar 1958; Hall and Pennal 1960; Letournel 1984; Sanders et al. 1993; Benirschke and Sangeorzan 1993). From reading these publications one could conclude almost anything one wished regarding the pathogenesis, the cause of pain, and the management of this fracture? Why should this particular fracture cause so much controversy and stir up so much emotion, when the management of the adjacent bone, the talus, has reached consensus mostly everywhere. This subject of os calcis fractures has developed an aura, almost a mystique.

What is the reason for this controversy? If we believe, as conventional wisdom would have it, that intra-articular fractures in major weight-bearing joints require anatomical reduction, internal fixation, and early rehabilitation to achieve excellent results, and since most displaced fractures of the os calcis enter a portion of the subtalar joint, the goals of treatment, namely, anatomical reduction, should be as for any other lower extremity joint. The problem is that the mechanism of injury, i.e., a fall from a height or a high-energy motor vehicle accident, causes a major soft tissue injury, not only to the deep structures such as the heel pad but also to the more superficial skin and soft tissues. Therefore, surgical solutions in the past have lead to a high number of complications, including amputation, clearly an unacceptable outcome for a closed fracture. Also, even in those cases where anatomical reduction has been obtained and no complications have ensued, many of the patients have continued to complain of pain. This raises the question of what causes the pain?

The pain may be caused by the intra-articular component causing secondary arthritis, residual deformity causing lack of a plantigrade foot, widening of the heel causing impingement at the lateral malleolus to all soft tissue structures, especially the peroneal tendon, and injury to the heel pad.

As in many intra-articular fractures of the lower extremity, in spite of improvement of technology, satisfactory outcomes elude us in many patients. The prognosis depends not only on the treatment, but also on the injury itself. As in other articular fractures, the injury pattern within the joint may be relatively simple with a single fracture line or markedly comminuted with virtual destruction of the articular surface. This is as true in the os calcis as it is in the acetabulum or in the pilon. The AO classification of articular fractures progressing from the more simple A to the grossly shattered C type has been developed to address this problem. As yet we have no satisfactory classification in the os calcis which addresses the comminution and severity factor. As in the acetabulum, the classification is more anatomical.

This is the reason why the literature is so confusing, since it invariably compares apples and oranges. In an early publication, Cotton and Henderson (1916) took an extremely pessimistic view of conservative or nonoperative care. In 1942, Bankart wrote that "the results of crushed fractures of the os calcis are rotten." In 1958, Lindsay and Dewar, in reporting on an extremely large series from the Ontario Workmen's Compensation Board, concluded that nonoperative care gave far superior results with fewer complications. Gissane introduced the percutaneous Gissane spike especially for tongue-type fractures, thereby elevating the joint. Bohler (1931) and the Viennese school recommended closed reduction and percutaneous pin fixation, followed by a cast. Based on the principle of stable internal fixation of articular fractures, surgeons have been searching for an operative panacea for this fracture. Operative fracture care was reported by Palmer (1948),whose surgical techniques mimic closely those used today. Gallie (1943) and Hall and Pennal (1960) advocated primary arthrodesis following reduction of the heel width as the treatment of choice in severely comminuted os calcis fractures. Recently, Benirschke and Sangeorzan (1993), Sanders et al, (1993), and others have advocated open reduction and internal fixation. Unfortunately, the early literature compares severely displaced with not so severely displaced fractures and is confusing. The more recent literature has attempted to use anatomically based classifications, but these rarely reflect the amount of comminution and the actual operability of the fracture.

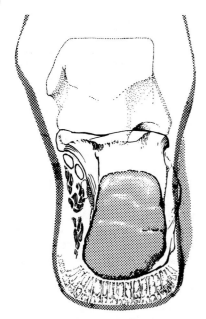

Fig. 24.1. Soft tissues – heel pads. The calcaneus is a subcutaneous bone along its medial and lateral border. The heel pad, composed of encapsulated cushions of fat separated by fibrous tissue, is important surgically; since, in a fall from a height, the most important mechanism of injury for the calcaneus, the fibrous bands may rupture, dissipating the fat and destroying the "cushion mechanism"

Fig. 24.2 a–c. Bony anatomy. **a** The articulation between the calcaneus as seen on its superior surface and the undersurface of the talus is complex. The joint has three facets, the largest being the posterior facet, the middle facet and the anterior facet. **b,c** Their relationship is also noted in the drawing from the lateral aspect (**b**) and the axial view (**c**), the view commonly seen on radiographs. Note also the relationship of the posterior tibial tendon to the sustentaculum from which arises the spring ligament

In the next decade, prospective randomized trials which are already underway, carefully classifying the fractures and documenting the operative versus nonoperative management, may answer the questions that have eluded us in the past. One large prospective randomized multicenter Canadian trial is in the final stage of data collection (Buckley et al. 1995). Preliminary studies have shown that there may be little difference between the operative and the nonoperative group in patient outcome.

24.2 Anatomy

The major feature of the anatomy of the os calcis is its soft tissue cover. The bone which takes the entire load of weight-bearing is basically subcutaneous except on the heel pad. Since virtually all os calcis fractures are caused by a fall from a height or a direct impact such as a motor vehicle accident, the distal portion of the os calcis is driven proximally, spreading the proximal bone against the underlying subcutaneous tissues. The soft tissue injury is, therefore, highly significant and may lead to many of the problems with surgical intervention. Furthermore, the heel pad is a complex structure made up of fatty tissue held firmly by fibrous connections to bone (Fig. 24.1). This heel pad may also be disrupted in os calcis fractures and may also represent a cause of late pain.

The bony anatomy is complex. The superior surface of the calcaneus has three articular surfaces: the posterior facet articulates with the talus and is separated from the anterior and middle facets by the tarsal canal and tarsal sinus; the middle one third of the calcaneus supports the posterior facet, and it is this area that is often impacted in a compression-type injury (Fig. 24.2 a,b).

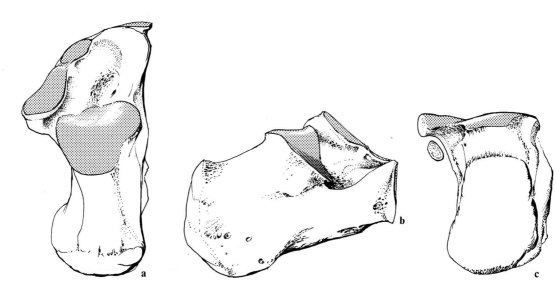

The anterior one third of the os calcis supports the middle and anterior facet. The articulation with the cuboid is also complex and saddle-like in shape. The sustentaculum tali articulates with the talus and is supported by the complex medial arch structures, including the insertion of the tibialis posterior tendon and the spring ligament, which are key soft tissues for the formation of the medial arch of the foot (Fig. 24.2 c). The fractures through the sustentaculum tali are a constant feature of all os calcis fractures and, if not anatomically restored, will interfere with the medial arch. Thus, it can be seen that this complex anatomical structure may make restoration of the anatomy extremely difficult, especially if the articular fracture is comminuted.

Both the lateral and medial walls of the os calcis are subcutaneous. The lateral wall is flat and is an ideal area for internal fixation, but with its subcutaneous location, as on the anterior tibia, may lead to complications (see Fig. 24.1).

The medial wall contains the dense bone of the sustentaculum, as well as the posterior tibial tendon. The posterior tibial nerve and artery are in close association with the medial wall and the area of the primary fracture through the sustentaculum. These complex structures on the medial side make open reduction in this area relatively hazardous.

Internally, the os calcis contains compression and tensile trabeculae. The central portion of the middle third is fairly weak cancellous bone, especially weak in compression.

Fig. 24.3 a–c. Mechanism of injury. **a** The axial view shows that the main fragment of the calcaneus is driven upward in a fall. The medial fragment containing the sustentaculum is held in place by the strong spring ligament and is a constant fragment in virtually all calcaneal fractures. **b** Viewed from the superior surface the displacement of the major fracture line and the rotation of the heel into varus is shown. **c** On the lateral view two constant patterns emerge: the so-called tongue type in which the fracture line exits posteriorly, leaving the joint surface depressed but intact, and the joint depression type in which the posterior facet of the calcaneus is driven into the main body through two primary fracture lines as illustrated

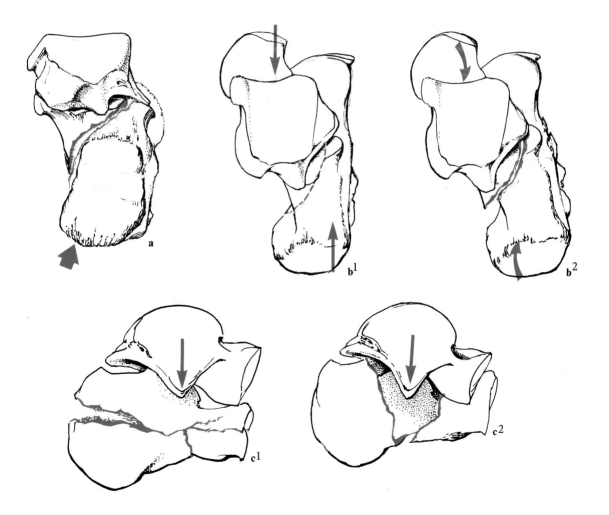

24.3 Pathoanatomy (Mechanism of Injury; Fig. 24.3)

As previously mentioned, most fractures of the os calcis are caused by a direct axial load either from a fall from a height or a motor vehicle accident. Following axial loading, there may also be a rotational element, especially in varus. As the axial load is applied to the hindfoot, the lateral progress of the talus is driven into the angle of Gissane, dividing the os calcis into two fragments. The constant medial fragment containing the sustentaculum tali remains in its anatomical position because of its strong soft tissues. The remainder of the talus rotates. The main rotation of the tuberosity is medial, but a thin

fragment of the lateral wall is often sheared and rotates laterally. As the axial load continues, secondary fracture lines occur. These may involve the joint itself in a single or in multifragments, or the fracture line may be a single horizontal line resulting in a so-called tongue-type fracture described by Essex-Lopresti (1993). Since the permutations and combinations of fracture lines beyond the primary fracture line are endless, many fracture classifications have resulted in none being accepted worldwide.

As the central portion of the posterior facet impacts into the underlining cancellous bone, the lateral wall is driven directly under the fibula, causing impingement to the soft tissues in that area.

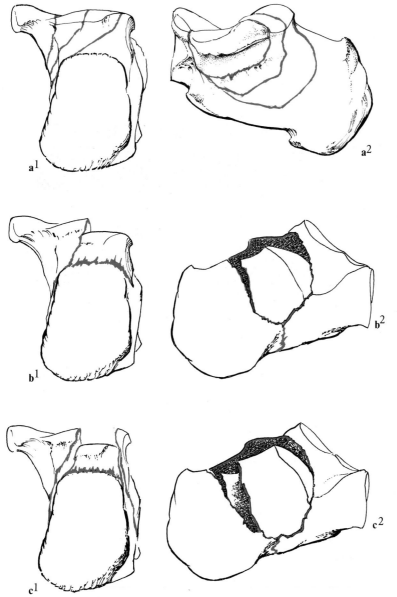

Fig. 24.4 a–c. Classification. The most widely used classification is based on the number of fragments especially seen on computed tomography (CT). The constant fragment is the sustentaculum which remains anatomical to the undersurface of the talus. The primary fracture line may be through the sustentaculum only, or may be more laterally placed through the joint, as noted on the axial drawing (**a¹**) and the lateral drawing (**a²**).
b¹,b² In the three-part configuration the sustentacular fragment is the same but the joint is depressed ususally through a tongue type mechanism leaving the lateral wall intact.
c¹,c² In the four-part fracture, the most common, the sustentaculum fragment is noted, the joint depression fragment noted, and the lateral wall is fractured as a separate fragment and displaced laterally under the fibula, thereby impinging the peroneal tendon. This most common pattern may be much more complex and contain other fracture lines going forward into the calcaneal cuboid joint. Therefore, there may be more than four parts, which ultimately makes any classification extremely difficult

24.4 Classification

None of the present classifications are fully accepted and, since they are anatomically based, they are all only a part of the decision making, which must also involve the soft tissues and the patient. The most commonly used classification involves two-part, three-part, and four-part configurations (Letournel 1984; Sanders et al. 1993; Tscherne and Zwipp 1993).

In the two-part configuration, the continuation of the fracture line through the sinus tarsae behind the interosseous ligament separates the sustentaculum tali. The sustentaculum remains in anatomical alignment with the talus, while the remainder of the os calcis rotates (Fig. 24.4 a).

In the three-part configuration, many secondary fracture lines are possible, but all involve separation of the posterior facet fragment from the main body of the os calcis. The fracture line may exit through the tuberosity (tongue type) or may involve the posterior facet itself with marked impaction and flattening of the angle of Gissane (Fig. 24.4 b).

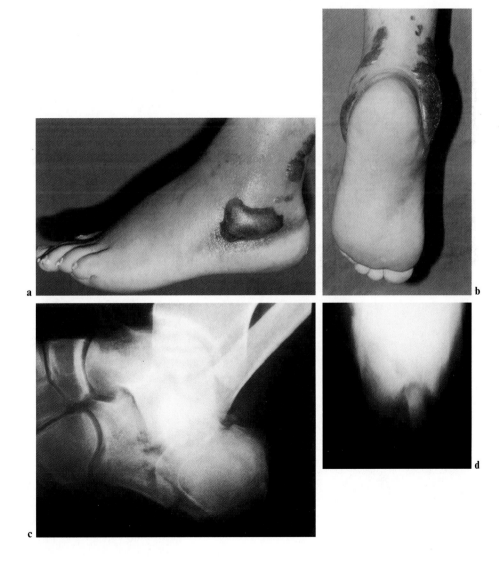

Fig. 24.5 a–d. Effect of soft tissue injury on decision making. The importance of the soft tissue injury in decision making cannot be overemphasized. Because the calcaneus is a subcutaneous bone and because the mechanism of injury often displaces the lateral fragment directly under this subcutaneous tissue, local ischemia may be produced in the skin, resulting in fracture blisters as noted in the photograph from the lateral (**a**)and posterior (**b**) views. The radiographic appearance is noted on the oblique (**c**) and axial (**d**) radiographs. The only safe approach here, if operative intervention was deemed important, would be the posterolateral approach since this area of skin is intact. In this case a nonoperative approach was taken with a good outcome

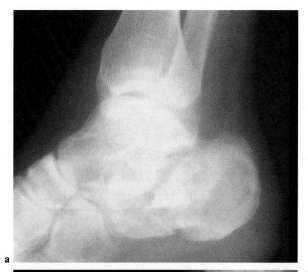

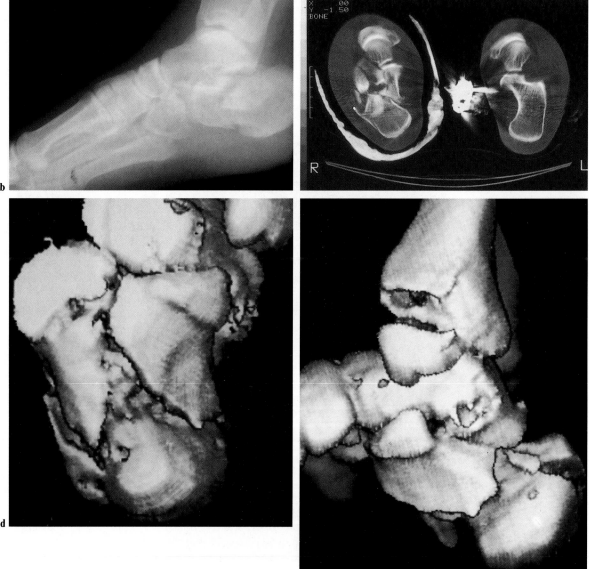

Fig. 24.6 a–e. Radiographic investigation includes standard radiographs and computed tomography (CT). **a,b** The standard radiographs include a lateral (**a**), oblique (**b**), and an axial view, which is difficult to obtain in a painful swollen foot. **c** CT examination has largely eliminated the need for an axial view since it gives the same projection in much greater detail. **d,e** Three-dimensional CT gives an overview of the fracture pattern. In **d**, the primary fracture lines are seen in the axial view; in **e**, note the associated medial malleolar fracture

In the four-part fracture, which may actually involve more than four parts, there is an additional fracture of the lateral wall of the os calcis with marked displacement, often causing impingement of the soft tissues of the fibula. The fracture lines often extend forward into the cuboid articulation (Fig. 24.4 c).

Variations of this classification have been described by many authors, including subtypes in each. I believe the next decade will bring general agreement on a classification which is not only anatomical, as noted above, but will also contain information about the state of the articular surface of the posterior facet versus the state of the calcaneus itself. For example, a four-part fracture with a shattered articular surface will have a vastly different prognosis than a four-part fracture of the tongue type, in which the main portion of the posterior facet is intact and can be surgically reconstructed.

Other important classification variables include whether fractures are closed or open and whether they are displaced or undisplaced.

24.5 Assessment

Assessment of a patient with an os calcis fracture needs to be both clinical and radiographic. The surgeon must determine whether the os calcis fracture is isolated or whether it is part of a polytrauma situation. The management of the patient will vary greatly depending on the above. Axial loads often produce spinal injuries as well as intra-abdominal rupture to solid viscera such as liver and spleen.

Clinical Assessment

Local examination looking for wounds or major soft tissue injury is imperative. As the subcutaneous bone strikes the thin subcutaneous tissue and skin laterally and medially, trauma and devascularization of skin may occur. This may lead to fracture blisters (traumatic bullae) and even skin necrosis (Fig. 24.5 a–d). If skin incisions are made through this traumatized devascularized area, skin necrosis often occurs and unfavorably alters the prognosis. Other injuries in the foot may lead to a compartment syndrome in the foot, which must be watched for. Neurovascular assessment is imperative.

24.5.1 Radiographic Assessment

Most of the fracture lines can be clearly seen on the plain radiographic views, which should include a lateral view, two oblique views to see the relationship to the remainder of the hindfoot and midfoot, and an axial view

(Fig. 24.6 a–e). The axial view is extremely important in determining the number of primary and secondary fracture lines and will clearly show the sustentaculum primary fracture line. However, in a badly injured patient with swelling, a good axial view is difficult to obtain.

Under these circumstances a computed tomography (CT) examination taken in the coronal plane will clearly show the state of the sustentaculum, the number of fracture lines, and the displacement in the posterior articular facet (Fig. 24.6 c). CT examination is invaluable in planning any operative approach and also in decision making as to whether surgery can achieve the objective of stable internal fixation and anatomical reduction.

Three-dimensional CT reconfigurations (Fig. 24.6 d, e) may also help in planning the surgical procedure, although the coronal CT is most valuable. CT in the plane of the plantar surface is also useful in seeing the fracture lines entering the midfoot.

24.6 Decision Making

As in all fractures, decision making will depend on fracture factors as assessed by the radiographic study and patient factors assessed by history and physical examination.

24.6.1 Fracture Factors

The causes of pain are related to deformity, articular damage to the posterior facet, widening of the heel causing impingement on the lateral malleolus, and disruption of the heel pad. If we believe that articular fractures in the lower extremity are best treated by anatomical reduction, stable fixation, and early motion, then it follows that any fracture that is displaced, that deforms and widens the os calcis, especially with the lateral fragment impinging on the lateral malleolus, and also depresses and alters the articular surface of the posterior facet is an indication for operative intervention. The aim of surgery is the correction of the deformity and the reconstruction of the articular surface, which will allow the narrowing of the heel.

However, there are fractures that will defy even the most expert surgeon because of the degree of comminution of the joint surface. Technological advances in the coming decades, especially with biological glues, may alter our present perception. However, at this time, if faced with radiographs and CT scans that show multifragments within the joint which are irreparable, the surgeon may choose nonoperative treatment, external fixation, or primary arthrodesis in the reduced position, as advocated by Hall and Pennal (1960).

··

24.6.2 Patient Factors

Having considered the pathoanatomy of the fracture using the various imaging techniques, the surgeon then needs to examine the patient factors, which include the age of the patient, the general medical state, the presence or absence of polytrauma, and especially the local factors such as fracture blisters, which may preclude an operative approach. Older patients with osteopenic bone, especially until the ultimate prognosis is clarified by prospective studies, may be best treated nonoperatively.

Fig. 24.7 a, b. Posterolateral approach to the calcaneus. The posterolateral approach may be used for patients in whom minimal internal fixation is desirable, with or without external fixation. The patient is placed in the prone position or in the lateral position, slightly tilted into prone. **a** The incision is made lateral to the Achilles tendon, making certain to protect the sural nerve. The incision is extensile as it may be extended further distally, becoming a posterolateral approach to the entire os calcis. **b** Deep dissection is along the lateral and superior aspect of the os calcis, by dissecting with a periosteal elevator under the Achilles tendon with the foot in the plantar flexed position. The subtalar joint may be seen and even the medial sustentacular fragment. Limited internal fixation may be inserted from the posterolateral to anteromedial aspect of the os calcis, as illustrated in this case

The other major factor is the state of the soft tissues. If there is obvious impingement of the bone against the soft tissues making the situation worse, the surgeon may choose to use an external fixator on the medial aspect from the tibia to the os calcis to correct some of the deformity and thereby the impingement. Otherwise, the patient should be splinted in a well-padded bandage with a posterior splint and the limb elevated. Surgery should not be attempted until the soft tissues allow this to be done safely.

Therefore, final decision making must include a careful assessment of the soft tissues and the fracture pattern. If the soft tissue injury is not severe, surgery, if indicated, may proceed, but if the soft tissue injury is severe, surgery must be delayed or alternate forms of treatment used.

··

24.7 Treatment

··

24.7.1 Nonoperative Treatment

If nonoperative management is chosen, the treatment should be aggressive. The limb should be elevated, swelling kept to a minimum by icing or other techniques, and early active exercise encouraged. Since these fractures

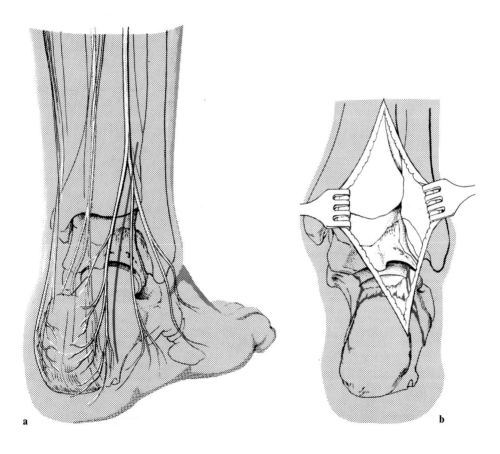

a   b

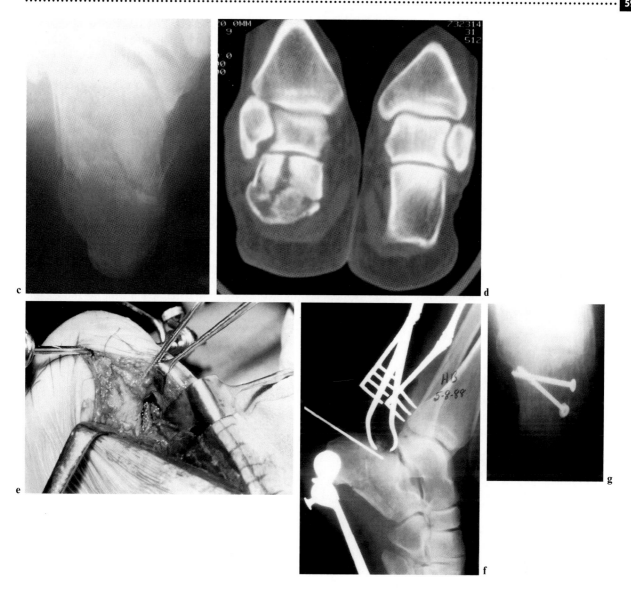

Fig. 24.7. c,d The axial view (**c**) and computed tomographic (CT) image (**d**) of a 49-year-old man who fell from a fence. **e** The patient was placed prone and a posterolateral incision made. **f** The intraoperative view showing a temporary traction pin in the distal fragment and a view of the subtalar joint is noted. **g** The final result on the axial view shows excellent restoration of the subtalar joint with minimal internal fixation

often compress cancellous bone, severe pain is often not a feature. The patients can safely and quickly restore excellent motion to the ankle and the other distal joints of the foot. It is often surprising how quickly the severe pain disappears in what is seemingly a severe injury. It is unclear whether results of aggressive nonoperative care are better than those of casting, but is suggested by the literature (Carr et al. 1989; Rowe et al. (1963); Lindsay and Dewar 1958). After early aggressive care, the patients

should be ambulated with crutches and very slight weight-bearing, with gradual restoration of full weight-bearing as pain disappears, usually at 8–12 weeks. I personally do not use a cast in patients with os calcis fractures that are being treated nonoperatively.

24.7.2 Operative Treatment

24.7.2.1 General Aspects

Timing. The most important decision to be made is the timing of surgery. There is a suggestion that extremely early surgery reducing the widened heel will allow better healing of soft tissues. This has not been tested by trials and rarely are patients taken to the operating room that quickly. In most cases, the surgery is delayed until some revascularization of the subcutaneous tissues and skin has occurred and any fracture blisters have resolved. This may require 5–14 days; obviously, the longer the surgeon waits, the more difficult it is to deal with the fracture operatively.

The incisions must be made away from major areas of fracture blisters, and the handling of skin and soft tissues must be meticulous and atraumatic. Prophylactic antibiotics are used.

24.7.2.2 Specific Aspects

a) Open Reduction and Internal Fixation

Surgical Approaches
Several operative approaches have been described for achieving anatomical reduction. These include the posterolateral, medial and lateral approaches.

Posterolateral Approach. The posterolateral incision (Gallie 1943)), allows the surgeon to see the posterior aspect of the medial primary fracture by dissecting behind the Achilles tendon and over the top of the talus (Fig. 24.7). In addition, the surgeon can see directly to the subtalar joint and easily fix a subtalar compression, especially of the tongue type. However, the posterior approach does not allow visualization of the anterolateral aspect of the os calcis unless the incision is carried around laterally.

Medial Approach. The medial approach has been advocated by McReynolds (1982), and others (Fig. 24.8). This approach is fraught with the danger of dissection in the area of the posterior tibial artery and nerve. However, its main advantage is direct anatomical reduction of the primary fracture line and fixation with a small two-hole plate or a staple. This medial approach has been used as a limited approach in conjunction with the more commonly used lateral approach or has been used as the primary incision with elevation of the main fracture done blindly.

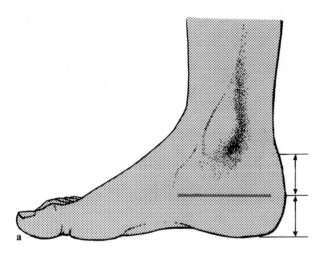

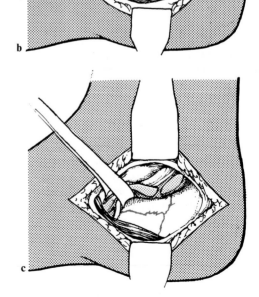

Fig. 24.8 a–c. Medial approach. **a** The skin incision may be transverse or oblique. The main problem in this approach is the proximity of the neural vascular bundle to the medial sustentacular fracture. **b** The localization of the neurovascular bundle is noted. **c** After retraction the main fracture fragments, especially the sustentacular fragment, can be seen

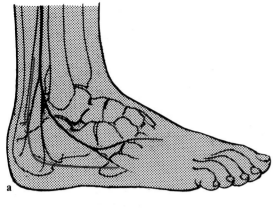

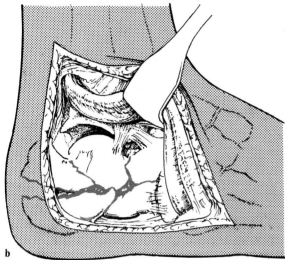

Fig. 24.9 a–c. Lateral approach to the calcaneum. The lateral approach to the calcaneum is now the most widely used approach for three- and four-part calcaneal fractures. **a** The skin incision curves along the posterior aspect of the calcaneum to its inferior aspect as shown. No skin flaps are raised. **b** The incision is taken directly to bone, as noted in the drawing. and by subperiosteal dissection, the bone is exposed. Note the raising of the peroneal tendons in their sheath, which allows entrance to the subtalar joint. This extensile approach allows anatomical reduction of the fragments on the lateral aspect and also visualization into the subtalar joint. **c** Screws and plates can be applied

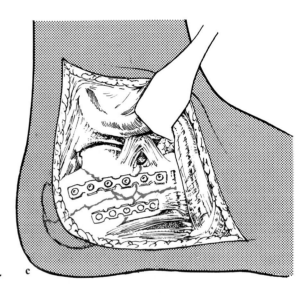

Lateral Approach. The lateral approach to the os calcis was favored by Palmer (1948) and Letournel (1984) and was modified by Benirschke and Sangeorzan (1993). It is now the most commonly used approach, either solely or in association with external fixation and/or a limited medial approach (Fig. 24.9). The advantage of this approach is excellent exposure of the tuberosity, the lateral wall, and the posterior facet of the subtalar joint, as well as the calcaneal cuboid joint. Its main disadvantage is that the sustentaculum fragment is not directly seen and reduction can only be performed indirectly.

The patient is placed in the lateral position, and an L-shaped incision is made. The incision is carried directly to the bone with great care not to raise the skin flaps. The periosteum is dissected along the lateral border of the os calcis, exposing all the fracture lines. The sural nerve must be protected at the proximal and distal end. When the entire lateral wall of the os calcis is exposed, retraction of the flap may be obtained with two Kirschner wires into the talus. The calcaneal cuboid joint also requires exposure in most cases.

Reduction and Fixation

The first step in reduction is to reduce the sustentacular fragment by placing a Schantz pin in the tuberosity, applying traction and translation medially (Fig. 24.10 a). Proximal fixation is obtained by Kirschner wires from posterolateral to anteromedial into the sustentaculum. The position should be checked on an image intensifier or plain radiographs. Restoration of the sustentaculum fragment anatomically reduces the medial wall and allows visualization of the subtalar joint by elevation of the lateral fragment. The fragments within the subtalar joint are then gently elevated and reduced to the sustentaculum (Fig. 24.10 b). In a tongue-type fracture, this is relatively easy, but if many fragments are present multiply K wires must be used. Once restoration of the joint has been obtained, a large gap may be seen beneath the reduced facet. This gap may be filled with cancellous bone graft from the iliac crest, allografts, or other bone substitutes (Fig. 24.10 c). When stability has been obtained, the lateral wall is replaced and the articular fragments fixed with small-fragment 3.5-mm screws into the sustentaculum.

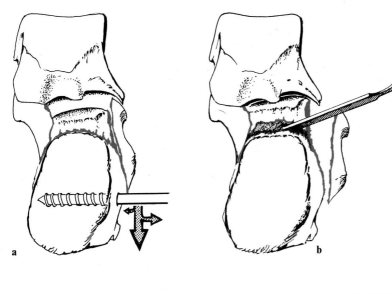

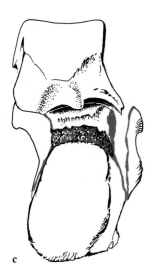

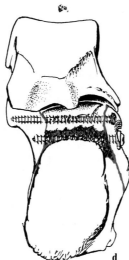

Fig. 24.10 a–d. Reduction and internal fixation techniques.

a Application of traction. It is helpful to insert a Schantz pin into the tuberosity fragment either through the tuberosity connected to a stirrup (see Fig. 24.6) or temporary connected to a frame the upper pin in the tibia.

b With the lateral fragment retracted the depressed joint fragment is elevated using a periosteal elevator.

c This often leaves a large gap under the depressed fragment which may require bone grafting with a cancellous bone block or a bone substitute bone block.

d The lateral fragment is then reduced and fixed with lag screws into the sustentaculum fragment. Cannulated screws are helpful. A view of the joint surface will ensure anatomical reduction if possible. If the soft tissues allow, buttress plates are used, either 3.5-mm reconstruction plates

Cannulated screws may be used for this procedure (Fig. 24.10 d).

The final stage is a buttress plate along the lateral aspect of the os calcis (Fig. 24.10 e). This is commonly a 3.5-mm reconstruction plate, but thinner H-type plates have been developed so as not to impinge on the thin soft tissues and skin in that area. The plate must not be overcontoured to allow varus or valgus deformation of the heel when the screws are tightened.

At the end of the procedure, an image intensifier check or axial radiographs must be done to ensure anatomical reduction (see Fig. 24.6). The skin flap is closed using atraumatic techniques over suction drains.

b) Primary Subtalar Arthrodesis

If the surgeon finds the fragments within the posterior facet of the os calcis to be too comminuted and irreducible, one option is a primary subtalar arthrodesis following the open reduction, as advocated by Hall and Pennal (1960). The first step is identical, i.e., reduction of heel width, restoration of the medial fracture, and fixation of the main body. If the articular cartilage is multifragmented, it can be removed and a large bone block inserted across the joint, as advocated by Gallie (1943; Fig. 24.11). The external fixator, first used to distract the joint, is then returned to the compressed mode to allow early healing. The results of this procedure have been satisfactory (Hall and Pennal 1960).

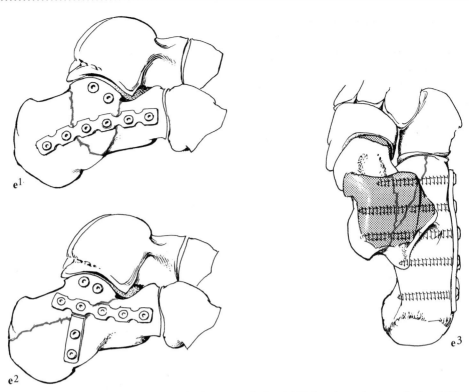

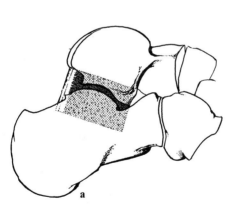

Fig. 24.10. e¹ or a combination of 3.5-mm reconstruction plates with 1/3 semi-tubular plates (**e¹**). I prefer the 1/3 semi-tubular plate because it is thin and does not interfere with soft tissue healing as much. Special H plates have also been designed. The axial view is noted in **e³**

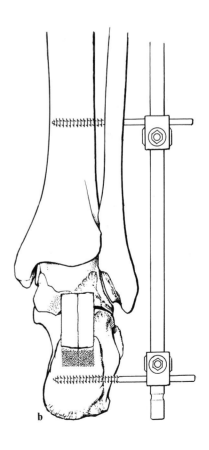

Fig. 24.11 a,b. Primary subtalar fusion. Posterior approach. As advocated by Pennal and Hall (1960) a primary subtalar fusion is indicated when the articular surface is so comminuted that reconstruction becomes impossible. Under these circumstances the internal fixation progresses as described in Fig. 24.10. In other words, reduction of the fracture diminishing the heel width is extremely important in this primary arthrodesis. Therefore, after insertion of the Schantz pin into the tuberosity and exposure of the subtalar joint posteriorly, the comminuted fragments of bone are removed to the intact portion of the calcaneus. An autogenous bone graft taken from the iliac crest is inserted as demonstrated in the lateral (**a**) and posterior (**b**) view. Stability is maintained by placing the external fixator in a slightly compressive mode

c) External Fixation and Minimal Internal Fixation

Another alternative in fractures in which comminution of the subtalar joint is marked or the lateral skin injury does not allow internal fixation is a combination of minimal internal fixation of the medial sustentacular fragment through a small approach and an external fixator placed on the lateral aspect from the tibia to the tubercle of the os calcis (Fig. 24.6). This will again restore height and reduce the width to the os calcis, and should a late subtalar joint reconstruction be required, it can be done on an anatomically reduced os calcis as opposed to one which has a continuing deformity and a nonplantigrade foot.

24.8 Postoperative Care

Postoperative care in all operative procedures is important and will vary from case to case depending on the soft tissue injury, the state of the wound, and the adequacy of the internal fixation. In general, the patient is placed in a well-padded soft bandage with a posterior plaster slab at 90°. The drains are removed at 24–36 h. When active restoration of dorsiflexion is obtained, the entire bandage and cast can be removed at 3–5 days, and early active motion encouraged if the surgeon is certain that the fixation is stable. If the surgeon is concerned about the stability of the fracture, then cast immobilization needs to be kept on for 8–12 weeks until the fracture is healed. Under ideal circumstances a night splint is used to keep the ankle at 90°, and during the day the patient is encouraged to exercise. Very slight weight-bearing with crutches is continued for 6–8 weeks, with progressive weight-bearing for 12 weeks.

24.9 Prognosis and Results

At present patients with an os calcis fracture must be told that the prognosis with respect to complete and normal return to function is uncertain. The final chapter has yet to be written and, in my opinion, it is doubtful whether a final chapter will ever be written because of the many variables in this and other intra-articular fractures in the lower extremity. Recent reports of operative treatment in expert hands have still shown variable outcomes with a relatively high incidence of complications. Letournel (1984), using a lateral approach in 99 patients, reported 56% good or very good results, and 44% fair or bad results. He reported three infections and six technical failures. Sanders et al. (1993), using lateral approaches in 120 cases, found the clinical results inversely proportional to the degree of comminution of the subtalar joint. In other words, the personality of the fracture with respect to joint comminution was more important than the treatment (Fig. 24.12). A total of 73% of patients with mild- to moderate comminution had excellent or good results, while only 9% with severe comminution had good to excellent results. They concluded that there might be indications for primary subtalar arthrodesis. Zwipp et al. (1988), using a combination of approaches in 157 patients, again found a direct correlation between fracture severity and clinical outcome. They reported 8.5% marginal necrosis of the wound and 2% deep infection.

Benirschke and Sangeorzan (1993) have reiterated the above results with 2% deep infection and skin necrosis in 10%. They report 70% of patients to be satisfied with the surgical outcome. It is clear that even in the hands of the above experts surgical outcomes remain uncertain and may not be better than nonoperative care considering the complications. In this particular fracture, as in most lower-extremity articular fractures, surgical technique is always extremely important. Whether these realistic results can be improved upon will depend somewhat on the expertise of the surgeons.

Ultimately, multicentered prospective clinical trials matching like groups of cases treated operatively and nonoperatively are required, like the one presently being pursued in many Canadian centers (Buckley et al. 1995). It is equally as important for the group being treated surgically that they be treated in an expert fashion, because

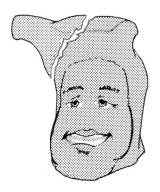 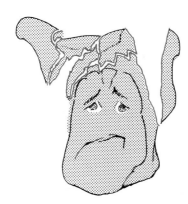

Fig. 24.12 a,b. The personality of fractures of the calcaneum. As in other joint injuries, calcaneal fractures may have a *good* personality (**a**) if there is a large single fracture through the joint and no comminution of articular cartilage, or a poor personality (**b**) with multifragmentation of the joint surface, widening of the heel, and poor soft tissues

the results of poor surgery are worse than the results of good nonoperative care. Therefore, in this particular trial, the surgeons involved have to demonstrate a minimum volume of cases to show competency.

24.10 Conclusions

I believe that at this stage in development individual decision making is imperative. Correction of deformity, restoration of the articular surface of the subtalar joint, stable fixation, and early motion are extremely desirable and may be obtained in many patients. However, patient factors such as age, general medical state, the presence or absence of other life-threatening injuries, and especially compromised soft tissues may preclude surgery. The surgeon and the patient must honestly discuss all of these factors and come to a decision together based on realistic expectations and our present knowledge.

As is so often the case in lower-extremity joint fractures, we have increased our ability to restore the anatomy, but are often defeated by the biology. The development of biological glues, which allow healing of articular cartilage, and other technical advances in the next decade may tip the balance in favor of the operative approach.

References

Bankart (1942) Fractures of the os calcis. Lancet 2:175

Benirschke SK, Sangeorzan BJ (1993) Extensive intraarticular fractures of the foot. Clin Orthop Relat Res 292:128–134

Bohler L (1931) Diagnosis, pathology and treatment of fractures of the os calcis. J Bone Joint Surg13:75–89

Buckley RE, Van de Guchte R, Stewart R (1995) Clinical and X-ray/CT correlates of displaced intra-articular calcaneal fractures Presented at the Canadian Orthopaedic Association Annual Meeting, Halifax, 6 June 1995

Carr JB, Hamilton JJ, Bear LS (1989) Experimental intraarticular calcaneal fractures: anatomic basis for a new classification. Foot Ankle 2:81

Cotton, FJ, Henderson FF (1916) Results of fractures of the os calcis. Am J Orthop Surg 14:290–298

Essex-Lopresti P (1993) The mechanism, reduction-technique, and results in fractures of the os calcis. Clin Orthop 290:3–16

Gallie WE (1943) Subastragalar arthrodesis in fractures of the os calcis. J Bone Joint Surg 25A:731

Hall MC, Pennal GF (1960) Primary subtalar arthrodesis in the treatment of severe fractures of the calcaneum. J. Bone Joint Surg [Br] 42:336–343

Letournel E (1984) Open reduction and internal fixation of calcaneal fractures. In: Spiegel P (ed) Topics in orthopaedic surgery. Aspen, Baltimore, p 173

Lindsay WRN, Dewar FP (1958) Fractures of the os calcis. Am J Surg 95:555

McReynolds IS (1982) The case for operative treatment of fractures of the os calcis. In: Leach RE, Hoaglund FT, Riseborough EJ (eds) Controversies in orthopaedic surgery. Saunders, Philadelphia, p 232

Palmer I (1948) The mechanism and treatment of fractures of the calcaneus: open reduction with the use of cancellous grafts. J Bone Joint Surg 30A:2

Rowe CR, Sakellarides HT, Freeman PA et al (1963) Fractures of the os calcis: a long term follow-up study of 146 patients. JAMA 184:920–923

Sanders R, Fortin P, DiPasquale T et al (1993) Operative treatment in 120 displaced intraarticular calcaneal fractures: results using a prognostic computed tomography scan classification. Clin Orthop 290:87–95

Zwipp H, Tscherne H, Walker N (1993) Calcaneal fracture. In: Tscherne H, Schatzker J (eds) Major fractures of the pilon, the talus, and the calcaneus: current concepts of treatment. Springer, Berlin Heidelberg New York, pp 153-174

25 Injuries of the Midfoot and Forefoot

D.J.G. STEPHEN

25.1 Fractures of the Navicular

25.1.1 Anatomy

The tarsal navicular bone has a concave articular surface for proximal articulation with the talus and a convex articular surface – with three facets – for distal articulation with the three cuneiforms. A fourth facet may be present to allow articulation with the cuboid. The navicular – with its position in the medial longitudinal arch of the foot – acts as a keystone for vertically applied forces at the arch (Eichenholtz and Levine 1964). Owing to the fact that most of the surface of the navicular is covered by articular cartilage, only a small area is available for vascular access (Torg et al. 1982; DeLee 1986). Torg et al. showed with microangiographic studies that the central third is relatively avascular compared to the inner and outer thirds. The blood supply enters the dorsal and plantar surfaces, as well as via the tuberosity (Sarrafian 1983). Sarrafian has shown that there are direct branches entering the dorsal surface from the dorsalis pedis artery, while the medial plantar artery gives branches to the plantar surface. An anastomosis of these two arteries supplies the tuberosity. Therefore, similar to the talus, the vascular supply plays a critical role in determining outcomes after injuries to the navicular.

25.1.2 Treatment

Dorsal lip avulsion fractures were the most common navicular fracture in a series by Eichenholtz and Levine (1964), accounting for 47% of the total. The mechanism of injury involves acute plantar flexion with inversion, and the talonavicular ligament avulses a small proximal dorsal fragment (DeLee 1986). If the fragment is small and extra-articular, symptomatic treatment is successful in the vast majority of cases (Giannestras and Sammarco 1975; DeLee 1986); care must be taken to exclude an associated midtarsal injury and, if present, immobilization for 6 weeks is indicated (Watsom-Jones 1955). If the fragment is large or more symptomatic, a short-leg walking cast is applied for 3–4 weeks

(Giannestras and Sammarco 1975). Open reduction and internal fixation is indicated when the avulsed fragment contains a significant portion of the articular surface (Hillegass 1976). For chronic or missed cases, delayed excision is indicated for large symptomatic bony prominences (Giannestras and Sammarco 1975; Hillegass 1976; DeLee 1986).

Acute eversion of the foot results in increased tension in the posterior tibialis tendon, causing an avulsion of the tuberosity (Giannestras and Sammarco 1975; DeLee 1986). Small or minimally displaced fragments are treated symptomatically in short-leg cast for 4–6 weeks. Indications for fixation of the avulsed tuberosity include involvement of a significant portion of the articular surface and displacement of the fragment. Sangeorzan et al. (1989) recommends operative fixation for displacement of 5 mm or more, which indicates incompetence of the posterior tibialis tendon. Tuberosity fractures are approached through a medial incision over the navicular prominence (DeLee 1986; Sangeorzan et al. 1989), and fixation may be enhanced with a soft tissue washer. Although nonunions of navicular tuberosity fractures occur, they are usually asymptomatic (Giannestra and Sammarco 1975). If a painful nonunion results, either fixation of large fragments or excision of small fragments is recommended (Giannestras and Sammarco 1975; DeLee 1986).

Fractures of the navicular body are the least frequent, occuring as a result of direct or indirect force (DeLee 1986). The exact mechanism of fractures due to an indirect force is controversial, but involves a combination of forced plantar flexion and abduction of the midfoot (DeLee 1986) This mechanism can result in displacement of the fracture fragments, damage to articular surfaces, extensive ligamentous disruption, and possibly osteonecrosis of the navicular. The fragments may be displaced into the medial or dorsal aspects of the foot. These displaced fragments must be reduced anatomically to restore articular congruity and to prevent shortening of the medial column of the foot. Shortening of the medial column can result in varus midfoot deformities, leading to degenerative arthritis.

Radiographic evaluation of suspected navicular body fractures requires three views of the foot: anteroposterior, lateral, and oblique projections, with computed

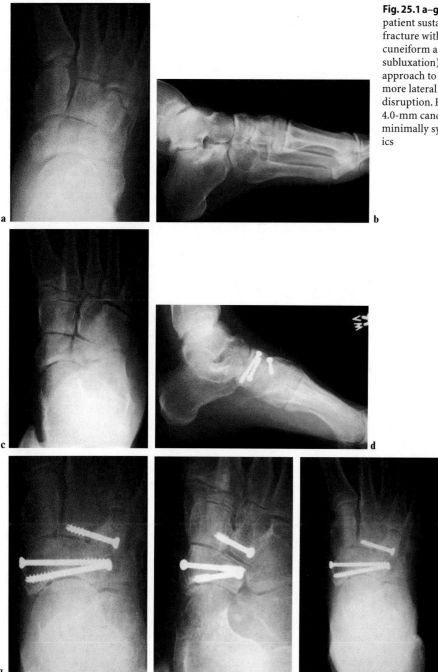

Fig. 25.1 a–g. In a motor vehicle accident, the patient sustained multiple injuries. Navicular fracture with disruption of middle and lateral cuneiform articulation (midfood fracture-subluxation). Combined dorsomedial approach to navicular and dorsal approach to more lateral navicular fracture and cuneiform disruption. Fixation with cannulated 3.5- and 4.0-mm cancellous lag screws. At 6 months minimally symptomatic with custom orthotics

tomography (CT) scanning reserved for comminuted fragments. Biplanar tomograms can be useful to further evaluate the number and position of fragments, as well as involvement of surrounding joints.

Navicular body fractures are approached through a medial incision that is between the tibialis posterior, and anterior tendons, centered over the navicular (Sangeorzan 1993). A second dorsal incision may be needed,

which is made in the region of the extensor digitorum longus. Sangeorzan et al. (1989) have classified navicular body fractures by the degree and direction of displacement, the number of articular fragments, the alignment of the forefoot, and any associated injuries. Type 1 fractures split the navicular in the coronal plane (parallel to plantar aspect of the foot), and the dorsal fragment is less than 50 % of the body. In a type 2 fracture, the fracture line passes from dorsolateral to plantarmedial. The major fragment is dorsomedial, leaving a smaller, often comminuted lateral fragment. There can be medial displacement of the larger medial fragment, which can cause shortening of the medial column of the foot. Type 3 fractures have increased comminution, with extension into the calcaneonavicular joint, making anatomical reduction difficult. There can be lateral displacement of the foot, with subluxation of the calcaneocuboid joint.

Undisplaced fractures of the navicular body are treated in a non-weight-bearing cast for 6–8 weeks, followed by longitudinal arch supports. All displaced fracures require anatomical reduction through medial and often dorsal incisions. When there is extensive comminution, restoration of any shortening of the medial column can be achieved by use of a mini external fixator into the talus and the first metatarsal (Sangeorzan et al. 1989; Sangeorzan 1993), analogous to its use in cuboid fractures (see Fig. 25.2). This can also be used as an indirect reduction technique. If the fragments are large, cannulated 3.5-mm or 4.0-mm screws are used to achieve stable fixation (Fig. 25.1). Bone graft may be required to fill defects resulting from cancellous impaction or after articular elevation. In cases with extensive comminution, screws can be passed from the larger navicular fragments into the second or third cuneiform bones or the cuboid bone. These screws are then removed after healing. The mini external fixator can be left in place to augment the reduction and stabilize the medial column until healing. A short-leg cast is worn postoperatively for 6–8 weeks, and weight-bearing is not initiated until union is evident radiographically and clinically.

In rare cases of extensive comminution or extensive articular damage, a primary fusion may be indicated. The use of the mini external fixator and a tricortical bone graft is essential to restore the length of the medial column of the foot. There is no agreement on the extent of the primary fusion (Dick 1942; Day 1947; Garcia and Parkes 1973). Some authours base their decision on the site of articular damage and limit the fusion to either the talonavicular or the naviculocuneiform joints (Garcia and Parkes 1973; DeLee 1986). Based on cadaveric studies, Day (1947) recommends a triple arthrodesis plus fusion of the naviculocuneiform joints. In the acute stage, we would recommend fusion of the most severely involved joint(s), and not a triple arthrodesis.

Complications include loss of fixation because of premature weight-bearing and/or poor bone quality and osteonecrosis of the navicular. Revascularization of the navicular can occur. In those cases where collapse or degenerative arthritis occurs, a fusion is indicated if conservative measures such as custom-molded insoles or rocker-bottom shoes fail. Determining the site and extent of the fusion can be difficult, and often

diagnostic blocks (with floroscopic guidance) can be of use in determining the involved joints. The defect resulting from débridement of the avascular bone is filled with tricortical bone graft and augmented with cancellous chips. The joints to be fused are débrided of any remaining articular cartilage and fixed with cancellous screws. A non-weight-bearing cast is worn for 6–8 weeks followed by a weight-bearing cast for another 6 weeks.

25.2 Fractures of the Cuboid

Isolated fractures of the cuboid are rare, occuring most frequently as a result of direct crushing force or by a fall onto a plantar flexed foot in eversion (Wilson 1933; McKeever 1950). The fracture can be an avulsion or can involve the entire body of the cuboid. Often fractures of the cuboid occur in association with fractures of the cuneiform bones, the calcaneus, or the bases of the lateral metatarsals (Chapman 1978). They can be associated with tarsometatarsal or midtarsal dislocations or subluxations (Garcia and Parkes 1973). The fracture of the cuboid body is often called a "nutcracker fracture," as it is caught between the fourth and fifth metatarsals and the calcaneus (Hermel and Geshon-Cohen 1953). This type of fracture can result in shortening of the lateral column of the foot. Radiographic evaluation includes anteroposterior, lateral, and oblique views; if more information is required, biplanar tomograms or CT scans can be obtained.

Undisplaced or avulsion fractures are treated by a short-leg weight-bearing cast for 4–6 weeks (Giannestras and Sammarco 1975). Care must be taken to assess the other joints of the midtarsal region; if an injury is suspected, longitudinal arch supports are used after the period of immobilzation. The indications for operative treatment are impacted (nutcracker) fractures that result in articular incongruity or subluxation. The surgical approach is made just dorsal to the peroneus brevis tendon, in a longitudinal fashion, just proximal to the tubercle of the fifth metatarsal. If the lateral column is shortened as a result of cuboid impaction, a mini external fixator is used with pins into the calcaneus and the fifth metatarsal (Fig. 25.2). Disimpaction can be enhanced by placing small K wires (0.045 or 0.062 mm) in the distal and proximal extent of the cuboid and then using a small lamina spreader to restore length (Sangeorzan and Swiontkowski 1990; Sangeorzan 1993). The resulting defect is filled with tricortical bone graft. To maintain this reduction a one-quarter, one-third tubular or mini-fragment plate is used (Sangeorzan and Swiontkowski 1990). Occasionally, fixation into the calcaneus and/or the fifth metatarsal is required (see Fig. 25.2). Postoperatively, patients are placed in a well-

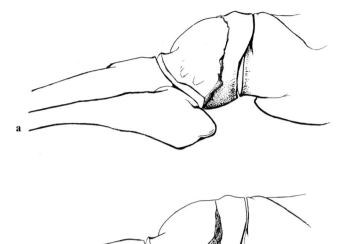

Fig. 25.2. a Cuboid (nutcracker) compression fracture, **b** restoration of length of lateral column with mini-external fixator, mini-fragment plate and bone graft. Note interrupted lines indicating possible extension of plate to include fifth metatarsal and calcaneus

padded posterior splint, which is converted to a non-weight-bearing cast when swelling has decreased. Weight-bearing is not initiated for 6–8 weeks, and – depending on the radiographic and clinical findings – patients are allowed protected weight-bearing for another 4–6 weeks. Complications include injury to the sural nerve at the time of operative treatment and degenerative arthritis of the calcaneocuboid or metatarsocuboid joints.

25.3 Fractures of the Metatarsals

25.3.1 Anatomy

During the stance phase, each of the lesser metatarsals supports an equal load, with the first metatarsal taking twice this amount (Shereff 1990). Displacement of metatarsal fractures is rare unless there is a significant injury to the intrinsic muscles or the strong intermetatarsal ligaments. However, metatarsal neck fractures are the exception (Anderson 1977). Displacement of the metatarsal head–neck (distal) fragment can occur. The cause for this is the plantar-proximal deforming force caused by the flexors and extensors to the toes. Any displacement (dorsal or plantar) alters the loading patterns of the foot, leading to metatarsalgia (plantar) or transfer metatarsalgia (dorsal) (Shereff 1990). There is an extensive anastomotic network in the region of the bases of the metatarsals supplied by branches of the dorsalis pedis and plantar arteries. The termination of the dorsalis pedis artery is the first dorsal metatarsal artery.

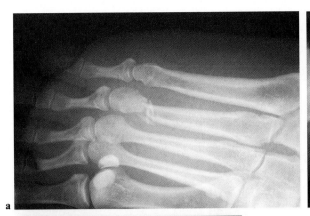

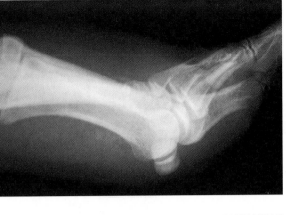

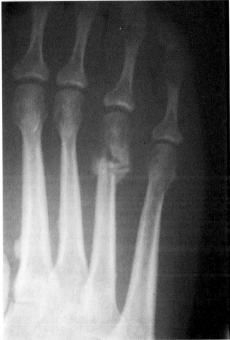

Fig. 25.3 a–c. Patient fell, sustaining fourth metatarsal neck. Treatment consisted of "buddy-taping" to third toe. At 2 months, patient is asymptomatic

25.3.2 Treatment

A direct force (crush) is usually responsible for fractures of the second, third, and fourth metatarsals, often causing multiple fractures (Garcia and Parkes 1973; DeLee 1986). An indirect force, such as twisting of the foot (inversion), often causes fractures of the fifth metatarsal (Giannestras and Sammarco 1975). Patients often have multiple injuries as a result of motor vehicle accidents, resulting in missed or neglected metatarsal fractures. Therefore, care must be taken to evaluate swelling, pain, and/or deformity in the region of the forefoot. Radiological evaluation includes anteroposterior, lateral, and oblique views centered over the forefoot.

Undisplaced fractures of the metatarsal shaft or neck (Fig. 25.3) can be treated with a postoperative shoe or a well-molded short-leg cast to allow early weight-bearing. Fractures of the first metatatarsal require correction of dorsal or plantar displacement. Comminuted fractures of the first metatarsal can result in a shortened first ray, leading to second transfer metatarsalgia. The length must be restored, either by closed means (finger traps) and percutaneous K wire fixation to the second metatarsal or by open reduction and internal fixation via a dorsomedial incision (DeLee 1986; Fig. 25.4). Fixation can be obtained by K wires or by small- or minifragment screws. Intra-articular fractures of the first metatarso-cuneiform joint must be reduced anatomically – either by closed or open reduction. In comminuted fractures of this joint, primary fusion may be indicated (Fig. 25.5). If displaced fractures of the lesser metatarsals can be reduced by closed reduction, percutaneous intramedullary K wire fixation, or cross fixation to an adjacent metatarsal is performed. If there is persistent plantar prominence of the head of the fractured metatarsal due to plantar–dorsal displacement, open reduction and internal fixation via a dorsal incision is indicated, with an intramedullary K wire or minifragment plate (see Fig. 25.7). Postoperatively, patients are immobilized in a well-padded splint, until decreased swelling permits

610 •••

Chapter 25   **Injuries of the Midfoot and Forefoot**

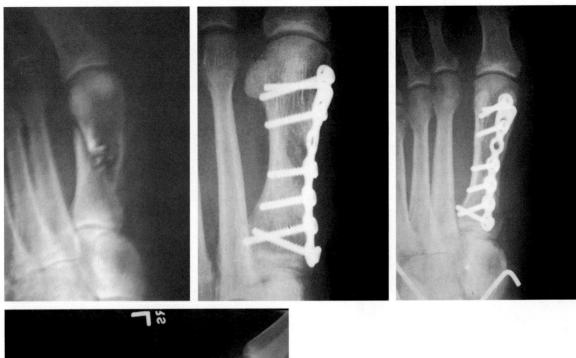

a - c

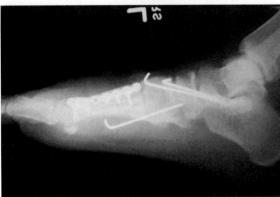

d

Fig. 25.4 a–d. Lawnmower injury. Patient sustained open, shortened, comminuted, first metatarsal shaft fracture. Treatment consisted of débridement of wound and fixation with 2-mm minifragment blade plate. Patient returned for second débridement of wound and delayed primary closure. Patient at 4 weeks with healed wound, mobilizing in postoperative shoe

Fig. 25.5 a–g. Motor vehicle accident. Patient sustained first metatarso-cuneiform fracture-subluxation. Consistent plantar fragment from first metatarsal allows dorsal subluxation of first metatarsal shaft. Fixation via dorsomedial approach. The long metaphyseal extension allows lag screw to plantar fragment restoring congruity of first metatarso-cuneiform joint. At 4 months there are only minimal symptoms ▶

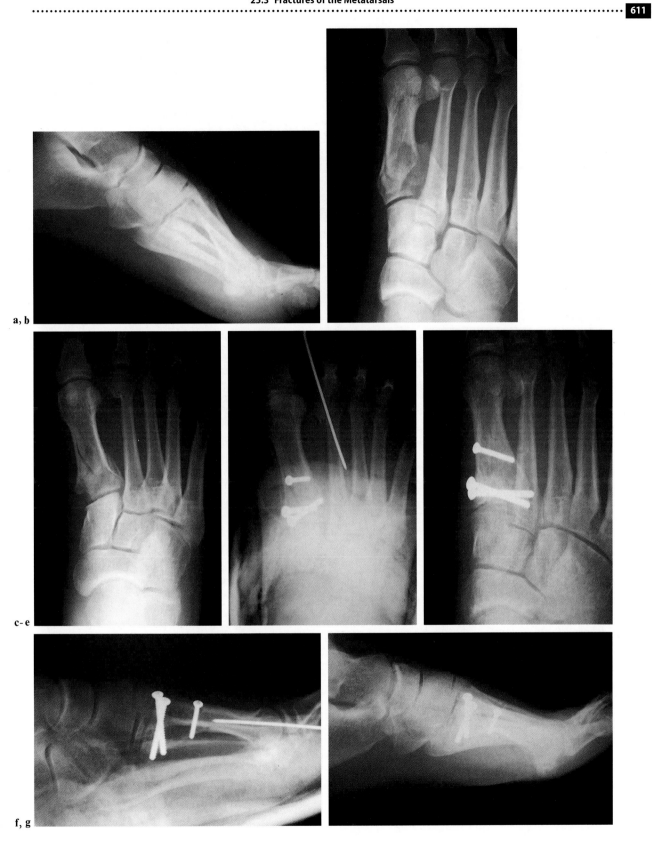

a, b

c- e

f, g

612 ·

Chapter 25   **Injuries of the Midfoot and Forefoot**

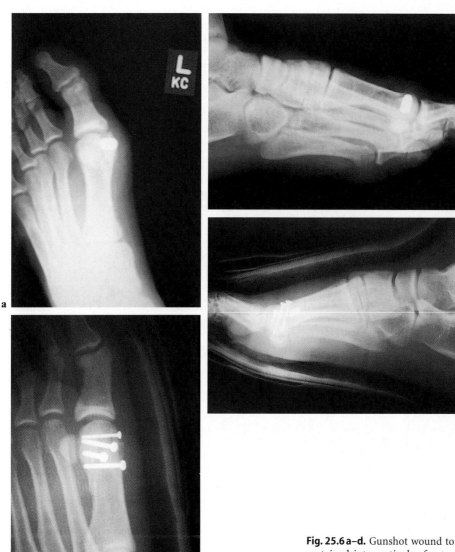

Fig. 25.6 a–d. Gunshot wound to first metatarsal head. Patient sustained intra-articular fracture at the metatarsophalangeal joint. Treatment consisted of limited débridement of wound, excision of bullet fragments, and internal fixation with minifragment screws

application of a non-weight-bearing short-leg cast. Depending on the severity and number of injuries, a weight-bearing cast (or commercially available removable walker) is applied at approximately 4–6 weeks and is worn for another 4–6 weeks. Any K wires are removed at approximately 4–6 weeks. A custom-molded arch support is worn after cast removal.

Metatarsal head fractures may be large enough to render the metatarophalangeal joint unstable. If closed reduction is successful, the injured toe is buddy-taped to an adjacent toe. If there is persistent displacement and instability, open reduction via a dorsal incision is indicated. Internal fixation is acheived by means of K wires,

minifragment or small Herbert screws (Fig. 25.6). Metatarsal neck fractures require assessment of any plantar or dorsal displacement of the metatarsal head, as this causes metatarsalgia if left unreduced (see arrow in Fig. 25.7 c). Sesamoid views often help this determination. Closed reduction is attempted by longitudinal traction (finger traps) and pressure below the metatarsal head (DeLee 1986). If this is successful, a short-leg cast with a toe plate is applied. If there is persistent plantar prominence, open reduction via a dorsal incision is indicated. The dorsal capsule is split longitudinally with care being taken to protect both neurovascular bundles. A K wire is inserted retrogradely through the metatarsal

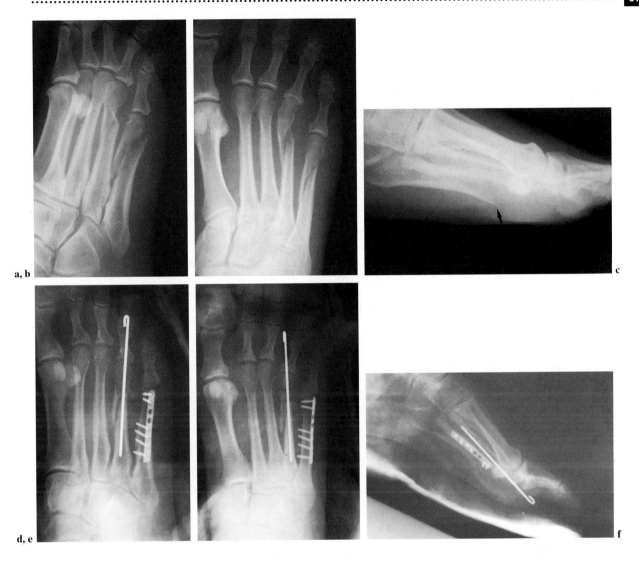

a, b

c

d, e

f

head and out of the plantar surface of the foot. The fracture is then reduced, and the K wire is advanced down the metatarsal shaft. A well-molded weight-bearing cast or a postoperative shoe is applied, and the K wires are removed at 3 weeks.

Fig. 25.7 a–f. Inversion injury. Patient sustained fifth metatarsal shaft and fourth metatarsal neck fractures. Treatment consisted of non-weight-bearing short leg cast. At 3 weeks there is shortening and dorsal displacement with plantar metaphyseal "spike" of fifth metatarsal (arrow in **c**). Operative fixation of the fifth metatarsal with a 2-mm plate, through a dorsolateral approach. Also open reduction of the fourth metatarsal neck because of lateral angulation. Postoperative films at 3 weeks

25.3.3 Fractures of the Proximal Fifth Metatarsal

Anatomy

The proximal fifth metatarsal has been divided into three zones (Fig. 25.8; Smith et al. 1992; Lawrence and Botte 1993). *Zone 1* is the area of the tuberosity and includes the insertion of the peroneus brevis tendon and the calcaneometatarsal ligamentous branch of the plantar fascia. Fractures in this zone usually extend into the metatarsocuboid joint. *Zone 2* includes the more distal tuberosity, with fractures extending into the articulation between the fourth and fifth metatarsals. There are strong dorsal and plantar intermetatarsal ligaments in this area (Dameraon 1995). *Zone 3* starts just distal to these ligaments and extends distally approximately 1.5 cm into the diaphysis. The nutrient artery to the fifth metatarsal enters medially in the middle third of the bone, dividing into a short proximal branch and a longer distal branch (Shereff et al. 1991; Smith et al. 1992). There are a significant number of very small metaphyseal vessels at each end of the bone. Fractures to the proximal diaphysis can disrupt the proximal branch of the intraosseous nutrient vessel, inerfering with the blood supply to the distal portion of the proximal fragment of the fifth metatarsal. The tuberosity obtains additional extraosseous blood supply from soft tissue attachments.

Fractures of the fifth metatarsal base are not only the most common metatarsal fracture, but also create the most confusion with regard to their treatment (Lawrence and Botte 1993; Dameron 1995). Sir Robert Jones reported a fracture of the fifth metatarsal metadiaphysis (zone 2), occuring in his own foot while dancing (Jones 1902). He also described more distal fractures (zone 3). It is now accepted that in the majority of cases, fractures in zone 3 are stress fractures (Kavanaugh et al. 1978; Dameron 1995).

The tuberosity of the fifth metatarsal extends lateral and proximal to the cuboid and is of variable size. The tendon of the peroneus brevis has a wide insertion on the dorsolateral aspect of the base of the fifth metatarsal and is often held responsible for avulsing a portion of the tuberosity after an inversion injury (Anderson 1983; Dameron 1995). However, numerous other structures have been implicated, including the adductor digiti quinti, the lateral portion of the plantar fascia, the abductor ossei metatarsi quinti, and the flexor minimi digiti brevis (Carp 1927; DeLee 1986; Lawrence and Botte 1993; Dameron 1995).

Clinical and Radiological Diagnosis

The clinical history is one of inversion of the foot, with resultant pain at the base of the fifth metatarsal. The most useful radiograph is the oblique projection, which allows assessment of the size of the fragment, the degree of displacement, and any articular involvement. It is important not to confuse this fracture with an apophysis within the proximal fifth metatarsal. The line of this apophysis runs parallel to the axis of the shaft and is extra-articular. There may be sesamoids in the tendons of the peroneus longus (os peroneum) or peroneus brevis (os vesalianum). Smooth, sclerotic surfaces help to differentiate these accessory bones from fractures.

Treatment

Zone 1 fractures begin laterally on the tuberosity and extend proximally entering the metatarsocuboid joint. This area is cancellous bone, with an excellent blood supply (Smith et al. 1992). The mechanism of injury is an inversion injury causing an avulsion by the peroneus brevis tendon and/or the lateral portion of the plantar aponeurosis (DeLee 1986; Dameron 1995; Fig. 25.9). The vast majority of these fractures heal with only symptomatic treatment with a postoperative wooden sole shoe and weight-bearing as tolerated. A persistent radiolucent line, suggestive of a delayed union or a nonunion, is rarely symptomatic. If there is chronic pain refractory to conservative measures, excision of small fragments or fixation of larger fragments is then considered.

Zone 2 fractures begin more distal on the tuberosity, entering the articulation between the fourth and fifth metatarsal. These injuries are more symptomatic, often requiring a short-leg weight-bearing cast. There is often more comminution of the fracture. The recovery period for these fractures is often prolonged, remaining symptomatic for several months.

Zone 3 fractures occur in the metadiaphysis, distal to the strong intermetatarsal ligaments. Fractures in this

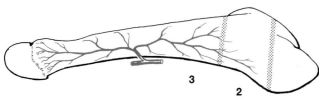

Fig. 25.8. Zones of the fifth metatarsal (from Donovan 1995)

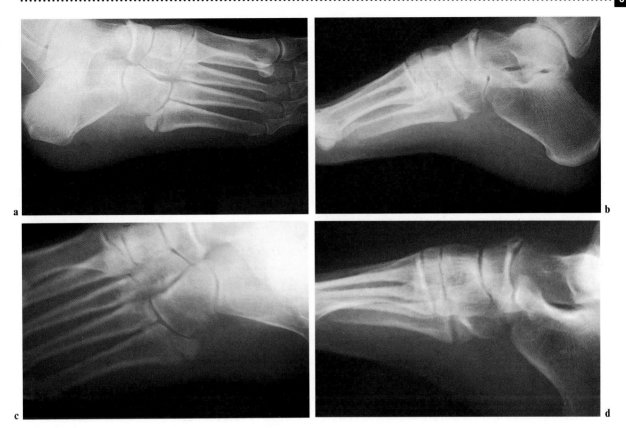

Fig. 25.9 a–d. Inversion injury. Patient sustained avulsion of fifth metatarsal tuberosity. Treatment in wooden sole operative sandal. At 3 months patient is asymptomatic

zone are usually stress fractures, occurring in competitive athletes involved in running and jumping with sharp turns, such as in basketball. These fractures have a high risk of delayed union and nonunion, especially with even mild continued activity (Carp 1927; Dameron 1995). There is often a history of 2–3 weeks of ankle or foot pain, requiring treatment. Radiological evaluation during this period reveals subperiosteal reaction with new bone formation at the area of maximal tenderness. If there are no changes seen on plain films, a technetium bone scan may show increased uptake in this region. At this stage – prior to fracture – modification of activity and symptomatic treatment is usually successful. If there is an obvious fracture, and the patient needs to resume his or her activities early (either athletic or employment), this is a relative indication for surgical management. If there is no urgency, the patient can be treated in a short-leg weight-bearing cast. Although controversial, there is no evidence that refraining from weight-bearing improves the outcome in zone 3 fractures (Lawrence and Botte 1993; Dameron 1986).

The fifth metatarsal shaft is triangular and often bowed, making percutaneous placement of the screw difficult (Anderson 1983). The patient is placed either in the lateral decubitus position or with the effected limb tilted up approximately 45°. A 2–3 cm dorsolateral incision is made, with retraction of the peroneus brevis tendon (Dameron 1995). Image intensification and the use of a cannulated system aids the placement of the cancellous compression screw. Some authors recommend exploring the fracture site if there is any preexisting sclerosis and supplementing the fixation with bone grafts (DeLee 1986). There is no weight-bearing for approximately 2–3 weeks, followed by the use of a weight-bearing cast for 4–6 weeks. The decision for further immobilization or return to graduated activities is based the clinical and radiological evaluations. Dameron (1995) recommends the use of a functional wrap-around thermoplastic brace for approximately 4–6 weeks after the cast is removed, especially if the patient is returning to high-risk activities. Arangio's review of the literature (Arangio 1993) reports that for acute fractures treated without fixation there is 38% incidence of delayed union and a 14% incidence of nonunion. Supplemental bone graft is indicated in those cases with a persistent gap at a nonunion site (despite screw compression) or in those in which the site is opened.

25.4 Fractures of the Phalanges

Fractures of the phalanges are most often caused by direct impact on the toe (Fig. 25.10). This may involve dropping a heavy object onto the toe or "stubbing" the toe onto a hard surface. Of the hallux phalanges, the proximal one is most commonly fractured (Chapman 1978). The distal phalanx is often comminuted and/or dislocated when it is injured. A fracture of the proximal phalanx of the lesser toes is commonly caused by an abduction force, as seen when the toes are struck on a coffee table. Fractures of the proximal phalanx tend to angulate plantarward as a result of the action of the toe extensor, flexor, and intrinsics. Angulation of the middle and distal phalanges depend more on the direction of the force (DeLee 1986).

Undisplaced fractures of the hallux or lesser toes can be treated with taping and immediate weight-bearing. The taping is continued for 2–4 weeks, until the pain subsides. Displaced fractures of the hallux, especially with involvement of the interphalangeal or metatarsophalangeal joint, require reduction and fixation. Closed reduction can be attempted with axial traction (finger traps). If this is successful in reducing the fracture, percutaneous K wire fixation is undertaken. A walking cast with a toe plate is applied for 4–6 weeks, followed by a postoperative shoe for another 4–6 weeks. The K wires are removed at 4–6 weeks. If open reduction is required, especially for intra-articular fractures, swelling guides the timing of surgery. Often a delay of 7–10 days is required to allow resolution of the swelling. K wires or minifragment screws can be utilized, and the

postoperative management is followed as for percutaneous fixation.

Fractures of the hallux sesamoids can be caused by indirect or direct trauma. Direct trauma, such as a crush injury, is more common. The typical history involves a fall from a height landing on the forefoot (DeLee 1986). This impacts on the sesamoids (especially the tibial one), causing a fracture (Garcia and Parkes 1973). The tibial (medial) sesamoid is fractured much more frequently than the fibular (lateral) sesamoid (Garcia and Parkes 1973). Indirect trauma occurs when the hallux is forcibly hyperextended (Chapman 1978). The sesamoids elevate the first metatarsal head during weight-bearing and also serve to increase the mechanical advantage of the flexor hallucis brevis tendon (DeLee 1986). The abductor hallucis and the medial head of the flexor hallucis brevis insert onto the medial (tibial) sesamoid. The tendon of the adductor hallucis and the lateral head of the flexor hallucis brevis insert onto the lateral (fibular) sesamoid. In addition to routine views of the foot, a "skyline" or axial view of the sesamoids is obtained. A fractured sesamoid must be differentiated from a bipartite sesamoid and osteochondritis dissecans of the sesamoid – the former has smooth, sclerotic edges, while the latter shows fragmentation and irregularity. The initial treatment of a sesamoid fracture involves a short-leg weight-bearing cast, followed by a metatarsal pad behind the head of the first metatatarsal. Symptoms may persist for 4–6 months, and therefore patients must be aware of the possibility of prolonged disability (DeLee 1986; Feldinqu et al. 1970). If significant pain and disability persists more than 6 months after the initial injury, excision of the fractured sesamoid is indicated. DeLee (1986)

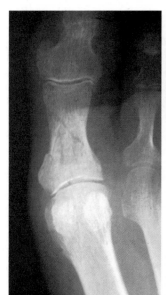 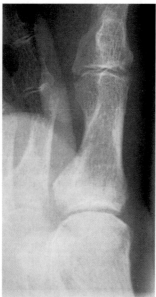

Fig. 25.10 a, b. Crush injury to great toe. Patient sustained undisplaced, comminuted fracture of the proximal phalanx. Treatment consisted of "buddy-taping" to second toe and postoperative shoe. At 6 weeks, patient was asymptomatic

a   b

prefers a medial longitudinal incision for the tibial sesamoid and a dorsal incision between the first and second metatarsal heads for the fibular sesamoid. Complete excision of the fractured sesamoid should be avoided. Removal of the smaller, or comminuted fragment is preferred.

25.5 Tarsometatarsal (Lisfranc) Fracture-Dislocations

25.5.1 Anatomy

The tarsometatarsal joint has intrinsic stability as a result of the shape of the bones and their relationship to one another in this area (DeLee 1986; Arntz and Hansen 1988). The first to third metatarsals articulate with their respective cuneiform bones, the second has separate facets for the medial and lateral cuneiform bones, and the forth and fifth metarsals articulate with the cuboid. The long second metatarsal is recessed between the medial and lateral cuneiform bones. This forms the keystone of the metatarsal arch and is the key to reduction of dislocations in this area. The medial three metatarsals have a trapezoidal shape and form the well-known Roman arch configuration (Jeffreys 1963; DeLee 1986; Arntz and Hansen 1988) Numerous authors have noted that no significant dislocation of the metarsals can occur without disruption of the second metatarsal (DeLee 1986; Arntz and Hansen 1988). The well-developed interosseous ligament between the second metatarsal and the medial cuneiform bone is known as the Lisfranc ligament (Jeffreys 1963). This ligament often avulses a fleck of bone from the second metatarsal with injuries in this area (Chapman 1978). Dorsal, plantar, and interosseous ligaments add to the inherent bony stability. The plantar ligaments are stronger than the dorsal ligaments and are further supported by the plantar fascia, intrinsic muscles, and peroneus longus (Chapman 1978; DeLee 1986). This accounts for the fact most dislocations are dorsal (Fahey and Murphy 1965). Although there are no interosseous attachments between the first and second metatarsals, the first is attached to the medial cuneiform bone by strong capsular ligaments and is reinforced medially by the anterior tibial tendon and plantolaterally by the peroneus longus tendon (DeLee 1986). The dorsalis pedis artery supplies an anastomotic branch to the plantar arch, between the bases of the first and second metatarsals. This can be injured in Lisfranc dislocations and can cause significant hemorrhage with compartment syndrome (Gissane 1951). The vascularity of the foot is not at risk unless there is an injury to the posterior tibial or the lateral plantar artery.

25.5.2 Mechanism and Classification

The mechanism of injury can either be direct (crush) or indirect (axial load in equinus or twisting of the forefoot) (Jeffreys 1963; Giannestras and Sammarco 1975; DeLee 1986; Arntz and Hansen 1988). The most common indirect mechanism is an axial load of the fixed forefoot, with the foot in equinus (Arntz and Hansen 1988). Motor vehicle or motorcycle accidents account for 50%–67% of these injuries (Arntz and Hansen 1988; Myserson 1989; Vuori and Aro 1993). However, low-energy traumas, such as a stumble or fall, can account for up to 33% of the total of injuries to the Lisfranc complex (Vuori and Aro 1993). Myerson (1989) states that 81% will be in patients with multiple injuries. Twisting injuries – such as in equestrians – occur with the forefoot abducted on the tarsus (DeLee 1986; Artnz and Hansen 1988). The mechanism of injury (most commonly a high-energy injury) can result in concommitant compression fractures of the cuboid, fractures of the bases of the metatarsals (the second metatarsal being most common, as mentioned above), or navicular fractures (Vuori and Aro 1993). The two mechanisms (axial load vs twisting) produce the deformities which form the basis for commonly described classifications (Hardcastle et al. 1982; DeLee 1986; Myerson 1989; Vuori and Aro 1993). The metatarsals can displace together (homolateral dislocation or total incongruity) or be split apart (divergent). There can also be isolated disruptions (partial incongruity), with the first metatarsal being displaced medially – alone or together with a variable portion of the medial or middle cuneiform bones. The lateral metatarsals (variable number) can also be displaced in an isolated fashion. Crush injuries follow the direction of the force and are usually directed from the dorsal surface plantarward, resulting in plantar displacement (Arntz and Hansen 1988).

25.5.3 Clinical and Radiological Diagnosis

Injuries to the Lisfranc complex may be overlooked in patients that have multiple life-threatening injuries or in patients with trivial injuries such as a misstep (Vuori and Aro 1993). The initial diagnosis of these injuries may be missed in as many as 20%–35% of cases (Gooses and Stoop 1983; Vuori and Aro 1993). Prompt diagnosis and treatment prevent long-term deformity and disability (Myerson et al. 1986). There can also be spontaneous reduction of the subluxation or dislocation, making the diagnosis difficult (Chapman 1978, DeLee 1986 Arntz and Hansen 1988).

The typical clinical deformity is forefoot abduction and equinus, with prominence of the medial tarsal area (Fahey and Murphy 1965). Gross swelling of the foot may

618 ·

Chapter 25   Injuries of the Midfoot and Forefoot

be present, and compartment syndrome must be ruled out (Myerson 1987).

The routine views of the foot – anterioposterior, lateral, and 30° obliques – form the basis of the radiographic evaluation. The oblique view provides the most information on the tarsometatarsal area. The medial border of the fourth metatarsal aligns with the medial border of the cuboid, and the medial borders of the second metatarsal and middle cuneiform bones are parallel (Stein 1983). The first and second intermetatarsal spaces should be parallel with the respective interspaces between the cuneiform bones (Stein 1983), and the first metatarsal should be perfectly aligned with the medial cuneiform bone. Finally, there should be no dorsal subluxation at the tarsometatarsal joint on the lateral projection. Often, the only finding is the presence of a small avulsion fracture from the second metatarsal base caused by the Lisfranc ligament (Arntz and Hansen 1988). In this situation or if there is a clinical suspicion, then weight-bearing (or stress) views should be obtained. If there is more than 2 mm at the first intermetatarsal space, then subluxation is present and requires treatment (Trevino and Baumhauer 1993).

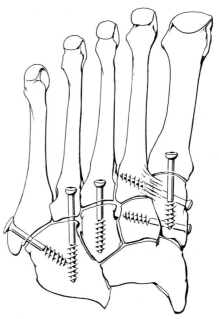

Fig. 25.11. Lisfranc (tarsometatarsal) injuries. The sequence of screw placement and number of screws depends on the injury pattern. The goal is to restore normal anatomical relationships at the tarsometatarsal joint(s). The relationship between the first metatarsal and medial cuneiform and second metatarsal and medial (and middle) cuneiform is the *key* to accurate reduction

25.5.4 Treatment

The goal of treatment is a stable, painless, plantigrade foot (Arntz and Hansen 1988). This goal is acheived by anatomical reduction and, if required, stable internal fixation (Hardcastle et al. 1982; DeLee 1986; Myerson et al. 1986; Arntz and Hansen 1988). Nondisplaced injuries with normal weight-bearing radiographs are best treated with a short-leg, non-weight-bearing cast for 6 weeks. If there is more than 1–2 mm of displacement at any portion of the Lisfranc complex, anatomical reduction is required (DeLee 1986; Myerson et al. 1986; Arntz and Hansen 1988; Trevion and Baumhauer 1993). Closed reduction and percutaneous screw fixation can be attempted, but infolding of soft tissue such as the anterior tibial or peroneous longus tendons or the avulsed Lisfranc ligament (most common) may make anatomical reduction impossible (Jeffreys 1963).

Open reduction is the best method of acheiving an anatomical reduction. Swelling may dictate a delay in open reduction of up to 7–10 days, during which time immobilzation and elevation is required. A longitudinal dorsal incision is made over the second metatarsal (see Fig. 25.1), which allows access to the first, second, and third rays (Arntz and Hansen 1988; Trevion and Baumhauer 1993). A second incision over the fourth ray may be utilized to gain access to the fourth and fifth rays. The dangers involve injury to the dorsalis pedis artery, the sensory branches of the deep peroneal nerve (medial incision), and the sensory branches of the superficial

peroneal nerve (lateral incision) (Arntz and Hansen 1988; Trevino and Baumhauer 1993). Contraindications to open reduction may include preexisting peripheral vascular disease, more than 6 weeks from the injury, or the presence of neuropathy (Trevino and Baumhauer 1993).

A variety of techniques have been described to achieve anatomical reduction and stable internal fixation (Fig. 25.11; Myerson 1987; Arntz and Hansen 1988; Trevino and Baumhauer 1993). Cannulated screws help to simplify the procedure, as the guidewires can be used for temporary reduction during the procedure. Alternatively, small 0.062-mm K wires can be used and then replaced with small-fragment screws. The first step is stabilization of the first ray, including the the first metatarsocuneiform and the naviculocuneiform joints. The wire is placed retrograde from the first metatarsal, approximately 1.5–2.0 cm from the joint, and directed in a plantar direction. A small trough is made in the first metatarsal to serve as a countersink. After temporary stabilization of the first ray with the guidewire, the Lisfranc complex is reduced and stabilized. Any loose avulsion fragments or interposed soft tissue is removed, and reduction forceps are used to reduce the second metatarsal to the medial cuneiform bone, and the medial to middle cuneiform bone. Again, guidewires (or 0.062-mm K wires) for the 4.0-mm cannulated system are used. Intraoperative fluoroscopy helps to simplify the procedure, but plain radiographs can be used. If there is felt to be anatomical restoration of these joints, then the wires are replaced with partially threaded 4.0-mm cancellous screws. If there is disruption of the lateral three rays, then a similar procedure is undertaken with sequential reduction of the tarsometatarsal articulations, followed by insertion of the screws. If there is a compression fracture of the cuboid or a fracture of the navicular, treatment is also carried out.

A well-padded, postoperative splint is applied and converted to a short-leg, non-weight-bearing cast when swelling permits. Weight-bearing is not initiated for 6–8 weeks (Arntz and Hansen 1988; Trevino and Baumhauer 1993). Protected weight-bearing is continued for another 6 weeks. Screw removal is controversial, both with regard to the timing and the necessity of it (Arntz and Hansen 1988; Trevino and Baumhauer 1993). Screw breakage can occur with unprotected weight-bearing, but removal should be delayed until approximately the fourth month to allow soft tissue healing (Arntz and Hansen 1988).

Post-traumatic arthritis may occur following injuries to the Lisfranc complex (Sangeorzan et al. 1990). If con-

servative measures – including: custom-molded longitudinal arch supports, anti-inflammatory medications, and activity modifications – fail, then tarsometatarsal arthrodesis is required. Further investigations, including biplanar tomograms and diagnostic injections, may be required to identify affected joints. The procedure is carried out in a similar fashion to that described for open reduction, with the addition of débridement of the affected joints and cancellous bone graft if indicated.

25.6 Compartment Syndromes of the Foot

Crush injuries, forefoot and midfoot fractures (and/or dislocations), and fractures of the calcaneus can increase the risk of compartment syndrome in the foot (Myerson 1988; Manoli 1990). The typical clinical findings found with compartment syndromes in the lower leg and forearm are less reliable in the foot (Ziv et al. 1989). Extreme swelling may increase the suspicion, but usually invasive compartment measurement is required for definitive diagnosis. There is debate as to the exact number of fascial compartments in the foot, but Myerson has shown there are at least nine compartments (Myerson 1988; Manoli and Weber 1990). Generally, three incisions – two dorsal and one medial – are utilized to gain access to the foot compartments (Fig. 25.12; Manoli 1990: Manoli and Weber 1990). A 6-cm incision is made medially, approximately 4 cm from the posterior aspect of the heel and 3 cm from the plantar surface, and is slightly concave plantar to follow the contour of the plantar surface of the foot (Manoli 1990). The fascia over the abductor hallucis is released (medial compartment), and this muscle is reflected plantar or dorsal to expose the medial intermuscular septum. This septum is opened to expose the lateral plantar nerve and vessels in the region of the quadratus plantae muscle, which is in the calcaneal compartment (deep central). This compartment has been shown to communicate with the deep posterior compartment of the lower leg

Fig. 25.12. Compartments of the foot (cross-section at midfoot, proximal metatarsals). There are nine compartments: the medial, central, lateral, and four interossei compartments. There is also a proximal calcaneal compartment (hindfoot) which communicates with the deep posterior compartment of the leg. In the medial compartment are abductor hallucis *(ABH)* and flexor hallucis brevis *(FHB)*; in the superficial central compartment the flexor digiroum brevis *(FDB)*, in the deep portion the quadratus plantae *(QP)*, and in the deep forefoot the adductor hallucis *(ADH)*; in the lateral compartment the abductor digiti quinti *(ABDQ)* and flexor digiti quinti brevis *(FDQB)*; and in the interossei compartment three plantar *(P1–P3)* and four dorsal *(D1–D4)* Note neurovascular bundle between *FHB* and *QP*

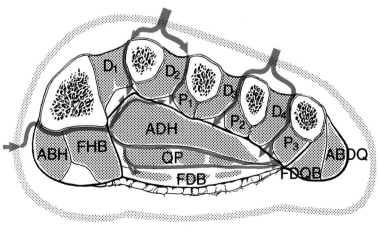

(Manoli and Weber 1990). The superficial central compartment containing the flexor digitorum brevis is opened by staying superficial to the abductor hallucis fascia. Then the lateral compartment (abductor digiti quinti) is released by retracting the flexor digitorum brevis plantarward. Two dorsal incisions are made, over to the second and fourth metatarsal shaft and just lateral to the fourth. Each of the four interosseous compartments is released. The adductor hallucis compartment is released by dissecting along the medial border of the second metatarsal in a subperiosteal fashion. If the patient has underlying fractures, the incisions may be modified depending on the exposure required for internal fixation. The wounds are left open, and sterile dressings are applied. The wounds can be closed or skin-grafted when swelling permits, usually within 7 days.

References

Anderson JE (1983) Grant's atlas of anatomy, 8 th edn. Williams and Wilkins, Baltimore

Anderson LD (1977) Injuries of the foot. Clin Orthop 122:18–27

Arangio GA (1983) Proximal displaced fractures of the fifth metatarsal (jones fractures): two cases treated by cross pinning with review of 100 cases. Foot Ankle 3:293–296

Arntz CT, Hansen Jr ST (1988) Fractures and fracture-dislocations of the tarsometatarsal joint. J Bone Joint Surg 70A: 173–181

Carp L (1927) Fracture of the fifth metatarsal bone with special reference to delayed union. Ann Surg 86:308–320

Chapman MW (1978) Fractures and dislocations of the ankle and foot. In: Mann RA (ed) DuVries surgery of the foot, 4 th edn. Mosby, St Louis

Dameron TB (1995) Fractures of the proximal fifth metatarsal: selecting the best treatment option. J Am Acad Orthop Surg 3:110–114

Day AJ (1947) The treatment of injuries to the tarsal navicular. J Bone Joint Surg 29:359 366

DeLee JG (1986) Fractures and dislocations of the foot. In: Mann RA, Coughlin MJ (eds) Surgery of the foot and ankle, 6 th edn, vol 2. Mosby, St Louis

Dick IL (1942) Impacted fracture-dislocation of the tarsal navicula. Proc R Soc Med 35:760

Donovan T (1995) J Am Assoc Orthop Surg 3

Eichenholtz SN, Levine D (1964) Fractures of the tarsal navicular bone. Clin Orthop 34:142

Fahey JJ, Murphy JL (1965) Dislocations and fractures of the talus. Surg Clin North Am 45:79–102

Feldinau F, Pochaczevsky R, Hecht H (1970) The case of the wandering sesamoid and other sesamoid afflictions. Radiology 96:275–284

Garcia A, Parkes JC (1950) Fractures of the foot. In: Giannestras NJ (ed) Foot disorders: medical and surgical management, 2 nd edn. Lea and Febiger, Philadelphia

Giannestras NJ, Sammarco GJ (1975) Fractures and dislocations in the foot. In: Rockwood CA Jr, Green DP (eds) Fractures, vol 2. Saunders, Philadelphia

Gissane W (1951) A dangerous type of fracture of the foot. J Bone Joint Surg 33B:535–538

Gooses M, Stoop N (1983) Lisfranc fracture-dislocations: etiology, radiology, and results of treatment. Clin Orthop 176:154–162

Hardcastle PH, Reschauer R, Kutscha-Lissberg E et al (1983) Injuries to the tarsometatarsal joint: incidence, classification, and treatment. J Bone Joint Surg 64B:349–356

Hermel MB, Gershon-Cohen J (1953) The nutcracker fracture of the cuboid by indirect violence. Radiology 60:850

Hillegass RC (1976) Injuries to the midfoot: a major case of industrial morbidity. In Bateman JE (ed) Foot science. Saunders, Philadelphia

Jeffreys TE (1963) Lisfranc's fracture-dislocations: a clinical and experimental study of tarso metatarsal dislocations and fracture-dislocations. J Bone Joint Surg 45B:546–551

Jones R (1902) Fractures of the base of the fifth metatarsal bone by indirect violence. Ann Surg 35:697–700

Kavanaugh JH, Brower TD, Mann RV (1978) The Jones fracture revisited. J Bone Joint Surg 60A:776–782

Lawrence SJ, Botte MJ(1993) Jones fractures and related fractures of the proximal fifth metatarsal. Foot Ankle 14:358–365

Lindholm R (1961) Operative treatment of dislocated simple fractures of the neck of the metatarsal bone. Am Chir Gynaecol Tenn 50:328–331

Manoli A II (1990) Foot fellows review: compartment syndromes of the foot: current concepts. Foot Ankle 10/6:340–344

Manoli A II, Weber TG (1990) Fasciotomy of the foot – an anatomical study with special reference to release of the calcaneal compartment. Foot Ankle 10:267–275

McKeever FM (1950) Fractures of the tarsal and metatarsal bones. Surg Gynecol Obstet 90:735–745

Myerson M (1987) Acute compartment syndromes of the foot. Bull Hosp Joint Dis Orthop Inst 47:251–261

Myerson MS (1988) Experimental decompression of the fascial compartments of the foot. The basis for fasciotomy in acute compartment syndromes. Foot Ankle 8:308–314

Myerson M (1989) The diagnosis and treatment of injuries of the Lisfranc joint complex. Orthop Clin North Am 20:655

Myerson MS, Fisher RT, Burgess AR et al (1986) Fracture-dislocations of the tarsometatarsal joints: end results correlated with pathology and treatment. Foot Ankle 6:225–242

Sangeorzan BJ (1993) Navicular and cuboid fractures. In: Myerson M (ed) Current therapy in foot and ankle surgery. Mosby, St Louis

Sangeorzan BJ, Swiontkowski MF (1990) Displaced fractures of the cuboid. J Bone Joint Surg 72B:376–378

Sangeorzan BJ, Benirschke SK, Mosca V et al (1989) Displaced intra-articular fractures of the tarsal navicular. J Bone Joint Surg 71A:1504–1510

Sangeorzan BJ, Veith RG, Hansen ST (1990) Salvage of Lisfranc tarsometatarsal joint by arthrodiesis. Foot Ankle 10:193–200

Sarrafian SK (1983) Anatomy of the foot and ankle. Saunders, Philadelphia

Shereff MJ (1990) Fractures of the forefoot. Instr Course Lect 29:133–140

Shereff MJ, Yang QM, Kummer FJ et al (1991) Vascular anatomy of the fifth metatarsal. Foot Ankle 11:350–353

Smith JW, Arnoczky SP, Hersh A (1992) The intraosseous blood supply of the fifth metatarsal: implications for proximal fracture healing. Foot Ankle 13:143–152

Stein RE (1983) Radiological aspects of the tarsometatarsal joints. Foot Ankle 3:286–289

Torg JS, Pavlov H, Cooley LH et al (1982) Stress fractures of tarsal navicular. J Bone Joint Surg 64A:700–712

Trevino SG, Baumhauer JF (1993) Lisfranc injuries in current therapy in foot and ankle surgery. In: Myerson M (ed) Current therapy in foot and ankle surgery. Mosby, St Louis, pp 233–238

Vuori JP, Aro HT (1993) Lisfranc joint injuries: trauma mechanisms and associated injuries. J Trauma 35/1:40–45

Watson-Jones R (1955) Fractures and joint injuries, 4th edn, vol 2. Williams and Wilkins, Baltimore

Wilson PD (1933) Fractures and dislocations of the tarsal bones. South Med J 26:833

Ziv I, Mosheiff R, Zeligowski A, Liebergal M, Love J, Segal D (1989) Crush injuries of the foot with compartment syndrome: immediate one-stage management. Foot Ankle 9: 285–289

Subject Index

Springer-Verlag
and the Environment

We at Springer-Verlag firmly believe that an international science publisher has a special obligation to the environment, and our corporate policies consistently reflect this conviction.

We also expect our business partners – paper mills, printers, packaging manufacturers, etc. – to commit themselves to using environmentally friendly materials and production processes.

The paper in this book is made from low- or no-chlorine pulp and is acid free, in conformance with international standards for paper permanency.